Current Progress in Veterinary Science

Current Progress in Veterinary Science

Edited by Gerardo Bailey

SYRAWOOD
PUBLISHING HOUSE
New York

Published by Syrawood Publishing House,
750 Third Avenue, 9th Floor,
New York, NY 10017, USA
www.syrawoodpublishinghouse.com

Current Progress in Veterinary Science
Edited by Gerardo Bailey

International Standard Book Number: 978-1-68286-697-9 (Hardback)

Cataloging-in-Publication Data

Current progress in veterinary science / edited by Gerardo Bailey.
p. cm.
Includes bibliographical references and index.
ISBN 978-1-68286-697-9
1. Veterinary medicine. 2. Medicine. 3. Animal health. 4. Animals--Diseases. I. Bailey, Gerardo.
SF745 .C87 2019
636.089--dc23

Printed in China.

TABLE OF CONTENTS

Preface

The world is advancing at a fast pace like never before. Therefore, the need is to keep up with the latest developments. This book was an idea that came to fruition when the specialists in the area realized the need to coordinate together and document essential themes in the subject. That's when I was requested to be the editor. Editing this book has been an honour as it brings together diverse authors researching on different streams of the field. The book collates essential materials contributed by veterans in the area which can be utilized by students and researchers alike.

The area of medicine related to the maintenance of health of all non-human animals and the treatment and prevention of diseases they are prone to, is known as veterinary science. It covers medicinal, clinical, scientific and technological aspects of animal diseases. Veterinary science has applications in diverse areas of livestock management and animal health. This book strives to provide a fair idea about this discipline and to help develop a better understanding of the latest advances within this field. It elucidates new techniques and their applications in a multidisciplinary manner. The various sub-fields of veterinary science along with technological progress that have future implications are glanced at in this book. It will prove immensely beneficial to professionals and students involved in this area at various levels.

Each chapter is a sole-standing publication that reflects each author´s interpretation. Thus, the book displays a multi-facetted picture of our current understanding of application, resources and aspects of the field. I would like to thank the contributors of this book and my family for their endless support.

Editor

Comparison Effect of Alcoholic and Non-Polar Extract of Persian Gulf Sea Cucumber (*Holothuria leucospilota*) on Steroid Hormones Levels in Molly Fish (*Poecilia sphenops*)

Fahimeh Golestani[1], Tahereh Naji[1]* and Homayoun Hosseinzadeh Sahaifi[2]

[1]*Department of Basic Sciences, Faculty of Pharmacy, Pharmaceutical Sciences Branch, Islamic Azad University (IAUPS), Tehran, Iran*
[2]*Iranian Fisheries Science Research Institute, Agricultural Research, Education and Extension Organization, Tehran, Iran*

Abstract

Background: sea cucumber is important aquatics with nutritional and medical properties.

Aim: So, the aim of this study was to determine comparison effect of alcoholic and non-polar extract of Persian Gulf sea cucumber on steroid hormones levels in Molly fish.

Methods: A total 210 Molly fish were randomly divided into 7 experimental groups (n=30). In Group 1, fish kept as control (without injection). In Group 2, fish injected with ethanol (100 mg/kg, i.m.) for 20 days. In Group 3, fish injected with hexane (100 mg/kg, i.m.) for 20 days. In Groups 4-5, fish injected with alcoholic extract of Persian Gulf sea cucumber (AEPGSC, 100 and 200 mg/kg, i.m.) for 20 days, respectively. In Groups 6-7, fish injected with non-polar extract of Persian Gulf sea cucumber (NPEPGSC, 100 and 200 mg/kg, i.m.) for 20 days, respectively. In all groups, the injection was given on alternate days. Then 24 h after the last injection, fish euthanized using PI_{222} (Pars Imen Daru, Tehran, Iran). The biometric indexes body length (cm) and weight (g) were determined. Then the gonads carried out and the body mass homogenized, body testosterone (ng/ml), β-estradiol (ng/ml), cholesterol (mg/dl) and germ cell index (mm) were determined.

Results: According to the results, injection of AEPGSC and NPEPGSC significantly diminished body β-estradiol levels (ng/ml) in the Moly fish compared to control group (P=0.012). Injection of AEPGSC (200 mg/kg) and NPEPGSC (100 and 200 mg/kg) significantly diminished body testosterone (P=0.000) and cholesterol (P=0.003) levels in the Molly fish.

Conclusion: these results suggest Persian Gulf sea cucumber extract has an effect on the production of steroid hormones in Molly fish.

Keywords: Persian Gulf sea cucumber extract; Germ cells division; Testosterone; 17-β estradiol; Molly fish

Introduction

Sea cucumbers are abundant worm-like and soft-bodied echinoderms found in nearly every marine environment [1]. To date approximately 1400 living species of sea cucumbers have been identified worldwide including Persian Gulf [2]. Based on the analysis it is reported sea cucumber is cholesterol-free and contains approximately 55% protein and 15% mucopolysaccharides, saponins and collagen peptides [3]. Sea cucumbers are aquatic creatures and have nutritional and therapeutic properties on human health [4]. It is reported polysaccharides isolated from sea cucumbers have anticoagulant, antitumor and immune modulating activity [5]. Recently it is reported polysaccharide derived from sea cucumbers have anti-hyperlipidemic effects [6]. It is reported injection of sea cucumber extract decreased serum total cholesterol and improved lipid metabolism in rats fed high-cholesterol diet [7]. On the other hand, it is known, saponins has effect on lipid metabolism [7]. For instance, aqueous extract of Malaysian sea cucumber (*Stichopus chloronotus)* minimize lipid biosynthesis [8].

Recently interests increased for curative effects of the biological components on reproduction where saponin significantly affects reproduction in animals [9]. The negative effect of saponins on animal reproduction is well documented [9] however controversial reports exist. Recently, Delghandi Moghadam et al. [10] studied effect of Persian Gulf sea cucumber (*Holothuria leucospilota*) on maturation of mice oocyte and granulosa cells. Based on their report, sea cucumber saponin enhanced follicle growth in mice, but precise mechanisms still unclear [10]. The saponin of sea cucumber suppressed pancreatic lipase and inhibiting triglyceride and cholesterol absorption in rat [7]. It is known that cholesterol is the main structure of sex steroid hormones which decrease cholesterol levels impair gonad estradiol, estrogen (E_2) and testosterone production [11].

Holothuria leucospilota are commercially important aquatics in the Persian Gulf and Oman Sea. These aquatics have important composition and medical properties [2] but there is no information about the biological activity of *Holothuria leucospilota* on sex hormone levels. Based on the literature, the sea cucumber has properties to diminish body lipid and cholesterol profile [6] as well because of correlation between cholesterol level and sex hormone biosynthesis [10], the hypothesis of the current study was to determine possible curative or adverse effect in the *Holothuria leucospilota* extract on

***Corresponding author:** Tahereh Naji, Associate of Professor, Department of Basic Sciences, Faculty of Pharmacy, Pharmaceutical Sciences Branch, Islamic Azad University (IAUPS), Tehran, Iran
E-mail: shahin.hassanpour@yahoo.com

steroid hormones levels in Molly fish. So, the aim of the current study was to determine comparison effect of alcoholic extract Persian Gulf sea cucumber extract (AEPGSC) and non-polar Persian Gulf sea cucumber extract (NPEPGSC) on steroid hormones levels in Molly fish (*Poecilia sphenops*).

Material and Methods

Sample preparation

Samples of Persian Gulf sea cucumber *(Holothuria leucospilota)* were collected from Persian Gulf, at the depth of 25-30 meters in 2016. Then samples transported and stored at -20°C in laboratory of Fisheries, Department of Pharmacology, Islamic Azad University, Tehran, Iran.

Persian Gulf sea cucumber extract

In this study two extracts type of Persian Gulf sea cucumber were done. The AEPGSC obtained using ethanol and NPEPGSC by hexane. The sea cucumber sample (2000 g wet weight) was cut into small pieces (1 cm), they were put in freeze dried until the tissue was dry (150 g dry weight). Extracts of powder sea cucumber were obtained by using three different solvents including: n-hexane, diethyl ether and methanol. After 24 hours of exposure in n-hexane, the extract was concentrated under low pressure at 30°C by rotary evaporation. The diethyl ether extract was ready after 48 h, and then the solvent was removed by rotary evaporation at 35°C. The methanol extract was ready after 72 h then the solvent was removed by rotary evaporation at 40°C. Ether-methanol was formed by adding Ether in order to separate the methanol-aqueous extract, then the upper phase was separated by separating funnel. The upper phase was combined by n-butanol and aqueous extract was separated by separating funnel. Each extract was shaken by mechanical shaking at room temperature (25°C). All processes were carried out on dark condition. Finally, both crude extracts were kept in freezer.

Study protocol

A total 210 Molly fish (*Poecilia sphenops*) (3 ± 0.2) were randomly divided into 7 experimental groups (n=30). The fish were kept in 2 m^3 tanks with a flow-through circuit, suitable aeration and filtration system and natural photoperiod. The water temperature ranged from 25.1 to 27.8°C. The environmental parameters, mortality and food intake were recorded daily.

In Group 1, fish kept as control (without injection).

In Group 2, fish injected with ethanol (100 mg/kg, i.m.) for 20 days (given on alternate days).

In Group 3, fish injected with hexane (100 mg/kg, i.m.) for 20 days (given on alternate days).

In Group 4, fish injected with AEPGSC (100 mg/kg, i.m.) for 20 days (given on alternate days).

In Group 5, fish injected with AEPGSC (200 mg/kg, i.m.) for 20 days (given on alternate days).

In Group 6, fish injected with NPEPGSC (100 mg/kg, i.m.) for 20 days (given on alternate days).

In Group 7, fish injected with NPEPGSC (200 mg/kg, i.m.) for 20 days (given on alternate days).

The doses for the extracts were used based on the previous reports [12-14] and our pilot studies (un-published).

Tissue extract and hormone assay

Then 24 h after the last injection, fish euthanized using PI_{222} (Pars Imen Daru, Tehran, Iran). The biometric indexes body length (cm), weight (g) and germ cell index (mm) were determined. Then the gonads carried out and the body mass homogenized. Then, body testosterone (ng/ml), β-estradiol (ng/ml) and cholesterol (mg/dl) were determined using commercial ELISA or colorimetric detecting kits [15].

Statistical analyses

Effect of AEPGSC and NPEPGSC was analyzed by repeated measure two-way analysis of variance (ANOVA) using SPSS 16.0 for Windows (SPSS, Inc., Chicago, IL, USA). Data is presented as mean ± SEM. For treatment showing a main effect by ANOVA, means compared by Tukey-Kramer test. P<0.05 was considered as significant differences between treatments.

Results

The comparison effect of AEPGSC and NPEPGSC on steroid hormones (testosterone, β-estradiol and cholesterol) levels in Molly fish (*Poecilia sphenops*) is presented in Figures 1-4. As seen in Figure 1, i.m. injection of AEPGSC and NPEPGSC significantly diminished body β estradiol levels (ng/ml) in the Molly fish compared to control group (P=0.012; F=4.126). However, there was no significant difference on body β estradiol levels (ng/ml) using different levels of the AEPGSC (100 and 200 mg/kg) and NPEPGSC (100 and 200 mg/kg) compared to ethanol (100 mg/kg) and non-polar base (100 mg/kg) (P>0.05).

As seen in Figure 2, only i.m. injection of AEPGSC (200 mg/kg) and NPEPGSC (100 and 200 mg/kg) significantly diminished body testosterone levels (ng/ml) in the Molly fish (P=0.000; F=16.868). However, administration in the ethanol (100 mg/kg), non-polar base (100 mg/kg), AEPGSC (100 mg/kg had no significant effect on body testosterone levels (ng/ml) compared to control group (P>0.05).

The effect of i.m. injection of AEPGSC and NPEPGSC on body cholesterol levels (mg/dl) is presented in Figure 3. According to the results, injection of the AEPGSC (100 and 200 mg/kg) significantly decreased body cholesterol levels in the Moly fish compared to control group (P=0.003; F=6.041). As observed in Figure 4, injection of AEPGSC and NPEPGSC had no effect on GIS in Molly fish compared to control group (P>0.05).

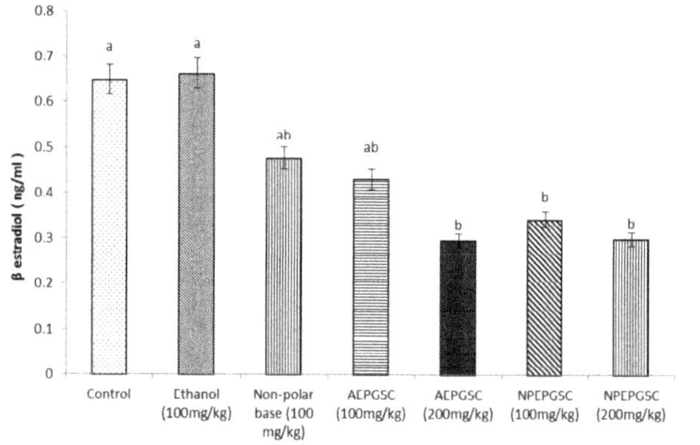

Figure 1: The effect of i.m. injection of AEPGSC and NPEPGSC on body β estradiol levels (ng/ml) compared to control group in Molly fish. i.m.: intramuscular, alcoholic extract Persian Gulf sea cucumber extract: AEPGSC, non-polar Persian Gulf sea cucumber extract: NPEPGSC. There are significant differences between groups with different superscripts in a column (a and b; P<0.05).

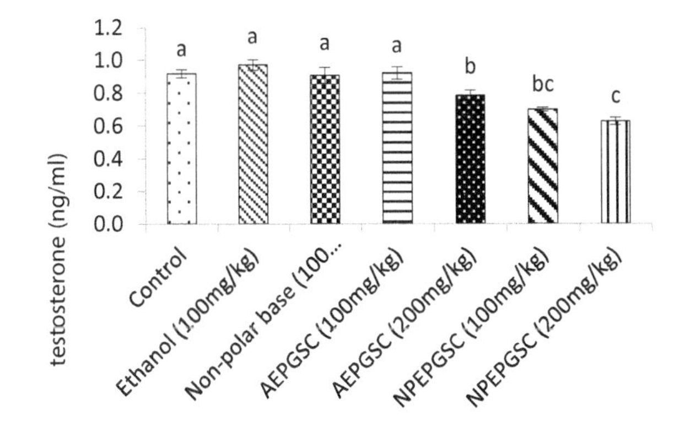

Figure 2: The effect of i.m. injection of AEPGSC and NPEPGSC on body testosterone levels (ng/ml) compared to control group in Molly fish. i.m.: intramuscular, alcoholic extract Persian Gulf sea cucumber extract: AEPGSC, non-polar Persian Gulf sea cucumber extract: NPEPGSC. There are significant differences between groups with different superscripts in a column (a, b and c; P<0.05).

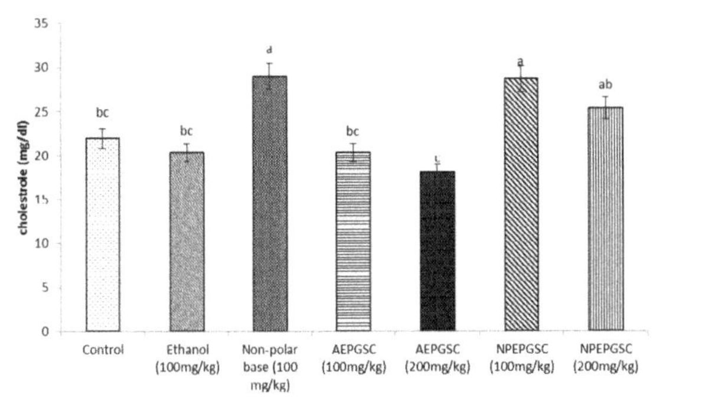

Figure 3: The effect of i.m. injection of AEPGSC and NPEPGSC on body cholesterol levels (mg/dl) compared to control group in Molly fish. i.m.: intramuscular, alcoholic extract Persian Gulf sea cucumber extract: AEPGSC, non-polar Persian Gulf sea cucumber extract: NPEPGSC. There are significant differences between groups with different superscripts in a column (a, b and c; P<0.05).

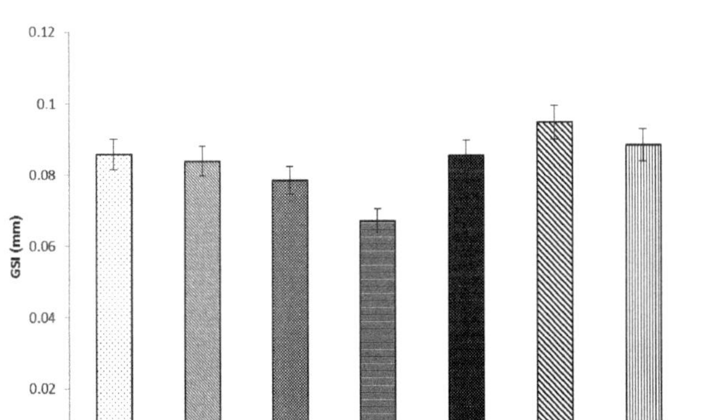

Figure 4: The effect of i.m. injection of AEPGSC and NPEPGSC on GIS (mm) compared to control group in Molly fish. i.m.: intramuscular, alcoholic extract Persian Gulf sea cucumber extract: AEPGSC, non-polar Persian Gulf sea cucumber extract: NPEPGSC, GSI: germ cell index. P<0.05 was considered as significant differences between treatments.

Discussion

During the past decade, growing attention has been centered towards discovery of novel drugs from marine organisms due to containing pharmacologically bioactive compounds. To our knowledge this is the first report on effect of AEPGSC and NPEPGSC. According to the results, injection of AEPGSC and NPEPGSC had no effects on body length and weight in the Molly fish while injection of the AEPGSC decreased body cholesterol levels in the Moly fish. Dry sea cucumber contains approximately 20 mg/g glucosylceramide. It is reported dietary sea cucumber contacting glucosylceramide decreased liver cholesterol and triglyceride compared to glucosylceramide free sea cucumber in mice but not affect body weight [16]. As observed in our study AEPGSC and NPEPGSC had no effect on body weight in Moly fish which was in agreement with previous reports. Fish have also been shown to exhibit stress reactions to the presence of saponins in water [9]. Bureau et al. [17] observed that saponins damaged the intestinal mucosa in rainbow trout and Chinook salmon at dietary levels above 1.5 g/kg. Polysaccharides can act as stimulators of bile acid synthesis and circulation and increasing the fecal excretion of bile acids so that fewer bile acids return to the liver [16]. On the other hand, antioxidant activity of polysaccharides might play major role in modify LDL formation but there is also increasing evidence to support the idea [18].

Herein, Injection of AEPGSC and NPEPGSC diminished body β-estradiol and testosterone levels in the Moly fish. To the best of our knowledge, there are no reports on the effects of Persian Gulf sea cucumber on reproductive hormones in Moly fish. Most of surveys have been reported about terrestrial saponin compounds. The negative effects of terrestrial saponins on animal reproduction have been introduced these bioactive compounds as abortifacient metabolites [9]. Injection of the saponin-rich extracts from *Combretodendron africanum* into female rats blocked the oestrous cycle [18]. Also, saponins directly inhibits the steroidogenesis genes and suppresses the proliferation of follicle-stimulating hormone-modulated granulosa cells in the mice ovarian follicle via similar mechanism as saponin-induced proliferation of tumor cells [9]. The same reports exist for male animals which lower Gonad-somatic index observed in male tilapia receiving a continuous supply of dietary saponin [19]. Despite the direct mechanism for reported results is not elicited but presumably interactions exist between saponins and steroid receptors given the similarities between the basic chemical structures of saponins and steroid hormones [20]. Presumably saponins block the expression of the genes coding for androgen receptors and 5-areductases that converts testosterone into the dihydrotestosterone [21].

As reported the saponins and polysaccharides are the main bioactive compounds in the sea cucumber [5] which decreased serum cholesterol in rats [7]. These results suggest Persian Gulf sea cucumber extract has impairs steroid hormone synthesis in Molly fish. So, the observed results might because of the bioactive components in the *Holothuria leucospilota*. However, there was no previous report on effect of sea cucumber on testosterone, β-estradiol and cholesterol in moly fish. So, further researches needed to determine accuracy of the results and the possible molecular and cellular mechanisms for effect of AEPGSC and NPEPGSC on steroid hormones levels in Molly fish. Also, because of differences in sex hormone generation between marine and human, further researches needed to determine administration of sea cucumber for human clinical trials.

References

1. Haider MS, Sultana R, Jamil K, Lakht Z, Tarar OM, et al. (2015) A Study on proximate composition, amino acid profile, fatty acid profile and some mineral contents in two species of sea cucumber. J Anim Plant Sci 25: 168-175.

2. Farjami B, Nematollahi M, Moradi Y, Nazemi M (2014) Derivation of extracts from Persian Gulf sea cucumber (*Holothuria leucospilota*) and assessment of its antifungal effect. Iranian J Fisheries Sci 13: 785-795.

3. Awaluddin A (2001) Pharmaceuticals. In: The Encyclopedia of Malaysia: The Seas. Ong JE, Gong WK (eds.). Editions Didier Millet, Kuala Lumpur, pp: 18-19.

4. Mamelona J, Pelletier E, Girard-Lalancette K, Legault J, Karboune S, et al. (2007) Quantification of phenolic contents and antioxidant capacity of Atlantic sea cucumber, *Cucumaria frondosa*. Food Chem 104: 1040-1047.

5. Guo LY, Wang L, Zou XY, Liu ZY, Liu XY, et al. (2009) Antitumor and immunomodulating effects of *Apostichopus japonicus* polysaccharides (AJPS) in tumor-bearing mice. Chinese J Microecol 21: 806-808.

6. Liu X, Sun Z, Zhang M, Meng X, Xia X, et al. (2012) Antioxidant and antihyperlipidemic activities of polysaccharides from sea cucumber *Apostichopus japonicas*. Carbohydrate Polymers 90: 1664- 1670.

7. Hu XQ, Xu J, Xue Y, Li ZJ, Wang JF, et al. (2012) Effects of bioactive components of sea cucumber on the serum, liver lipid profile and lipid absorption. Biosci Biotechnol Biochem 76: 2214-2218.

8. Althunibat OY, Hashim RB, Taher M, Daud JM, Ikeda MA, et al. (2009) *In vitro* antioxidant and antiproliferative activities of three Malaysian sea cucumber species. Eur J Sci Res 37: 376-387.

9. Francis G, Kerem Z, Makkar HPS, Becker K (2002) The biological action of saponins in animal systems: a review. Br J Nutr 88: 587-605.

10. Moghadam FD, Baharara J, Balanezhad SZ, Jalali M, Amini E (2016) Effect of *Holothuria leucospilota* extracted saponin on maturation of mice oocyte and granulosa cells. Res Pharm Sci 11: 130.

11. Cabas I, Chaves-Pozo E, García-Alcázar A, Meseguer J, Mulero V, et al. (2013) The effect of 17α-ethynylestradiol on steroidogenesis and gonadal cytokine gene expression is related to the reproductive stage in marine hermaphrodite fish. Marine drugs 11: 4973-4992.

12. Ridzwan BH, Leong TC, Syed I (2003) The antinociceptive effects of water extracts from sea cucumbers *Holothuria leucospilota* Brandt, *Bohadschia marmorata vitiensis* Jaeger and coelomic fluid from *Stichopus hermanii*. Pak J Biol Sci 6: 2068-2072.

13. Esmat AY, Said MM, Soliman AA, El-Masry KSH, Badiea EA (2013) Bioactive compounds, antioxidant potential, and hepatoprotective activity of sea cucumber (*Holothuria atra*) against thioacetamide intoxication in rats. Nutr 29: 258-267.

14. Dakrory AI, Fahmy SR, Soliman AM, Mohamed AS, Amer SAM (2015) Protective and Curative Effects of the Sea Cucumber *Holothuria atra* Extract against DMBA-Induced Hepatorenal Diseases in Rats. BioMed Research International 2015: 563652.

15. Bligh EG, Dyer WJ (1959) A rapid method for total lipid extraction and purification. Can J Biochem Physiol 37: 911-917.

16. Hossain Z, Sugawara T, Aida K, Hirata T (2011) Effect of dietary glucosylceramide from sea cucumber on plasma and liver lipids in cholesterol-fed mice. Fish Sci 77: 1081-1085.

17. Bureau DP, Harris AM, Cho CY (1998) The effects of purified alcohol extracts from soy products on feed intake and growth of chinook salmon (*Oncorhynchus tshawytscha*) and rainbow trout (*Oncorhynchus mykiss*). Aquaculture 161: 27-43.

18. Li HP, Zhang MM, Ma GJ (2010) Hypolipidemic effect of the polysaccharide from Pholiota nameko. Nutr 26: 556-562.

19. Francis G, Makkar HPS, Becker K (2001) Antinutritional factors present in plant-derived alternate fish feed ingredients and their effects in fish. Aquaculture 199: 197-227.

20. Menzies GS, Howland K, Rae MT, Bramley TA (1999) Stimulation of specific binding of [3H]-progesterone to bovine luteal cell-surface membranes: specificity of digitonin. Mol Cel Endocrinol 153: 57-69.

21. Liu WK, Xu SX, Che CT (2000) Anti-proliferative effect of ginseng saponins on human prostate cancer cell line. Life Sci 67: 1297-1306.

2

Major Animal Health Constraints of Market Oriented Livestock Development in Sidama Dale District Southern Region Ethiopia

Abdulhakim Albe[1], Teka Feyera[1] and Kefyalew Gebeyew[2*]

[1]*College of Veterinary Medicine, Jigjiga University, Jigjiga, Ethiopia*
[2]*College of Dry Land Agriculture, Department of Animal and Range Science, Jijiga University, Ethiopia*

Abstract

Background: Knowing the status of major problems that constrain livestock development no doubt contributes to initiating projects that can help improve productivity and market success of Ethiopian farmers; aiming at contributing to reduction in poverty of the rural poor through market oriented agricultural development. The objective of this study is to characterize the livestock production system and investigating the major livestock health problems in the area.

Methodology: Purposive sampling method was used to select 60 households from four peasant association (PA). A structured questionnaire was prepared and the heads of selected households were interviewed to collect data on production system characteristics and the importance of livestock health problems. Focus group discussion was also made with key respondents from each PA and the participants described the major husbandry problems in their area.

Results: The results revealed that mixed crop-livestock production system is the predominant system and animals are kept in very limited grazing land. The livestock herd was dominated by poultry (36.4%), goat (19.51%), sheep (19.13%) and cattle (18.94%) while the cattle herd was dominated by cows (39.27%) and oxen (12.87%). The main roles of poultry in the area are for egg production (43.79%), sale (29.76%) and meat production (26.43%). The main role of cattle in the farming system is as a source of traction power (41.7%) for crop production while small ruminants as source of income (100%). Equines were used as pack and transport animals. The livestock feeding was mainly based on natural pasture (100%). In cattle; blackleg, mastitis, Lumpy Skin Disease (LSD) and calf diarrhea were the most important diseases. Ectoparasite and GIT parasitosis were the most important diseases in small ruminants. Colic and respiratory problems were considered important in equine. In poultry, Newcastle disease was the most devastating disease. Most of the respondents complained that animal feed followed by water shortage is serious problem in the livestock sector. Modern veterinary medicaments (95%) were known and used by most of the farmers, but traditional medicines were also used to a considerable extent (5%).

Conclusion: Emphasis should be given in the animal health delivery to maximize health service coverage of the area and Detail epidemiological studies on major economically important diseases of livestock is recommended to be under taken.

Keywords: Animal; Health; Constraints; Livestock; Dale; Survey

Introduction

Livestock in the Greater Horn of Africa is vital resource in promoting development. They provide 20-30% of the Gross Domestic Product (GDP), and at the farmer level as much as 70% of cash income is generated from livestock [1]. Livestock are used by humans to provide a wide range of products and services. Foods derived from animals are important source of nutrients [2] that provide a critical supplement and diversity to staple plant-based diets [3,4].

Ethiopia has one of the largest livestock population in Africa with the estimated domestic animal number of 52.13 million cattle, 24.2 million sheep, 22.6 million goat, 2.5 million camels, 44.89 million poultry, 1.96 million horses, 0.37 million mules and 6.4 million donkeys [5]. Ethiopia's great livestock potential is not properly exploited due to different factors such as traditional management system, limited genetic potential, lack of appropriate disease control policy and lack of appropriate veterinary services [6]. Animal diseases are considered as a major health problem and cause a significant economic loss in countries where livestock production is an important segment of the agricultural practice [7].

Infectious animal diseases that are endemic, or common in a region, generate a variety of significant adverse economic consequences. Most directly, mortality, morbidity, barrenness, and miscarriage in production animals reduce technical efficiency. Costly treatments and altered management practices to ameliorate these losses also reduce profitability [8]. Diseases have numerous negative impacts on productivity and fertility of herds (losses due to mortality and morbidity, loss of weight, depressed growth, poor fertility performance, decrease physical power and the likes [9]. Thus, knowing the status of major problems that constrain livestock development no doubt contributes to initiating projects that can help improve productivity and market success of Ethiopian farmers; aiming at contributing to reduction in poverty of the rural poor through market oriented agricultural development [10]. Therefore, this research intended to characterize the livestock production system in the selected peasant associations of the Dale Districts and to provide baseline information on the major animal health constraints that contribute to poor livestock productivity in the area.

***Corresponding author:** Kefyalew Gebeyew, Lecturer, College of Dry Land Agriculture, Department of Animal and Range Science, Jijiga University, PO Box 1020, Jijiga, Ethiopia, E-mail: kefyalewgebeyew@yahoo.com

Materials and Methods

Description of study area

The study was conducted in Dale District which is located between 6°27'00" - 6° 51'00" N latitude and 38°00'00" -38°37'00"E longitude in Sidama Zone, Southern Nations Nationalities and Peoples (SNNP) Regional State of Ethiopia. This District is one of the 21 District in the Zone covering a total area of 1,494.63 km^2 with the altitude range of 1100 m to 2650 m (from low lands in the west to the highlands in the east) and at about of 320 km south of Addis Ababa [11]. The main livestock species in the District are cattle, goats and sheep. The livestock resources are cattle - 225,698 (82,666 local cows and 1584 crossbred dairy animals, 80% are in urban and peri-urban areas); sheep - 30,152; Goats - 31,443; Poultry - 218,923; Horses - 2,498; Mules - 431; Donkeys - 16,321; Beehives - 10,949.

Study protocol

Sampling procedure and sample size: A purposive selection method has been done to select the peasant associations based on accessibility to transport and difference in geographical location. Accordingly, four peasant associations (PAs) namely; Arada, gejaba, Mesincho and Shefin were purposely selected as study sites. From each PA 15 households were randomly selected which then made a total of 60 households to be included in the study. All livestock (Cattle, sheep, goat, equine) and poultry owned by selected respondents were considered as study animals, consequently, there were a total of 1597 animals sampled constituting 303 cattle, 312 goats, 306 sheep, and 91 equine and 585 poultry.

Data collection

Questionnaire survey: A detailed questionnaire was designed to generate information related to animal production (demographic features of respondents and their land use pattern, livestock herd size, livestock function, feeding practice and availability, management systems such as watering, housing, breeding and record keeping, labor use and livestock marketing) with particular emphasis on major livestock health problems in the area and measures taken by the farmers against livestock diseases and trend of using modern veterinary services. The questionnaire was pretested before its full implementation and adjusted for clarity to shorten the time it takes while administering and minimize recall bias and it was filled directly by interviewing randomly selected farmers from different villages of the four PAs.

Focus group discussion

The focus group discussion was done with 10 key respondents from each PA identified by PAs development agents. Points considered during the discussion were disease occurrence and trend for the last few years and constraints of livestock production. The major livestock problems such as major diseases, major feed types in the area, and other issues on livestock production have been raised for discussion to collect basic information. Consultation of the District veterinary professional to identify the major livestock health problems in their area and about the health services coverage of the District. The cases were classified by species in to diseases affecting cattle, goat, sheep and equine.

Data analysis

The data collected were entered in to MS-Excel 2000 computer program. The analysis and summarization of the data was made using simple descriptive statistics.

Results

Demographic and land holding features of respondents

Demographic feature of respondents showed that most of the interviewees (81.7%) were male and the rest female (18.3%). Their educational back ground indicated that 56.7% (n=34) were literate, 33.4% (n=20) are primary school, 23.3% (n=14) are secondary school and above, 20% (n=12) had illiterate knowledge and 23.3% (n=14) had religious knowledge (Table 1). Respondent's family size proportion showed 158 (44.8%) and 194 (55.2%) have family members less or equal to 15 years of age and greater than 15 years of age, respectively. The average family size was 5.87 persons from which more than half (55.2%) was above 15 years old.

The vast majority (90%) and majority of the farmers (73.3%) had their own crop land and grazing land, respectively. The average total land size owned by households was 1 ha and about 90% of the respondents had their own crop land where as some 6.7% of the respondent's uses ranted cropland. On the other hand, average crop and grazing land per household were 0.8183 and 0.125 ha respectively. The average privately owned crop land size was 0.016 ha and none of them owned private grazing land at all (Table 2).

Livestock inventory and composition

The average herd size and composition of cattle, sheep, goats, equines and poultry per households' are presented in Table 3. Poultry comprise the largest proportion of the livestock herd (n=585, 36.4%), and followed by goat (n=312, 19.51%), Sheep (n=306, 19.13%), cattle (n=303, 18.94%), lastly Equines (n=91, 5.67%) in their order of appearance. Cows (39.27%) dominate the most shares of cattle herd size followed by calves (24.3%). In the case of sheep and goats, the flock is comprised primarily of ewe and doe respectively. In goats doe's represent 102 (32.6%) and in Sheep ewe's proportion were 99 (32.3%). The equine herd is very much dominated by donkeys taking 70.32% of the share of which mature male donkeys are the predominant ones 57.8%.

Purpose of keeping livestock

The most important product of cattle was milk (100%). There were also households producing meat (46.7%), and hides (20%) from cattle. Milk was consumed as raw by 80% of the respondents and regarding

Variable	N	Category	Frequency (Proportion)
Sex	60	Male	81.7
		Female	18.3
Educational Status	60	Illiterate	20.0
		Religious	23.3
		Literate	56.7
		primary school	33.4%
		≥ Secondary school	23.3%
Family size	60	<15 years	44.8
		=> 15 years	55.2

Table 1: Demographic and land holding features of respondents.

Land use pattern	Mean	Minimum	Maximum
Cropland owned (ha)	1.1	4 (0.2 ha)	3 (2 ha)
Crop land contracted (ha)	0.5	56 (0 ha)	4 (1 ha)
Fallow land owned (ha)	0.15	10 (0.1 ha)	7 (0.2 ha)
Grazing land owned (ha)	0.3	13 (0.1 ha)	5 (0.5 ha)
Total (ha)	2.05		

Table 2: Mean maximum and minimum values of land holdings in the sampled households.

√		Number	Range	Minimum	Maximum	Proportion from livestock herd	Proportion from species herd
	cattle						N=303
√	Calve male	26	1	1	2	1.62	8.5
√	Calve female	48	2	1	3	3.00	15.8
√	Heifers	32	3	1	4	2.00	10.5
√	Dry cow	38	3	1	4	2.37	12.5
√	lact. cow	81	3	1	4	5.07	26.7
√	Oxen	39	1	1	2	2.44	12.8
√	Bulls	39	1	1	2	2.44	12.8
	Goat						N=312
√	Kid male	21	1	1	2	1.31	6.7
√	Kid female	17	2	1	3	1.06	5.4
√	Yearling	46	2	1	3	2.88	14.7
√	Doe	102	4	1	5	6.38	32.6
√	Goat castrated	24	2	1	3	1.50	7.6
√	Buck	102	4	1	5	6.38	32.6
	Sheep						N=306
√	Lamb male	24	2	1	3	1.50	7.8
√	Lamb female	27	1	1	2	1.69	8.8
√	Yearling	49	1	1	2	3.06	16.0
√	Ewe	99	3	1	4	6.19	32.3
√	Sheep castrated	14	1	1	2	0.87	4.5
√	Ram	93	3	1	4	5.82	30.3
	Donkey						N=64
√	Young donkey	18	1	1	2	1.12	28.1
√	Mature female donkey	9	0	1	1	0.56	14.0
√	Mature male donkey	37	1	1	2	2.31	57.8
	Horse						N=27
√	Young horse	5	1	1	2	0.31	18.5
√	Mature female horse	1	0	1	1	0.06	3.7
√	Mature male horse	21	1	1	2	1.31	77.7
	Poultry						N=585
√	Young	236	19	1	20	14.7	40.3
√	Mature female	183	5	1	6	11.4	31.2
√	Mature male	166	5	1	6	10.3	28.3

Table 3: Herd size of livestock per household.

meat, 19.7% consumed raw form. Most of the households consumed egg in boiled/cooked form (91.7%) and 8.3% of the respondents consumed raw. The most important purpose of cattle was provision of traction power (41.7%). Goats (85%) and sheep (86.7%) were kept for sale and meat production (58.3%) and (56.7%) for both goats and sheep respectively. Donkeys were kept solely for loading (100%) and horses for transportation (100%) purposes.

Livestock management

Housing: Some of the respondents (10%) house comprises different species of animals within one house, which is separated from their own (main) house; and 90% of the respondent's house comprises the same species of animals in different houses, which are separated their own (main) home. Regarding breeding, most of the respondents (73.3%) use uncontrolled natural mating and only 26.7% of the respondents use selected bulls (controlled natural breeding) to reproduce cattle.

Water source: In the study site, they have water sources for watering animal like rivers, streams, ponds and well. Majority of the livestock water source were river (40.2%), well (27.3%), stream (18%), and pond (14.3%). These water sources are not available throughout the year. They encounter shortage of water mostly during the dry season especially from January to March (winter) seasons.

Feed resources and feeding practices

Natural pasture (100%) and Stover (65%) were the most frequently used feed resources in the study area. The respondents also reported that feed availability depends on seasons. Feed shortage is the main problem especially during dry season in the study area to maintain market oriented livestock development extension. Natural pasture was more available in the wet season (100%). Most of the farmers supplement livestock with minerals (51.7%) and availability of minerals is most of the time during the wet season about (95%) (Table 4). Among the interviewed farmers, 23.3% had communal grazing land and (73.3%) of interviewed farmers used grazing land on year round basis.

Livestock culling criteria and disposal of cadaver and abortion materials

The most common reasons of culling livestock mentioned by farmers were poor productivity (33.3%), old age (25.5%), diseased (22%) and infertility (19.1%) were also mentioned by farmers. Majority of the respondents (77.7%) said that dead animals, after birth fluids and aborts were simply thrown away in the nature. Giving to scavenger animals (dogs and hyena) (13.3%) also mentioned as a disposing means, and burring (9%) to some extent.

Feed resource	Frequency (Proportion) of farmers	Availability	
		Dry season	Wet season
Natural pasture	100 (60)	0	100 (60)
Stover	65 (39)	18.3 (11)	81.7 (49)
Cultivated pasture	81.7 (49)	16.7 (10)	83.3 (50)
Minerals	51.7 (31)	5 (3)	95 (57)

Table 4: Major livestock feed resources in the study areas.

Health problems identified by respondents at survey

The information generated through the questionnaire survey and focus group discussion indicated that diseases are one of the most important limiting factors of livestock keeping in the area. They also indicated that the disease dynamics is aggravated by many factors like, inadequate veterinary service, season, agro-ecological and minimum attention to animal health by government and non-government bodies. Scarcity and shortage of livestock feed are also known to be limiting factors to animal production by making animals unproductive and susceptible to many diseases. Livestock owners were asked to describe five important diseases, which affect animal species in the study area (cattle, sheep, goats and equines) and prioritize them based on their relative degree of importance. Respondents described diseases in their local names (Table 5). These local names were given their veterinary equivalent name based on, the symptoms mentioned and discussions with veterinarians in the area. According to the District animal health professionals, the main problems affecting the livestock keeping in order of appearance is shortage of feed/ grazing land, water shortage and diseases respectively. Lack of transport followed by lack of drugs and vaccines are the major problems faced in the treatment of livestock and the drugs that are available are costly in the District because of that owners use traditional healers. Furthermore, the respondents reflected that they need to have the knowledge how to improve feed shortage, e.g., using cultivated pasture and they had comments like, the drug that the animal health professional use privately is not the correct drug, but drug like soft drinks.

Occurrence of abortion in the last two years

About 38.3% of the farmers encountered abortion in the past two years. The most frequent abortion occurred in bovine (39.1%), caprine (26.1%) and ovine (34.7%). Mostly abortions occurred in early and late gestation period. The season's encountered abortions are autumn and summer

Control measures against livestock diseases

Although the majority of the farmers on the study area have access to modern veterinary service (95%), a considerable proportion of respondents, 48.3%, use traditional healer for many different abnormalities, and diseases conditions such as infectious diseases, parasitic diseases and non-infectious cases. From the proportion of respondents who use traditional healer, infectious cases (51.7%) are the most treated using traditional medicament followed by parasitic cases (48.22%). Modern treatment is given in the Yirgalem veterinary clinic at Yirgalem town; there was no other private veterinary clinic in the area and there were only private drug shops. From the proportion of respondents who use modern veterinary services, 40.32% mentioned transport/ distance to the veterinary clinic as a main problem faced when they want to treat or vaccinate their animals. Drugs and vaccine shortage and Lack of modern clinical services were mentioned by 41.86%, and 17.81% of the respondents respectively.

Veterinary service

95% of the respondents have an access to modern veterinary service and 5% have no access to modern veterinary service. Cost of treatment and vaccination and proportion of respondents is described in Table 6. The survey also indicated that 31.7% (N=19) of the respondents reported to the government body when outbreak /diseases were encountered.

Discussion

Characteristics of the livestock production system

This survey showed that mixed-livestock production is the most practiced production system in the area. Shortage of land is mentioned to be one of the constraints for the livestock development in the area, since food crop cultivation is given first priority. Poultry are the dominant livestock species present in the area. Cattle, Sheep and goats also comprised a good proportion of the livestock species. The farmers kept cattle mostly for milk, meat and traction power although the yield of the local cattle is not significant, which is not exceeding the house hold consumption according to Ref. [12]. Use of local bulls for breeding is the primary option for most farmers (73.33%). This figure is more or less similar to the survey report of Ref. [12], conducted in Alaba District which reported that 75% use local bulls for breeding. This may be attributed to shortage of AI service coverage in the area. Based on the result of this study livestock diseases and their consequences have severe impact on the small holder farmers' livelihood directly and indirectly. Animal diseases have also been indicated as public health hazards [13]. It is also indicated that major constraints to alleviate animal health problems include low quality and inadequate animal health services, minimum attention to the services, low and/or no private sector involvement, moreover, the animal health of the District is also exacerbated by different factors like feed and water shortage, poor management, dirty water, traditional treatment practices.

Animal health problems

Cattle: Black leg was one of the most mentioned infections of cattle's as described in the in Table 5. All of the respondents describe black leg to affect all age and sex groups of cattle except calves. Although the degree varies as found in heifer, cows and bulls as found in this study. This is consistent with that described by Radostits et al. [14] regarding the diseases incidence that is high when calves reach the susceptible age group which is largely confined to young stock between the age of 6 months and 2 years. Black leg was also reported to be the most important infectious diseases with a prevalence rate of 20% in the north part of Ethiopia by Leggess [15]. Furthermore the diseases were claimed to be the leading cattle health problem together with anthrax in Ginchi water shade areas as reported by Eshete et al. [16].

Mastitis was also the second most important disease affecting cows as mentioned by 33.33% of the interviewed farmers. Cows are at risk of acquiring mastitis when there is improper milking and poor udder health management like preventing teat from lesion causing agent like tick infestation [17]. Mastitis was one of the most economically important multi-causal infections of cows in the study area. Mastitis is economically the single most important diseases of the dairy cattle. It reduces milk yields, profit and the quality of milk and milk products in all dairy producing countries of the world and premature culling [18]. There is also culling due to diseases caused low production (milk); that was described by Mungube [19] who reported annual mastitis culling rate of 7.23% due to milk loss.

The result of this study revealed that Lumpy Skin Disease (LSD) was the most mentioned skin disease by respondents. Especially in

Name of the disease	Local name	No of farmers described the disease as					Overall Rank
		1st	2nd	3rd	4th	5th	
Calves							
• Calf diarrhoea	*Siittu deeo*	25	20	6	4	5	1
• Black leg	*Lammootta*	17	31	6	3	3	2
• Mite	*Bijajo*	9	15	26	8	2	3
Cow							
• Black leg	*Lammootta*	21	17	9	7	6	1
• Mastitis	*Gadansa*	20	19	21	0	0	2
• LSD	*Qada*	19	31	4	3	3	3
Ox							
• Black leg	*Lammootta*	24	16	12	6	2	1
• LSD	*Qada*	26	15	10	9	0	2
• Tick infestation	*Deere*	10	30	17	3	0	3
Shoat							
• Ectoparasite	*Gobbayidi irkiraano*	30	15	8	5	2	1
• GIT parasite	*Godowu gido irkirano*	19	31	6	3	1	2
• Respiratory problem	*Folate amanyoti qara*	11	29	13	5	2	3
Equine							
• Wound	*Mada*	27	23	6	4	0	1
• Colic	*Game*	22	17	15	3	3	2
• Respiratory problem	*Folate amanyoti qara*	11	20	14	9	6	3

Table 5: Major diseases of livestock mentioned by sampled farmers.

Degree of cost	Treatment		Vaccination	
	Frequency	Percentage	Frequency	Percentage
Expensive	28	46.7	19	31.7
Moderate	27	45.0	36	60.0
Cheap	5	8.3	5	8.3

Table 6: Response to cost of treatment and vaccination at the study area.

cow, (16%) has got the third diseases affecting cows. This is followed by in heifer (15%) which has got the third rank from the list of diseases affecting heifer groups [20]. Also report similar result (7%) incidence in Yerer water shade, Adaliben District. The disease is known to affect the body condition and work output of the affected cattle and decreased milk yield as indicated by different authors [14,17]. All age groups (except calves) and both sex are mentioned by respondents in this study to be affected by LSD.

In the present study, calf diarrhea is mentioned by farmers as a serious health problem affecting calf. Calves could be infected by environmental bacteria such as *Eshershicia coli*, *Salmonella* species as well as virus like Rota virus, Corona virus, and feed change. The importance of calf diarrhea was also reported by previous authors [21]. Several factors affect the health and vigor of calf in the early period of calf hood. Among these factors inadequate feeding of colostrums, farm hygiene and environmental conditions are the most important.

Sheep and goat

Parasitic diseases in small ruminants were found to be high which was responded by the farmers during interview and contact of veterinary professional. Among the parasitic diseases, endoparastic infestation comprises more than half of the reported cases. This could be attributed to overgrazing of infested pasture and low use of antihelmenthics. Which also agrees (15%) with the report of Abraha [22].

In sheep and goats, respiratory problems which is characterized by nasal discharge and coughing and subsequently death in some cases was mentioned by farmer as the first most important disease. The same result was reported by Mekonnen [23] in Arsi highlands. The clinical signs are suggestive of pasteurellosis which are in agreement with the signs of pasteurellosis described by Gilmour [24].

Equine

Wounds are amongst one of the commonest health concerns to afflict working donkeys in many countries [25]. In addition, the study on donkey in Ethiopia has demonstrated that back sores and wounds are the most commonly observed health problem. Unfortunately, carts, wounds, punctures and lacerations are a fact of life when one has mules and donkeys. The potential cause of equine wounds are almost endless: punctures from sharp object like metal and glass; shear wounds from barbed wire sticks; collusion injuries from falling or running in to the object and entrapment, such as getting a leg hung up in a rope or in a cattle are major cause of injury [26].

Wounds in working donkeys are seen on the leg, girth, tail, saddle and wither regions [26]. These wounds are often caused by a combination of poorly fitting and designed tack or harnesses, beating with sticks and improper management practices. One approach to decrease the prevalence of wounds is through educations of donkey users. Ethiopian farmers have themselves identified a need for greater knowledge through training [27].

Colic (abdominal pain) is an important and frequently occurring disease in the area according to the respondents both in the group discussion and questionnaire survey. All owners of equines listed this disease problem as the second most important. This is attributed to poor management, especially poor care of the teeth, heavy infestation rate of houses with the red worms, restricted access to water, feeding of equine with feeds that their intestine is not able to digest. The causes of this disease sign are numerous in number among these are impaction [28], spasmodic colic, intussusceptions, vulvulus torsion, strangulation, tympany, colitis and verminous cases. The third important equine health problem in this study was respiratory disease complex. Three to eight percent incidence rate of respiratory disease complex was reported by Rose [28].

The first most important equine health problem causing death and decreased work output in this study was respiratory disease complex. 3-8% incidence rate of respiratory disease complex was reported by Rose [28]. In another study in central Ethiopia, 57% and 43% incidence rates were reported for males and females, respectively [29]. It could be associated with high temperature and aridity of some parts of the District.

Poultry

Focus group discussion and interviewees strongly complained that Newcastle disease (NCD) is a very important chicken disease. It was also reported by Dessie [30] that NCD was the single major health constraint which causes heavy mortality and morbidity to village chicken and affects productivity of the system in the country. This could be due to poor hygienic conditions of the backyard raising condition, selling or low attention to treat sick chicken and receive no vaccination at all. Its frequency in the District is related to absence of control and prevention methods to reduce its economic impact. Salmonellosis and coccidiosis were also among the mentioned diseases by veterinary professional in Yirgalem veterinary clinic.

Conclusion

Diseases and feed shortage were the problem of livestock development extension programs in the study area. Blackleg, Mastitis, LSD and Calf diarrhea were the most important diseases of cattle. Wound, colic and respiratory disease complex were considered as the most important constraints of equine health. Modern veterinary medicaments were known and used by most of the farmers, but traditional medicines were also used to a significant extent. Therefore, Emphasis should be given in the animal health delivery to maximize health service coverage of the area. Livestock owners must receive basic training regarding animal diseases prevention, modern techniques in animal husbandry and management skills which can fit to the local situation, and Detail epidemiological survey on major economically important diseases of livestock is recommended to be under taken.

Competing Interest

The authors declare that they have no competing interest.

Authors' Contributions

AA conceived the study, designed and conducted all laboratory experiments; analyzed and interpreted experimental results. TF and KG participated in the proposal, study design and manuscript preparations. All authors read and approved the final manuscript.

Acknowledgements

The author's heart fully appreciation is to Jigjiga University for funding the cost of research work. Most truthful thanks go to all my friends and family, Sidama District Agriculture office staffs for their valuable assistance during data collection work of this study.

References

1. Ndikima S, Suth J, Kamadi R, Ossera S, Marambi R, et al. (2000) Coping mechanisms and their efficiency in disaster-prone pastoral system of greater horn of Africa. Effect of the 1995-1997 draught and the 1997-1998 ELNINO rains and response of pastorals and livestock. International Livestock research Institute (ILRI), Nairobi, Kenya. pp: 2-4.
2. Givens DI (2010) Milk and meat in our diet: good or bad for health? Animal 4: 1941-1952.
3. Murphey SP, Allen LH (2003) Nutritional importance of animal source foods. J Nutr 133: 3893-3897.
4. Randolph TF, Schelling E, Grace D, Nicholson CF, Leroy JL, et al. (2007) Invited review: Role of livestock in human nutrition and health for poverty reduction in developing countries. J Anim Sci 85: 2788-2800.
5. Central Statistics Authority (2012) Federal Democratic Republic of Ethiopia. Agricultural sample survey on livestock and livestock production (Private peasant holdings), Statistical Bulletin No. 532, Addis Ababa, Ethiopia 2: 9-20.
6. Genet M, Tadesse G, Basaznew B, Mersha C (2012) Pathological Conditions Causing Organ and Carcass Condemnation and Their Financial Losses in Cattle Slaughtered in Gondar, Northwest Ethiopia. Afr J Basic Appl Sci 4: 200-208.
7. Fekadu A, Legesse E, Tesfaye D (2012) The Cause, Rate and Economic Implication of Organ Condemnation Cattle Slaughtered at Jimma Municipal Abattoir, Southwestern Ethiopi. Global Veterinaria 9: 396-400.
8. Bennett R, Ijpelaar J (2005) Updated Estimate of the cost Associated with thirty four Endemic Livestock Diseases in Great Britain: A note. J Agric Econ 56: 135-144.
9. Central Agriculture Census Commission (2003) Ethiopian Agricultural Sample Enumeration, Land Use 2001-2002 (1994 E.C), Addis Ababa, Ethiopia. pp: 29-43.
10. https://ipmsethiopia.wordpress.com/
11. Central Statistics Authority (2003) Ethiopian Agricultural Sample Enumeration, 2001/2002. Southern Nation Nationalities and Peoples Region. Statistical report on livestock and farm implements. Addis Ababa, Ethiopia. pp: 35-43.
12. Mekonnen K (2007) Major animal health problems of market oriented livestock development in Alaba Woreda, Southern Nations Nationalities and people's region. DVM thesis, FVM, Addis Ababa University, Debrezeit, Ethiopia. p: 21.
13. Assegid W (2000) Constraints to livestock and its products in Ethiopia: Policy implications. DVM Thesis, FVM, Addis Ababa University, Debrezeit, Ethiopia.
14. Radostits DM, Blood DC, Gay CC (1994) Veterinary Medicine. A Text book of diseases of cattle, sheep, pigs, goats and horses. 8th edition. London, Bailliere Tindal, pp: 748-785.
15. Leggess G (1996) Livestock Health Conditions in Central Tigray. In: Rural Exploratory Studies Processing of a Workshop. Oyhus AO, Gebru G (eds). Agricultural University of Norwegian (AUN). pp: 85-100.
16. Eshete G, Yami A, Baars R (2002) An assessment of feed resources, their management and impact on livestock productivity in Ginchi watershed area. MSc Thesis Presented to School of Graduate Studies of Haramaya University, Haramaya, Ethiopia.
17. Quinn PJ, Carter ME, Markey B, Carter GR (1994) Clinical veterinary microbiology. Wolfe publishing, London. pp: 175-179.
18. Radostitis OM (2001) Heard health: Food animal production medicine. 3rd edition. WB Saunders Company, USA, pp: 1-45.
19. Mungube E (2001) Management and Economics of dairy cow mastitis in the urban area of Addis Ababa. MSc Thesis, Faculty of Veterinary Medicine, Addis Ababa University, DebreZeit, Ethiopia.
20. Tesfahiwot Z (2004) Major health problems of livestock in the Yerer watershed, Adaliben woreda, South Eastern Shoa, DebreZeït, Ethiopia. DVM Thesis, Faculty of Veterinary Medicine, Addis Ababa University, DebreZeit, Ethiopia.
21. Busato A, Steiner L, Martin SW, Shoukri MM, Gaillard C (1997) Calf health in cow-calf herds in Switzerland. Prev Vet Med 30: 9-22.
22. Abraha G (2007) Major animal health problems of market oriented livestock development in Atsbin Womberta woreda, Tigray Regional State. DVM Thesis, Faculty of Veterinary Medicine, Addis Ababa University, DebreZeit, Ethiopia.
23. Mekonnen T (2000) An epidemiological study on ovine pasteurellosis in Arsi, South East Ethiopia. DVM Thesis, Faculty of Veterinary Medicine, Addis Ababa University, DebreZeit, Ethiopia.
24. Gilmour NJL (1993) Pasteurelosis: The Disease. In: Pasteurelosis in Animal Production. ACIAR Proceedings 43: 79-83.
25. Nengomasha E, Jell N, Pearson RA (1995) Phenotypic characteristics of working donkeys in Western Zimbabwe. In: Proceedings of the ATNESA workshop 'Meeting the challenges of animal traction', December 4-8 1995, Karen, Ngong Hills, Kenya.
26. Martin Curran M, Feseha G, Smith DG (2005) The impact of access to animal health services on donkey health and livelihoods in Ethiopia. Trop Anim Health Prod 37 Suppl 1: 47-65.
27. Tesfaye A, Martin Curran M (2005) A longitudinal survey of market donkeys in Ethiopia. Trop Anim Health Prod 37 Suppl 1: 87-100.
28. Rose RJ, Hodgson DR (2000) Manual of equine practice. 2nd edn. WB Saunders, USA, pp: 187-292.
29. Alemnesh W (2004) Investigation in the Occurrence of Strangles in Four Woreda of Central Ethiopia. DVM Thesis, Faculty of Veterinary Medicine, Addis Ababa University, Debrezeit, Ethiopia.
30. Dessie T, Jobre Y (2004) A review of the importance and control of Newcastle disease in Ethiopia. Ethiopian Veterinary Journal 8: 71-81.

Identification of Commonly Used Anthelmintic Drugs and Evaluation of their Utilization in University of Gondar Veterinary Clinic

Chalachew Kassahun[1], Ahmed Adem[1], Mebrie Zemene[1]*, Gashaw Getaneh[2] and Kassahun Berrie[1]

[1]*Department of Veterinary Pharmacy, Faculty of Veterinary Medicine, University of Gondar, Gondar, Ethiopia*
[2]*Department of Biomedical Science, Faculty of Veterinary Medicine, University of Gondar, Gondar, Ethiopia*

Abstract

A retrospective study was conducted from March, 2016 to June, 2016 in University of Gondar veterinary clinic to identify commonly used anthelmintic drugs and to assess the pattern of anthelmintic utilization. Data on 557 anthelmintics was collected from case registration books written for the last two years and three months (from January 01, 2014 to March 30, 2016). Out of the total anthelmintics (557), 285 (51.2%) albendazole, 214 (38.4%) ivermectin, 24 (4.3%) mebendazole, 22 (3.9%) fenbendazole, 7 (1.3%) triclabendazole, 4 (0.7%) tetramizole and 1 (0.2%) praziquantel were utilized. 44.3% of the anthelmintics were prescribed to treat diseases that were tentatively diagnosed as nonparasitic cases. Out of the total anthelmintics utilized, 253 (45.4%) were given for bovine. 227 (40.8%) and 330 (59.2%) of the anthelmintics were prescribed for young and adult animals respectively. 395 (70.0%) and 167 (30.0%) of the anthelmintics were also given for animals with poor body condition and good body condition, respectively. 9.5%, 34.6%, 31.8%, and 24.1% of the anthelmintics were utilized in winter, spring, summer and autumn, respectively. 513 (92.1%) of the anthelmintics were prescribed to treat diseases that were diagnosed empirically. The remaining 44 (7.9%) were prescribed based on definitive (laboratory- supported) diagnosis. The total number of anthelmintics was prescribed by generic name. Out of the total anthelmintics, 385 (69.1%) were prescribed in combination with other drugs. The findings had shown that problems of correct diagnosis, repeated use of the same class of anthelmintics for long period and prescription of anthelmintics for nonparasitic diseases. Therefore, sound veterinary diagnosis before considering the use of anthelmintics and rotation of anthelmintics between classes should be practiced.

Keywords: Anthelmintics; Retrospective study; Utilization

Introduction

In Ethiopia, animals are important sources of income for rural communities whose livelihood is largely based on livestock production [1]. However, animal production in the country is hindered by many factors including animal health constraints, inadequate nutrition and poor husbandry systems [2]. Studies in different parts of the country have shown that helminth parasites are major problems in animal production, causing mortality and production losses [3-5]. The control of parasitic helminths in domestic animals relies largely on the use of anthelmintic drugs. But inappropriate and indiscriminate use of anthelmintic leads to the emergence of anthelmintic resistance, treatment failure and increase in mortality and morbidity [6].

Most failures during anthelmintic therapy may occur when the parasite is unknown and anthelmintic drugs are administered empirically. To avoid these problems, confirmatory diagnosis and selection of the right anthelmintic should be applied [7]. Irrational use of drugs in veterinary medicine as well as the need for control of their use becomes even bigger problem when used on food producing animals. In this case, there is the possibility that minimal quantities of drugs and their metabolites (residues) which remain in edible tissues or in animal products (meat, milk, eggs, honey) induce certain harmful effects in humans as potential consumers of such food [8]. When drugs are used to improve the productivity of food animals that are intended for human consumption, then there is possibility for producing adverse effects on humans. To prevent this risk, it is necessary to use drugs rationally, i.e., to use them only when they are really indicated, in the right way, at the right time, in the right dose and respecting withdrawal period [7].

Unsound use of anthelmintics in veterinary practice, for both food producing and companion animals, favors the development of either intrinsic or acquired anthelmintic resistance. Anthelmintic drug resistance is a growing problem, and indeed developing new drugs may not be the solution for this problem. Some of the common causes that contribute to the development of anthelmintic resistance are unnecessary use of anthelmintic drugs, inappropriate dose, inadequate duration of therapy, use of irrational drug combinations [9].

Globally, more than half of all medicines are prescribed, dispensed or sold improperly, and 50% of human patients fail to take them correctly. This is more wasteful, expensive and dangerous, both to the health of the individual patient and to the population as a whole that magnifies the problem of misuse of anthelmintic agents [7]. In Ethiopia, improper utilization of anthelmintic drugs has been reported by Beyene et al. [10] in Bishoftu, Central Ethiopia. The study conducted by Melaku et al. [11] from January to September, 2011 in North Gondar also revealed that anthelmintic drugs are quite commonly but improperly utilized in the area. There is no recent published report on the utilization of commonly used anthelmintics to control helminths of animals at university of Gondar veterinary clinic in particular and in north Gondar in general.

***Corresponding author:** Mebrie Zemene, Lecturer, Department of Veterinary Pharmacy, Faculty of Veterinary Medicine, University of Gondar, Gondar, Ethiopia
E-mail: zemenemebrie@gmail.com

Therefore, the objectives of the study were:

- To identify the commonly used anthelmintics in University of Gondar veterinary clinic
- To assess the pattern of anthelmintic utilization in University of Gondar veterinary clinic

Materials and Methods

Study area and period

The study was conducted from March, 2016 to June, 2016 in University of Gondar Veterinary Clinic, Gondar, North West Ethiopia, which is located at 739 km North West of Addis Ababa. Gondar is situated at 12.3-13.8°N, latitude and 35.3-35.7°E longitude and an altitude of 2200 meter above sea level. Farmers near to Gondar town practice a mixed crop-livestock farming system [12].

Study design

A retrospective survey was carried out to identify commonly used anthelmintic drugs and to assess the pattern of anthelmintic utilization in University of Gondar veterinary clinic. The study was conducted on anthelmintic drugs utilized in University of Gondar veterinary clinic from January 01, 2014 to March 30, 2016 for the treatment of animal's patients. All anthelmintic drugs utilized from January 01, 2014 to March 30, 2016 were assessed.

Data collection

Data was collected retrospectively from case registration books in University of Gondar Veterinary Clinic. The specific data necessary to the study was recorded for each anthelmintic drug and was entered into a data record form. For this particular study, data on 557 anthelmintics that contain the treated animal's characteristics (age and body condition), disease diagnosis (name, empiric or physical clinical examination and confirmatory laboratory tests used), prescribed anthelmintics (type, naming (generic or brand), other combined drugs prescribed and route of administration were collected from case books written for the last two years and three months (from January 01, 2014 to March 3, 2016).

Data analysis

All data in the record form was entered into Microsoft Excel spread sheet and descriptive statistics (Percentage) was computed. The data was analyzed using Statistical Package for Social Sciences (SPSS) version 16 statistical software.

Results

Commonly used anthelmintics

A retrospective data was collected on a total of 557 anthelmintics utilized in University of Gondar veterinary clinic from January 1, 2014 to March 30, 2016 and analyzed. Out of the total anthelmintics (557), 285 (51.2%) albendazole, 214 (38.4%) ivermectin, 24 (4.3%) mebendazole, 22 (3.9%) fenbendazole, 7 (1.3%) triclabendazole, 4 (0.7%) tetramizole and 1 (0.2%) and praziquantel were utilized (Table 1). 44.3% of the anthelmintics were prescribed to treat diseases that were tentatively diagnosed as nonparasitic cases (Table 2).

Anthelmintic utilization based on species, age, body condition of animals and season

Based on species of animals, out of the total anthelmintics utilized, 253 (45.4%) were given for bovine (Table 3). 227 (40.8%) and 330 (59.2%) of the anthelmintics were prescribed for young and adult animals, respectively (Table 3). 395 (70.0%) of the anthelmintics were also given for animals with poor body condition. The remaining 167(30%) were prescribed for animals with good body condition. The study indicated that the maximum anthelmintic use was observed in spring. The minimum anthelmintic use was also observed in winter (Table 3).

Anthelmintic utilization by type of diagnosis and prescription

The type of diagnosis, anthelmintic prescription and combination were also assessed. Among all anthelmintics utilized, 513 (92.1%) were prescribed to treat diseases that were diagnosed empirically, without getting correct definitive (laboratory- supported) diagnosis. The remaining 44 (7.9%) were prescribed based on definitive (laboratory-supported) diagnosis. The total number of anthelmintics was prescribed by generic name. Out of the total anthelmintics, 385 (69.1%) were prescribed in combination with other drugs (multivitamin, oxytetracycline, procaine penicillin, etc.) (Table 4).

Discussion

The study revealed that anthelmintic drugs are quite commonly but improperly utilized in the clinic. Three group of anthelmintics namely benzimidazoles (Albendazole, fenbendazole, mebendazole and triclabendazole), imidazothiazole (tetramisole and levamisole) and macrocyclic lactone (Ivermectin) were used. Other alternative anthelmintics were not available. Utilization of limited group of drugs for a long period may favour the development of resistance [13]. Benzimidazoles group of anthelmintics especially albendazole was the most commonly used in the clinic. Similar findings were also reported by Melaku et al. [11] in North Gondar, Niguse et al. [14] in eastern part of Ethiopia and Kumsa et al. [15] in the Southern part of Ethiopia. This might be due to easy access of albendazole in the country and its broad spectrum nature. Benzimidazoles have been developed as broad-spectrum anthelmintic agents [16,17] also reported similar scenarios in Cuba.

The percentage of anthelmintics prescribed by generic name in the present study is 100% (Table 4), which is in line with the standard derived to serve as ideal (100%) [18] In the study conducted by Beyene et al. [10] in Bishoftu indicated the percentage of drugs prescribed by generic name for animal subjects was 90.1%, which is lower than the current finding. A national baseline study on drug use indicators in Ethiopia in September 2002 also showed the percentage of drugs

Anthelmintics	Frequency	Percentage (%)
Albendazole	285	51.2
Ivermectin	214	38.4
Mebendazole	24	4.3
Fenbendazole	22	3.9
Triclabendazole	7	1.3
Tetramizole	4	0.7
Praziquantel	1	0.2

Table 1: Percentage of anthelmintic utilized in University of Gondar veterinary clinic from January 01, 2014 to March 30, 2016.

Characteristics	Frequency	Percentage (%)
Diseases treated		
Lungworm infection	69	12.4
GIT parasitism	177	31.8
Non- parasitic diseases	247	44.3
Ectoparasite infestation	64	11.5

Table 2: Percentage of anthelmintic utilized based on animal diseases diagnosed in University of Gondar veterinary clinic from January 01, 2014 to March 30, 2016.

Characteristics	Frequency	Percentage (%)
Species		
Bovine	253	45.4
Equine	62	11.1
Ovine	166	29.8
Caprine	16	2.9
Canine	60	10.8
Age		
Young	227	40.8
Adult	330	59.2
Body condition		
Good	167	30.0
Poor	395	70.0
Season		
Winter	53	9.5
Spring	193	34.6
Summer	177	31.8
Autumn	134	24.1

Table 3: Percentage of anthelmintic utilized based on species, age, body condition and season in University of Gondar veterinary clinic from January 01, 2014 to March 30, 2016.

Characteristics	Frequency	Percentage (%)
Type of diagnosis		
Tentative	513	92.1
Definitive	44	7.9
Anthelmintic prescription		
Generic name	557	100
Trade name	0	0
Anthelmintic combination		
Only anthelmintic	172	30.9
Anthelmintic combined with other drugs	385	69.1

Table 4: Percentage of anthelmintic utilized based on types of diagnosis, anthelmintic prescription and combination in University of Gondar veterinary clinic from January 01, 2014 to March 30, 2016.

prescribed by generic name for human subjects was 87% [19], which is lower than the present finding (100%). In the study conducted in 12 developing countries (human subject), the percentage of generic drugs prescribed was low in Nigeria (58%) and Sudan (63%) but encouraging in Tanzania (82%) and Zimbabwe (94%) [20,21].

Though the primary purpose of veterinary drugs is to safeguard the health and welfare of animals [22], 44.3% anthelmintics were prescribed irrationally to treat diseases that were tentatively diagnosed as nonparasitic cases (Table 2). This may be due to unavailability of diagnostic aids for confirmatory tests, inadequate recognition of the disease and to make the treatment more broad anthelmintics can be given in combination with other drugs. Additionally, 92.1% of anthelmintics in university of Gondar veterinary clinic were utilized to treat diseases that were tentatively diagnosed without getting correct laboratory supported diagnosis (Table 4). These reveal the presence of irrational anthelmintic use. This may be due to inadequate recognition of the disease, unavailability of diagnostic aids for confirmatory tests, and absence of a right drug. The four main reasons of irrational anthelmintic prescribing are inadequate recognition of infections that lead to prescription of unnecessary drugs, inappropriate choice of route, dose and duration of anthelmintics [23].

In the present study, the percentage of anthelmintic utilization among different species of animals was highest in bovine (45.4%), followed by ovine (29.8%), equine (11.1%), canine (10.8%) and caprine (2.9%), respectively (Table 3). This may be due to the difference in feeding habits. In this study, the rate of anthelmintic utilization in adult animals (59.2%) was higher than in young (40.5%) (Table 4). The lower rate of anthelmintic utilization in younger animals could be most likely due to the tradition of keeping young animals homestead than letting them to travel distance in search of grass, which could be due to fears for wild predators and young animals are unable to walk long distances in search of grass. The rate of anthelmintic utilization in animals with poor body condition (70%) was higher than in animals with good body condition (30%) (Table 3). This variation might be associated to limited immunological response of animals with poor body condition for parasite infections. In fact the poor body condition could be due to the parasite itself or other diseases or nutritional problems. Whatever the cause, there is compromised immune response to infection in poor body condition animals that increases vulnerability to worms [24].

The study indicated the effect of season on anthelmintic utilization in different seasons. The highest utilization was observed during the spring season (Table 3). This could be ascribed to the fact that the high moisture content during these seasons that leads to increased development of larvae and abundant pasture, thus resulting in increased contact between the host and parasites. The lowest utilization rate was also found in winter (Table 3). The probable reason may be due to decreased infection of helminths due to the unfavorable environmental factors for the development and growth of most helminths species [25,26]. Most of the helminths species are susceptible to desiccation in dry climatic conditions that results from the high temperature at which even eggs fail to develop into infective stage [3,27,28].

In this study the high percentage of anthelmintics were prescribed in combination with other drugs (Table 4) such as oxytetracyclin, procaine and penicillin. This may be due to inadequate recognition of the disease, unavailability of diagnostic aids for confirmatory tests and prescribers' belief that better therapeutic efficacy of combined drugs.

Conclusion and Recommendations

The study revealed that anthelmintic drugs are quite commonly but improperly utilized in the clinic. There was high percentage of anthelmintic use in adult, poor body conditioned and bovine species of animals. The highest utilization was also observed during the spring season. Moreover, there was good anthelmintic prescription by generic name. However, limited group of anthelmintics were utilized. Benzimidazole group of anthelmintics especially albendazole was the most commonly used in the clinic. The finding of anthelmintic prescription showed that there were problems of correct diagnosis. Anthelmintics were prescribed irrationally to treat diseases that were tentatively diagnosed as nonparasitic cases. Additionally, anthelmintic drugs were utilized to treat diseases that were tentatively diagnosed without getting correct laboratory supported diagnosis.

Based on the above conclusions the following recommendations are forwarded:

- Adequate diagnostic aids for confirmatory diagnosis should be available/full-filled in the clinic.
- Sound veterinary diagnosis must be carried out before considering the use of anthelmintics.
- Awareness should be created on the use of anthelmintics to avoid using anthelmintics for nonparasitic diseases.

Frequent and repeated use of anthelmintics from the same class, over an extended period of time may favour the development of resistance so rotation of anthelmintics between classes should be practiced.

References

1. Metaferia F, Cherenet T, Gelan A, Abnet F, Tesfay A, et al. (2011) A Review to Improve Estimation of Livestock Contribution to the National GDP. Ministry of Finance and Economic Development and Ministry of Agriculture. Addis Ababa, Ethiopia.
2. Tembely S, Lahlou-Kassi K, Rege JE (1998) Breed and season effects on the peri-parturient rise in nematode egg output in indigenous ewes in a cool tropical environment. Vet Parasitol 77: 123-132.
3. Negassa A, Rashid S, Gebremedhin B (2011) Livestock production and marketing in Ethiopia. Ethiopian Support Strategy Program II (ESSP II) Working Paper 26. International Food Policy Research Institute, Washington, D.C., USA.
4. Abebe W, Esayas G (2001) Survey of ovine and caprine gastro-intestinal helminthosis in eastern part of Ethiopia during the dry season of the year. Rev Med Vet 152: 379-384.
5. Biffa D, Jobre Y, Chakka H (2006) Ovine helminthosis, a major health constraint to productivity of sheep in Ethiopia. Anim Health Res Rev 7: 107-118.
6. Taylor MA, Coop RL, Wall RL (2007) Veterinary Parasitology. 3rd edn. Blackwell Publisher, Ltd., UK, pp: 195-198.
7. Ćupić V, Dobrić S, Antonijević B, Čelebićanin S (2011) The significance of rational use of drugs in veterinary medicine for food safety. Tehnologija mesa 52: 74-79.
8. Sanders P (2007) Veterinary drug residue control in the European Union. Technologija mesa 1: 59-68.
9. AAVP (2005) Anthelmintic Resistance: An Examination of its Growing Prevalence in the US cattle herd. Executive Summary of the 2005 Anthelmintic Resistance Roundtable. pp: 1-8.
10. Beyene T, Endalew D, Tolossa Y, Feyisa, A (2015) Evalution of rational use of veterinary drugs especially antimicrobials and anthelmintics in Bishoftu, Central Ethiopia. BMC Res Notes 8: 482.
11. Melaku A, Bogale B, Chanie M, Fentahun T, Berhanu A (2013) Study on the utilization and efficacy of commonly used anthelmintics against gastrointestinal nematodes in naturally infected sheep in North Gondar, North-Western Ethiopia. Academic Journals 7: 679-684.
12. CSA (2007) Census Central Statistics authority. Ethiopian agricultural enumerations. Result for Amhara region.
13. Papadopoulos E (2008) Anthelmintic resistance in sheep nematodes. Small Rumin Res 76: 99-103.
14. Niguse A, Shimelis D, Feyera T (2014) Epidemiology and Chemotherapy of Gastrointestinal Parasites of Sheep in and Around Jigjiga, Eastern Ethiopia. Eur J Biol Sci 6: 46-53.
15. Kumsa B, Debela E, Megersa B (2010) Comparative efficacy of Albendazole, Tetramisole and Ivermictin against gastrointestinal nematodes in naturally infected goat in Ziway Oromia Regional state (South Ethiopia). J Anim Vet Adv 9: 2905-2911.
16. Brunton L, Goodman LS (2008) Goodman and Gilman's Manual of Pharmacology and Therapeutics. McGraw-Hill Professional, Pp: 697-709.
17. Arece J, Mahieu M, Archimède H, Aumont G, Fernández M, et al. (2004) Comparative efficacy of six anthelmintics for the control of gastrointestinal nematodes in sheep in Matanzas, Cuba. Small Rumin Res 54: 61-67.
18. Isah AO, Ross-Degnan D, Quick J, Laing R, Mabadeje AFB (2004) The development of standard values for the WHO drug use prescribing indicators. International conference on improving use of medicines (ICIUM). INRUD-Nigeria1, Support Group 2; DAP-WHO3. Nigeria.
19. EPA (2003) Assessment of the Pharmaceutical Sector in Ethiopia. Addis Ababa, Ethiopia.
20. Bimo D (1993) Report on Nigerian field test. INRUD News. 1992; 3: 9-10. How to investigate drug use in health facilities. Geneva: WHO, p: 74.
21. WHO (2002) Promoting rational use of medicines: core components. WHO Policy and perspectives on medicine. Geneva.
22. Cannavan A (2004) Capacity Building for Veterinary Drug Residue Monitoring Programmes in Developing Countries. Joint FAO/WHO Technical Workshop on Residues of Veterinary Drugs without ADI/MRL - Bangkok, 24-26 August 2004.
23. Pallares R, Dick R, Wenzel RP, Adams JR, Nettleman MD (1993) Trends in antimicrobial utilization at a tertiary teaching hospital during a 15 year period (1978-1992). Infect Control Hosp Epidemiol 14: 376-382.
24. Sykes AR (2010) Host immune responses to nematodes: benefit or cost? Implications for future development of sustainable methods of control. R Bras Zootec 39: 376-382.
25. Andrews SJ (1999) The life cycle of *Fasciola hepatica*. In: Fasciolosis. Dalton JP (ed). CAB, Wallingford, pp: 1-29.
26. Lima WS (1998) Seasonal infection pattern of gastrointestinal nematodes of beef cattle in Minas Gerais State-Brazil. Vet Parasitol 74: 203-214.
27. Banks DJD, Singh R, Barger IA, Pratap B, Le Jambre LF (1990) Development and survival of infected larvae of *Haemonchus contortus* and *Trichostrongylus colubriformis* on pastures in a tropical environment. Int J Parasitol 20: 155-160.
28. Waruiru RM, Mutune MN, Otieno RO (2005) Gastrointestinal parasite infections of sheep and goats in a semi-arid area of Machakos District, Kenya. Bull Anim Health Prod Afr 53: 25-34.

4

Urinalysis - A Diagnostic Factor for Urolithiasis and Prognostic Factor for its Recurrence in Young Ruminants

Mohsin Ali Gazi[1]*, Makhdoomi DM[1], Mir SA[2] and Sheikh GN[3]

[1]*Division of Surgery and Radiology, Sheri Kashmir University of Agricultural Sciences and Technology Kashmir, Jammu and Kashmir, India*
[2]*Division of Pharmacology and Toxicology, Sheri Kashmir University of Agricultural Sciences and Technology Kashmir, Jammu and Kashmir, India*
[3]*Division of Epidemiology and Preventive Medicine, Sheri Kashmir University of Agricultural Sciences and Technology Kashmir, Jammu and Kashmir, India*

Abstract

The experiment was a completely randomized block design with 6 groups awarded different treatments including 17 rams, 12 bucks and 113 calves. Animals clinically manifesting urolithiasis from field were merely screened as stone and non-stone formers. All replicates were run under different clinical situations with the objectives to screen calves as stone formers and non-stone formers and to ascertain recurrence risk due to residual fragments in future, and estimate urine biochemical analysis to ascertain a diagnostic factor for urolithiasis and prognostic factor for its recurrence that would help to evolve prophylactic protocol. Crystal formation indicated that urine was sufficiently saturated which support the formation and growth of uroliths. The, male calves showing numbers of crystals with a concomitant inflammatory process are at risk for calculi formation. Alterations in Urinary Calcium Phosphorous and Magnesium cannot be fixed as a diagnostic or prognostic value for detection of uroliths forming animals to a fear degree of accuracy. Urinalysis is simple and reliable test to confirm urinary tract disease and identify pathophysiology mechanisms associated with the underlying cause.

Keywords: Urolithiasis; Ruminants; Bovines; Calves

Introduction

Urinalysis is a screening and/or diagnostic tool as it can help detect substances or cellular material in the urine associated with different metabolic and kidney disorders. It is widely and routinely to detect any abnormalities that require follow up. The Clinical manifestation of urolithiasis in Ovine and caprine are remarkably different than in bovines. They may show Partial obstruction and complete obstruction with ruptured urinary bladder and hence demand different surgical protocols ranging from amputation of urethral process, Cystorehexsis and tube cystotomy/Bladder marsupialisation depending upon the diverse clinical situations. In sheep and goats abdominal ultrasound, may be useful for the diagnosis and prognosis of this disease [1,2] to detect stones of different shapes and sizes [3].

Between Year 2011 and 2013, over 106 calves were treated who were suffering from urolithiasis; there was a dramatic increase in the prevalence during these years from overall 9.6% to 14.02% in 2013. Since 2008, the frequency of urolithiasis in calves has increased more than 8-fold. This reversion in urolith prevalence is continuing. Despite the difficulty of obtaining samples from dysuric patients and the urgency to provide therapy, it importantly requires collection prior to therapy to arrive at accurate interpretation of results. The method of collection, the duration and method of storage are essential to fully interpret results. The present clinical study was undertaken to predict the animals manifesting clinical urolithiasis in future and to ascertain the possibility of urolithiasis recurrence by examining crystal load in urine of the animals post treatment.

Materials and Methods

The study was conducted on clinical cases presented for surgical treatment of urolithiasis at Veterinary Clinical Complex Shuhama Kashmir, for a period of one year. Calves aged between 3 to 18 months and sheep and goat manifesting urolithiasis formed the subject for the study. An attempt has been made to find out the probable cause of the Urolithasis and to ascertain the recurrence of the disease.

Anamnesis

Anamnesis included previous history eliciting information about the previous treatment, nutritional history, related to type of feed, change of feed present ailment and symptoms. The clinical examination was done, where the status of the eyeballs, visible mucous membranes, smell of breath, was recorded. Much emphasis was laid for urinary conduct examination regarding, presence of calculi in the palpable part of urethra right from external urinary orifice pre scrotal, post scrotal and ischial part of urethra, pattern of urination, bladder distension, ruptured and intact bladder, degree of abdominal distension and abdominal thrill on the basis of which grouping of animals was done. This experiment was a completely randomized block design with 113 calves, 17 rams and 12 bucks. All the rams and bucks and 33 calves were clinically manifesting urolithiasis. 80 calves from field were merely screened as stone and non-stone formers. There were 6 groups awarded different treatments. All replicates were run in as presented, under different clinical situations with the objectives to screen calves as stone formers and non-stone formers and to ascertain recurrence risk due to residual fragments in future, and estimate urine biochemical analysis to ascertain a diagnostic factor for urolithiasis and prognostic factor for its recurrence that would help to evolve prophylactic protocol.

Grouping of animal

The animals were divided into six groups as under: 33 calves were divided into three groups as, **Group A** (n=12). The calves showing

***Corresponding author:** Mohsin Ali Gazi, Division of Surgery and Radiology, Sheri Kashmir University of Agricultural Sciences and Technology Kashmir, Jammu and Kashmir, India, E-mail: mohsingazi9975@gmail.com

crouching Posture, Slight tenderness of abdomen, urinary thrill and hairs on body stood erect. **Group B** (n 12) includes the calves with uraemic breath, mild conjuctival congestion, recumbency, fluid thrill in abdomen. **Group C** (n 9), the calves were flexic with severe conjunctival congestion and massive bilateral distension. Sheep with ruptured urinary Bladder were put in **Group D** (n=9) and those with intact Urinary Bladder were grouped as **Group E** (n=8). The caprine cases were grouped as **Group F** (n=6) as low risk Group and **Group G** (n=6) high risk Group

Urine sample collection

In apparently healthy animals the samples were collected in the wide mouth plastic vials as soon the animals voided urine or preputial massage was done to collect the sample. In other cases Cystocentesis was performed a site, 5 inch lateral and parallel to the penile urethra using a 6 inch long spinal needle. After collection of sample the needle was withdraw and the site was mopped and urine was processed for urinalysis. In general from day 0, day 7, after surgery, urine was collected from the catheter (Figure 1). After the urinary catheter was removed normal spontaneous urine was collected through the preputial opening.

In 30 cases, urine samples were collected during laprocystotomy. Those samples collected in clinical complex were immediately processed for screening while those urine samples collected from the field were preserved using 1 drop of 40% formaldehyde to 30 ml urine and were processed for screening within 24 hours using urine analyzer (Urine analyzer - Uri-plus 200 Crest Biosystems, Division of coral clinical systems, Alto Santa Cruz complex P.O, Goa-403 202, India).

Screening of animals as stone formers and non-formers

In present study we used digital urine analyzer for speedy evaluations and that would bypass laborious laboratory procedures. 50 urine samples from 30 calves, 13 bucks and 7 rams were subjected to screening by urine analyzer. In case, where analyzer was not available the screening was done as per method of Teotia [4]. The urine sample was being collected in urine collecting bag. Each sample was filtered through Whatman filter paper No 1 to remove any crystalline material and mucous etc. 50 ml of the urine were taken in a 100 ml beaker. The pH was adjusted to 6.00 and four drops of chloroform were added to prevent growth of bacteria. Glass fibers of 0.05 mm diameter were suspended with a thread in the center of the urine sample. Calcium chloride (0.1 ml) and sodium oxalate solution (0.1 ml) was diffused in the urine by means of filter paper wicks. The glass fibers got coated with silver nitrate for 30 minutes. The fibers were counter stained with Safranin solution for a period of 2 to 3 minutes. The presences of the crystals on the fiber under microscope were screened as positive for stone formation. The animals were screened for crystal urea/ urolithiasis up to 8 weeks using urine analyzer.

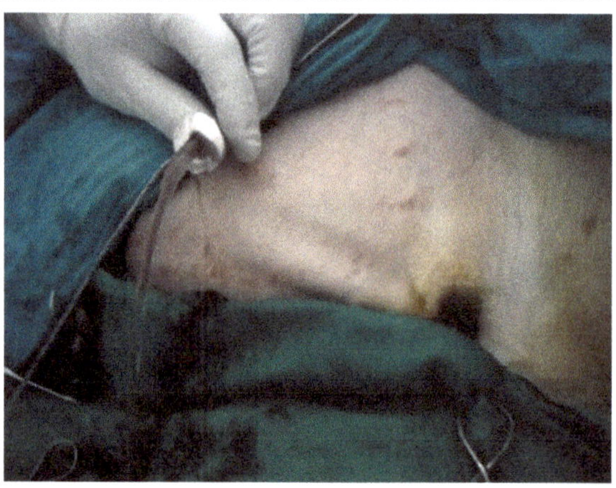

Figure 1: Collection of urine sample in a calf.

Crystal estimation of urine

After the institution of surgical treatment (different for different animals), the screening of urine for presence of crystal load was done at, 24 and 72 post-operative hour, and on the date of normal restoration of urine flow / at the time of removal of catheter post-operatively. This was followed at 2, 4, 6 and 8 weeks.

Biochemical analysis of urine

The urine samples were filtered using Whatman filter paper no 1 to remove any crystalline material and mucous etc. The samples were centrifuged and the supernatant taken for the estimation of Calcium [5], Phosphorus and Magnesium [6], using diagnostic kits (Miles India limited, Baroda Gujarat state, India).

Results

A record of anamnesis of the present study revealed two things in common. All the animals whether calves, sheep or bucks were in pre-ruminant stage and were fed rations pre maturely. The ration offered included rice bran, rice straw or commercial feeds either alone or in combination. 60% bovine calves and 40% caprine and ovine kids had received previous treatment which included diuretic injections. The rest others had been given steroids, analgesics or tranquilizers.

Stone former and non-stone former

A total of 113 calves were subjected to screening as stone former and non-stone former. The fresh samples (n=33) were screened for presence and absence of crystals. 100 percent cases were positive for presence of different forms of crystals. The degree of positivity ranged 48.48% as highly (16 out of 33) +++, 30.30% moderately positive (10 out of 33) ++ and 21% mildly positive (7 out of 33) +, differentiated as having crystals. Out of 80 samples collected from field, subjected to screening as stone and non-stone formers by method as described by Teotia [4], 41.25% (34) were confirmed as positive and 58.75% cases were confirmed as negative. Among positive cases, 20 cases (58.82%) were highly positive "+++". 8 cases (23.52%) were moderately positive "++" and 6 cases (17.64%) were mildly positive "+".

Out of 67 stone former positive cases 21 (31.34%) were presented to our University hospital with clinical manifestations of urolithiasis for treatment within span of 8-12 weeks (Table 1). In some cases the urine showed heavy crystal load even after operation for some time.

An average of measurements taken in quadruplicate over 2 collections both pre and post-operative collections periods (Table 2) revealed that the crystal score was positive in all the groups under study, however the score was statistically non-significant in all other groups except group A, where it was 23.10 and decreased post operatively to 12.80 with a mean of 2.75. The score however decreased significantly after surgery but the animals continued to show the crystal score positive due to the residual effect of the preexisting cause. As for the number of the crystals counted group A recorded highest (278.6) followed by groups D (237.4), C (229.00) and G (212.7).

Patterns of crystals in urine

The results of the present study reveal that the types of the crystals varied in different species of animals. In calves crystals were triple Phosphate, Calcium/Amorphous Phosphate, calcium Carbonate, Calcium oxalate, Uric acid and mostly the calculi were Silica ++ to ++++. The shape of crystals was Prismatic, coffin lid shaped, star and elongated rod shaped, feathery or fern like (Table 2).

In sheep the type of crystals are calcium oxalate, triple Phosphate and Uric acid which shaped Spherical granules, amorphous rosette shaped, a cluster of 1 to 4 while in bucks hexagonal struvite type of crystal were seen (Table 3). The detailed microscopic examination of sediment revealed organized sediments +++, erythrocytes four cases of calves, 2 sheep and two bucks each, leucocytes (2-4/hpf) in calves and occasional in sheep and Bucks, epithelial cells casts (10-12/hpf), in calves and 6-8/hpf in Sheep and bucks each, glucose was negative in all the cases of all the species of animals, and casts and in general RBC (0-4/hpf) were observed during microscopic examination of urine.

Urinary calcium phosphorous and magnesium

The results of urinary calcium, phosphorous and magnesium (mmol/liter) in urine before and after surgery at various intervals of obstructive urolithiasis in different Groups are presented in Table 4. There was significant ($p<0.05$) increase in the urinary calcium levels from the day of admission of the animals for treatment to the phase of recovery. The urinary calcium levels at day zero were lower than normal in all the groups from A1 to G group viz., 4.91, 4.81, 5.43, 7.02, 4.58, 4.91, 4.85 and 4.84 m moles/litre. By 24th post treatment hour, there was recovery toward normal in the levels and by 72 post-surgical hour till restoration of normal urine flow irrespective of the severity of disease, the urinary calcium was within the physiological range. The severity of the disease affected significantly ($P>0.05$). There was significant ($p<0.05$) increase in the urinary calcium levels from the day of admission of the animals for treatment to the phase of recovery. At day zero, there was increase in urinary phosphorous levels with the severity of disease in all the groups under study. However, 24 and 72 post-surgical hour and at the time of removal of catheter, the variability levels in urinary phosphorous among different groups was varying significantly ($P>0.05$). With the advancement of post-treatment period, there was significant ($p<0.05$) decreasing trend in the urinary phosphorous levels within normal range on restoration of free urine flow irrespective of the severity of the disease. The postoperative observations of urinary phosphorous were almost reverse to the calcium levels and postoperative lowering of urinary phosphorous was observed in the animals of all groups at all the postoperative intervals. On the day of hospitalization, the urinary magnesium levels were high depending upon duration of disease in all the groups under study. However, at 24th and 72 post-surgical hour till the time of removal of catheter, the variability levels in urinary magnesium among different groups was varying significantly ($P>0.05$). With the advancement of post-treatment period, there was significant ($p<0.05$) decrease in the urinary magnesium levels within normal restoration of urinary flow.

Residual effect of urolithiasis

The incidence of recurrence clinically at 2nd week post operatively included two animals from calves, one am. In 4th post operative week, the recurrence cases included two calves one ram and two bucks. In 6th week one calf was reported with the recurrence (Table 5).

Discussion

The diagnosis of urolithiasis is based on a complete anamnesis and physical examination, and may be complemented by laboratory tests (of blood and urine), ultrasonography and radiography of the urinary tract [1,7]. In present study 75% calves had received diuretics and all such animals had ruptured urinary bladder which has not been evaluated in urolithiasis with calcium oxalate uroliths calves so for. Cystocentesis consists in the transabdominal collection of urine from the urinary bladder (Figure 3), under ultrasonographic control (Figure 4). It may increase the patient's comfort and temporarily alleviate bladder distension in turn reducing the risk of necrosis and rupture, but bladder leakage and subsequent uroperitoneum must be

Total Cases 113	Stone Formers	67	59.29%
	Non-Stone Formers	46	40.70%
	Cases presented from Stone Formers	21	31.34%
Fresh Cases 33	Cases +ve	33	100%
	Mild	07	21.22%
	Moderate	10	30.30%
	High	16	48.48%
Field Cases 80	Cases +ve	34	48.48%
	Mild	06	17.64%
	Moderate	08	23.52%
	Severe	20	58.82%
	% Cases presented for Urolithiasis among non-stone formers	21/34	61.75%

Table 1: Screening of animals from University Hospital and Field as stone and non-stone formers.

Crystal Score (1-5)							
Collection	A	B	C	D	E	F	G
Pre Collection	2 3.10	2.40	2.33	2.75	2.15	2.37	2.54
Post Collection	1 2.80	2.20	1.76	2.50	1.63	2.16	1.98
Mean	2.75	2.80	2.04	2.63	1.89	2.35	2.18

Number of Crystals Counted

Pre Collection	278.6	196.2	229.3	237.4	156.8	181.4	212.7
Post Collection	132.5	103.5	43.8	118.0	28.6	72.9	73.6
Mean	205.6	49.8	136.5	177.7	92.7	127.2	143.2

Table 2: Showing Crystal Score (1-5) and number of crystals.

Species	Type of crystals	Shape of crystals
Calves	Triple Phosphate	Prismatic, coffin lid shaped, star and elongated rod shaped, feathery or fern like
	Calcium/Amorphous Phosphate, calcium Carbonate , calcium oxalate, Uric acid Silica ++ to ++++	Spherical Granules amorphous, rosette shaped A cluster of 1 to 4.
Sheep	Calcium oxalate Triple Phosphate Uric acid	Square envelop coffin lid Diamond shaped
Goat	Cystine Struvite,	Hexagonal shaped

Table 3: Patterns of crystals in urine of Calves Sheep and Goats.

Period		Groups							Mean
		A_1 (N=12)	B (N=12)	C (N=9)	D (N=9)	E (N=8)	F (N=6)	G (N=6)	
0 hour	Ca	4.91	5.43	7.02	4.58	4.91	4.85	4.84	5.17
	P	6.65	6.93	7.64	5.37	5.79	4.33	4.85	6.03
	Mg	3.95	6.96	3.47	4.38	2.63	4.15	4.50	4.41
3 hour	Ca	4.78	5.39	9.33	4.60	5.99	6.85	5.00	5.70
	P	6.56	5.70	7.04	5.34	5.69	4.28	4.81	5.74
	Mg	3.92	6.69	8.75	5.06	6.25	7.82	7.80	6.43
24 hour	Ca	5.04	5.56	9.48	6.42	7.07	6.86	7.06	6.56
	P	6.17	6.48	7.21	5.06	5.38	4.25	4.39	5.67
	Mg	4.15	6.84	8.61	5.04	6.20	7.51	7.70	6.40
72 hour	Ca	6.28	6.67	10.25	6.94	6.99	7.56	6.48	7.10
	P	6.13	6.45	6.49	4.75	5.11	4.05	3.63	5.34
	Mg	3.92	6.53	8.60	4.18	5.99	7.33	7.41	6.03
Restoration	Ca	9.11	8.24	10.73	7.85	8.51	7.47	6.66	8.36
	P	5.65	5.48	5.59	4.74	4.74	3.49	3.39	4.86
	Mg	3.37	5.75	6.91	3.26	5.99	6.82	6.78	5.26
Mean	Ca	6.02	6.27	9.36	6.08	6.69	6.56	6.00	
	P	6.21	6.21	6.79	5.05	5.34	4.08	4.21	
	Mg	3.86	6.56	7.27	4.38	5.41	6.73	6.84	

Table 4: Mean Values of Urinary Calcium, phosphorous and magnesium (m mol/litre) in urine before and after surgery at various intervals of obstructive Urolithiasis in different groups.

Animals	2 weeks	4 weeks	6 Weeks	8 Weeks	Animals Screened at 8 weeks	% +ve
Calves 84	2	2	1	Nil	69 **(18)**	26.08%
Sheep 17	1	1	Nil	Nil	15 **(5)**	33.33%
Goat 12	Nil	2	Nil	Nil	9 **(2)**	22.22%

The values in Brackets indicate positive cases

Table 5: Recurrence of urolithiasis up to 2 months due to residual effect.

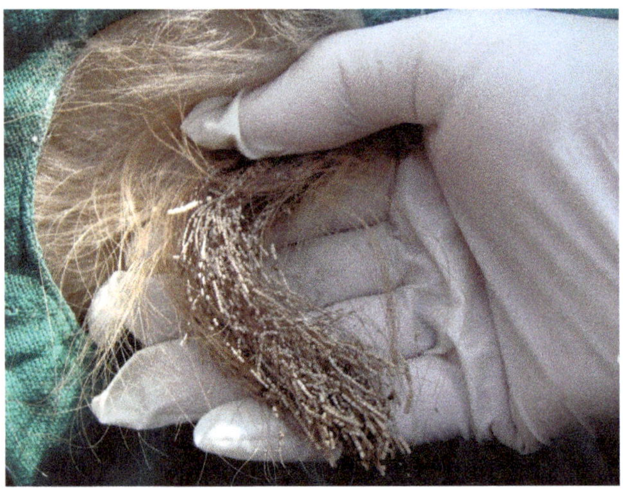

Figure 2: Calf screened a stone former manifesting clinical urolithiasis after 6 weeks the calculi are adhered to preputial hairs as garlands.

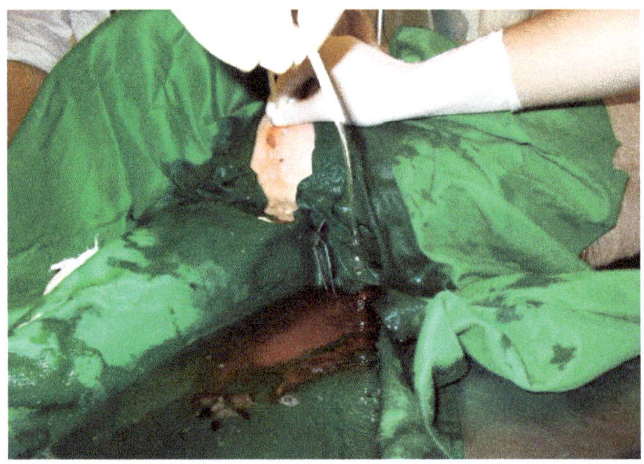

Figure 3: Catheterization in calf.

anticipated and managed [8]. It may also be indicated while postponing surgery [9]. Rakestraw et al. [10] reported a foul-smelling abdominal fluid and multiple adhesions between the loops of the small intestine and between the small intestine and bladder in a goat suffering from obstructive urolithiasis that had a history of repeated cystocentesis.

A total of 113 calves were subjected to screening as stone former and non-stone former by method as described by Teotia [4]. Out of 67 stone formers 21 (31.34%) were presented for treatment to our Hospital with clinical manifestations of urolithiasis. In a study on clinical urolithiasis in calves Khan [11] recorded that screening can be a good index for prediction of urolithiasis cases up to the accuracy of 54 per cent. The percentage could be more. Teotia [4] demonstrated screening of animals as stone former and non-stone former and reported 60% accuracy. Hence it could be concluded that screening using a urine analyzer has an accuracy of 100%, besides it is less invasive, instant, less time consuming and has no chances of error, hence should be a preferred method for the screening of animals for urolithiasis over Teotia [4] wherever the facility is available.

The crystal load and crystal score in all the groups was maximum on the day of presentation and subsequently declined after surgery due

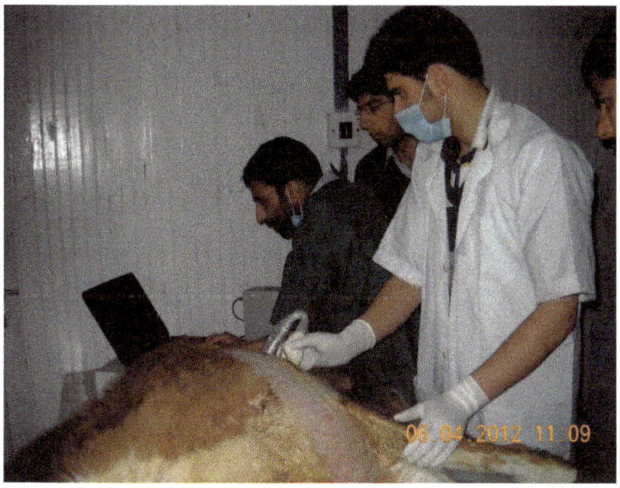

Figure 4: Ultrasonography in progress.

elimination of crystal via urine due to more formation of such crystals. The crystal score decreased significantly after surgery but the animals continued to show the crystal score positive due to the residual effect. The crystal number is of greater significance than crystal shape and size [12]. The types of the crystals vary in different species of animals and crystalluria was an indicator to evaluate the patient for uroliths. Crystals also form as a consequence of disease processes that alter urine composition.

Animals were presented for screening as stone and non-stone formers. In calves the positive percentage was 26.08, in Rams 33.33 and in Bucks the positive percentage was 22.22% (Figure 2), in study in Srinagar city Khan [11] reported an recurrence percentage of 54.28 5 in calves treated for urolithiasis at different intervals of disease

Biochemical analysis of urine

The improvement in the calcium range, decrease in phosphorous and magnesium levels towards normalcy could be due to regain of appetite, discontinuation of ruminant ration seems a reason in absence of detailed acid-base study. The inverse effect of the elevated calcium level in the blood has been reported by Singh et al. [13] and Khan [11]. Stewart et al. [14] and Crook and Robbins [15] reported high urinary excretion of phosphorus, and low urinary calcium excretion in lambs which readily developed phosphatic calculi. Crook and Robbins [15] demonstrated that lambs which developed urolithiasis had higher serum levels and lower urinary excretions of magnesium ($p<0.05$) then unaffected animals. Increased dietary magnesium has also been shown to increase the incidence of calculi in feedlot lambs even at a normal Ca to P ratio, but especially in the presence of high urinary phosphorus [16,17].

Goats of various breeds and purposes have been documented with urolithic stone problems in captivity [18]. These stones often occur when a mainly concentrate diet is presented to the goats, with a high phosphorus content. Normal healthy ruminant species have very low urinary phosphorus excretion; due to phosphorus recycling mechanisms. Any excess phosphorus absorbed will be re-secreted into the digestive tract as saliva and lost in the faces. High grain, low roughage diet decreases the formation of saliva, resulting in excess phosphorus excretion into the urine [3].

From the present study it could be concluded that the urinalysis is a simple and reliable test to confirm urinary tract disease and identify path physiologic mechanisms associated with the underlying cause. Crystal formation indicates that urine is sufficiently saturated such that it could support the formation and growth of uroliths of that respective mineral type. If sufficient numbers of crystals are present, with a concomitant inflammatory process, male small ruminants are at risk for calculi formation. Alterations in Urinary Calcium Phosphorous and Magnesium cannot be fixed as a diagnostic or prognostic value for detection of uroliths forming animals to a fear degree of accuracy. The recurrence due to residual effect was 26.08% calves the positive percentage was, 33.33% in Rams and in 22.22% Bucks. Screening revealed 59.29% non-stone former, 40.70% stone former from which 61.75% animals manifested urolithiasis within 2 months (Table 5). The Pre and post collections showed crystal load in urine in all the groups was maximum on presentation day and subsequently declined irrespective of the severity of the clinical manifestations however some cases showed crystals even after operation for some time. The crystals varied from triple Phosphate, calcium/amorphous phosphate, calcium Carbonate, calcium oxalate to uric acid in different species under study. In the present study on the day of admission varying degree of dehydration was present in all the animals, which could have raised the relative concentration of urinary mineral solutes and increased the likelihood of their precipitation.

References

1. Monoghan ML, Boy MG (1990) Diseases of the Renal System-Ruminant Renal System. In: Large Animal Internal Medicine. Smith BP (ed.). Mosby, USA, pp: 895-899.
2. Braun U, Schefer U, Föhn J (1992) Urinary tract ultrasonography in normal rams and in rams with obstructive urolithiasis. Can Vet J 33: 654-659.
3. Belknap EB, Pugh DG (2002) Diseases of the urinary system. In: Sheep and Goat Medicine. Pugh DG, Baird AN (Eds.). W. B. Saunders Company: Philadelphia.
4. Teotia G (1975) Screening of calves as normal and stone formers. Veterinary Record 128: 234-238.
5. Kaser M, Stekol JA (1979) A critical study of the Carr-Price reaction for the determination of β-carotene and vitamin A in biological materials. Transl Res 28: 904-909.
6. Amardor E, Urban J (1977) Simplified serum phosphorus analyses by continuous flow UV- spectrophotometry. Clinical Chemistry 18: 601-604.
7. Radostitis OM, Blood DC, Gray GC, Hinchcliff KW (2000) Veterinary Medicine: A Textbook of the Diseases of Cattle, Sheep, Pigs, Goats, and Horses. Bailliere Tindall, London, pp: 1877.
8. Makhdoomi DM, Gazi MA (2012) Obstructive Urolithiasis - A Review. Vet World 6: 233-238.
9. Van Metre D (2004) Urolithiasis. In: Farm Animal Surgery. Fubini SL, Ducharme NG (Eds.) WB Saunders, New York, pp: 534-547.
10. Rakestraw PC, Fubini SL, Gilbert RO, Ward JO (1995) Tube cystostomy for treatment of obstructive urolithiasis in small ruminants. Vet Surg 24: 498-505.
11. Khan AM (2010) Surgical management of Urolithiasis in calves with possible role of calcium, phosphorous and magnesium shift in blood, urine and calculi. Thesis submitted to Sheri Kashmir University of Agricultural Sciences and Technology Kashmir in partial fulfilment of MVSc degree.
12. Clark P, Swenson CL, Osborne CA, Ulrich LK (1999) Calcium oxalate crystalluria in a goat. J Am Vet Med Assoc 215: 77-78.
13. Singh J, Singh AP, Peshin PK, Singh M, Sharma SK (1983) Studies on the effects of total nephrectomy in sheep. Can J Comp Med 47: 217-221.
14. Stewart SR, Emerick RJ, Pritchard RH (1991) Effects of dietary ammonium chloride and variations in calcium to phosphorus ratio on silica urolithiasis in sheep. J Anim Sci 69: 2225-2229.
15. Crookshank HR, Robbins JD (1962) A reciprocal relationship between the

urinary excretion of magnesium and phosphorus in wether lambs. Nature 396: 1343.

16. Bezeau LM, Bailey CB, Slen SB (1961) Silica urolithiasis in beef cattle IV. The relationship between the pH and buffering capacity of ash of certain feeds, pH of urine and urolithiasis. Can J Anim Sci 41: 49-54.

17. Larson BL (1996) Identifying, treating and preventing bovine urolithiasis. Vet Med 91: 366-377.

18. Kimberling CV, Arnold KS (1983) Diseases of the urinary system of sheep and goats. Vet Clin North Am Large Anim Pract 5: 637-655.

Effect of Perch Height and Position on the Usage in Enriched Colony Housing Systems for Laying Hens

Helen Louton[1]*, Elke Rauch[1], Sven Reese[2], Michael Erhard[1] and Shana Bergmann[1]

[1]Department of Veterinary Sciences, Chair of Animal Welfare, Ethology, Animal Hygiene and Animal Husbandry, Faculty of Veterinary Medicine, LMU Munich, Veterinaerstraße 13/R, 80539 Munich, Germany

[2]Department of Veterinary Sciences, Chair of Anatomy, Histology and Embryology, Faculty of Veterinary Medicine, LMU Munich, Veterinaerstraße 13, 80539 Munich, Germany

Abstract

In order to determine the utility of different perches in enriched colony housing systems for laying hens, the use of perches and an effect of the type and location in the system was examined in this behavioral study. Laying hens of the line Lohmann Selected Leghorn were housed in four different enriched colony housing systems which differed particularly in the alignment and arrangement of the functional areas. For analysis, perches were grouped into three types: low, low underneath the drinking trough and high. To evaluate the use of the perch types, video recordings were taken for 48 hours during three observation periods. These recordings were analyzed hourly at daytime and twice at nighttime. Through scan sampling, the overall number of hens using the perches and the fraction of hens per meter on a specific perch type were assessed. At nighttime, an average 62% of the laying hens used the perches. On average, 24% of the laying hens used the perches at daytime, with no significant difference between the different systems. Low perches that were not installed underneath the drinking trough were less commonly used than high perches. However, the hens used low perches that were positioned underneath the drinking trough more than other perch types during the day. At nighttime, high perches were used frequently and, depending on the system, more than the low perches. It should be considered that the hens used the low perches underneath the drinking trough during the day not to rest but rather to have better access to the drinking trough. It can be recommended that a sufficient number of high perches should be offered, so that all hens have access to these obviously preferred perches. If perches are installed underneath the drinking trough, it should be considered if additional perch space should be offered.

Keywords: Layers; Laying hens; Enriched cage; Perch

Introduction

The enriched colony housing system for laying hens was introduced in 2006 as an alternative to the conventional cage, which was prohibited in Germany as of January 1st, 2010. In the year 2010, when the pullets of the presented study hatched, 18.2% of the laying hens in Germany were housed in an enriched colony housing system [1]. The German "Order on the Protection of Animals and the Keeping of Production Animals" [2] was amended and published on August 22nd, 2006 and last changed on February 5th, 2014. Due to procedural errors, the German federal constitutional court (BVerfG) declared in October 2010 that §13b of this German order, which regulates the keeping of laying hens in enriched colony housing systems, was unconstitutional [3]. It was therefore legitimate to execute the §13b until March 31st, 2012 as a transitional period. Since then, the respective district veterinary offices must evaluate these housing systems during regular animal welfare inspections to assure that the following rules are observed:

Each laying hen must have a minimum absolute usable area of 800 cm^2 in the enriched colony housing system. Additionally, for 10 hens a litter area of at least 900 cm^2, as well as a nest of at least 900 cm^2 and a perch space of 15 cm per hen must be supplied additionally. At least two perches at different heights in the housing system must be installed for one group, so that an undisturbed rest is possible for all hens at the same time. In order to determine the utility of these necessary perch types, the use of three perch types (low, low underneath the drinking trough and high) and an effect of the location of the perch in the enriched colony housing system was examined in this comparative behavioral study.

Studies have shown that caged laying hens use perches and that perches allow hens to show species-specific resting behavior and increase the well-being of laying hens [4,5]. Many factors are known to influence the use of perches in housing systems by laying hens, with the characteristics of the perch itself such as the diameter and shape [6,7], the material [8,9] and the height being crucial [10,11]. However, genetic differences between the hens also may influence the use of different perches [12]. Furthermore, the size of the flocks was shown to influence the choice of different perch heights [13]. In studies examining the acceptance and use of perches in furnished cage systems at daytime, authors reported that hens spent about 25 to 47% of the daytime on perches [4,14,15]. Rönchen et al. [16] observed 10 to 24% of laying hens on perches in several trials in studies with laying hens in furnished cages, small group systems and modified small group systems. Telle [17] and Hergt [18] recorded 10 to 16% on perches at daytime in the same housing systems as used in this study. In cage-free housing systems, higher uses of perches are reported during the day by Carmichael et al. [19], with 47% of the laying hens perching in an aviary system. Duncan et al. [4] observed that the placement of the

***Corresponding author:** Helen Louton, Department of Veterinary Sciences, Chair of Animal Welfare, Ethology, Animal Hygiene and Animal Husbandry, Faculty of Veterinary Medicine, LMU Munich, Veterinaerstrasse 13, 80539 Munich, Germany
E-mail: h.louton@lmu.de

perch (e.g., near the drinking or food trough) in the system strongly influenced the use. At night time authors observed 81 to 99% of the laying hens on perches in enriched cage systems [14,15,20]. In aviary systems, Plattner [21] found a very high variety in the use of perches by laying hens during the night, ranging from 17 to 100% of the hens on a perch, depending on the farm.

Studies on perching behavior and the prevalence of hens on different perches in enriched colony housing systems according to the German legislation are rare. In this study, the perching behavior of laying hens in four different enriched colony housing systems was observed. The overall use and the use of the three perch types were investigated in order to assess the use of the perch types and an effect of the location of the perch in the housing system of four enriched colony housing systems which are used in practice.

Materials and Methods

Animals

This study was performed in the course of a joint research project to refine and optimize the enriched colony housing system for laying hens. Hens of the layer line Lohmann Selected Leghorn (LSL) and Lohmann Brown (LB) were housed in four different enriched colony housing systems (system A=Big Dutchman, Type KV 1500 a-D40; system B=SALMET International GmbH, Type 4000/735; system C=SALMET International GmbH, Type FC-S 715/725; system D=TESO Ten Elsen GmbH & Co. KG, Type 206-740). System A and B were stationed in one barn at the Institute for Poultry education and applied research in Kitzingen, Germany. The systems C and D were located in two separate barns at the Ludwig-Maximilians-University in Munich, Germany. The hens of all four systems hatched on the 24th of June 2010, were not beak trimmed and reared in cage systems at the Kommanditgesellschaft Geflügelzuchtbetriebe Gudendorf-Ankum, GmbH Co, Ankum, Germany. On the 27th of October, at the age of 17wk and 6d, the hens were randomly housed in the four enriched colony housing systems A to D with alternating filling of the layer lines (LSL and LB) in the cage units. The systems differed particularly in size and alignment of the functional areas nest, dust bath, and perches (Figure 1). In system A, 40 hens per cage (stocking density: 800 cm^2/hen, 720 hens in total, 360 of each layer line) were housed with two low perches (L1, L2; 10 cm distance to cage floor) on the side of the cage unit, one low perch (L3; 8 cm distance to cage floor) in the middle underneath the drinking trough and two high perches (H1, H2; 30 cm distance to cage floor) between each side perch and the middle perch. A total of 18 cages, stacked in two levels were stationed in one barn together with the system B. In system B, 33 hens were housed per cage (stocking density: 800 cm^2/hen, 792 hens in total, 396 of each layer line) with four low perches (L1, L2, L3, L4; 8-16 cm distance to cage floor) and one high perch (L1; 30 cm distance to cage floor). In total, 24 cages of the system B were stacked in two levels and two rows. In system C, 50 hens were housed per cage (stocking density: 880 cm^2/hen, 300 hens in total, 150 of each layer line) with four low perches (L1, L2, L3, L4; 13-18 cm distance to cage floor) and two high perches (H1, H2; 27 cm distance to cage floor). Six cages of the system C were stacked in three levels. All perches in systems A, B and C were made of galvanized metal. In system D, 40 hens were housed per cage (stocking density: 800 cm^2/hen, 480 hens in total, 240 of each layer line) with two low plastic perches (L1, 7 cm distance to cage floor; L2, 9 cm distance to cage floor) in the middle of the cage underneath the drinking trough and one high perch of galvanized metal (H1, 25 cm distance to cage floor). The system D was constructed of two rows of cages on two levels with three cages in each row. In all of the observed systems, only

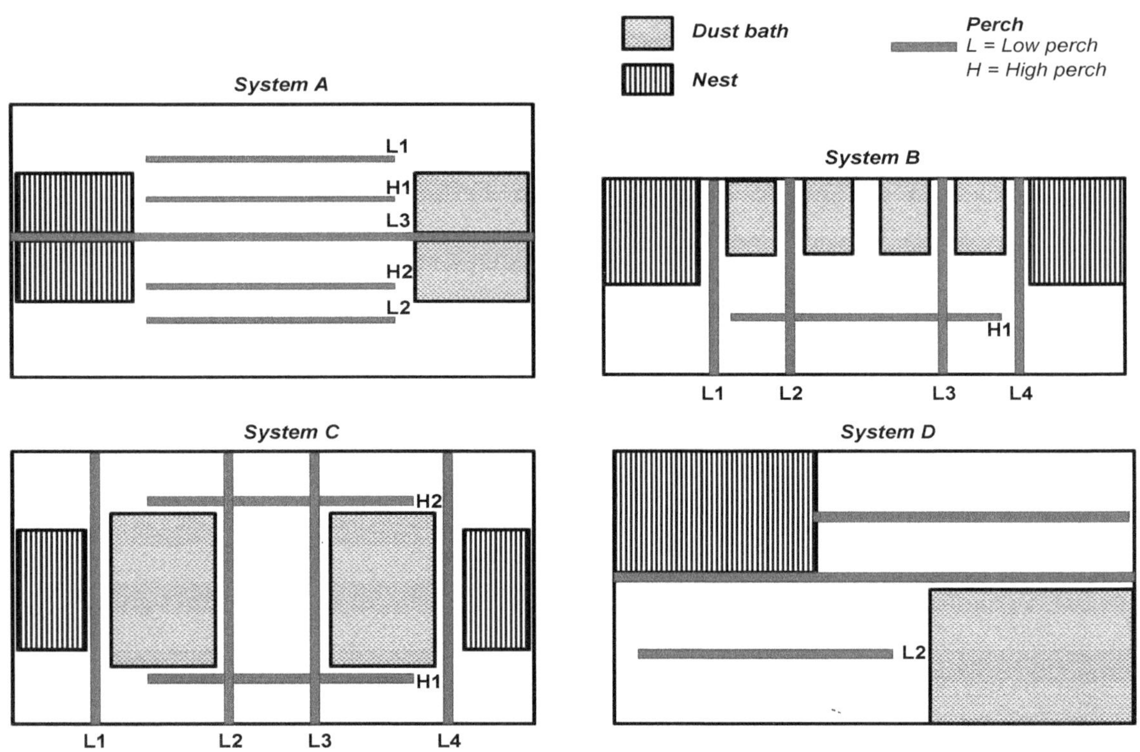

Figure 1: Functional areas dust bath, nest and perches in the four observed enriched colony housing systems A to D considering high and low perches. The presentation is not to scale.

artificial lighting was used with a 14 h daylight period (4 AM-6 PM). The hens were fed with conventional layer feed of three phases during the laying period (Korngold LAM 41° from 18th until 47th week of age, Korngold LAM 40° from 48th until 63rd week of age, and Korngold LAM 38° from 64th until 70th week of age; BayWa AG, Bockhorn, Germany). The management of the farms was consistent to ensure randomization.

Behavior observations

For behavior observations, video recordings with infrared cameras of the type VTC-E220IRP with IR-LED (Santec Security Solutions/ Sanyo Video AG, Ahrensburg, Germany) were taken for 48 hours during three observation periods (OPs) within the laying period (first OP: 24-25 weeks of age; second OP: 47-48 weeks of age; third OP: 63-64 weeks of age). By this, the observation periods were evenly distributed throughout the laying period. Because of technical reasons, only hens of the strain Lohmann Selected Leghorn were observed. The video signals of the cameras were transferred to encoder boxes (Indigo Vision 8000, Indigo Vision, Inc., Edinburgh, UK). Network cables connected the encoder boxes with Switchports (AT-FS 708 Switch, Allied Telesis, Inc., USA), that were connected to a computer. The software used was Indigo Vision Control Center (Version 3.16.09, Indigo Vision, Inc., Edinburgh, UK).

In systems A (33 hens per unit) and B (40 hens per unit) four randomly chosen cage units, in system C three randomly chosen cage units (50 hens per unit) and in system D (40 hens per unit) six randomly chosen cage units were observed by video recordings (three cage units in the third observation period in system D). The scan sampling method by Martin and Bateson [22] was used to determine the use of the perches and prevalence of hens on specific perches. Using this method, a group of hens is observed at time points determined prior to the observation in order to assess the use of the functional area perch. The first time point determined in this study was 30 minutes after the beginning of the daytime and then a sampling followed hourly during the day and twice within the night. Thereby, the absolute number of hens on the different perches was counted in hourly intervals at daytime (4:30 AM to 5:30 PM) and twice at nighttime (8:30 PM and 1:30 AM). For the overall use of perches, the total number of hens standing or sitting with both legs on any perch was related to the total number of hens in the cage.

Statistical analyses

The determined frequency of perch use was presented as percentage of the number of hens per meter perch per unit. A Chi-Square-Test was used to analyze the differences between the four different housing systems at day and nighttime as well as between the different observation periods (Excel Tool by ACOMED Statistics, Leipzig, Germany) [23]. The absolute numbers of hens on different perches and at different times of the day was documented. To analyze the frequency of hens on the perch types, grouped into three categories (low, low underneath the drinking trough and high), the number of hens on one meter of a specific perch was related to the total number of hens in the particular unit (system A n=4 units; system B n=4 units, system C n=3 units, system D n=6 units, last OP n=3 units). The frequency of hens on the different perch types was calculated as arithmetic means of the perch use during the day and night time in the observed units (14 observations times during the day, two at night). A t-test was used to calculate significant differences in the frequency of hens on the different perch types as well as the different housing systems. A correction for multiple testing was performed according the Bonferroni and Holm-method. The statistical level was set at $P<0.05$. Additionally a Cohen d was calculated to quantify the effect of different housing systems and perch types. Cohen [24] refers to a small, medium and large effect if d is 0.2, 0.5 or 0.8 respectively.

Results

At daytime, an average of 23.9% of the laying hens used the perches in the enriched colony housing systems (Table 1). The average perch use at daytime varied, and ranged from the lowest usage of 17.4% in system A to the highest use of 29.9% in system B. In the first (24-25 weeks of age) and third (63-64 weeks of age) observation periods, there were no significant differences between the four different systems ($P>0.05$). In the second (47-48 weeks of age) observation period, the perches in system A were used significantly less than those in system D ($P \leq 0.05$).

At nighttime, the hens showed a more frequent use of perches with an average of 62.1% (Table 1). The range of the average use was between 53.2% (first observation period, system C) and 71.6% (third observation period, system A).

In system A, five perches were installed in the housing system, two low perches at the sides, one low perch in the middle (underneath the drinking trough) and two high perches between the low ones (Figures 1). A difference in the use of these perches was observed particularly during the daytime (Figure 3). At daytime, the low perch in the middle underneath the drinking trough was used more often than the low ($P \leq 0.001$, d=7.61) and the high perches in this housing system ($P \leq 0.01$, d=4.54). Even though the low perches were used less than the high perches during the daytime of all OPs, this was only significant in the third OP ($P=0.028$, d=3.91).

In system B, there was no notable effect of the perch height on the use of the perches at day- or nighttime in all observation periods (Figures 2 and 3).

At daytime (Figure 3), even though there was an effect of the perch height on the use of the perches visible in the system C, this was not significant in any of the observation periods ($P>0.05$, OP1 d=3.23, OP 2 d=2.77, OP 3 d=3.09). At nighttime in the second and third observation periods (Figure 2), the high perches were used more often than the low perches (OP 2 $P=0.005$, d=13.11; OP 3 $P=0.019$, d=7.21).

	OP	Layer on perch (%) during Night time (min/max)	Layer on perch (%) during Daytime (min/max)
System A	1	55.8 (51.3/58.8)	17.8 (10.0/31.3)
	2	60.8 (47.5/71.8)	17.4 (7.5/30.8)
	3	71.8 (65.0/80.3)	25.6 (10.0/55.0)
	Average	62.8 (47.5/80.3)	20.3 (7.5/55.0)
System B	1	69.9 (59.1/78.8)	26.4 (13.6/39.4)
	2	59.9 (40.9/75.0)	26.0 (13.6/40.6)
	3	59.4 (48.5/72.6)	29.9 (16.7/46.8)
	Average	63.1 (40.9/78.8)	27.4 (13.6/46.8)
System C	1	53.2 (38.0/68.0)	19.1 (6.0/36.0)
	2	63.2 (56.0/69.0)	21.3 (5.2/39.0)
	3	64.9 (58.0/72.9)	24.0 (7.1/36.7)
	Average	60.4 (38.0/72.9)	21.5 (5.2/39.0)
System D	1	66.2 (42.5/86.3)	24.7 (2.5/41.3)
	2	54.0 (40.9/64.1)	29.7 (7.4/51.5)
	3	66.1 (51.3/74.3)	29.2 (13.2/51.5)
	Average	62.1 (40.9/86.3)	27.9 (2.5/51.5)

Table 1: Average percentage (%), minimum and maximum of laying hens per meter perch in systems A to D at night time and day time in the three observation periods. OP=Observation Period (1=First observation period, 24-25 weeks of age; 2=Second observation period, 47-48 weeks of age; 3=Third observation period, 63-64 weeks of age).

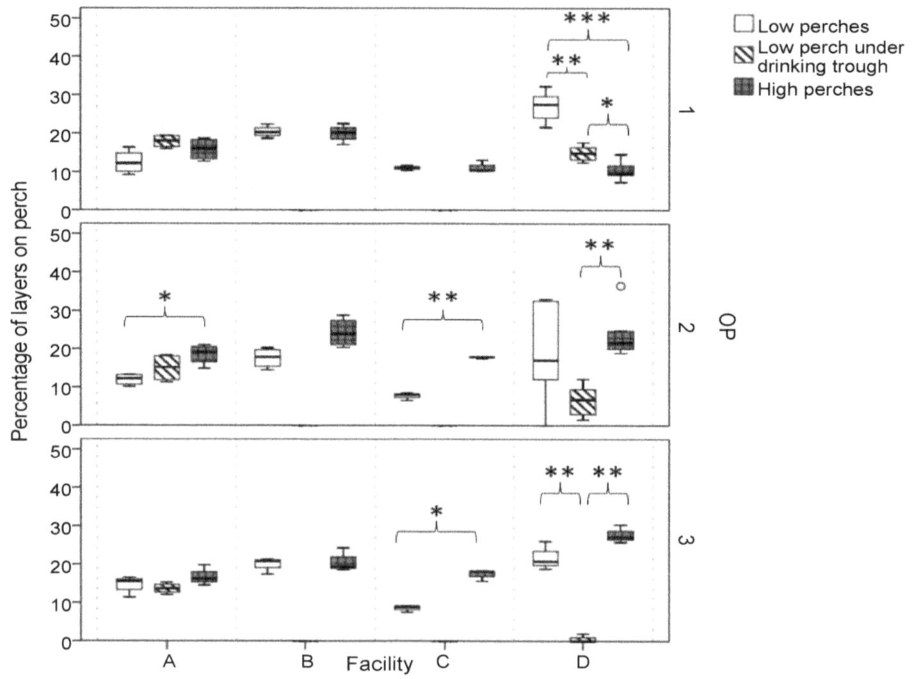

Figure 2: Average percentage (%) of layers per meter of the three perch types low, low under the drinking trough and high, in systems A to D at night time in the three observation periods. OP=Observation period (1=first observation period, 24-25 weeks of age; 2=Second observation period, 47-48 weeks of age; 3=Third observation period, 63-64 weeks of age). *:p-value<0.05, **:p-value<0.01, ***:p-value<0.001.

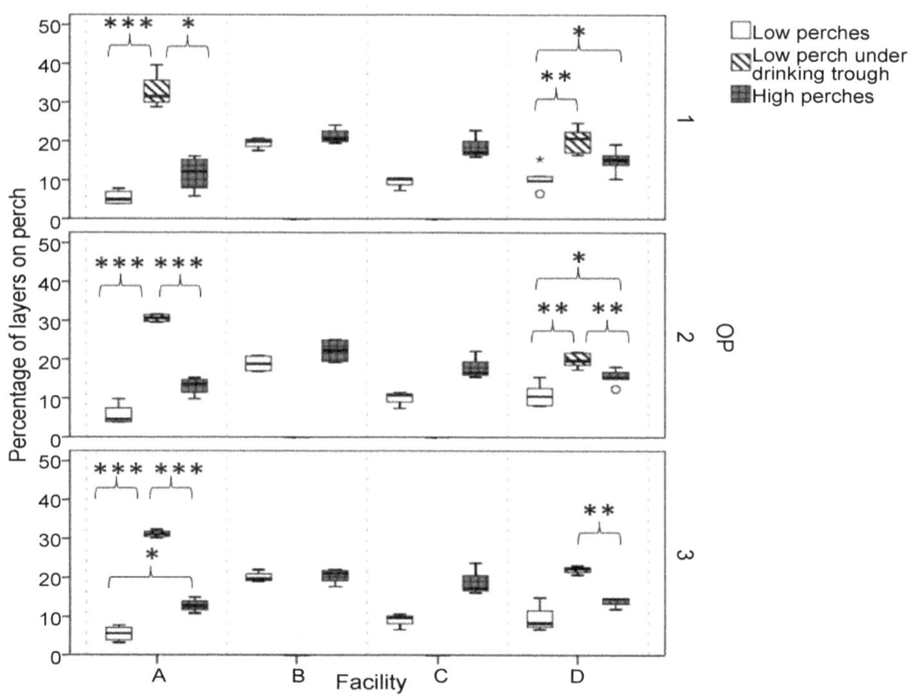

Figure 3: Average percentage (%) of layers per meter of the three perch types low, low under the drinking trough and high, in systems A to D at daytime in the three observation periods. OP=Observation period (1=first observation period, 24-25 weeks of age; 2=Second observation period, 47-48 weeks of age; 3=Third observation period, 63-64 weeks of age). *:p-value<0.05, **:p-value<0.01, ***:p-value<0.001.

In system D (Figure 3), the low perch in the middle of the system underneath the drinking trough was used more often than all other perches at daytime in all observation periods. The frequent use of this perch was especially determined by hens that used the perch to reach the drinking trough. The high perch was used more frequently at daytime in all observation periods compared with the low perch located at the side of the system (OP 1 $P=0.046$, d=1.62; OP 2 $P=0.049$, d=1.82). The prevalence of hens on specific perches at nighttime in system D changed from the first to the third observation period (Figure 2). In the first observation period, the low perch in the middle of the system underneath the drinking trough and the low perch were used ($P<0.05$) more frequently than the high perch. In the second and third observation periods, the low perch in the middle of the system underneath the drinking trough was used less than the low and high perch.

Discussion and Conclusions

In the four enriched colony housing systems tested in our study, an average of 23.9% of the hens were observed sitting or standing on the perches at daytime. The observed average use of perches, ranging from 17.4 to 29.7%, differed between housing systems and observation periods, we suggest that this was caused because the number of hens on perches was influenced by the number of hens in other functional areas (food trough, dust bath, nest) showing other behavior than resting.

An average of 62.1% of the hens in this study used the perches at nighttime. The average ranged between 53.2 and 71.6%. Thus, 28.4 to 46.8% of the hens in the observed enriched colony housing systems did not use the perches during the night. Other authors reported a high variability in the use of perches, with 60 to 99% of laying hens resting on perches in furnished cage systems at nighttime [4,14,18]. Telle [17] observed only 26 to 67% laying hens on a perch at nighttime. The fact that not all of the hens in this study used a perch at night could be explained by the preference of hens for specific perches, causing an "overcrowding" on specific perches and thus insufficient space for all of the hens on these perches. Similar observations were done by authors analyzing behavior of laying hens in an aviary systems, in which by laying hens preferred perches were overcrowded and others in the same housing system in contrast not used by the hens [25]. Since 28.4 to 46.8% of the hens did not use a perch at night, even though hens are highly motivated to perch [26], it should be discussed, if the provided perch space of 15 cm per hen is sufficient or if more space, especially on high perches, should be provided.

Analysis of the usage of individual perch types at daytime showed that not only the height but also the location of the perch had an effect. If provided, low perches underneath the drinking trough in the middle of the housing systems (systems A and D) were used by the highest proportion of hens. Similarly, Duncan et al. [4] observed that perches near drinking troughs or feeding areas were used frequently at daytime. Perches are installed to provide hens with an area for resting. However, if hens can use them to reach a water resource, the increased movement on and near these perches can deplete their original function as rest areas.

Other low perches in the systems that were not installed underneath the drinking trough were less commonly used than the high perches at daytime. These observations are to some extent in contrast to those described by other authors. Blokhuis [27] observed a frequent use of low perches at daytime, especially for short naps and grooming behavior. Rönchen et al. [16] and Hergt [18] reported a more frequent use of low perches than high perches at daytime in enriched colony housing systems. Rönchen et al. [16] explained the lesser use of high perches by the inappropriate design, the position in the cage system and the insufficient distance to the ceiling of the cage. In this study, low perches were used more than high perches at daytime only if they were installed underneath a drinking trough. The use of and the preference for high perches was interpreted as an anti-predator behavior by several authors [11,28]. Also, Struelens and Tuyttens [7] observed a more frequent use of high perches if the distance to the ceiling of the cage was at least 19 to 24 cm. The high perches in this study all had a minimum distance of 29 cm to the ceiling.

At nighttime, the use of perches differed in the different housing systems and the observation periods. In system A, the differences were only marginal and a systematic prevalence of hens on specific perches was not visible at nighttime. In system B, no differences in terms of frequency in the use of specific perches could be observed, neither at daytime nor at nighttime. In system C in the second and third observation period, more hens were observed on the high perches compared to the low perches during the night observation. These results agree with findings of Schrader and Müller [11] and Struelens and Tuyttens [7] who observed that the height of perches influenced their use and that hens preferred to rest on high perches. In system D, the prevalence of hens on specific perches at nighttime changed from the first to the third observation period, which is, with progressing laying period and age of the hens. The low perch in the middle of the system underneath the drinking trough that was used frequently at the beginning of the laying period was avoided in the third observation period, when more hens were observed on the high perch. We conclude that the hens first had to learn to hold on to the relatively slippery, round high perch which was made of galvanized metal in contrast to the low perch in this system made of plastic. A systematic comparison of the housing systems A to D is not feasible, because of differences in the number of hens per cage and available perch types in the cages. This is due to the reason, this study was conducted to assess the use of perches in enriched colony housing systems under conditions used in practice.

In this study, the number of hens using a specific perch type was applied as a measure to assess the use of perches. Pickel et al. [10] recommended considering the quality of rest (balance movements) as an additional important factor. By applying this method, it should be possible to explain why the hens did not use the high perch in system D at the beginning of the laying period. Furthermore, the hens in our study had been raised in a conventional cage system without any access to perches, which is another factor that might influence the later use of perches. As shown by Heikkilä et al. [29], it seems to be important that laying hens have early access to perches, as hens used these more often once they were older if they had learned the use at a younger age. However, in this study we aimed to observe hens as they are housed in practice and the pullets for cage systems in practice are raised without perches.

In conclusion, the results showed that laying hens in enriched colony housing systems used the provided perches. However, a fraction of the hens (28.4 to 46.8%) did not use the perches at night time; we suggest that this was observed because they preferred specific perches and areas of the cages, which were already occupied by other hens. The use of the perches varied, depending on the daytime as well as the type of the perch (low, low underneath the drinking trough, high). There was a high frequency of hens on high perches in the observed housing systems, not only at nighttime but under specific circumstances also at daytime. Perches installed underneath the drinking troughs were used frequently at daytime. It should be considered that the hens used these perches not to rest but rather to have better access to the drinking trough. Since the perches of all systems were used and a system-related influence in the overall use was not observed, it seems that the use of perches is a basic need and as observed by other authors, hens show a high motivation to perch at night [26]. It has been shown by other authors that perches allow the hens to show species-specific-resting behavior [4,5]. Considering the results of this study, it can be recommended that a sufficient number of high perches should be offered, so that all hens have access to these obviously preferred perches. It should be considered if additional perch space should be offered if perches are installed underneath the drinking trough and it should be reconsidered if the required perch space of 15 cm per hen is sufficient.

Acknowledgements

This project was supported by funds of the Federal Ministry of Food and Agriculture (BMEL) based on a decision of the Parliament of the Federal Republic of Germany via the Federal Office for Agriculture and Food (BLE, Grant number 2813600507) under the innovation support program.

References

1. Destatis (2015) Statistisches Bundesamt. Fachserie 3, Reihe 4.2.3.
2. https://www.bigdutchman.com/en/nc/poultry-production/news/dictionary/dchar/g/term/standing-heat.html
3. https://www.bundesverfassungsgericht.de/SharedDocs/Entscheidungen/DE/2010/10/fs20101012_2bvf000107.html
4. Duncan ET, Appleby MC, Hughes B (1992) Effect of perches in laying cages on welfare and production of hens. Br Poult Sci 33: 25-35.
5. Olsson IA, Keeling LJ (2000) Night-time roosting in laying hens and the effect of thwarting access to perches. Appl Anim Behav Sci 68: 243-256.
6. Muiruri HK, Harrison PC, Gonyou HW (1990) Preferences of hens for shape and size of roosts. Appl Anim Behav Sci 27: 141-147.
7. Struelens E, Tuyttens FAM (2009) Effects of perch design on behaviour and health of laying hens. Animal Welfare 18: 533-538.
8. Scott GB, MacAngus G (2004) The ability of laying hens to negotiate perches of different materials with clean or dirty surfaces. Animal Welfare 13: 361-365.
9. Struelens E, Tuyttens FA, Duchateau L, Leroy T, Cox M, et al. (2008) Perching behaviour and perch height preference of laying hens in furnished cages varying in height. Br Poult Sci 49: 381-389.
10. Pickel T, Scholz B, Schrader L (2010) Perch material and diameter affects particular perching behaviours in laying hens. Appl Anim Behav Sci 127: 37-42.
11. Schrader L, Müller B (2009) Night-time roosting in the domestic fowl: the height matters. Appl Anim Behav Sci 121: 179-183.
12. Faure JM, Jones RB (1982) Effects of sex, strain and type of perch on perching behaviour in the domestic fowl. Applied Animal Ethology 8: 281-293.
13. Chen DH, Bao J, Meng FY, Wei CB (2014) Choice of perch characteristics by laying hens in cages with different group size and perching behaviours. Appl Anim Behav Sci 150: 37-43.
14. Appleby MC, Smith SF, Hughes BO (1993) Nesting, dust bathing and perching by laying hens in cages: effects of design on behaviour and welfare. Br Poult Sci 34: 835-847.
15. Abrahamsson P, Tauson R, Appleby MC (1996) Behaviour, health and integument of four hybrids of laying hens in modified and conventional cages. Br Poult Sci 37: 521-540.
16. Rönchen S, Scholz B, Hamann H, Distl O (2010) Use of functional areas, perch acceptance and selected behavioural traits in three different layer strains kept in furnished cages, small group systems and modified small group systems with elevated perches. Eur Poult Sci 74: 256-264.
17. Telle M (2011) Verhaltensbeobachtungen bei der Kleingruppenhaltung von Legehennen (LSL). Dissertation, Dr. Med. Vet., Ludwig-Maximilians Universität München, Munich, Germany.
18. Hergt F (2007) Vergleichende Untersuchung zum Verhalten von Legehennen in Klein- und Großvolierenhaltung. Dissertation, Dr. Med. Vet., Ludwig-Maximilians-Universität München, Munich, Germany.
19. Carmichael NL, Walker AW, Hughes BO (1999) Laying hens in large flocks in a perchery system: influence of stocking density on location, use of resources and behaviour. Br Poult Sci 40: 165-176.
20. Appleby MC, Walker AW, Nicol CJ, Lindberg AC, Freire R, et al. (2002) Development of furnished cages for laying hens. Br Poult Sci 43: 489-500.
21. Plattner C (2016) Behaviour of non-beak-trimmed laying hens in alternative housing systems with a special focus on the pecking behaviour. Dissertation, LMU München: Faculty of Veterinary Medicine, Munich, Germany.
22. Martin P, Bateson P (2007) Measuring Behaviour, an Introductory Guide. Cambridge University Press, Cambridge, UK.
23. Acomed (2013) Chi-Quadrat-Test (Vierfelder-Tafel).
24. Parker RI, Hagan-Burke S (2007) Useful effect size interpretations for single case research. Behav Ther 38: 95-105.
25. Campbell DL, Makagon MM, Swanson JC, Siegford JM (2016) Perch use by laying hens in a commercial aviary. Poult Sci.
26. Olsson IAS, Keeling IJ (2002) The Push-Door for Measuring Motivation in Hens: Laying Hens are Motivated to Perch at Night. Animal Welfare 11: 11-19.
27. Blokhuis HJ (1984) Rest in poultry. Appl Anim Behav Sci 12: 289-303.
28. Newberry RC, Estevez I, Keeling LJ (2001) Group size and perching behaviour in young domestic fowl. Appl Anim Behav Sci 73: 117-129.
29. Heikkilä M, Wichman A, Gunnarsson S, Valros A (2006) Development of perching behaviour in chicks reared in enriched environment. Appl Anim Behav Sci 99: 145-156.

The Utilization of the SDS-PAGE Salivary Protein Profiles for Clustering Analysis of Bali Cattle (*Bos sondaicus/javanicus*) and the *Taurine* or *Zebu* Cross Breeds in North Lombok District, Indonesia: A Preliminary Study

Masri Junihardy, Maskur M, Soegeng Prasetyo, Muhamad Ali and Sulaiman N Depamede*

Postgraduate Study Program of Management and Livestock Resources, Faculty of Animal Science, Mataram University, Jalan Majapahit 62 Mataram, NTB-83125, Indonesia

Abstract

The main aim of this study is to investigate the salivary protein profile of Bali cattle (*Bos sondaicus/javanicus*) and their crossbred descendents with *Bos taurus* or *Bos indicus* in the country side farm of North Lombok District, Indonesia. A total of 52 samples of saliva collected from Bali cattle, a mix of Bali cattle and taurine or zebu cattle, and a pure taurine dairy cattle, were investigated through SDS-PAGE. Intra and inter specific relationships were estimated using Jaccard's similarity and Euclidean distance index. Dendograms based on cluster analysis, and hierarchical analyses using Ward's method were developed. It was revealed that cluster analyses of salivary proteins in the range of 17-45 kDa were able to be classified and disengaged from the breed or species in the population in this study. It can thus be concluded that saliva has a good prospect as an alternative biological material for phylogenetic studies in the population. It is explicable that further verification using molecular genetics technology, should be carried out before the concept is decided to be put into daily practice.

Keywords: *Bos sondaicus/javanicus*; *Bos indicus*; *Bos taurus*; Saliva; Dendogram

Introduction

Bali cattle (*Bos sondaicus/javanicus*) are an indigenous cattle breed of Indonesia, domesticated form of wild banteng [1,2]. These cattle are of beef cattle type, with relatively small body size, weighing about 250-350 kg, although there are cattle that also weigh up to 600-800 kg [3]. Farmers in Indonesia like to keep these cattle because they are easy to handle, have high adaptability, and are resistant to adverse conditions [4].

In the late 1970s or early 1980s, efforts to improve the quality of Bali cattle have been carried out through artificial insemination programs, or by the introgression of superior bulls of taurine and zebu breeds such as Simmentals, Herefords, Limousines and Brahman Angus or Brangus [5].

In further developments, many farmers are interested in the descendants of crossbred cattle, due to the increase in size. After more than three decades, certain regions in Indonesia seek to refine the local cattle, including Bali cattle to preserve them as the native cattle breed [6]. For these reasons, a screening method in the field or on farm is needed. There are some relationship analysis studies based on morphological phenotypes of body size or physical characteristics, which have been carried out to screen the local cattle breed from the cross cattle breed in a population. In addition, genetic information through DNA blood analysis has also been used as a gold standard. However, the latter, is admittedly still too expensive for farmers.

In the last decade, saliva has been used as an alternative biological material for studying the physiological status of the animal [7], as well as to compare one animal species to another [8]. An advantage of using saliva is that saliva is taken by a non-invasive procedure compared to blood which is taken invasively. This enables farmers, especially in the countryside, to agree for their cattle to be used as research subjects.

Based on these considerations, we have conducted a preliminary study on comparing the salivary protein profiles to analyze whether the protein profiles can be used as indicators of genetic relatedness between Bali cattle and the taurine or zebu crossbreed descendants in a community farm in North Lombok District, Indonesia.

Materials and Methods

Determination of subjects

The main material of this study is saliva, which is isolated from healthy, non-pregnant adult cattle, maintained by farmers in North Lombok District (~1200 m above sea level, masl) in Lombok Island, Indonesia (Figure 1). The cattle were fed King grass and the local roughages available around the farm mixed with rice bran twice a day, while the drinking water supplied *ad libitum*. A total of 23 cattle, selected by purposive sampling were used, consisting of Bali cattle, and cattle of taurine or zebu cross breeds. The type of cattle was determined based on physical characteristics from each type of cattle breed. Bali cattle are easily distinguished from taurine (*Bos taurus*) or zebu cattle (*Bos indicus*). Their coat color is very distinctive, usually reddish-brown, except for a clearly defined white area on the hindquarters that extends along the belly, and also white socks reaching from the hooves to just above the hocks compiled by Lindell [9].

Saliva was collected and treated as described previously [10] from oral cavity of the cattle, using disposable plastic pipettes. About 5-10 ml of saliva collected in disposable glass tubes containing preservative/bactericidal (0.2% v/v NaN_3) were placed in a cool box containing ice and immediately taken to the laboratory for further treatments.

***Corresponding author:** Sulaiman Ngongu Depamede, Postgraduate Study Program of Management and Livestock Resources, Faculty of Animal Science, Mataram University Jalan Majapahit 62 Mataram, NTB-83125, Indonesia
E-mail: depamede@gmail.com (or) sulaiman_n@unram.ac.id

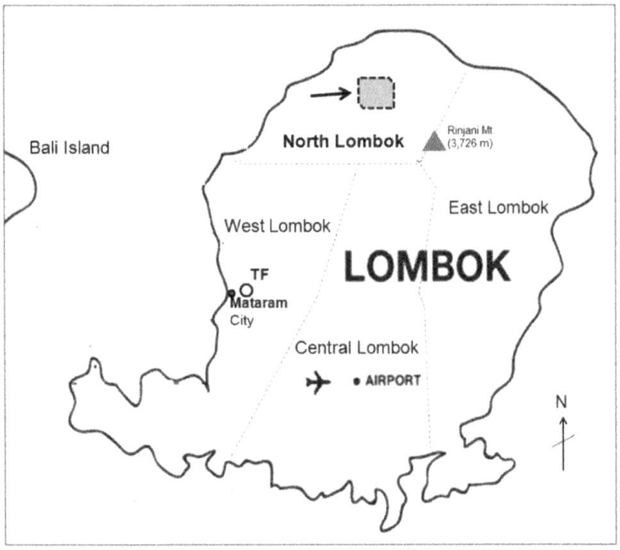

Figure 1: Map of Lombok, Indonesia, showing the location of the farm (arrow) in North Lombok District, and the Teaching Farm of Mataram University located in West Lombok District (TF, open circle) where the saliva samples were collected.

As a comparison, salivary profiles of 28 Bali cattle reared in the Teaching Faculty of Animal Science, Mataram University, West Lombok District were used as representation of the native local Bali cattle. These cattle do not have blood relations with those cattle in the study site in North Lombok District, and have never been crossed with other breeds. In addition, salivary profiles of Friesen Holstein cattle, as a representation of *Bos taurus* was also included (Courtesy: Dr. Wheeler TT, AgResearch Centre, Hamilton, NZ).

Sample preparation, protein estimation and SDS-PAGE profiling

In the laboratory, the saliva was centrifuged at 3000 rpm, 4°C, for 5 minutes, and the supernatant was aliquoated, and frozen at -80°C. Salivary protein concentration was determined using a NanoDrop 2000cSpectrophotometer (Thermo Fisher Scientific, USA) at a wavelength of 280 nm. All samples were further diluted with phosphate buffered saline at pH 7.4 and brought to a 1 mg/ml concentration. Electrophoresis was carried out under denaturing conditions in a discontinuous 1-D SDS-PAGE system using 12.5% acrylamide according to Laemmli [11], performed at a constant voltage of 100 V. Each sample was mixed with loading buffer and loaded at 10 µg per well after boiling for 4 minutes at 100°C. As a molecular weight standard, a protein molecular marker also ran along with the saliva samples according to the manufacture's instruction (Intron, Biotechnology). Gels were stained using Coomassie brilliant blue dye R-250 (Sigma, Aldrich), scanned and documented for analyzing purposes.

Band scoring and analysis

The banding patterns of the gel were analyzed manually and molecular weight values for various bands were calculated based on its relative migration distance or retardation factor (Rf), plotted into a graph as suggested by [12]. Interpolating the value from this graph then gave the molecular weight of the unknown protein band. The process was carried out with the assistance of Microsoft Office Excel 2007.

In this study salivary protein between the species in the region of 17-45 kDa molecular weights were preferred for analyzing due to some specific markers for bovine saliva that have been found in that range [10,13-15]. Only the unambiguous bands were scored or coded for the presence (scored 1) or absence (scored 0) of each saliva sample. Furthermore, similarity matrixes based on Jaccard's coefficient [16] were created for each group breed of cattle. Cattle of each group with Jaccard's similarity coefficient value of ≥ 0.75 were merged. With these values, dendograms were generated based on cluster analysis with Jaccard's and Euclidean similarity distance. In addition, a cluster tree was also elaborated using Ward's method. Tabulation and analyzing data were carried out using Excel Microsoft Office for Windows in combination with PAST (Paleontological Statistics) software package [17].

Results and Discussion

Morphological determination of the cattle used in this study

This study used local Bali cattle (*Bos sondaicus/javanicus*) and taurine or zebu crossbred cattle. The taurine or zebu crossbred cattle were introduced at the location of this study about 20-30 years ago. Some representations of photographs of the cattle, is presented in Figure 2. It is clear that, there are morphological differences between the local Bali cattle (Figure 2a) and the crossbreed cattle. Unfortunately, there is no good recording at the farm level, but from the farmers' testimony, it was informed that the cattle that they raise are the results of crossbreeding process. Furthermore, they named the cattle as Simbal after the Simmental and Bali cross (Figure 2b), Brangbal after the crossing of Brangus × Bali cattle (Figure 2c), Limbal for descendants crossing of Limousine and Bali cattle (Figure 2d), while Herbal is the nickname for the results of cross-breeding between Hereford and Bali cattle (Figure 2e).

SDS-PAGE salivary protein profiles

SDS-PAGE analysis had resulted about 7-12 protein bands for the salivary proteins of cattle in this study as presented in Figures 3a and 3b. Of the various bands obtained, in general, it appears that there are inter and intra-specific relationships between individual cattle. Of those bands generated, the bands with estimated molecular weight (Mr) between 17 and 45 kDa were selected. This is because that molecular weight range meets the requirements of manual calculation procedure based on Rf, as suggested by Hames [12]. Furthermore, as stated in the methods, from the 52 samples used, the individual cattle of the same breed that had homolog salivary protein profile were aligned and merged according to Jaccard's similarity value of ≥ 0.75. As a result, a total of 29 out of the 52 samples were developed (Table 1).

It can be seen in Table 1 that there are some predominant markers found in nearly all subjects (i.e., assigned as 1), namely proteins of 17 kDa, 18 kDa and 21 kDa. These protein markers are possibly in line with the peptides reported by Depamede [10] in Bali cattle saliva known as predicted zymogen granule protein 16 homologue (G3MZ19) with a nominal mass (Mr) 17.708 kDa, and Pancreatic adenocarcinoma upregulated factor-like (FINZ8) with a relative molecular weight (Mr) of 22.091 kDa. Furthermore a phylogenetic tree based on Bali cattle G3MZ19 gene has also been reported [15].

Phylogenetic analysis

In connection with the possibility of utilizing the salivary protein profiles to differentiate and determine relationships between local Bali cattle (*Bos sondaicus/javanicus*) and the descendant crossbreed between Bali cattle (*Bos sondaicus/javanicus*) and *Bos taurus* (Simbal,

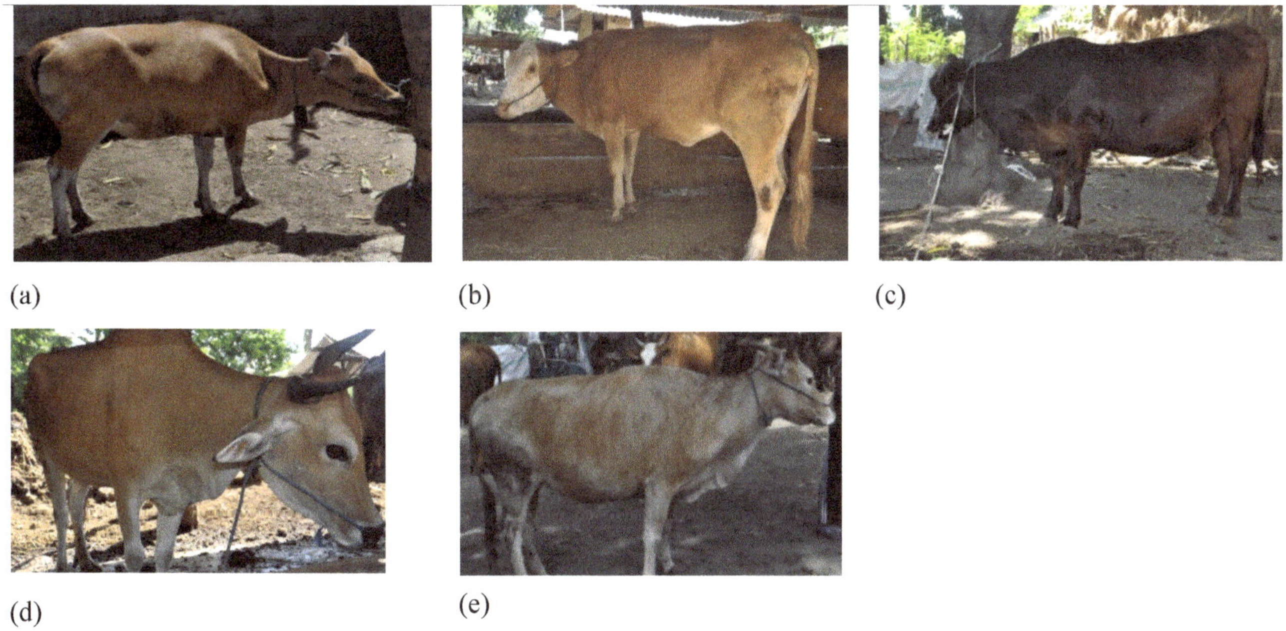

Figure 2: Representation of cattle used as source of saliva in this study reared by the farmers in Lombok North District (LND). Name of the type of species or breeds was based on the name given by the farmer. (a) Local Bali cattle; (b) Simbal: Simmental × Bali cattle crossbreed; (c) Brangbal: Brangus × Bali cattle crossbreed; (d) Limbal: Limousine × Bali cattle crossbreed; (e) Herbal: Hereford × Bali cattle crossbreeds.

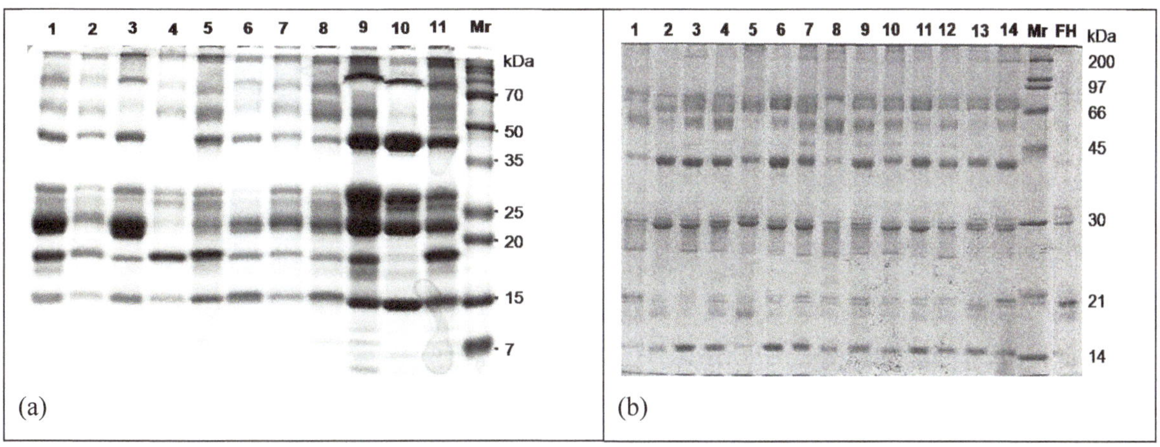

Figure 3: (a) Representation of protein profiles of Bali cattle saliva collected from Local Farm at North Lombok District (1-11). Simbal (1-2), Brangbal (3-5), Brahbal (6-8), Bali cattle (9-11). Mr: molecular weight marker. The protein profiles showing inter and intra specific relationships. (b) Representation of protein profiles of Bali cattle saliva collected from Teaching Farm (1-14) and a New Zealand dairy cattle saliva (FH). Mr: molecular weight marker.

Table 1: Molecular weight values for various bands of cattle salivary proteins based on SDSPAGE analysis after synchronization according to Jaccard's similarity distance within each cattle breed group.

No.	MW (kDa) / Sample Code	45	39	37	36	30	29	28	25	21	20	18	17
1.	Bal-KLU.01	1	0	0	1	0	0	0	0	1	0	1	1
2.	Bal-KLU.02	0	0	0	1	0	0	0	1	1	1	1	1
3.	Brahbal.01	0	0	0	1	0	0	0	1	1	0	1	0
4.	Brahbal.02	0	0	0	1	0	0	0	1	1	1	0	1
5.	Brahbal.03	0	0	1	0	0	0	0	1	1	0	1	0
6.	Brahbal.04	1	0	0	1	0	0	0	0	1	0	1	1
7.	Brangbal.01	0	0	0	1	0	0	0	1	0	1	1	0
8.	Brangbal.02	1	0	0	0	0	0	0	1	0	0	1	0
9.	Brangbal.03	1	0	1	0	0	0	0	0	1	1	0	1

10.	Herbal.01	1	0	0	1	0	0	0	1	1	0	1	1
11.	Herbal.02	0	1	0	0	0	0	0	0	1	1	0	1
12.	Herbal.03	1	0	1	0	0	0	0	1	1	0	0	1
13.	Herbal.04	0	0	1	0	0	0	0	0	1	0	1	1
14.	Limbal.01	1	0	0	1	0	0	0	0	1	1	0	1
15.	Simbal.01	0	0	0	1	0	0	0	1	0	1	1	0
16.	Simbal.02	1	0	0	1	0	0	0	1	1	1	1	0
17.	Simbal.03	0	0	0	1	0	0	0	0	1	1	0	1
18.	Simbal.04	0	0	1	0	0	0	0	0	1	1	0	1
19.	Bal. 1	0	1	0	0	0	0	1	1	1	0	1	0
20.	Bal. 7	0	1	0	0	0	0	0	1	0	0	0	0
21.	Bal. 10	0	1	0	0	0	0	1	0	1	0	0	0
22.	Bal. 11	0	1	0	0	0	0	1	0	0	0	1	0
23.	Bal. 14	0	1	0	0	0	0	0	1	1	0	1	0
24.	Bal. 15	0	1	0	0	0	0	1	0	0	0	1	0
25.	Bal. 17	0	1	0	0	0	0	1	1	1	0	0	0
26.	Bal. 19	0	1	0	0	0	0	1	1	0	0	1	0
27.	Bal. 21	1	1	0	0	0	0	0	0	0	0	1	1
28.	Bal. 24	0	1	0	0	0	0	1	0	0	0	1	0
29.	NZ. FH	0	0	0	0	1	1	1	0	1	1	0	0

No. 1-18: Cattle reared in NLD farm; **No. 19-28:** Cattle reared on Teaching Farm, Faculty of Animal Science, Mataram University. Bal-KLU: NLD-Bali cattle; Brahbal: Brahman × Bali cattle crossbreed; Brangbal: Brangus × Bali cattle crossbreed; Herbal: Hereford × Bali cattle crossbreed; Limbal: Limousine × Bali cattle crossbreed; Simbal: Simmental × Bali cattle crossbreed; Bal.: Bali cattle and **NZ. FH:** New Zealand Frisian Holstein cattle.

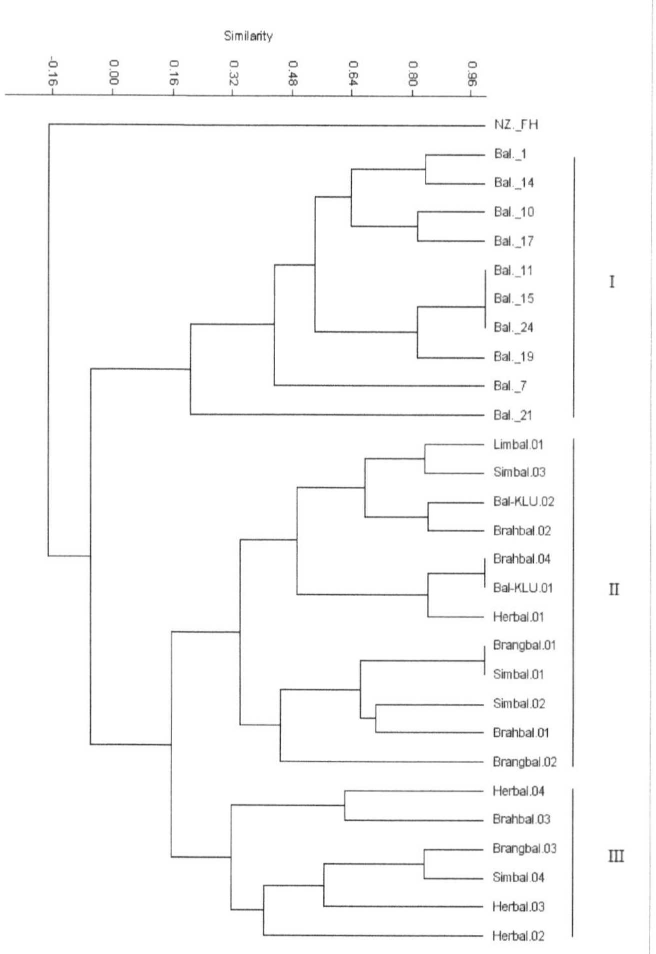

Figure 4a: A cluster analysis based on Jaccard similarity.

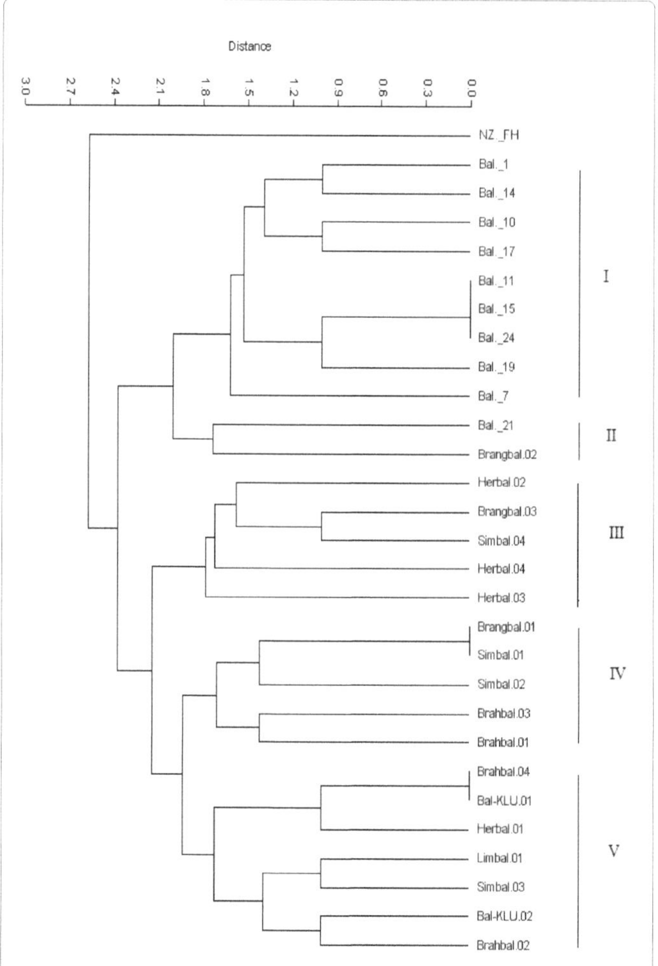

Figure 4b: A cluster analysis based on the Euclidean distance.

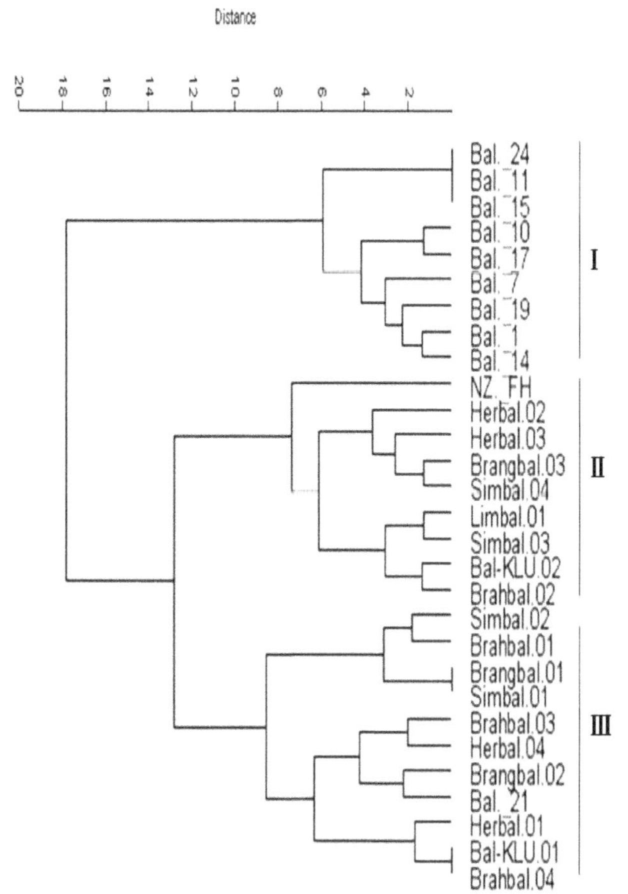

Figure 4c: Dendogram created by hierarchical cluster analysis of the data using Ward's method and Euclidean distance.

Herbal, and Limbal) or Zebu cattle/*Bos indicus* (Brangbal and Brahbal), the phylogenetic tree was constructed. Dendograms were constructed based on Cluster analysis with Jaccard's similarity and Euclidean distance matrix (Figures 4a and 4b) and hierarchical cluster based on Ward's method (Figure 4c).

The dendograms with Jaccard's similarity or Euclidean distance give only one major cluster i.e., the local breed (Bali cattle) and their crossbred descendants, with the New Zealand Friesian Holstein (NZFH) cattle in the out group position (Figures 4a and 4b). This is quite reasonable since NZFH is known as taurine dairy cattle, different from the others, which are of the beef type cattle. However, the dendogram that was generated based on hierarchical cluster analysis using Ward's method and Euclidean distance, gives two main clusters. Interestingly in this dendogram, NZFH dairy cattle is not in the out group position but fall into the group that consists of local crossbred cattle i.e., descendants of Brahman × Bali cattle crossbreeds (Brangbal) and Simmental × Bali cattle crossbreeds (Simbal).

If we observe closer, from all dendograms it can be clearly seen that the cattle in this study are grouped into orderly and organized clusters or sub clusters. It can be seen that all Bali cattle which were reared in the Teaching farm of Faculty of Animal Science, Mataram University fall into one sub cluster (I). The other sub clusters (II and III or II-V) consisted of the local cattle reared by the farmers at North Lombok District, the site of this study. The distribution pattern of the dendogram was in line with the nature of the samples. Bali cattle at the Teaching Farm were selected for research purposes based on the morphological characteristics of pure Bali cattle as compiled by [9]. On the other hand, the cattle reared by the farmers at the site of this study were of the progeny of crossbred between Bali cattle and *Bos taurus* or *Bos indicus* descendants. And this crossbreeding has been going on for a long time. It began with an artificial insemination program (late 1970s), and followed by the natural mating among descendent crosses without proper selection process conducted by farmers, which is quite a common practice in small holder farms [18,19].

Farmers carried out selection or cross mating their cattle, possibly without good management control. The crossbred cattle present until today, seem to be the cattle that have been able to survive better than others. The survival and distribution of the mixing crossbreds between imported breeds and the local breeds in North Lombok District is therefore quite reasonable since the district is a highland area (~1200 masl), which is suitable for the development of the offspring of crossbred cattle between native cattle (*Bos sondaicus/javanicus*) and the taurine or zebu descendant cattle [1,5,20].

In hierarchical analysis (Figure 4c) it can be clearly seen that New Zealand dairy cattle (NZFH) exist in cluster II, even though its position is separated from the local cross breed cattle. It is quite hard to explain about this, however we may speculate that the position of NZFH as representation of taurine cattle in this dendogram, strengthen the facts that cattle reared by the farmers at the site of this study were mixed crossbred cattle.

Overall, it can be seen that in general the lineage of the cattle in the site of the present study can still be traced based on their salivary protein profiles. In other words, saliva has potential prospect to be used as an alternative biological source to help the farmers examine their cattle descent. Especially for screening purposes on farms in which, taking blood samples is a serious concern. However obviously, it must be further followed by verification using molecular genetics technology, before it is decided to put it into daily practice.

Acknowledgments

SND was supported by the General Directorate of Higher Education, Ministry of Research, Technology and Higher Education, Republic of Indonesia through research competency grant (HIKOM Program) No. 61W/SPP-HIKOM/UN18.12/PL/2016. Bali cattle at the Teaching Farm, Faculty of Animal Science, Mataram University were provided by Dr. Dahlanuddin as part of an Australian Centre for International Agricultural Research (ACIAR)-funded collaborative project (LPS 2008-038).

References

1. Mohamad K, Olsson M, van Tol HT, Mikko S, Vlamings BH, et al. (2009) On the origin of Indonesian cattle. PLoS One 4: e5490.
2. Nijman IJ, Otsen M, Verkaar EL, de Ruijter C, Hanekamp E, et al. (2003) Hybridization of banteng (*Bos javanicus*) and zebu (*Bos indicus*) revealed by mitochondrial DNA, satellite DNA, AFLP and microsatellites. Heredity 90: 10-16.
3. Martojo H (2003) Indigenous Bali Cattle: The Best Suited Cattle Breed for Sustainable Small Farming in Indonesia. In: The Relationship between Indigenous Animals and Humans in APEC Region. Chang HL, Huang YC (Eds.). Chinese Society of Animal Science, Taiwan, pp: 21-36.
4. Martojo H (2012) Indigenous Bali cattle is most suitable for sustainable small farming in Indonesia. Reprod Domest Anim 47: 10-14.
5. Setyawan AD (2015) Review: genetic diversity of local and exotic cattle and their crossbreeding impact on the quality of Indonesian cattle. Biodiversitas 16: 327-354.
6. Purwantara B, Noor RR, Andersson G, Rodriguez-Martinez H (2012) Banteng and Bali cattle in Indonesia: status and forecasts. Reprod Domest Anim 47: 2-6.

7. Lamy E, Mau M (2012) Saliva proteomics as an emerging, non-invasive tool to study livestock physiology, nutrition and diseases. J Proteom 75: 4251-4258.

8. Lamy E, Da Costa G, Silva FC, Potes J, Coelho AV, et al. (2008) Comparison of electrophoretic protein profiles from sheep and goat parotid saliva. J Chem Ecol 34: 388-397.

9. Lindell IC (2013) Phenotyping of Bali cattle and interviewing farmers in Indonesia-a minor field study. Department of Animal Breeding and Genetics, Swedish University of Agricultural Sciences.

10. Depamede SN (2013) Proteomic Analysis of a 14.2 kDa Protein Isolated from Bali Cattle (Bos Sondaicus/Javanicus) Saliva Using Single Dimension Sodium Dodecyl Sulphate-Polyacrylamide Gel Electrophoresis and Matrix-Assisted Laser Desorption Ionization Time-of-Flight Tandem Mass Spectrometer. Ital J Anim Sci 12: e59.

11. Laemmli UK (1970) Cleavage of structural proteins during the assembly of the head of bacteriophage T4. Nature 227: 680-685.

12. Hames BD (1998) Gel electrophoresis of proteins: A practical approach. 3rd edn. Oxford University Press, Oxford, New York, USA.

13. Wheeler TT, Haigh BJ, McCracken JY, Wilkins RJ, Morris CA, et al. (2002) The BSP30 salivary proteins from cattle, LUNX/PLUNC and von Ebner's minor salivary gland protein are members of the PSP/LBP superfamily of proteins. Biochim Biophys Acta 1579: 92-100.

14. Wheeler TT, Haigh BJ, Broadhurst MK, Hood KA, Maqbool NJ (2011) The BPI-like/PLUNC family proteins in cattle. Biochem Soc Trans 39: 1006-1011.

15. Depamede SN (2015) Expression of the Fragment Gene of Predicted Zymogen Granule Protein (G3MZ19) Homologue in the Bali Cattle (Bos Javanicus) Based on MALDITOF/TOF.MS Analysis of Bali Cattle Saliva. J Vet Sci Technol 6: 260.

16. Real R, Vargas JM (1996) The probabilistic basis of jaccard's index of similarity. Systematic Biology 45: 380-386.

17. Hammer O, Harper DAT, Ryan PD (2001) PAST: Paleontological Statistic software package for education and data analysis. Paleontologica Electronica 4: 1-9.

18. Talib C, Siregar AR, Budiarti-Turner S, Diwyanto K (2003) Implementation of a breeding program for Bali cattle. Technical issues at national and regional levels. Strategies to improve Bali cattle in Eastern Indonesia. ACIAR proceedings 110: 82-85.

19. Talib C, Siregar AR, Diwyanto K (2003) Options for genetic improvement of Bali cattle-assessing the strengths and weaknesses of alternative strategies. Option 3. Expensive technologies and AI deleted. Strategies to improve Bali cattle in Eastern Indonesia. ACIAR proceedings 110: 76-78.

20. Mohamad K, Olsson M, Andersson G, Purwantara B, van Tol HTA, et al. (2012) The Origin of Indonesian Cattle and Conservation Genetics of the Bali Cattle Breed. Reprod Domest Anim 47: 18-20.

The Reproductive Behavior of Indian Leopards (*Panthera pardus fusca*)

Boon Allwin[1], Kalignan PA[2], Pradeep Nag BS[3], Gopikrishnan D[3] and Nishit S Gokarn[4]

[1]*Department of Wildlife Science, Madras Veterinary College, TANUVAS, Chennai, Tamil Nadu, India*
[2]*Zoo Veterinarian, Bannerghatta Zoological Park, Karnataka, India*
[3]*Department of Gynecology, Madras Veterinary College, TANUVAS, Chennai, Tamil Nadu, India*
[4]*Department of Surgery, Madras Veterinary College, TANUVAS, Chennai, Tamil Nadu, India*

Abstract

Leopards are very elusive and elegant cats and their reproductive behavior has been a challenging one to document. All behavioral observations were carried out after the daily cleaning activities of the zoo keepers, from a vantage point undisturbed and unhindered. The animals were observed for 2 hours at a frequency of 4 times a day. A total of 38 leopards were included in the study comprising of 33 animals (17 males and 16 females) from Bannerghatta National Park and 5 animals (3 males and 2 females) from Aringar Anna Zoological Park. The study focused on the mating behavior of leopards which was divided into pre-copulatory period, copulatory period and post-copulatory period, invariable of the number of animals, the total number of matings were regarded prime in this study. The behavioral oestrus periods were calculated as the difference from the day of the first observed behavioral signs shown by the animal to the last observed day of the oestrus signs. The inter-oestrus interval was calculated from the last day of the previous observed behavioral oestrus to the first day of the next observed behavioral oestrus. The behavioral indicators are documented and the findings are discussed.

Keywords: Leopard; Oestrus behavior; Sexual behavior

Introduction

The abundant growth in the human population has resulted in the extensive degradation of the wild life habitat, which poses main threat to the conservation of wild felids [1]. Conservation of these wild felids could be achieved only by reducing the human wild life conflict and by the proper and through understanding of their reproductive physiology [2]. However, the data regarding the quantification of the reproductive parameters requires a collection over multiple generations [3] which make the study laborious. Although enormous studies had been done exploring the reproductive behaviors and reproductive success in lions [4,5], cheetahs [6], tigers [7] and leopards, the basic behaviors of estrus and mating has not yet been elucidated in these wild felids which are essential for understanding the reproductive physiology of these species. Leopards have a wide range of distribution with the exception in the Himalayas and the desert regions. The elusiveness and behavioral flexibility of the leopards allow this species to survive near villages and human settlements. Although studies had been done on the behaviours of reproduction in male leopards [8], relatively few data are available for the reproductive behaviour in females. Hence the present was aimed to elucidate the estrus and mating behaviours of the leopards in captivity.

Study area

The entire study was carried out at two different geographical locations. The first at the Bannerghatta Biological Park, popularly known as BBP, has been an integral part of Bannerghatta National Park and emerged out as an independent establishment during the year 2002 (12.8009° N, 77.5777° E). The second at Arignar Anna Zoological Park (AAZP), Vandalur located 32 kms, South of Chennai on the eastern side of the Grand Southern trunk road (NH 45) (12.8781° N, 80.0859° E) in the Vandalur reserve forest of Kancheepuram district and is one of the biggest zoos in India extending over 510 hectares.

Study animals

A total of 38 leopards were included in the study comprising of 33 animals (17 males and 16 females) from Bannerghatta National Park and 5 animals (3 males and 2 females) from Aringar Anna Zoological Park. The study focused on the mating behavior of leopards which was divided into pre-copulatory period, copulatory period and post-copulatory period, invariable of the number of animals, the total number of matings were regarded prime in this study. All the animals in the study have attained sexual maturity and are considered adults.

Husbandry

The zoo keepers start their work by 08:30-09:00 hrs. The animals are either retained in the off-exhibit enclosure or let into the on-exhibit enclosures on a rotation basis after routine cleaning procedures. The animals were usually housed indoors in individual enclosures at night. The animals are not exhibited on Tuesdays when the zoo remains closed. All animals were fed a diet of raw beef with bones about 4-5 kg daily at around 16:30 hrs except on Tuesdays providing *ad libidum* water on all days. All the female animals had visual, auditory and/or olfactory communication with male con-specific. The animals are annually vaccinated against Feligen® and are dewormed quarterly.

Behavioral observations

General behavior: All behavioral observations were carried out after the daily cleaning activities of the zoo keepers, from a vantage point undisturbed and unhindered. The animals were observed for 2 hours at a frequency of 4 times a day. Initial periods of observation were spent in characterization of various behaviours as behavioral states and as behavioral events as defined by Martin and Bateson [9] and an ethogram were duly prepared. All observations were done

***Corresponding author:** Boon Allwin, Research Scholar, Department of Wildlife Science, Madras Veterinary College, TANUVAS, Chennai, Tamil Nadu, India
E-mail: boonallwin@gmail.com

with naked eye and with the aid of a pair of binoculars (10 × 50) when required. The timing was maintained using a digital stop watch.

The various macro-environment data viz. maximum and minimum temperature, rainfall, humidity, photoperiod were recorded for the study area on a daily basis. The temperature and humidity of the study animal houses were recorded on a daily basis as per standard procedures.

Behavioral events are those behavioral patterns that are of relatively short duration such as discrete body movements, vocalizations etc., which could be approximated as points in time. Behavioral states are those behavioral patterns that are of relatively long duration, such as prolonged activities or body postures.

For analysis, the behavioral states were broadly classified as resting behaviour and activity behaviour. The behavioral states like sleeping, lying, sitting, grooming were grouped under resting behaviour while walking, standing, stereotypic pacing were grouped under activity behaviour.

Oestrous behaviors: The animals were focally observed [10] for the occurrence of the 6 established feline signs characteristic of oestrus viz. vocalization, rubbing, rolling, urine marking, lordosis and mounting [11]. The observations were recorded on a specially designed check sheet in 1 minute blocks during each of the 60 minutes sampling period.

The behavioral oestrus periods were calculated as the difference from the day of the first observed behavioral signs shown by the animal to the last observed day of the oestrus signs. The inter-oestrus interval was calculated from the last day of the previous observed behavioral oestrus to the first day of the next observed behavioral oestrus.

Sexual behaviors: The sexual behaviors, when mating was allowed, were observed and recorded *in toto* (totally, entirely and completely). A qualitative description of the sexual act, pre- copulatory, copulatory and post copulatory behaviour was recorded. Quantitative measurement of the sexual behaviours with reference to total number of mating, the frequency of mating, the mating periods, inter-mating interval was also recorded.

Results

The entire findings of this study between Bannerghatta and Arignar Anna Zoological Park will be treated as the same unless and until specified.

Oestrus behavior

The following behavioral indicators of oestrus were observed and recorded during the course of this study.

Vocalization: The female leopards in oestrus were observed to have increased frequency of vocalization. This was further sub classified into 3 types.

- A long low sound like expelling air through the nostrils This was mainly the greeting call exhibited by both the sexes sounding like an expiratory grunt
- "Calling" - These were long loud vocalizations - which lasted more than 5 seconds. The calling was usually in bouts ≥ 5 per calling.
- "Moaning" - These were long vocalizations but not louder, sometimes also observed during the greeting between the sexes.

Rubbing: Rubbing of the face, flank and entire body against the walls, cage bars were observed. Rubbing was prominent when a male leopard was present in the adjacent cage. Rubbing also characteristically indicated a typical feline sexual behavior.

Crouching, rolling and position: Turning over and over on the back and writhing on the back was observed. Elevation of rear quarters and extension of back (lordosis), head rubbing, rolling presentation of vulva and constant lashing of the tail was well pronounced Rolling was almost always accompanied with a moaning vocalization. Sometimes rolling was not completed - "Quarter rolls and half-rolls".

Urine marking

Two types of urine marking were observed namely spraying of urine and squatted urination. The frequency of urine spraying was relatively increased during the oestrus period. The female leopard stood erect, tail raised and actively sprayed a small quantity of the urine onto the walls and cage bars. Urine spraying was found to be particularly more on the cage door when a male was housed adjacently. The leopard chose a specific spot for urination within the enclosure and held snarling head "a typical feline aggressive gait".

Flehmen

The male leopards were observed to sniff the walls, floors, cage bars and exhibited a snarling facial expression as how in any leopard will react in response to pain as markedly noted in other leopards with the ears positioned backwards

Vaginal discharge: Slight white mucus discharge was also observed during the oestrus.

Genital licking: Intermittent licking of genitalia was also a frequent feature during the oestrus period.

Mounting and lordosis

Apart from these indicators, the leopards were observed to be restless and constantly pacing and preferred a dark location inside the animal enclosure, Loss of appetite was also a regular feature. Standing and looking into the male's cage was also observed. Those leopards that exhibited the estrous behaviours were taken for the study. The behavioral oestrus periods and the inter-oestrus interval for the individual leopards as well as for the species as a whole are given in Table 1.

Sexual behavior

The various aspects of the sexual behaviour observed are presented below.

Mating behaviour

Pre-Copulatory behavior: It was observed that almost always it was the female who initiated the mating. The female was seen to greet the male with a long low sound and the male responded. The female showed an interest in the male, approached him and rubbed her face with that of the male head rubbing or flank rubbing. This initiated the male to move towards the female and she led him on with her tail raised and lashing from side to side (between 45° to 135°), after repeated rubs, tail lashes and tail rubs the female attained a typical lordosis posture presenting her to the male. Simultaneously the male approached the female from behind for mounting.

Copulatory behavior: The male Leopards mounted on the female and positioned themselves by arching his back and thrusting forward for intromission as typically seen in domestic felines. During this act both the male and the female exhibited a typical snarling expression. Following the intromission, the male emitted a characteristic prolonged

Leopard No.	Behavioural oestrous	Behavioural inter-oestrous interval
1	8	29
2	6	28
3	7	31
4	6	32
5	8	28
6	9	26
7	7	27
8	8	31
9	7	26
10	9	34
11	6	33
12	9	29
13	8	30
14	7	30
15	9	25
16	8	27
17	6	32
18	8	31
Mean ± SE	**7.56 ± 0.95**	**29.39 ± 0.62**

Table 1: The behavioral estrus periods and the inter-estrous interval for the individual leopards.

copulatory growl indicating the act of ejaculation, the duration of which varied, before leaning forward to grip the neck of the female

Post-Copulatory behavior: The male dismounted from female by jumping. Sometimes it was observed that the female gave a jerk to dislodge the male and tried to hit him with her paw with a growl. At times the jerk from the female was heavy and attempts to bite the male were clearly exhibited.

The male and the female seemed to exhibit different post copulatory behaviours. The female following the copulation engaged in one or more of the following behaviours: rolling, grooming, genital licking, lying sternal or lateral, walking or sleeping. The male on the other hand spent most of the time walking in the moat, lying, urine spraying and sleeping. Both the males and females were also observed to spend their post copulatory activity partly inside the water trough kept for watering within the enclosure.

After each mating, the animals took some time before they mated again. The inter-mating period or refractory period was calculated as the time from the previous dismount to the time of next successful mount. The refractory period was calculated to be 56.46 ± 0.15 minutes (n=45) on an average. The actual range extended from 0.93 minutes to 181 minutes.

Period of receptivity

This was calculated as the number of days permitted by female leopard for copulation by the male. In this study, the number of days was ranging from 6 to 9 days.

Mating time: This was calculated as the time from mounting to the time of dismounting. Successful mounts (in which intromission was present) were only considered for mating time. The average mating time was 40.38 ± 0.22 seconds (n=45) with the range extending from 12.36 to 80.03 seconds. The mating was observed only during the day time and since the animals were separated in the night. A total of 45 matings were observed during the entire study period and of these 26 (57.77%) took place in the forenoon session (9.30 AM-12.00 AM) while the remaining 19 (42.22%) took place in the afternoon session. (12.01-5.00 PM). There was not much interference during the feeding time and mating took place during the feeding time also.

Unsuccessful matings: Of the 72 approaches observed, only 45 (62.5%) resulted in successful matings. The remaining 27 (37.5%) were unsuccessful. The unsuccessful matings were either mounts with no intromission or just check rubbing, flank rubbing only. Of the 72 interactions involved 55 (76.38%) were initiated by the female while only 17 (23.61%) were initiated by the male.

Discussion

During the present study, apart from the established feline oestrus signs, the following observations were recorded - increase in activity behavior or restlessness, loss of appetite, "flehmen" and vaginal discharge previous studies by various authors [12-17] in tigers indicated that restlessness and pacing is a constant feature of oestrus as against the complete apathy females display during anoestrus which is characterized by resting quietly. It is noteworthy mention of Estep and Dewsbury [18] who stated that an increase in general activity manifested as increased locomotion, restlessness, or increased social interactions is coincident with oestrus in many species as observed in the present study. During this study, it was also observed that the oestrus signs observed and recorded in leopards include loss of appetite, lashing of tail, increase in activity behaviour and flehmen. Social behaviours like rubbing perineal area, lordosis, mounting, getting under, being mounted reported by Schmidt et al. [19].

Flehmen reaction, previously unreported in leopards was exhibited by 8 of the leopards out of 18 leopards during the alternate cycles individually. This detection was very rare and was not observed in the other leopard and in the same Leopard during subsequent cycles. Urine scent marking also was a less prominent sign as compared to that of tigers. Vocalization, rubbing, rolling were prominently associated with oestrus and varied from animal to animal with regards to the intensity of expression and rolling was almost always accompanied by a moaning sound.

Lashing of tail was observed in all the Leopards and this was prominent during its pacing when the male was near the adjacent cage door. This behavior was not observed in the absence of the male and it strongly suggests invitation for mating. Similar "lashing of tail" has been reported by Schaller [20] in lionesses.

The oestrus periods determined for the leopards was 7.55 ± 0.95 days (n=18, 6-9 days). This is in accordance with the earlier studies 3-14 days [21], 4-14 days [22], 4-11 days [23] and 7 days. The inter-oestrus period was found to be 29.38 ± 0.62 days (n=18, 26-34 days) in two leopards. This was in contradiction to the earlier reports by Sadlier [21]-43 days (13-112) and Schmidt et al. [19] 7-8 weeks and Wildt [8]-46 days. Felines normally being induced ovulators ovulation occur after 2-3 matings and the period of exhibiting estrus varies within the oestrus period. These felids show a gap known as the "oestral recess" for a period varying from 5-7 days. After this period typical signs of estrus were recorded and mating progressed. However it was beyond the scope of this study to understand the endocrine basis of such occurrences for which, the respective hormones have to be assessed.

Vaginal discharge

Vaginal discharge was observed in the study for the first time. Acharjyo et al. [13] stated that the external genitalia of tigress in oestrus was swollen which was coinciding with the findings of this study and 15 (83.33%) of the leopards exhibited these signs which can be a reliable indicator for assessing oestrus. While Feldman and Nelson [24] argued that the vulvar labiae of the female cats are relatively nonresponsive to oestrogen and they remain small and covered with hair during the proestrus and oestrus Vaginal discharge was well appreciated in 5 (27.77%) of the leopards under study during oestrus and hence this can be regarded as a indicator for oestrus in Leopards.

Urine marking was observed to be negatively correlated with oestrus by Kleiman [12] in Bengal tigers. However, in this study, urine marking was significantly associated and positively correlated with oestrus and was exhibited by all the leopards during the estrus period. There were individual variations in the intensity of expression. This is in accordance with Kleiman [12] who found that, in felids, individual females differ in the manner of displaying oestrus and that all females may occasionally exhibit these patterns at one time or another.

Sexual behavior of leopards

Mating behavior: Mating behavior has been earlier described by Acharjyo et al. [13] and by Palita et al. [17] in captive tigers of Nandankannan Biological Park, Orissa. The observations in this study concurred with the earlier reports. However, while Acharjyo et al. [13] states that mating was always initiated by the female tigress, it was not so in this study as 72 interactions involved 55 (76.38%) were initiated by the female while only 17 (23.61%) were initiated by the male. The neck grip was not always observed during the mounting but before dismounting, the male invariably gripped the neck of the female Schaller [20] in lions and Morris in cats contend that the neck bite before dismounting is actually a "behaviour trick" played by the male to protect himself from assault by the female after dismounting since the withdrawal of the penis causes considerable pain in the female as observed in the study. All cats have evolved a "freeze" reaction being taken by the neck bite and this temporary immobilization of the female allows the male to jump to safety. It was observed as in the earlier studies [13,17] that the penis remained outside for sometime after the post copulatory jumping and the raised tail condition observed while jumping is probably to maintain the balance of the body.

Mating time: The average mating time was 40.38 ± 0.22 seconds (n=45) with the range extending from 12.36 to 80.03 seconds. This varies from that of Acharjyo et al. [13] who reported 8-35 seconds, 0.5 to 3 minutes [14] and 7.35 seconds [17].

Inter-mating period: The inter-mating period was calculated to be the refractory period was calculated to be 56.46 ± 0.15 minutes (n=45) on an average. The actual range extended from 0.93 minutes to 181 minutes. Acharjyo et al. [13] reported the inter-mating period to vary from 20 minutes to several hours, while Palita et al. [17] gave the range of 2-70 minutes. The present observations were in coinciding correlation with these reports.

Post-copulatory behaviors: The post copulatory behaviors recorded in the present study were similar to those reported earlier [13,17].

Unsuccessful matings

Of the 72 approaches observed, only 45 (62.5%) resulted in successful matings. The remaining 27 (37.5%) were unsuccessful. The unsuccessful matings were either mounts with no intromission or just check rubbing, flank rubbing only [25]. Of the 72 interactions involved 55 (76.38%) were initiated by the female while only 17 (23.61%) were initiated by the male. This is in agreement with the observations of Acharjyo et al. [13] and Palita et al. [17].

Conclusion

The overall finding of this study was an effort to document the sexual behavior of this elusive feline, there is still paucity in the reproductive details of these cats. An elaborate study is essential with dedicated individual animals to understand more about their physiological, psychological governance.

References

1. Kitchener A (1991) The Natural history of wild cats. Comstock Publishing Associates, Ithaca, New York, USA.
2. Holt WV, Pickard AR, Rodger JC, Wildt DE (2003) Reproductive science and integrated conservation. Cambridge University Press, Cambridge, United Kingdom.
3. Clutton-Brock TH (1988) Reproductive success: Studies of individual variations in contrasting breeding systems. University of Chicago Press, Chicago, Illinois, USA.
4. Packer C, Herbst L, Pusey AE, Bygott JD, Hanby JP, et al. (1988) Reproductive success of lions. In: Reproductive Success. Clutton Brock TH (Editor). Univ. Chicago Press, Chicago, USA, p: 363383.
5. Meena V (2009) Variation in social organization of lions with particular reference to the Asiatic Lions *Panthera leo persica* (Carnivora: Felidae) of the Gir forest, India. Journal of Threatened Taxa 1: 158165.
6. Kelly MJ, Laurenson MK, FitzGibbon CD, Collins DA, Durant SM, et al. (1998) Demography of the Serengeti cheetah (*Acinonyx jubatus*) population: the first 25 years. J Zool 244: 473-488.
7. David Smith JL, McDougal C (1991) The Contribution of Variance in Lifetime Reproduction to Effective Population Size in Tigers. Conservation Biology 5: 484-490.
8. Wildt DE, Phillips LG, Simmons LG, Chakraborty PK, Brown JL, et al. (1988) A comparative analysis of ejaculate and hormonal characteristics of the captive male cheetah, tiger, leopard, and puma. Biol Reprod 38: 245-255.
9. Martin P, Bateson P (1995) Measuring Behaviour: An introductory guide. Cambridge University Press.
10. Altmann J (1974) Observational study of behavior: sampling methods. Behaviour 49: 227-267.
11. Michael RP (1961) Observations upon the sexual behaviour of the domestic cat (*Felis catus* L.) under laboratory conditions. Behaviour 18: 1-24.
12. Kleiman DG (1974) Patterns of behavior in hystricomorph rodents. In: The Biology of hystricomorph rodents: the proceedings of a symposium held at the Zoological Society of London on 7 and 8 June. Rowlands IW, Weir BJ (Eds.). Academic Press, UK.
13. Acharjyo LN, Mishra CG (1981) Some notes on the longevity of two species of Indian wild cats in captivity. Journal of the Bombay Natural History Society 78: 155-156.
14. Seager SWJ, Demorest CN (1986) Reproduction in captive wild carnivores. In: Zoo and Wild Animal Medicine. 2nd edn. Fowler ME, Miller RE (Eds.) W. B. Saunders, Philadelphia, USA, pp: 852-881.
15. Seal US, Plotka ED, Smith JD, Wright FH, Reindl NJ, et al. (1985) Immunoreactive luteinizing hormone, estradiol, progesterone, testosterone, and androstenedione levels during the breeding season and anestrus in Siberian tigers. Biol Reprod 32: 361-368.
16. Tilson R, Soemarna K, Ramono W, Sukumar R, Seal US, et al. (1994) Asian Elephant in Sumatra. Population and Habitat Viability Analysis. Minnesota: CBSG.
17. Palita SK, Patra AK, Patnaik MR (1996) Studies on the reproductive behaviours of tiger (*Panthera tigris* Linn.) in captivity. Readings in Behaviour, pp: 188-197.
18. Estep DQ, Dewsbury DA (1996) Mammalian reproductive behavior. In: Wild Animals in Captivity. Kleiman DG, Allen ME, Thompson KV, Lumpkin S (Eds.). University of Chicago Press, Chicago, USA, pp: 379-389.
19. Schmidt AM, Hess DL, Schmidt MJ, Lewis CR (1988) Serum concentrations of oestradiol and progesterone and frequency of sexual behaviour during the normal oestrous cycle in the snow leopard (*Panthera uncia*). J Reprod Fertil 82: 43-49.
20. Schaller GB (1972) The Serengeti lion. University of Chicago Press, Chicago, Illinois, USA.
21. Sadleir RMFS (1966) Notes on reproduction in the larger Felidae. International Zoo Yearbook 6: 184-187.

22. Desai JH (1975) Observations on the reproductive biology and early postnatal development of the panther, *Panthera pardus* L., in captivity. Journal of the Bombay Natural History Society 72: 293-304.

23. Acharjyo LN, Patnaik SK (1985) Observations on some aspects of reproduction among the panthers (*Panthera pardus*) of Nandan-Kanan Biological Park, Orissa. Indian Journal of Forestry 8: 8-14.

24. Feldman EC, Nelson RW (1996) Canine and feline endocrinology and reproduction. 2nd edn. WB Saunders Company, Philadelphia, USA.

25. Daniel JC (2009) The leopard in India: A natural history. Natraj Publishers, Dehra Dun, India, p: 228.

8

Practical Manual on Veterinary Clinical Diagnostic Approach

Ararsa Duguma*

Haramaya University, College of Veterinary Medicine, Ethiopia

Abstract

Veterinary clinical examination relies on knowledge of Anatomy, Physiology, Pathology and Animal behavior, skills in the methods and techniques of clinical examination, clinical sign and pathogenesis of the diseases which are the basic requirements for clinician in his/her good diagnostic approach. Disease problems in veterinary medicine are invariably presented to the clinician through the medium of the owner's complaint, which is a request for professional assistance by giving animal history. In any clinical examination procedures, it is necessary to employ some suitable means of restraint: physical, chemical or verbal, in order to be able to carry out the examination safely and without danger to the clinician or his assistants. Inspection, Palpation, percussion and auscultation are the commonly used methods of physical examination for assessing pathophysiological or anatomical abnormalities of given animal during clinical examination. The general clinical examination involves detailed consideration of physical body condition; conformation/shape; posture; gait; abnormal behavior; body temperature; pulse; and respiration of individual animal; whereas the regional or systematic clinical examination involves the application of the various clinical methods to the various regions or systems of the body. The system involved is identified and is then examined in greater detail using either a complete or a problem oriented examination. In addition to history taking and clinical examination; skills on techniques of laboratory sample collection and submission is an important consideration for further diagnosis, treatment and take practicable control and prevention measures on identified disease.

Keywords: Clinical examination; History taking; Physical method; Restraint; Sampling techniques

Introduction

In the investigation of any animal disease problem, the veterinarian must, of necessity, undertake a careful and thorough clinical examination with the object of recognizing the nature of the affection, so that effective treatment and, where practicable, control measures are adopted. The situation is rendered complex by the necessity to deal with a variety of species of domestic animals and birds. Increasing specialization on the part of practicing veterinarians will resolve some of the apparent problems thus presented. In general, however, the same principles may be applied in all cases to deal with the diverse difficulties that clinical diagnosis presents.

The organs or systems involved, the location, type of lesion present, the pathophysiological processes occurring and the severity of the disease can be deduced from the information gained during the clinical examination. Without a proficient clinical examination and an accurate diagnosis it is unlikely that the control, prognosis and welfare of animals will be optimized.

The success of clinical examination relies heavily on the knowledge of the clinician and usually assumes a single condition is responsible for the abnormalities. Many clinicians begin their examination by performing a general examination which includes a broad search for abnormalities [1,2]. The system or region involved is identified and is then examined in greater detail using either a complete or a problem oriented examination. For this sound knowledge of Anatomy, Physiology, Pathology and Animal behavior, skills in the methods and techniques of clinical examination, knowledge of etiology, clinical sign and pathogenesis of the diseases are the basic requirements for clinician to make diagnosis. This manual is a practical guideline for veterinary practitioner with the following objectives:

- Guide to apply methods of animal handling/restraint and ability to take history
- A guide for general and systemic physical clinical examination for further diagnosis, treatment and take practicable control and prevention measures on identified disease
- Having knowledge on preparation and administration of veterinary drugs
- Gives skills on veterinary laboratory sampling techniques

History Taking

Disease problems in veterinary medicine are invariably presented to the clinician through the medium of the owner's complaint, which is a request for professional assistance. For completeness and accuracy of history taking, the following points should be well considered (Patient data, Immediate/present history, past history, Management and Environment history).

Patient data

This data is essential for accurate identification of the patient and includes:

- Owner's name
- Owner's address: postal address, telephone, kebele, peasant association, etc.
- Species, breed, sex, age, name, ID No., body weight, etc.
- Description including color, marking, polledness, and other identification marks of patient

***Corresponding author:** Ararsa Duguma, Haramaya University, College of Veterinary Medicine, College of Veterinary Medicine, PO Box 138 Dire Dawa, Ethiopia, E-mail: ararsad@yahoo.com

Present history

This relates to the sequence of events associated with the period of time that the animal has been ill. Points to be focus in present history are:

- Duration of the disease: whether it is peracute, acute, subacute or chronic
- Clinical sign/symptoms: (appetite for food or drink, defecation, urination, respiration, sweating, physical activity, milk production, growth, gait, posture, voice, odour, etc.)
- The number of animals affected: (morbidity rate and mortality rate)
- Treatment given: determine whether any treatment has, in fact, been given before calling for assistance

Past history

In this respect, information should be obtained relating to the nature and timing of any previous illness which had affected the individual animal or group.

- Details regarding clinical features, diagnosis, treatments, morbidity and mortality rates, post mortem observations, laboratory test etc., should be obtained [3].
- Ascertain the system of animal replacement on the farm or in the home.
- If animal introduced from outside sources, further enquiries should be made concerning the health history and status of the source animals.

Management and environmental history

The examination of an animal must be accompanied by a consideration of its surroundings and circumstances.

Management:

- Nutrition,
- Livestock at pasture,
- Drinking water,
- Feeding methods/practice
- House space, satisfactory ventilation
- Proper management of milking cow and milking machine to avoid udder injury
- Breeding and Reproductive history
- Stocking rate/population density

Examination of the environment:

- Topography
- Soil type
- Ground surfaces
- Climatic conditions
- Environmental Hygiene
- An excessive buildup of feces and urine
- Quality of Floor

Methods of Restraint

Since animals often resist many of the clinical examination procedures, it may be necessary to employ some suitable means of restraint, in order to be able to carry out the examination safely and without danger to the clinician or his assistants. The methods available may be classified as:

- **Physical restraint** when various instruments are employed.
- **Chemical restraint** when drugs inducing varying degrees of sedation or immobilization are administered.
- **Verbal/Moral restraining** which can be more practiced by owner.

Physical restraint

It is important to perform all the physical manipulations in a quiet and gentle manner in order to carry out the examination safely without causing danger to the clinician or his assistants and to avoid disturbing the patient.

Restraining methods for equine, cattle, Pet animal, sheep and goats.

Training materials: open air clinic

Live animals

Rope, nose twitch, bull holder, crash etc.

Procedure:

Restraints of the equine:

- Twitch is applied to the upper or lower lip or to the ear
- Nose twitch
- Lifting the fore-leg and hind-leg by unaided hands or with Leg twitch
- A loop of strong cord or soft rope is applied to the appropriate part
- Two ropes one-person horse casting
- Two ropes four persons horse casting

Restraint of the cattle:

- The nasal septum is gripped between the thumb and one finger or with 'bull-holder
- Leg twitches are also employed
- One rope locking two horns on a post or tree
- One rope two person cattle casting
- Two ropes three person cattle casting

Restraint of sheep and goat:

- One person holds the neck of the sheep or goat by two hands
- One person stands beside the sheep or goat embracing the animal
- Small animals are restrained by placing them on a table in the upright, lateral or dorsal position

Pet animals

- Placing them on a table in the upright, lateral or dorsal position

- In the dog a tape muzzle or a leather muzzle is used

Chemical restraint

Drugs that is useful for this purpose includes:

- Acepromazine, Acetylpromazine, Chlorpromazine, Promazine and Trimeprazine; members of this group can be used in most species of animals.

Verbal/moral restraining

It is more practiced by owner e.g., feed provision, massaging, calling name of animal etc.

Physical examination methods

Objective

To apply general inspection, palpation, percussion and auscultation methods used to detect clinical signs of abnormalities.

Training materials

- Live animals (equine, cattle, sheep and goats)
- Pleximeter, hammer
- Stethoscope
- Gloves

Procedure

General inspection: It is done some distance away from the animal; sometimes go round the animal or herd/flock, in order to get the general impression about the case [4].

- Attention should be paid to the following items: (Behavior, Appetite, Defecation, Urination, Pasture, Gait, Body condition, Body conformation)
- Lesions on outer surface of the body can be observed: (Skin and coat, Nose, Mouth, Eyes, Legs and hoofs, Anus)

Palpation:

Objective: To detect the presence of pain in a tissue by noting increased sensitivity

Method: Use fingers, palm, back of the hand, and fist, in order to get the information about the variation in size, shape, consistency and temperature of body parts and lesions, e.g., the superficial lymph nodes.

The terms, which can be used to describe the consistency of parts during palpation, are:

- **Resilient**, when a structure quickly resumes its normal shape after the application of pressure has ceased (e.g., Normal rumen)
- **Doughy**, when pressure causes pitting as in edema
- **Firm**, when the resistance to pressure is similar to that of the normal liver (e.g., neoplasia/tumor)
- **Hard,** when the structure possesses bone-like consistency (e.g., Actinomycotic lesion)
- **Fluctuating**, when a wave-like movement is produced in a structure by the application of alternate pressure (e.g., hernia, hemorrhage/hematoma)
- **Emphysematous,** when the structure is swollen and yields on pressure with the production of a crepitating or crackling sound (e.g., Black leg) [5].

Percussion:

Objective: To obtain information about the condition of the surrounding tissues and, more particularly, the deeper lying parts. Percussion can examine the area of the subcutaneous emphysema, lungs, rumen and rump

Method: By means of striking a part of the body to be percussed

Immediate percussion: Using fingers or hammer directly strike the parts being examined.

Mediate percussion: Finger-finger percussion; Pleximeter-hammer percussion

The quality of the sounds produced by percussion is classified as:

Resonant: which is characteristic of the sound emitted by air containing organs, such as the lungs.

Tympanic: The sound produced by striking a hollow organ containing gas under pressure, e.g., tympanitic rumen or caecum.

Dull: Sound emitted by a solid organ like the liver or heart [6].

Modified percussion:

- **Ballottement percussion:** Used to detect late pregnancy in small ruminants, dogs and cats

Procedure: Apply a firm and interrupted push on the uterine region of the abdomen of small ruminants

Detection of rebound of floated material shows pregnancy

- **Fluid percussion:** Used to detect fluid in the abdomen

Procedure: Apply a push on one side of the abdomen, percussion on the other side

The presence of wave-like fluid movement shows accumulation of fluid in the abdomen, e.g., ascites [7].

Auscultation:

Objective: To listen the sounds produced by the functional activity of an organ located within a part of the body. This method used to examine the lung, trachea, heart and certain parts of the alimentary tract.

Direct auscultation:

Procedure: Spread a piece of cloth on the part to be examined using two hands to fix the cloth and keep your ears close to the body, then listen directly.

Indirect auscultation: Use stethoscope.

Procedure: Fix the probe of the stethoscope firmly on the part of the body to be examined and listen to the sounds produced by the functional activities of the body carefully.

Clinical Examination of the Patient

General physical examination

Temperature taking:

Materials:

- Live animals

- Thermometer
- Lubricant (soap or petroleum jelly), Antiseptics

Procedure:

- The places, which can be used to take temperature are rectum or vagina (approximately 0.5 degree centigrade higher in vagina).
- The thermometer should be sterilized by disinfectant (antiseptics) before use.
- It should be well shaken before recording of temperature to bring the mercury column below the lowest point likely to be observed in different species of animals.
- The bulb end of the thermometer should be lubricated with liquid paraffin or glycerin or soap especially in case of small pup and kitten.
- Insert the thermometer in a rotational way and gentle manner. Care should be taken so that the bulb of the thermometer remains in contact with the rectal mucous membrane.
- The thermometer should be kept in site for at least 3-5 minutes.
- Pull out the thermometer, clean it and read the number.
- Evaluation: Read the value to define and explain a state of fever, hypothermia, and febrile or non-febrile animals [8].

Pulse taking: Pulse can be adapted from the number of heart beats per minute by using stethoscope in less manageable animals. The rhythm of pulse should also be noticed while taking pulse.

Procedure:

- Place the digits on the artery to be examined
- Applying gentle pressure until the pulse wave can be detected
- Note the pressure or pulsation of the arteries felt on the finger digits
- Count the number of beats per minute (counting should be done at least for 30 seconds and multiplied by 2); notice the quality and rhythm of pulse (Table 1).

Materials

- Live animals
- Stethoscope
- Watch

Respiration taking

Materials:

- Live animals

S No	Species of animal	Site of pulse taking
1	Horse	External maxillary artery Transverse facial artery Median artery Great metatarsal artery
2	Cattle	Facial artery Median artery Middle coccygeal artery
3	Sheep/goat, dog, cat, pig, and calf	Femoral artery

Table 1: Site of pulse taking for different species of animals.

- Stethoscope
- Watch
- Gloves
- Crash

Method: The respiration rate is measured through counting of either contraction or expansion of the thorax and abdomen which can be observed during clinical examination

Procedure: A method for respiration rate taking includes:

- **Inspection:** Stand behind and to one side of the animal, and observe the movement of the thoracic and abdominal areas of the body.
- **Palpation:** Put one hand in front of the nostril, feel the exchange of the gas; or put one hand on the lung area or the thorax and feel the respiratory movements.
- **Auscultation:** Use stethoscope, listen to the respiration sound in the trachea or lung area.

Capillary Refill Time (CRT):

Method:

- This is taken by compressing the mucosa of the mouth or vulva to expel capillary blood, leaving a pale area
- Recording how long it takes for the normal pink color to return.
- In healthy animals the CRT should be less than 2 seconds.
- A CRT of more than 5 seconds is abnormal, and between 2 and 5 seconds may indicate a developing problem

Physical body condition: Body condition scoring is an important management practice used by producers as a tool to help optimize production, evaluate health, and assess nutritional status. Different scores can be given for individual animal and can further classified as normal, fatty, lean/thin, emaciation.

Condition Score 1: Very thin: This animal's skeletal structure is very prominent. Notice the deep depressions next to the spine, between the pelvis and rib cage, between the hooks and pins, and around the tail head.

Condition Score 2: Thin: The animal's skeleton is still very apparent. The individual spinous processes are clearly visible, but there is a small amount of fat tissue over the spine, hooks, and pins.

Condition Score 3: Medium (Normal body condition): The animal appears smooth over the spine, ribs, and pelvis and the skeletal structure can be easily palpated. The hooks and pins are still discernible, with a moderate, rather deep depression between the pelvis and rib cage, hooks and pins, and around the tail-head.

Condition Score 4: Fat: There are no spinous processes detectable, and no depression in the loin area, which gives the top-line of the animal a flat, tabletop appearance. The ribs can no longer be felt, and the pelvis can only be felt with firm pressure. The hooks and pins have a rounded appearance due to areas of fat covering.

Condition Score 5: Very Fat: The animal appears rounded and smooth with a square-shaped appearance, because of the amount of fat filling in the loin. The skeletal structure is no longer visible, and can only be palpated with excessive pressure

Normal demeanor: When, on being approached, an animal makes a normal response to external stimuli, such as movement and sound, the demeanor is said normal (bright). Normal reaction under these circumstances may consist of elevating the head and ears, turning towards and directing the attention at the source of stimuli, walking away and evincing signs of attack or flight.

Abnormal demeanor: Behavioral change/ response to external stimuli.

- Decreased response (depression): dull (apathetic); dummy state; comma.
- Excitation or increased response: apprehension (mildly anxious); restlessness; mania; frenzy.
- Posture: It denotes the anatomical configuration when they remain in stationary situation. How does it stand? How does it sit? How does it lie?
- Gait: It indicates about the locomotory process of an animal.
- Body conformation: shape and size of the different body regions relative to other regions

Regional or systematic clinical examination

Clinical Examinations of the head and neck region:

Objective: To identify pale and discolored mucus membranes; assess problems of oral cavity and deranged appetite. The following points are to be considered:

- Visible mucous membrane
- Eyelids, conjunctivae and eyes
- Nasal regions and nasal mucous membrane
- Prehension, mastication and deglutition
- Salivation
- Teeth eruption

Materials: Live animals, crash and glove

Procedure:

- Visible mucous membrane examined by visual inspection to note the presence of lesions, discharge, glaucoma, nystagmus.
- Examine the nose and nasal sinuses; lesions, discharges should be noted by percussion, palpation
- Examine the mouth and appetite; oral lesions, salivation, feed intake should be noted

Examination of skin and appendages: Structures or parts associated with skin as its appendages are hoofs, hairs, horns, quills, claws, nails, sebaceous glands and sweat glands.

Objective: Assessing the condition of skin and coat to identify clinical signs of skin lesions such as:

- Condition of the coat
- Elasticity of the coat
- Pruritus
- Primary and secondary skin lesions
- Dermatitis
- Hyperkeratosis or parakeratosis
- Presence of ectoparasites

Materials: Live animals, crash, glove

Procedure

Examine the skin and coat: grasp the skin of the upper part of the body and notice the elasticity, visual inspection of the condition of the coat and presence of skin lesions should be noted.

Examinations of the thoracic cavity:

Objective: to show the regional anatomy of the lungs and the heart, and perform physical examination of the lung and the heart area

Materials:

- Live animals
- Pleximetre and percussion hammer
- Stethoscope

Procedure:

Regional anatomy of the lungs -locate the lung area

The lung is located on the external surface of the thoracic region by forming an imaginary triangle by using the points at the angle of the scapula, olicranun process and the second intercostals space from the last.

Physical examination of the thorax (lung area)

- Inspection -note respiratory movements
- Palpation -check the presence of pain by applying pressure
- Percussion -notice resonant sound
- Auscultation -note bronchial sounds (trachea and anterior part of the lungs) and alveolar sounds (Figure 1)

Regional anatomy of the heart -locate the heart area

The heart is suspended by great vessels and located on the left median mediastinum of ventral thorax. The left side of the heart apex reaches the chest wall.

- In horse, heart is located between 2nd to 6th intercostals space
- In cattle, 3rd to 6th
- In camel, 3rd to 7th.

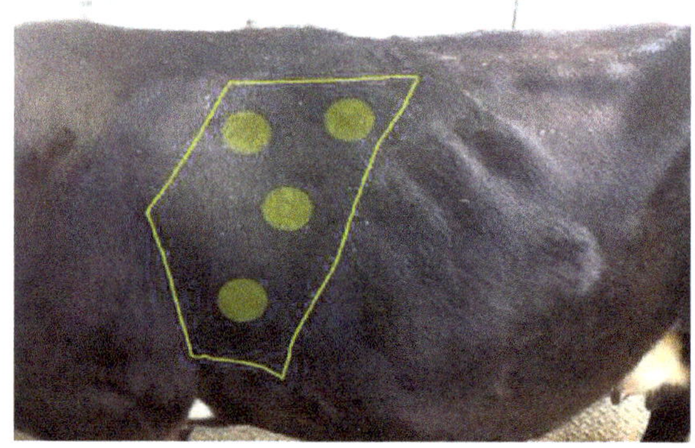

Figure 1: Anatomical location of lung in cow.

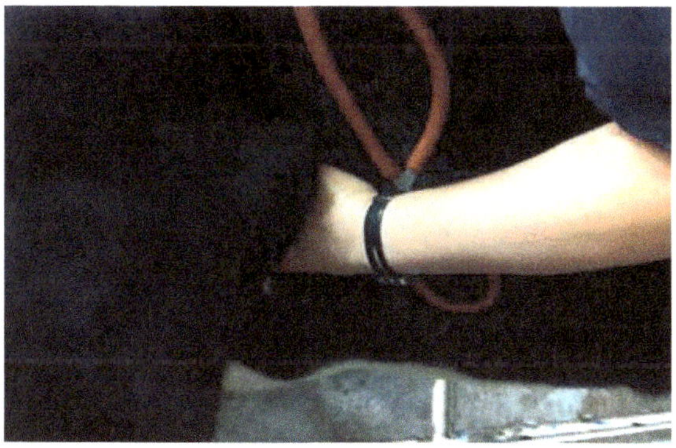

Figure 2: Auscultation to assess heart sound in cow.

After locating the heart the following should be noted through physical examination (palpation, percussion, auscultation)

- Heart rate
- Abnormal variation in heart rate
- Heart sounds
- Normal heart sounds (dub-lab)
- Adventitious heart sounds (murmurs)
- Pericardial frictional sounds
- Venous pulsation (jugular pulsation) (Figure 2)

Clinical examinations of the abdominal and associated digestive organs

Objective: to undertake clinical examination of the abdomen and identify disturbances of the digestive system.

Materials:

- Live animals
- Stomach tube
- Gloves
- Lubricant
- Trocar and cannula

Procedure: Applied anatomy of the abdominal region of animal

General clinical examination of the abdominal region

Clinical examination of the stomach and intestines

- **The examination of rumen** is performed by inspection, palpation, percussion and auscultation, stomach tube can be used as well. In bloat case, the left side would be bulged, and the motility would be decreased.
- **The examination of reticulum:** TRP by back grasp, below pole lifting, up and down hill leading, hand palpation
- **The examination of omasum:** done by exploratory puncture.

The examination of the displacement of abomasums is done by inspection, palpation, and auscultation.

The disorder of stomach can be detected by taking stomach contents sample: Insert the stomach tube or nasal tube after cleaning, disinfecting and lubrication or trocarisation (Figures 3 and 4)

- **Rectal examination of the internal abdominal structures:** cut and smooth the nail; wear shoulder long glove; lubricate; cone shape of the fingers; insert in rotating way; notice: the hand cannot open, or even grasp organs inside. It's necessary or possible to use tranquilizer to reduce the sensitivity of the rectum in horse. In bloat case, the pressure in the abdomen would be very high, so it would be difficult to insert the hand inside (Figure 5).

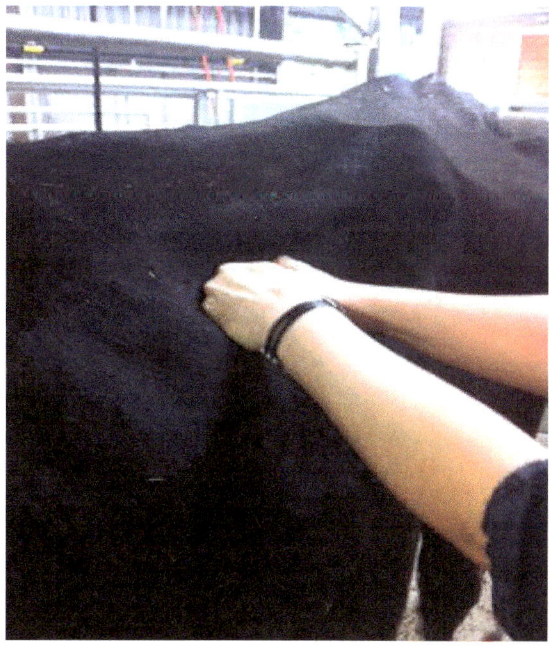

Figure 3: Feeling rumen contraction by palpation.

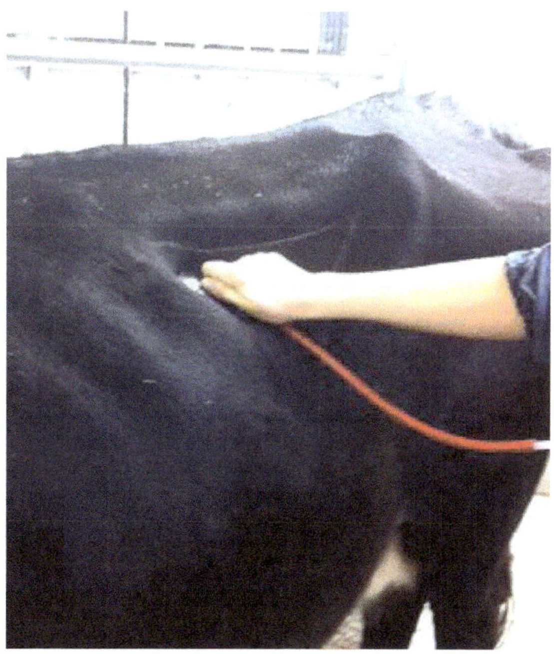

Figure 4: Auscultation of rumen contraction.

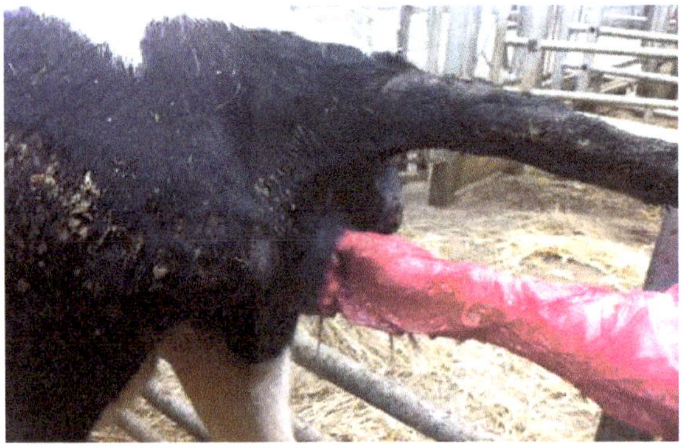

Figure 5: Rectal examination of cow.

- **Clinical Examinations of the Feces**

Objective: To see Character of the feces and abnormal constituents in feces

Procedure

- Observe the surface of the faeces, where mucus and blood always exists
- The colour of the faeces surface, the odour of the feces
- Fishy smell generally indicates bleeding, and abnormal constituents in feces

Examination of the urogenital system:

Objective: To identify the regional anatomy, undertake clinical and physical examination of urinary system and assess urinary abnormalities, perform clinical examination of female and male reproductive organs as well as the mammary glands and teats.

Materials:

- Live animals, milk
- Catheter
- Speculum and artificial light
- 0.1% potassium permanganate
- lubricant

Procedure:

Identify the anatomic structure of the kidney on live animal: the left kidney is located ventral of the transverse process of the 3rd to 5th lumbar vertebrae. The kidney can be examined by inspection, external palpation, rectal palpation, and urianalysis.

- The examination of the urinary bladder is performed by stimulating the sense of urination from the lower part between the two hind legs on small animals or rectal palpation on large animals. Attention should be paid to the paralysis of the bladder and retention of urine and rupture.
- Clinical examination of male genital organs- visual inspection and palpation are employed to examine the testes, prepuce and the penis after withdrawing from the prepuce.
- Here orchitis, cryptorchidism, scrotum hernia, obstruction of urethra by calculi, phimosis, paraphimosis, inflammation of the prepuce, testes and penis are noted.
- Clinical examination of female genital organs- visual inspection and palpation of the vaginal region, use of vaginal speculum to examine the inside of vagina and intrarectal examination of the cervix, uterus and ovaries would be performed
- Take the sample of urine examine through physical methods
- Fresh urine is collected with test tube after stimulating urination by palpating the perennial region or by inserting catheter
- Note how to insert catheter.
- Clinical examination of the mammary glands and teat- inspection and palpation to detect the presence of swelling and lesions on the teats/decrease in size and shape, any discharge, temperature of the udder, consistency, and pain reactions are performed
- Clinical examination of milk samples: after collecting the milk samples in clean test tubes one can apply different physical and laboratory examinations
- For the gross examination of the milk, the change of the color, odor, viscosity and flakes in the milk should be identified.

Examinations of the nervous and musculoskeletal system:

Objective: For examination and detection of clinical signs of various problems associated with the nervous and musculoskeletal systems

Materials: Live animals, Audiovisuals and pictures

Procedure:

The examination of the nervous system:

1. Observe the behavior of the animal

2. Note responses of the animal while applying different stimuli

- Examine the brain by corneal reflex, the pupil reflex
- Examine the spinal cord of the neck and thorax by withers reflex
- Examine the spinal cord of the back part by applying hoof stimuli and anus stimuli
- Move the animal to and from or uncomfortable position to examine the locomotors

3. Examine the joints long bones and different muscles: arthritis, dislocation of the joints, rickets or osteomalacia, muscular atrophy, central or peripheral origin paralysis

Examination of superficial lymphnodes of animals

Objectives: to compared each paired node for size and consistency with the contralateral node.

Method:

Grossly enlarged lymph nodes may have been seen during observation of the patient before it is handled. Observation and palpation is possible when the animal is restrained.

Anatomical Location of lymphnodes (LN):

- **Submandibular lymph nodes:** situated and are palpable on the medial aspect of the 'angle of the jaw' where the horizontal and vertical rami of the mandible meet. (Normal size is 1.5 to 2 cm)
- **Prescapular lymph nodes:** It lies subcutaneously and underneath the cutaneous muscle just anterior to the shoulder joint (Normal size 1 cm × 3.5 cm)

- **Axillary lymph nodes:** Found on each side of the chest in the armpit area. Normally only palpable in young calves without heavy muscling (Normal size 1.5 cm)
- **Popliteal lymph nodes:** These nodes are found surrounded by dense muscle tissue immediately behind the stifle. It found on each rear leg on the opposite side of the knee. They are relatively superficial and easy to feel (normal size 1-1.5 cm)
- **Inguinal lymph nodes:** These are usually palpable as a small group of fairly mobile and firm structures adjacent to the inguinal canal.(normal size 0.5 cm)
- **Supramammary lymph nodes:** These are normally readily palpated on the caudal aspect of the udder just above the upper limit of the mammary glandular tissue. (normal size 2.5 cm) (Figure 6)

Preparation and Administration of Medicaments

Drug dosage form

Oral dosage forms: Refers to administration of drug through the mouth. The most commonly used preparations are solid oral dosage forms such as tablets, capsules, granules, powder, paste and boluses etc.

Parentral dosage forms: the most common parentral dosage forms are stable aqueous solutions and subcutaneous implants.

External dosage forms:

- Ointment- semisolid preparation for external application.
- Cream- a viscous semisolid, consisting of oil in water emulsion or water in oil emulsion.
- Dusting powder e.g., popular antibacterial agent applied on animal wounds.
- Lotion- an aqueous solution or suspension for local application.
- Spray-a drug applied in liquid form by pressure.

Inhalation dosage forms: gaseous and volatile liquid anaesthetic agent (drugs), given by inhalation, e.g., Halothane

Routes of drug administration

Oral administration: There are large numbers of pharmaceutical preparations available for oral administration. Solid dosage forms (powders, tablet, capsules, pills, etc.) and liquid dosage forms (syrups, emulsion, mixture, drench, electrolytes, etc.)

Parenteral administration (IV, IM, SC, Id, epidural, subconjunctival): It refers to a drug administration by injection directly in to the tissue fluid or blood without having to cross the intestinal mucosa.

Intravenous route (IV): Gives swift, effective and highly predictable blood concentration and allows rapid modification of dose and is used for emergency treatment. In most animals (horse, cattle, sheep and goat) usually given through **jugular vein**, in pig-**ear veins**, in the dog and cat-**cephalic vein** and recurrent **tarsal vein**.

Intramuscular (IM) route: Absorption occurs either haematogenous or via lymphatic and is usually fairly rapid except for long acting preparation.

Subcutaneous (SC) route: Preferred when slow and continuous absorption of drug is required. The injected drug disperses through the loose connective tissues. They dissolve in tissue fluid before it can enter either capillaries or lymphatic.

Intradernal route (ID): Used for testing hypersensitivity test and for vaccination.

Epidural route: Refers to deposition of drug up on or outside the dura matter.

E.g., Introduction of local anaesthetics between the first and second coccygeal vertebra to eliminate straining.

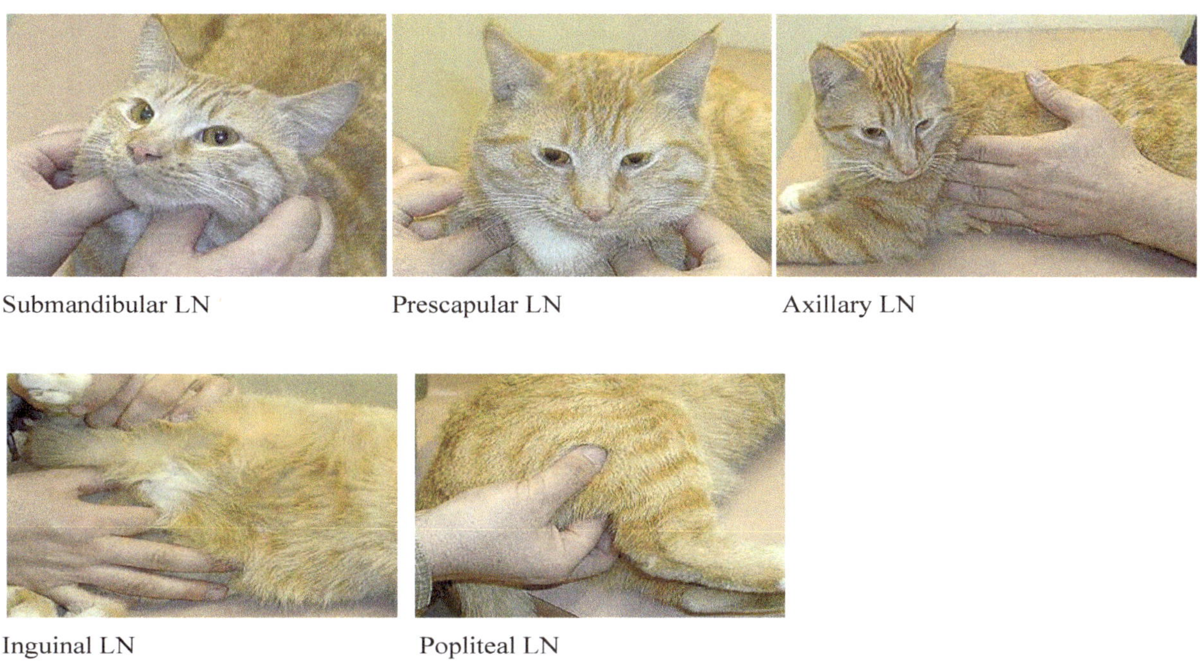

Figure 6: Anatomical location of superficial lymph node.

Subconjunctival: Disposition of a pharmaceutical preparation beneath the conjunctiva.

Topical or local application: It refers to external application of drug to the body surface for localized action at accessible site, such as skin, eyes, body orifices, body cavity.

Drug dose calculation

Dose is the quantity of the drug to be administered at one time and expressed in mg/kg or IU/kg.

$$Dose: \frac{Body\ weight \times Dose\ Rate}{Concentration}$$

E.g., A 5 kg cat needs an antibiotic at a dose of 15 mg/kg. The antibiotic comes in liquid form at concentration of 25 mg/ml how many ml do you give?

Solution:

$$Dose: \frac{5kg \times 15mg/kg}{25mg/ml} = 3ml$$

Veterinary Laboratory Sampling Techniques

Sample submission requirements

Ensure all information is completed and contains all relevant case details.

Labeling of specimens:

- Type specimen (e.g., Serum, whole blood, liver, brain, urine, etc.), whether preservative is used or not and type of preservative used.
- An identification of animals (e.g., tag, name, colors of hair coat, etc.) if specimens were collected from more than one animal.
- The names of the owner, if specimens from different cases are packed together in the same parcel.
- Date of collection.

Handling and transport of specimens

- The parcels should be securely packed in order to withstand rough handling and protect shipper and the environment
- Great care should be taken to ensure that the containers with specimens do not leak! (a sticky tape may be used)
- Use cotton wool, newspaper or other absorbent materials to soak up any leakage that, despite all the precautions, might occur.
- Small cooler (Styrofoam) boxes are preferred for shipping refrigerated specimens.

Collection of specimen

Whole blood:

- Aseptically bleed directly in to vacutainers containing EDTA or heparin preservatives
- Mix gently by rolling the tube
- Do not freeze but keep cool on ice

Serum:

- Use red topped vacutainer tubes for serology and mineral analysis
- After collecting the blood sample, the tube is left untouched at room temperature till clotting is complete
- The clot is then carefully removed and then Centrifuge or allow any remaining cells to settle
- Gently pour the clear serum into a fresh or sterile tubes or cryo-vials
- Care must be taken to keep the serum completely free from blood cells
- Keep refrigerated (or -20°C) if the serum stay longer at your laboratory/clinic before shipment

Blood smears:

- Remember to shake the blood gently while collecting blood to prevent clotting.
- Use clean, dry smears
- Take a small drop blood and place on right end of one slide about 1 cm from edge
- Place another glass slide (spreader) to the left of drop at 30° angle gently touching the drop
- Wait until blood has spread all way across the glass (spreader) slide
- Move spreader slide to the left quickly but smoothly
- Dry by waving in the air

Note:

- Use dry, non-greasy glass slides.
- Must be dried before wrapping in clean tissue paper.
- Protect from rain, flies, dust and abrasion.
- Submit at least 6 slides for a single case.
- Label smears clearly with pencil
- Pack individually.

Faeces:

- Should be fresh and free of soil and vegetation
- Collect direct from rectum
- Lubricate your finger after wearing glove and rotate for easy entrance without damage the mucous membrane
- Keep cool or use other preservation to prevent hatching and no need of preservation if needed for larva recovery

Skin scrapings:

- Should be sent dry and unpreserved in a plastic bottle.
- Scrape deep at the periphery of the lesion until blood oozes.
- If Ringworm is suspected, pull hair from edge of lesion with forceps and add to sample.

Skin biopsy:

- Cut about 1 cm square and deep enough to reach subcutaneous tissue.

- Preserve in 10% buffered formalin for histopathology
- Use ice for skin biopsies to be screened for viruses e.g., LSD and Orf.

Urine:

- Should be collected in clean and sterile bottles for bacteriological and hormone residues examination.
- 20 ml urine+1.5 ml 10% formal saline for leptospirosis
- 2.5% Boric acid can be used as a preservative if to be used for bacteriology
- Use faecal analysis bottles.

Pus:

- Swab aseptically and deep from the edge of the abscess.
- Put swab in commercial semi solid transport medium.
- Collect into a sterile syringe or test tube and keep refrigerated.

Fluids:

- This refers to fluids from joint, peritoneal, pleural, pericardial, cerebrospinal fluid, etc.
- Collect asceptically using a sterile needle and syringe/ vacatainers.
- Should be preserved on ice.

Milk:

- Ensure no antibiotic treatment was given prior to sampling
- Wash the teats with water
- Wash your hands and disinfect with 70% alcohol
- Dry off teats and disinfect with 70% alcohol
- Expel the foremilk then milk into a sterile bottle held almost horizontally to avoid dirt particles falling inside
- Submit within a short time while fresh
- Keep cool on ice.

References

1. Ballard B, Rockett J (2009) Restraint and Handling for Veterinary Technician and Assistants. Delmar, Cengage Learning, USA.
2. Frandson RD, Wilke WL, Fails AD (2009) Anatomy and Physiology of Farm Animals. 7th edn. Wiley-Blackwell, USA.
3. Jackson P, Cockcroft P (2002) Clinical Examination of Farm Animals. Blackwell Science, UK.
4. Kahn CM (2010) Merck Veterinary Manual. 10th edn. Whitehouse Station, Merck, NJ, USA.
5. Kelly WR (1974) Veterinary Clinical Diagnosis. 2nd edn. Bailliere Tindal & Casell, London, UK.
6. Radostits OM, Gay CC, Hinchcliff KW, Constable PD (2007) Veterinary Medicine: A textbook of the diseases of cattle, sheep, pigs and goats, horses. 10th edn. St. Louis: Saunders (Elsevier).
7. Riviere JE, Papich MG (2001) Veterinary Pharmacology & Therapeutics. 9th edn. Wiley-Blackwell, USA.
8. Chauhan RS, Agarwal DK (2008) Textbook of Veterinary, Clinical and Laboratory Diagnosis. 2nd edn. Jaypee Publishers, New Delhi, India.

The Restraint of Bovine Sperm Cell Motility Increases Survival: Role of Extracellular Calcium in the Phenomena

Ian Scott[1], Alfredo Ramirez-Reveco[3] and Jorge Parodi[1,2*]

[1]Laboratorio de Biología Celular Aplicada, Escuela de Medicina Veterinaria, Núcleo de Investigación en Producción Alimentaria, Facultad de Recursos Naturales, Universidad Católica de Temuco, Chile

[2]Laboratory Research and Education Tonalli Ltd., Chile

[3]Cryobiology and Spermatozoa Functionality Analysis Laboratory, Institute of Animal Sciences, Faculty of Veterinary Sciences, Universidad Austral de Chile, Valdivia, Chile

Abstract

Sperm cells are complex models for handling *in vitro*, their viability is limited, and their physiology is complex. The study of their properties is of great application in the animal production industry, to improve the selection of gametes, control pathologies and for the development of cryobiology protocols. It is therefore important to have viable and functional gametes. Consequently, it has been demonstrated that the increase of sperm cell mortality is related to the increase of the Reactive Oxygen Species (ROS), and ROS is secondary to normal metabolic processes of the cell, i.e., special motility. One of the processes where the mature sperm cells' main activity is the consumption of more energy, it is the flagellar movement through which high ATP consumption generates high quantities of ROS in the seminal plasma. There is evidence of strategies that lead to reduced metabolic activity for different variables (temperature, pH and other), the intention being that seminal plasma protects the sperm cells and reduces the mortality, and thus it is correct to suggest reducing mortality by reducing motility. It has to be considered that flagellar movement is a complex action that involves energy consumption, regulated by calcium. The phenomenon has not been fully characterized, but it is established that in certain mammalian models, the entry of calcium in specific channels such as CATsper or voltage-dependent channels is a signal for flagellar movement to occur. Reduce the motility of bovine spermatozoa using calcium channel blockers can increase cell survival and we hypothesized that: the general blockade of the calcium channel generated reduced the calcium entry into bovine sperm cells, restricting motility and increased survival of these cells. We propose to in the future explore whether the modulation of calcium channels in bovine sperm cells can reduce motility and increase the survival of these cells in experimental conditions, to reduce the mortality of the sample and improve laboratory manipulation.

Keywords: Sperm cells; Gametes; Seminal plasma

General Overview

"Mature sperm cells are complex cellular machines that control a series of steps and environments to reach their target, which is the oocyte, and fulfill the purpose of delivering their genetic material via fertilization. For this study, we highlight kinetic parameters of motility and the complex capacitation process, whose final step is characterized by acrosome reaction. Regarding the process of capacitation, in recent years the function of CatSper channels as regulatory elements has been demonstrated to be indirectly involved in modulating sperm motility and fertilization capacity, as well as calcium entry. Additionally, a recent study demonstrated that the CatSper channel is involved in the motility process but not so in the Acrosome Reaction (AR) [1]. Flagellar movement generates various changes such as ROS production, and these ROS increases may be able to explain the reduction of cell viability. Moreover, some sperm cell models can remain immobile for a period of time, as in the case of fish sperm cells. The activation process occurs and the cells become motile only when external signaling takes place (i.e., osmotic changes). These fish sperm cells show a long period without mortality and maintain cellular functions for days. Calcium regulation is important for the general cellular function. In mammalian sperm cells, a recent study described that there are two steps regulated by calcium entry: motility and AR. Motility generates metabolic changes and therefore our hypothesis is that regulation by calcium reduces motility and the cells' general metabolic state, leading to an increase in cell survival. Hypothesize that regulation the calcium flux, reduces the motility and the general metabolic state of the cells, leading to increased cell survival. Regulatory mechanisms, for calcium flux, are important for the conservation and manipulation of sperm cells. Because food production, especially that of animal protein, has increased in recent decades, reproductive processes must be controlled more efficiently. It is vital for the development of the food industry to study these processes, yet little is known about the cells involved and the conditions that must occur. Thus, we should study other species as a reference for the development and maintenance of sperm handling", taken from the Parodi 2014 review [2].

Sperm Cell Motility

Flagellar motion and motility generation for sperm cells is a highly demanding energetic process in which extracellular calcium has been shown to play a role at the onset of hyperactivation. Once the sperm enter the oviduct, they go through a process of called "hyperactivation" [3], characterized by high amplitude, asymmetrical beating pattern of the sperm tail (flagellum). These movements are associated with an increase in speed, a decrease in linearity and an increase in the amplitude of lateral head movement and whipping of the flagellum, all of which differ from what is observed in isolated ejaculated sperm [4,5].

***Corresponding author:** Jorge Parodi, Laboratorio de Biología Celular Aplicada Escuela de Medicina Veterinaria, Núcleo de Investigación en Producción Alimentaria, Facultad de Recursos Naturales, Universidad Católica de Temuco, Av. Las Mariposas S/N, Campus Dr. Rivas, Temuco, Chile, E-mail: jparodi@uct.cl

Various physiological stimuli such as calcium, cAMP, bicarbonate and metabolic substrates have been used for the initiation or maintenance of motility hyperactivation *in vitro*. In hamster sperm, calcium can be added to the medium to maintain hyperactivation and keep the sperm cells swimming [6]. Understanding of the various waves affecting motility is important for the comprehension of other phenomena, as in gamete selection, pathology control, the development of cryobiological protocols and overall viability of the sperm cells [2]. How this process is triggered has not been completely characterized, but some models have established the role of specific channels such as the CatSper, for example [7], or voltage-dependent calcium channels for maintaining motility [8]. The manipulation of calcium channel and its impact on the handling and conservation of sperm cells and has not been fully assessed. Calcium wave modeling and analysis has been performed on some sperm cells and suggests that depolarizing changes of the membrane may also induce calcium entry, which could be interpreted as a different signal from hyperactivation, mediated by CATsper. The complex model of sperm cell motility shows dependency on calcium and generates several compounds for live sperm cells' motility [9]. After ejaculation, once the sperm mixes with seminal plasma which exhibits a pH<7.0, there is an alkalizing effect on sperm cytoplasm [10], inducing sperm motility. Another important factor in sperm motility activation is an increase in cAMP levels, which is reported to activate protein kinase A (PKA) and cause phosphorylation on axonemal proteins Nevertheless, even though sperm may be motile, the fertilization capacity can be minimal and is reversed when the sperm undergo capacitation [11,12]. Once human spermatozoa have penetrated the cervical barrier and entered the uterine cavity, upon finding the oviductal epithelium they initiate the process of sperm capacitation, and calcium is key for triggering these phenomena [2]. In biological terms, capacitation can be seen as a priming process by which spermatozoa attain a level of heightened responsiveness to signals emanating from the cumulus-oocyte complex. One of the changes that signals the attainment of a capacitated state is the expression of hyperactivated motility [13]. This particular form of movement is characterized by the development of high-velocity, large-amplitude asymmetrical flagellar waves, and is thought to facilitate detachment of spermatozoa from the oviductal epithelium and penetration of the *Zona pellucida* (ZP), and is part of the complex function of capacitation [14].

Sperm Cell Mortality and Function

Handling procedures result in alterations in sperm that can cause premature sperm capacitation [15]. This process leads to the acrosome reaction and decreases the sperm's useful life. Loss of fertilization capacity results from the presence of large amounts of Reactive Oxygen Species (ROS) following ejaculation. Kirchhoff [16] and Alvarez [17] indicated that sperm produce and export ROS generated mainly by the mitochondria to the extracellular environment, secondary to the flagellar activity of the cells. The loss of sperm function, i.e., the fertilization capacity, results from the presence of high levels of ROS, either following ejaculation or secondary to high levels of motility. Kirchhoff [16] and Alvarez [17] have indicated that sperm produce and export ROS to the extracellular environment, in their majority generated by mitochondria and the product of the monovalent reduction of molecular oxygen during oxidative phosphorylation [16,17]. Mammalian sperm cells are described as having a one-hour period of viability and function with high motility and metabolism. In porcine sperm, when the temperature is reduced, conservation increases sample preservation time [18]. Further, in fowl, temperature regulates calcium influx [19], a process mediated by the channel TRPM8. These lines of evidence suggest the importance of temperature control during *in vitro* manipulation of sperm cells, which is correlated with changes during travel through the oviduct. Temperature is a key factor in sperm cell function and can be controlled *in vitro*. Thus, natural changes can be observed in the oviduct when the sperm cells are swimming toward the oocyte. In example the temperature are important for maintaining motility and increases the mortality in porcine sample [20] and changes in pH are important for generation of calcium signaling, in porcine sample for example [21]. Several process occurred to the spermatozoa, for example, survival regulation occurs in the epididymis and cell maturation [22]. In stallion semen, conservation of the mitochondrial function by exogenous molecules (antioxidants), is used to preserve viability [23] and can change same protein state phosphorylation for intracellular signaling, for example in porcine sperm [24]. Other models present evidence that the phosphorylation state can change calcium flux and induce capacitation, particularly in humans; and the function of PKA activity induces increased calcium entry [25]. For these reasons, recent reports have described how the extracellular solution and seminal plasm can regulate and prolong the function of the spermatozoa models [26]. The reduction of ROS to increase antioxidant molecules has a positive effect on the samples [27] and different solutions, with antioxidant may be employed to observe spermatozoa function *in vitro* conservation [28].

Sperm Capacitation

Fertilization is a unique and amazing process involving fusion of two morphologically distinct cells, the sperm and the oocyte. This process begins when the sperm begins to penetrate the oocyte envelope and plasma membrane, and ends with the exchange of maternal and paternal chromosomes, representing the formation of the zygote. The sperm must undergo functional changes since its genesis and subsequent maturation takes place during the epididymal transit. During capacitation, the sperm cell undergoes a series of biochemical and biophysical changes at the level of the cell membrane, cytoplasm and nucleus, which results in changes in motility patterns. The seminal plasma provides many molecules for spermatozoa survival and induces activation when the spermatozoa reach the oocyte and perform the acrosome reaction prior to the fertilization process [29]. Thus, displacement of capacitation-inducing factors in the sperm membrane, such as antioxidants, metal ions and peptides, increases the removal of cholesterol from the membrane and raises calcium levels through the activation of Ca channels and CatSper, leading to an increase in cAMP levels and phosphorylation of tyrosine residues [30,31]. The entire capacitation process, including hyperactivation, must be regulated by the entry of calcium to the cells, is described as one single step but our group suggested in a review, more complex process and includes entry of the calcium, increase of motility and Acrosome Reaction (AR) for a calcium wave [21], that the calcium wave concept was incorporated (Figure 1) and it was suggested that with a one calcium entry and motility increase and a second wave for AR, the process can be manipulated and the cells kept healthy [32,33]. The AR allows sperm to penetrate the physical barriers posed by the oocyte and, thus enabling delivery of genomic content. The capacitation process leads to the acrosome reaction and causes a decrease in the spermatozoa lifespan. A premature state of capacitation can be induced through sperm dilutions, which are a component of various treatments, and potentially lead to the removal of adsorbed proteins and other compounds present in the seminal plasma that are necessary to maintain sperm viability. Studies have shown that the addition of adequate amounts of seminal plasma in equine models can protect sperm by providing membrane stability when sperm are subjected to cryopreservation processes [34], high dilutions [35,36] or separation via flow cytometry [37].

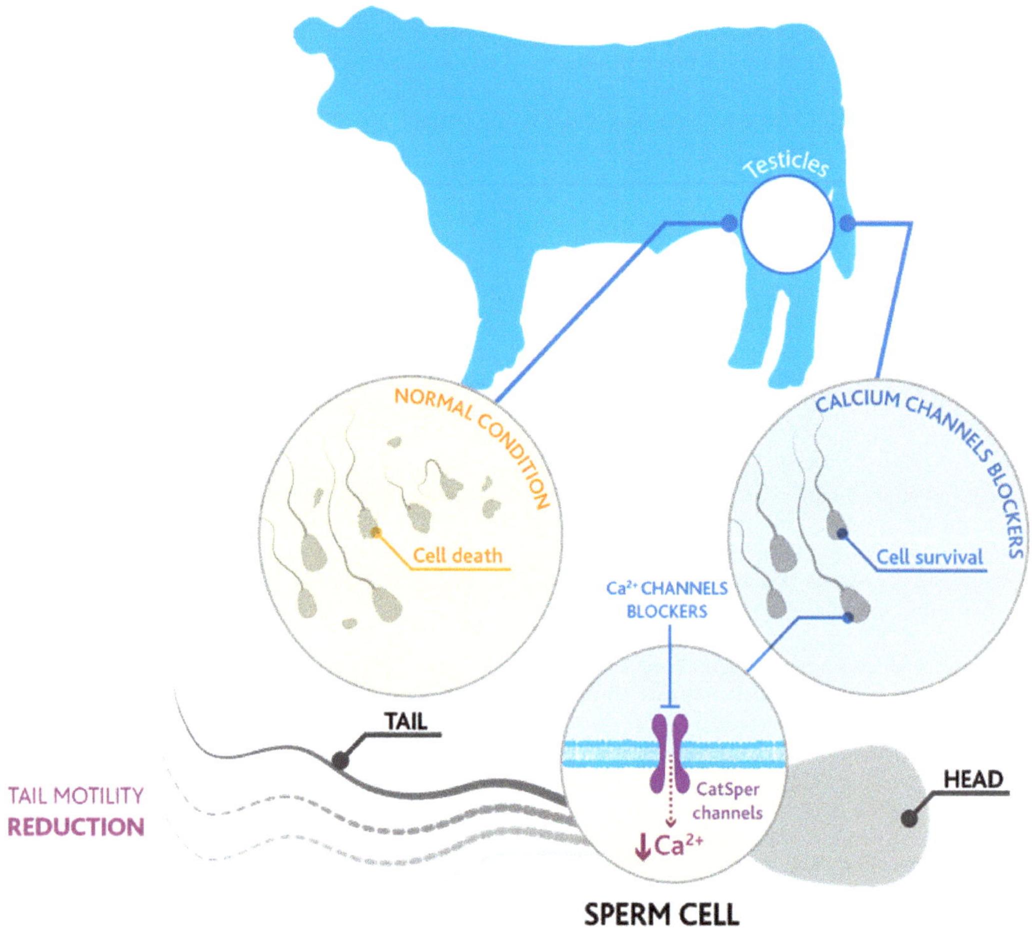

Figure 1: Motility reduction. The model summary the idea of the reduction of the motility by calcium channel blockers can reduce the mortality of the sperm cells under laboratory condition.

Calcium and Spermatozoa Function

We described previously that mammalian sperm acquire fertilizing ability through a process called capacitation. At the molecular level capacitation is a complex process involving the cAMP-dependent pathway, intracellular pH, calcium, and an increase in tyrosine phosphorylation. How these signaling systems interact during capacitation is not well understood [38]. A recent paper presented the biphasic effects of calcium in the spermatozoa function, in particular in the regulation of cAMP-dependent signaling. Using nominal zero calcium, spermatozoa incubated in this medium did not undergo PKA activation or the increase in tyrosine phosphorylation calcium. However, chelation with EGTA (ethyleneglycol acid-bis-(β-aminoethyl ether) N', N', N', N' tetra acetic acid) induced both cAMP-dependent phosphorylation and increased tyrosine phosphorylation and this suggests that calcium ions regulate sperm cAMP and tyrosine phosphorylation pathways in a biphasic manner [38] Some factors can induce a calcium wave and induce a separate calcium deposit, for example in boar semen [39] and hyperpolarization or when used bicarbonate activation signaling [40]. However, depolarization can induce calcium change and activation of the spermatozoa [41], which suggests that the regulation of calcium is important for the normal function of spermatozoa in general. The precedents of calcium are complex and depend on which stimuli are used, but are important described the exactly mechanism of regulation of this ion for understand the beginning of activation of spermatozoa. Regulation of the calcium and motility of the spermatozoa is a complex model that is not completely described and in example recent study on boar semen show differences in storage for regulated AR, supporting the idea that calcium and its effects effect depend on the storage used [42].

Plasma Membrane and Ion Channels

The plasma membrane is a lipoprotein interface that acts as a permeability barrier, allowing the cell to maintain a different composition in the intracellular medium from that of the extracellular medium. The most abundant components of the plasma membrane are phospholipids and proteins, which together form the fluid mosaic pattern [43]. Resting potential is a particular state of the membrane potential in which the sum of ion currents through the membrane is zero, due to the presence of transmembrane electrochemical gradients resulting from selective permeability to ions and secondary various structures, such as transmembrane channels, pumps and ion exchangers. From the resting potential, the excitation of cells can generate an action potential that allows the cell to respond to different stimuli. During this process, each ion tends to draw the membrane potential toward its own electrochemical equilibrium potential, by the Nernst Equation [44]. Ionic currents through channels not only determine transmembrane bioelectric phenomena related to the membrane potential but also modulate enzyme activity, metabolism and cellular genetics. Specifically, in sperm cells, the transmembrane ionic currents and their potential, among other factors, regulate the intracellular concentration of calcium and the genesis of second messengers. These factors are essential for fertilization-associated processes, such as sperm motility, capacitation and the Acrosome Reaction (AR) as present in the Parodi review [21].

The study of ion channels is therefore extremely valuable for understanding the electrophysiological processes and biological responses of both excitable cells and isolated cells. In particular, determining the roles of these channels in the mammalian sperm membrane is essential for understanding the processes involved in fertilization. The main tool for investigating the characteristics and distribution of ion channels in the plasma membrane is the patch-clamp technique [45,46], a high-resolution method currently used to determine the electrophysiological and pharmacological properties of the cell structure.

Kv Currents Identified in Sperm

A previous study revealed the presence of different types of potassium channels with varying localizations in relation to sperm morphology [47,48]. An example is the delayed rectifier K^+ type channel found in rat spermatogenic cells, which shows a trend that is independent of extracellular calcium and sensitive to blockade by tetraethylammonium chloride, TEA [47]. Based on these characteristics, we identified an inward rectifier K^+ channel referred to as Kir [48,49]. This channel is also regulated by the intracellular pH, with an acidic intracellular pH (6.3) inhibiting the current in spermatogenic cells, while a rising intracellular pH (7.4) significantly increases conductance in these cells. We further identified a third type of K^+ channel, designated mSlo3, which was cloned in rat spermatogenic cells and has been expressed in *Xenopus laevis* oocytes for biophysical analyses. Recent research using electrophysiological methods enabled detection of an output current from the sperm midpiece that is sensitive to TEA [50], and described the depolarization process regulating calcium entry.

Calcium Voltage Channels (CaV) Regulation during Capacitation

During capacitation, ionic channels are susceptible to being activated when a change occurs in the configuration of these channels and they are mediated by a change in the membrane potential. In untrained rat and bovine sperm, the membrane potential is between -10 and -50 mV [51,52]. Low voltage calcium is inactivated at these voltages and therefore does not respond to depolarizing stimuli. Analysis of the membrane potential of rat spermatozoa showed that only cells that maintain hyperpolarization are able to generate an increased flow of calcium secondary to contact with the ZP (likely secondary CaVs) and carry out the RA [53]. Capacitation, resulting in hyperpolarization, changes the configuration of the CAV in a manner that is open to the agonist-mediated ion flow only at a specific stage, thus avoiding early RA. Studies in sperm conducted using electrophysiological methods have demonstrated the role of calcium channel functional keys in the capacitation process, which are dependent on the membrane potential [52,54]. However, the complete mechanism underlying this phenomenon and its regulation via calcium entry is not completely understood. In this context, it was recently suggested that calcium entry occurs via depolarization and the regulation of motility, with a second entry event occurring due to pH regulation and depolarization, and this second calcium influx is mediated the AR [55]. These findings have led to new models in which not only the type of CatSper channel is responsible for this phenomenon [7], and which have further enabled the electrophysiological investigation of new phenomena such as depolarization, that are also involved in the regulation of these voltage-dependent calcium channels. The general hypotheses are present in Figure 1.

CatSper Channels

Four members of the CatSper (i.e., the English acronym for cationic sperm) channels have been described (CatSper1-4) in murine sperm [56,57]. These channels consist of 6 transmembrane domains (6TM1) that are voltage-dependent and calcium-permeable and appear to be found only in sperm cells. CatSper1 and 2 channels have been reported to be essential for sperm hyperactivation and fertility. However, reports concerning these channels still mainly result from studies of humans and mice [58]. These channels are describe modulate by progesterone and mostly explain the physiological change in the mammalian sperm as described by Darszon in his 2011 review [59]; however in 2014 the models are more complex and new actors are part of the sperm cells' functional regulation [21]. The mutant sperm cells cannot fertilize the eggs with an intact zone pellucid but can fertilize eggs whose outer layers have been enzymatically removed [57], suggesting changes in some cell functions. Male mice lacking CatSper2 are also infertile due to a lack of the hyperactivated motility required for penetration of the egg's extracellular matrix [60]. In a study of humans, sub fertile men with deficient sperm motility showed significantly reduced expression of CatSper1 [61]. Little is known about CatSper3 and CatSper4, but they appear to be involved in supporting sperm cell functions [58]. However, CatSper Channels explain in the entire model the sperm activity? It is accepted that CatSper channels' isoforms are responsible for cellular functions in the sperm, but more events need to coordinate for the process of fecundation — the AR, membrane stability, calcium signaling, mitochondrial function and more. However, these are not described in all models and there are other electrical phenomena can cooperate in the cellular events described in sperm by Darszon in his 2011 review [59], which presents a complete table of ion channels, indicating the presence of calcium channel voltage dependent and CatSper, but only in humans and murines [59]. This indicates a lack of complete localization of these channels, and of other mechanisms that may also alter intracellular calcium levels.

Regulation of Calcium in Spermatozoa

Calcium influx in nonexcitable cells regulates such diverse processes as exocytosis, contraction, enzyme control, gene regulation, cell proliferation, and apoptosis. The dominant Calcium entry pathway in these cells is mediated by the calcium channel and the store-operated one [62], intracellular complex in the spermatozoa, the way of calcium are store in these cells, regulated the function in the activation of the spermatozoa [63]. There is strong evidence that in sperm, though they lack an endoplasmatic reticulum, intracellular calcium stores are present which accumulate calcium through an adenosine-triphosphate (ATP)-dependent calcium pump [64] and the explain for intracellular flux calcium are part explain for acrosome store. Thus, through this mechanism, sperm are able to control acrosomal exocytosis. Since it is known that AR can be induced by the release of calcium from the internal calcium store, it has been suggested that these stores must be localized in the acrosomal region of the sperm head. Because the IP3-receptors are placed in the same region, this organelle seems to act as the calcium store [64] and is mobilized by IP3. The release of

Ca^{2+} from these internal stores elevates intracellular calcium to induce the AR in capacitated as well as in non-capacitated sperm, but only in the presence of extracellular calcium [65]. The mitochondrion is another way to explain the intracellular calcium store in spermatozoa [66]. The calcium is moved in faster manner by plasm membrane ATP-calcium depended pump, sodium/calcium antiport and calcium channel of mitochondrion [67]. Moreover, in general we still find a describe calcium channels in these organelles, mitochondrial calcium uptake is regulated by the Mitochondrial Calcium Uniporter (MCU), at least one non-MCU calcium channel and possibly a mitochondrial ryanodine receptor and two more mechanisms can mediate calcium outward efflux, the sodium dependent channels (mNCX) and the sodium independent calcium efflux [68].

Concluding Remarks

We suggest that complex regulation of calcium in the spermatozoa and extracellular calcium have important effects on the function of spermatozoa capacitation, however the differing storage of intracellular calcium needs to be controlled in order to develop a model that can explain how reduction of the function, particularly motility, by altered calcium movement can increase the survival of bovine spermatozoa. And generate the future question for research, does the general blockade of the calcium channel generate reduced the calcium entry into bovine sperm cells, restrain motility and increase survival of these cells?

Acknowledgements

This study was funded by a grant (MECESUP-UCT 0804) awarded to Jorge Parodi and partial support from Grant 412-455 "Fondo de investigación Interna" and http://www.journalrevisions.com/ for the final edition.

References

1. Sagare-Patil V, Vernekar M, Galvankar M, Modi D (2013) Progesterone utilizes the PI3K-AKT pathway in human spermatozoa to regulate motility and hyperactivation but not acrosome reaction. Mol Cell Endocrinol 374: 82-91.
2. Parodi J (2014) Motility, viability, and calcium in the sperm cells. Syst Biol Reprod Med 60: 65-71.
3. Ho HC, Suarez SS (2001) An inositol 1,4,5-trisphosphate receptor-gated intracellular Ca(2+) store is involved in regulating sperm hyperactivated motility. Biol Reprod 65: 1606-1615.
4. Suarez SS, Pacey AA (2006) Sperm transport in the female reproductive tract. Hum Reprod Update 12: 23-37.
5. Suarez SS (2008) Control of hyperactivation in sperm. Hum Reprod Update 14: 647-657.
6. Yanagimachi R (1994) Fertility of mammalian spermatozoa: its development and relativity. Zygote 2: 371-372.
7. Xia J, Reigada D, Mitchell CH, Ren D (2007) CATSPER channel-mediated Ca2+ entry into mouse sperm triggers a tail-to-head propagation. Biol Reprod 77: 551-559.
8. Benoff S, Chu CC, Marmar JL, Sokol RZ, Goodwin LO, et al. (2007) Voltage-dependent calcium channels in mammalian spermatozoa revisited. Front Biosci 12: 1420-1449.
9. Darszon A, Treviño CL, Wood C, Galindo B, Rodríguez-Miranda E, et al. (2007) Ion channels in sperm motility and capacitation. Soc Reprod Fertil Suppl 65: 229-244.
10. Hamamah S, Gatti JL (1998) Role of the ionic environment and internal pH on sperm activity. Hum Reprod 4: 20-30.
11. Harrison RA, Gadella BM (2005) Bicarbonate-induced membrane processing in sperm capacitation. Theriogenology 63: 342-351.
12. Chang MC (1951) Fertilizing capacity of spermatozoa deposited into the fallopian tubes. Nature 168: 697-698.
13. Aitken RJ (2006) Sperm function tests and fertility. Int J Androl 29: 69-75.
14. Ferramosca A, Zara V (2014) Bioenergetics of mammalian sperm capacitation. Biomed Res Int 2014: 902953.
15. Gómez MC, Catt JW, Gillian L, Evans G, Maxwell WM (1997) Effect of culture, incubation and acrosome reaction of fresh and frozen-thawed ram spermatozoa for *in vitro* fertilization and intracytoplasmic sperm injection. Reprod Fertil Dev 9: 665-673.
16. Kirchhoff C, Osterhoff C, Pera I, Schröter S (1998) Function of human epididymal proteins in sperm maturation. Andrologia 30: 225-232.
17. Alvarez JG, Agarwal A (2006) Development of a novel home sperm test - what are the limitations? Hum Reprod 21: 3029-3030.
18. Althouse GC, Wilson ME, Kuster C, Parsley M (1998) Characterization of lower temperature storage limitations of fresh-extended porcine semen. Theriogenology 50: 535-543.
19. Thomson MF, Wishart GJ (1991) Temperature-mediated regulation of calcium flux and motility in fowl spermatozoa. J Reprod Fertil 93: 385-391.
20. Tatemoto H, Ootaki K, Shigeta K, Muto N (2001) Enhancement of developmental competence after *in vitro* fertilization of porcine oocytes by treatment with ascorbic acid 2-O-alpha-glucoside during *in vitro* maturation. Biol Reprod 65: 1800-1806.
21. Magdalena Cuevas, Fernando Romero, Jorge Parodi (2013) Reactive oxygen species can alter physiological parameters of sperm; the future of macromolecules in boar semen dilutions. Porcine Res 3: 40-48.
22. Dacheux JL, Dacheux F (2013) New insights into epididymal function in relation to sperm maturation. Reproduction 147: R27-42.
23. Davila MP, Bucci D, Mari G, Vega FJP, Galeati G, et al. (2014) Stallion sperm requires intact mitochondrial function to bind heterologous oocytes. Reprod Domest Anim 49: 120-120.
24. Katoh Y, Takebayashi K, Kikuchi A, Iki A, Kikuchi K, et al. (2014) Porcine sperm capacitation involves tyrosine phosphorylation and activation of aldose reductase. Reproduction 148: 389-401.
25. Battistone MA, Alvau A, Salicioni AM, Visconti PE, Da Ros VG, et al. (2014) Evidence for the involvement of proline-rich tyrosine kinase 2 in tyrosine phosphorylation downstream of protein kinase A activation during human sperm capacitation. Mol Hum Reprod 20: 1054-1066.
26. Lee TH, Shih YF, Huang CC, Lee MS (2014) The effect of different synthetic serum supplementation for fertilization media on sperm capacitation in a short incubation perio. Fertility and sterility 102: e316.
27. Bateni Z, Azadi L, Tavalaee M, Kiani-Esfahani A, Fazilati M, et al. (2014) Addition of Tempol in semen cryopreservation medium improves the post-thaw sperm function. Syst Biol Reprod Med 60: 245-250.
28. Andrisani A, Donà G, Ambrosini G, Bonanni G, Bragadin M, et al. (2014) Effect of various commercial buffers on sperm viability and capacitation. Syst Biol Reprod Med 60: 239-244.
29. Anderson SH, Killian GJ (1994) Effect of macromolecules from oviductal conditioned medium on bovine sperm motion and capacitation. Biol Reprod 51: 795-799.
30. Aitken RJ, McLaughlin EA (2007) Molecular mechanisms of sperm capacitation: progesterone-induced secondary calcium oscillations reflect the attainment of a capacitated state. Soc Reprod Fertil Suppl 63: 273-293.
31. Pons-Rejraji H, Artonne C, Sion B, Brugnon F, Canis M, et al. (2011) Prostasomes: inhibitors of capacitation and modulators of cellular signalling in human sperm. Int J Androl 34: 568-580.
32. Rossato M, Di Virgilio F, Rizzuto R, Galeazzi C, Foresta C (2001) Intracellular calcium store depletion and acrosome reaction in human spermatozoa: role of calcium and plasma membrane potential. Mol Hum Reprod 7: 119-128.
33. Breitbart H (2003) Signaling pathways in sperm capacitation and acrosome reaction. Cell Mol Biol (Noisy-le-grand) 49: 321-327.
34. Ollero M, García-López N, Pérez-Pé R, Cebrián-Pérez JA, Muiño-Blanco T (1997) Surface changes of ram spermatozoa by adsorption of homologous and heterologous seminal plasma proteins revealed by partition in an aqueous two-phase system. Reprod Fertil Dev 9: 381-390.
35. Maxwell WM, Johnson LA (1999) Physiology of spermatozoa at high dilution rates: the influence of seminal plasma. Theriogenology 52: 1353-1362.

36. Centurion F, Vazquez JM, Calvete JJ, Roca J, Sanz L, et al. (2003) Influence of porcine spermadhesins on the susceptibility of boar spermatozoa to high dilution. Biol Reprod 69: 640-646.

37. Larsen J, Christensen K, Larsen JK, Jensen PØ, Gustavsson I, et al. (2004) High resolution DNA flow cytometry of boar sperm cells in identification of boars carrying cytogenetic aberrations. Theriogenology 62: 501-511.

38. Navarrete FA, García-Vázquez FA, Alvau A, Escoffier J, Krapf D, et al. (2015) Biphasic role of calcium in mouse sperm capacitation signaling pathways. J Cell Physiol 230: 1758-1769.

39. Rodriguez-Gil JE, Fernandez-Novell JM, Estrada E, Giaretti E, Rigau T, et al. (2014) Dynamics of separate calcium deposits during boar sperm *'in vitro'* capacitation and acrosome exocytosis. Reprod Domest Anim 49: 90-91.

40. Tardif S, Dubé C, Bailey JL (2003) Porcine sperm capacitation and tyrosine kinase activity are dependent on bicarbonate and calcium but protein tyrosine phosphorylation is only associated with calcium. Biol Reprod 68: 207-213.

41. Navarrete P, Martínez-Torres A, Gutiérrez RS, Mejía FR, Parodi J (2010) Venom of the Chilean Latrodectus mactans alters bovine spermatozoa calcium and function by blocking the TEA-sensitive K(+) current. Syst Biol Reprod Med 56: 303-310.

42. Yeste M, Fernández-Novell JM, Ramió-Lluch L, Estrada E, Rocha LG, et al. (2015) Intracellular calcium movements of boar spermatozoa during *'in vitro'* capacitation and subsequent acrosome exocytosis follow a multiple-storage place, extracellular calcium-dependent model. Andrology 3: 729-747.

43. Hasdemir U (2007) The role of cell wall organization and active efflux pump systems in multidrug resistance of bacteria. Mikrobiyol Bul 41: 309-327.

44. Hille B (1992) Ionic channels of excitable membranes. Sinauer Associates Sunderland, USA.

45. Neher E, Sakmann B (1976) Noise analysis of drug induced voltage clamp currents in denervated frog muscle fibres. J Physiol 258: 705-729.

46. Neher E, Sakmann B, Steinbach JH (1978) The extracellular patch clamp: a method for resolving currents through individual open channels in biological membranes. Pflugers Arch 375: 219-228.

47. Hagiwara S, Kawa K (1984) Calcium and potassium currents in spermatogenic cells dissociated from rat seminiferous tubules. J Physiol 356: 135-149.

48. Darszon A, Acevedo JJ, Galindo BE, Hernández-González EO, Nishigaki T, et al. (2006) Sperm channel diversity and functional multiplicity. Reproduction 131: 977-988.

49. Muñoz-Garay C, De la Vega-Beltrán JL, Delgado R, Labarca P, Felix R, et al. (2001) Inwardly rectifying K(+) channels in spermatogenic cells: functional expression and implication in sperm capacitation. Dev Biol 234: 261-274.

50. Marconi M, Sánchez R, Ulrich H, Romero F (2008) Potassium current in mature bovine spermatozoa. Syst Biol Reprod Med 54: 231-239.

51. Clapham DE, Montell C, Schultz G, Julius D, International Union of Pharmacology (2003) International Union of Pharmacology. XLIII. Compendium of voltage-gated ion channels: transient receptor potential channels. Pharmacol Rev 55: 591-596.

52. Darszon A, Nishigaki T, Wood C, Treviño CL, Felix R, et al. (2005) Calcium channels and Ca2+ fluctuations in sperm physiology. Int Rev Cytol 243: 79-172.

53. Arnoult C, Kazam IG, Visconti PE, Kopf GS, Villaz M, et al. (1999) Control of the low voltage-activated calcium channel of mouse sperm by egg ZP3 and by membrane hyperpolarization during capacitation. Proc Natl Acad Sci USA 96: 6757-6762.

54. Wennemuth G, Westenbroek RE, Xu T, Hille B, Babcock DF (2000) CaV2.2 and CaV2.3 (N- and R-type) Ca2+ channels in depolarization-evoked entry of Ca2+ into mouse sperm. J Biol Chem 275: 21210-21217.

55. Escoffier J, Boisseau S, Serres C, Chen CC, Kim D, et al. (2007) Expression, localization and functions in acrosome reaction and sperm motility of Ca(V)3.1 and Ca(V)3.2 channels in sperm cells: an evaluation from Ca(V)3.1 and Ca(V)3.2 deficient mice. J Cell Physiol 212: 753-763.

56. Quill TA, Ren D, Clapham DE, Garbers DL (2001) A voltage-gated ion channel expressed specifically in spermatozoa. Proc Natl Acad Sci U S A 98: 12527-12531.

57. Ren D, Navarro B, Perez G, Jackson AC, Hsu S, et al. (2001) A sperm ion channel required for sperm motility and male fertility. Nature 413: 603-609.

58. Clapham DE, Garbers DL (2005) International Union of Pharmacology. L. Nomenclature and structure-function relationships of CatSper and two-pore channels. Pharmacol Rev 57: 451-454.

59. Darszon A, Nishigaki T, Beltran C, Treviño CL (2011) Calcium channels in the development, maturation, and function of spermatozoa. Physiol Rev 91: 1305-1355.

60. Quill TA, Sugden SA, Rossi KL, Doolittle LK, Hammer RE, et al. (2003) Hyperactivated sperm motility driven by CatSper2 is required for fertilization. Proc Natl Acad Sci U S A 100: 14869-14874.

61. Nikpoor P, Mowla SJ, Movahedin M, Ziaee SA, Tiraihi T (2004) CatSper gene expression in postnatal development of mouse testis and in subfertile men with deficient sperm motility. Hum Reprod 19: 124-128.

62. Parekh AB, Penner R (1995) Activation of store-operated calcium influx at resting InsP3 levels by sensitization of the InsP3 receptor in rat basophilic leukaemia cells. J Physiol 489: 377-382.

63. Witte TS, Schäfer-Somi S (2007) Involvement of cholesterol, calcium and progesterone in the induction of capacitation and acrosome reaction of mammalian spermatozoa. Anim Reprod Sci 102: 181-193.

64. Breitbart H (2002) Intracellular calcium regulation in sperm capacitation and acrosomal reaction. Mol Cell Endocrinol 187: 139-144.

65. Publicover SJ, Barratt CL (1999) Voltage-operated Ca2+ channels and the acrosome reaction: which channels are present and what do they do? Hum Reprod 14: 873-879.

66. Breitbart H, Rubinstein S, Gruberger M (1996) Calcium efflux mechanism in sperm mitochondria. Biochim Biophys Acta 1312: 79-84.

67. Lubart R, Friedmann H, Levinshal T, Lavie R, Breitbart H (1992) Effect of light on calcium transport in bull sperm cells. J Photochem Photobiol B 15: 337-341.

68. Hoppe UC (2010) Mitochondrial calcium channels. FEBS Lett 584: 1975-1981.

Fecal Microbial Communities of Overweight and Obese Client-Owned Dogs Fed Cooked Bean Powders as Assessed by 454-Pyrosequencing

Alison N Beloshapka[1], Genevieve M Forster[3], Hannah D Holscher[1], Kelly S Swanson[1,2]* and Elizabeth P Ryan[3,4]

[1]*Department of Animal Sciences, University of Illinois, Urbana, IL, USA*
[2]*Division of Nutritional Sciences, University of Illinois, Urbana, IL, USA*
[3]*Department of Clinical Sciences, Colorado State University, Fort Collins, CO, USA*
[4]*Department of Environmental and Radiological Health Sciences, Colorado State University, Fort Collins, CO, USA*

Abstract

Dry beans are consumed around the world and contain a multitude of health benefits, some of which may be related to the gut microbiome. The objective of this study was to evaluate the effects of feeding a 25% cooked Navy Bean (NB) or Black Bean (BB) powder on the fecal microbiota of overweight and obese companion dogs undergoing calorically restricted weight loss, compared to dogs fed an iso-nutrient control diet using 454 pyrosequencing. A double-blinded, placebo-controlled, three-arm clinical trial was conducted. Thirty client-owned, clinically healthy, overweight or obese, adult, male and female dogs of diverse breeds were randomized to one of the three isocaloric, nutritionally complete weight loss diets containing either 0% bean powder (placebo-control); 25% cooked BB powder; or 25% cooked NB powder and calorically restricted to achieve weight loss of up to 2% body weight/wk. for 4 wks. Fresh fecal samples were collected from each dog immediately after completing the 4-wk diet intervention and weight loss phase. Fecal genomic DNA was extracted and used to create 16S rRNA gene amplicons, which were subjected to 454-pyrosequencing. Predominant bacterial phyla present in all dogs included Firmicutes, Fusobacteria, Actinobacteria, Proteobacteria, and Bacteroidetes. Predominant fecal bacterial genera included *Clostridium*, *Blautia*, *Fusobacterium*, and undefined *Lachnospiraceae*. Fecal undefined *Ruminococcus* were greater ($P<0.05$) in dogs fed BB compared to dogs fed the control diet. Client-owned dogs with various dietary and environmental exposures, ages, and breeds were evaluated for fecal microbiota changes during short-term weight loss on different diets. A high variability in fecal microbiota was observed in this free living dog population, leading to few differences among treatments. The gut microbiota may be an area for investigation during long-term weight loss in companion animals, but such studies require a higher level of dietary control and larger sample sizes.

Keywords: Black beans; Caloric restriction; Canines; Gut microbiota; Navy beans; Obesity; Weight loss

Abbreviations: BB: Black Bean; BW: Body Weight; GI/GIT: Gastrointestinal/Gastrointestinal Tract; NB: Navy Bean; BCS: Body condition score

Introduction

Dry common beans (*Phaseoulis vulgaris* L.), also referred to as pulse grains, are an excellent source of protein, carbohydrates, dietary fiber, vitamins, minerals, and phytochemicals [1,2]. Consumption of beans and bean-containing products have been previously studied in humans, rats, and mice [1,3-9]. Consumption of these foods are associated with numerous health benefits, primarily observed in humans, including weight loss promotion, decreased risk of cardiovascular disease, cancers, diabetes, osteoporosis, hypertension, gastrointestinal (GI) disorders, and reduced blood cholesterol [1,3-9]. The health benefits of bean consumption may be, in part, due to the non-digestible carbohydrates they contain and the consequent impact they have on the gut microbiome composition and function [7,10]. Because obesity continues to be a major issue in the U.S. for companion animals, with an estimated 30-50% of pet dogs considered overweight or obese [11], investigating the potential for bean consumption to support healthy weight control in companion dogs is warranted.

The canine colon is densely populated with microorganisms, approximately 10^{11} to 10^{12} colony forming units/mL of digesta [12]. The gut microbiome has a number of roles pertaining to overall host health including to: (1) develop and maintain GI immunity, (2) contribute to fecal biomass and ultimately aid in laxation, (3) produce organic acids, which provide energy for GI epithelial cells and induce apoptosis in pre-cancerous cells, (4) improve mineral absorption, and (5) inhibit pathogen adhesion to GI epithelia [13-16]. Predominant bacterial phyla present in the canine GI tract (GIT) include Firmicutes, Bacteroidetes, Proteobacteria, Fusobacteria, and Actinobacteria and dietary intervention is known to alter GI microbiota numbers and/or activity [17-23].

Recently, we reported that consumption of navy bean- and black bean-containing diets supported body weight (BW) reduction and modulated serum lipid concentrations in calorically restricted overweight and obese dogs [24]. Because the microbiota have been linked with improved metabolic status in humans and animal models [25,26], we evaluated the fecal microbiota in companion dogs after short-term caloric restriction. The purpose of this study was to determine the effects of cooked bean powder-containing diets on the fecal microbiota of overweight and obese dogs when compared to dogs fed an isocaloric, nutrient matched control diet using 454-pyrosequencing.

***Corresponding author:** Kelly S Swanson, Department of Animal Sciences, University of Illinois, 1207 W. Gregory Drive, Urbana, IL 61801, USA
E-mail: ksswanso@illinois.edu

Dog ID	BCS[1]	Age	Sex	Baseline Breeds[2]
O_C1	6	6	F	Dalmatian
O_C2	7	6	M	Labrador Retriever Mix
O_C3	7	4	F[3]	Saint Bernard
O_C4	7	7	F	Labrador Retriever
O_C5	7	7	M	Corgi
O_C6	6	5	F	Australian Shepherd
O_C7	7	3	M	Mixed - unknown
O_C8	8	7	F	Labrador Retriever Mix
O_C9	9	6	F	Golden Retriever
O_C10	8	7	F	Border Collie
O_BB1	8	5	F	Keeshond
O_BB2	6	3	F	Basset Hound
O_BB3	8	7	M	Australian Cattle Dog
O_BB4	9	5	F	Border Collie Mix
O_BB5	7	2	F	Boston Terrier Mix
O_BB6	9	3	M	Shih Tzu
O_BB7[4]	7	5	F	Pit Bull
O_BB8	7	5	M	Australian Cattle Dog
O_BB9	8	6	F	Australian Cattle Dog
O_BB10	8	2	M	Australian Shepherd Mix
O_NB1	7	6	M	Airedale mix
O_NB2	7	2	M	Border Collie Mix
O_NB3	7	4	F	Boston Terrier
O_NB4	7	8	F	Labrador Retriever
O_NB5	8	4	M	Dachshund
O_NB6	9	4	M	Dachshund
O_NB7	6	5	M	Australian shepherd
O_NB8	7	6	F	Australian shepherd
O_NB9	7	2	F	Boxer
O_NB10	8	5	M	Karelian Bear Dog Mix

[1]BCS, body condition score
[2]As reported by owner
[3]Intact female
[4]Only provided a fecal sample at wk. 0 and was not included in the microbiome analysis

Table 1: Body condition score, age, sex, and breed of overweight or obese dogs prior to beginning study diets for weight loss

Materials and Methods

Animals and diets

The Colorado State University (CSU) Institutional Animal Care and Use Committee approved all animal procedures prior to experimentation. The study design, animal procedures, and complete inclusion/exclusion criteria are described in detail by Forster et al. [24]. Briefly, thirty client-owned, clinically healthy, overweight or obese, male and female adult dogs were recruited for the study and written informed owner consent was obtained. Each dog was assessed by the study clinician and assigned a BCS on a 9 point scale [27]. Dogs were classified as overweight with BCS of 6-7/9 and obese with BCS of 8-9/9. A summary of the baseline characteristics for each dog, including BCS, age, sex and breed can be found in Table 1. These dogs were monitored by a veterinarian at the CSU Veterinary Teaching Hospital throughout the study, including weekly BW checks and biweekly physical exams, BCS monitoring, and blood collection as reported in Forster et al. [24]. Additionally, a medical observation form was completed by the owner at weeks 2 and 4 of the study in order to report any adverse effects or changes in the dogs' health and behavior, including vomiting, diarrhea, flatulence, fecal score (5-point scale), energy level, and diet acceptance [24].

Dogs were randomized based on BCS to one of three isocaloric, macro- and micronutrient matched weight loss diets: (1) placebo-control diet (0% bean powder); (2) BB diet; or (3) NB diet. The BB and NB diets included cooked BB or NB powder at 25% of the diet (Vegefull, ADM Edible Bean Specialties, Decatur, IL, USA). Before being ground into powder, the beans are washed, soaked, cooked, and dehydrated. Diets were formulated to meet nutritional recommendations and regulatory standards [28,29]. All 3 diets were manufactured and processed in the same location under the same conditions (ADM Alliance Nutrition Feed Research Pilot Plant, Quincy, IL, USA; Applied Food Biotechnology Plant, St. Charles, MO, USA). Canines were calorically restricted with all study diets for a target weight loss of 2% BW/wk. Dog owners and study clinician were blinded to the assigned diet group during the study. Dogs were equally distributed and randomized to diet groups by sex and BCS (Figure 1).

Fecal DNA extraction and Pyrosequencing

One fresh fecal sample was collected from each dog at baseline and after 4 wks. of consuming the study diet. Owners were instructed to collect each sample within 5 hrs. of defecation. Samples were immediately frozen at -20°C and stored at -80°C until analysis. Genomic DNA was extracted from fecal samples using the PowerLyzer™ PowerSoil® DNA Isolation Kit (MO BIO Laboratories, Inc., Carlsbad, CA, USA) according to the manufacturer's instructions. Extracted DNA was quantified using a Qubit® 2.0 Fluorometer (Life Technologies, Invitrogen, Grand Island, NY, USA) and DNA quality was measured using E-Gel® electrophoresis (EX 2% agarose, Invitrogen, Life Technologies™, Grand Island, NY, USA). Amplification of a 600-bp sequence in the V4-V6 variable region of the 16S rRNA gene was done using barcoded primers as previously described [30,31]. PCR amplicons of all samples were further purified using AMPure XP beads (Beckman-Coulter, Inc., Indianapolis, IN, USA) to remove smaller fragments. The quality of the DNA was assessed before sequencing using 2100 Bioanalyzer (Agilent Technologies, Santa Clara, CA, USA). Finally, the DNA amplicons were combined in equimolar ratios to create a DNA pool that was used for pyrosequencing. Pyrosequencing of the PCR amplicons was performed on a GS PicoTiterPlate (PTP) at the W. M. Keck Center for Biotechnology at the University of Illinois using a 454 Genome Sequencer and FLX titanium reagents (Roche Applied Science, Indianapolis, IN, USA).

Bioinformatics and statistical analyses

Sequence data analysis was performed with QIIME 1.8.0 [32]. Read quality was assessed and found to decrease at 420 bases, so all sequences were truncated after position 420 [33]. Sequences were then demultiplexed and quality filtered with split_libraries.py with default parameters. Resulting sequences were clustered into operational taxonomic units (OTU) using closed-reference OTU database (97% similarity threshold) then quality was filtered [34]. The dataset was rarified to 2,572 OTU for analysis of diversity and species richness. Weighted and unweighted UniFrac distances between all samples were visualized using principal coordinates analysis (PCoA) and performed to evaluate differences in microbial communities among treatment groups.

Data are presented as percentage of sequences at each taxonomic level and were analyzed using the type 3 method of the mixed models procedure of SAS (version 9.4, SAS Institute Inc., Cary, NC, USA). The main fixed effect of diet was analyzed. Proc Univariate was used to test for homogeneity of variance and normality. Means were separated using a protected least squares difference with a Tukey adjustment to control for multiple comparisons. A probability of P<0.05 was accepted as being statistically significant and P≤0.10 accepted as trends. Due to differences in baseline diets and consequent microbial populations among animals, statistics were applied and reported to test for dietary effects with 4 wk. data only (control vs. BB vs. NB).

Results

Dogs were randomized to one of three dietary interventions. The three diets contained approximately 28% crude protein, 8.5% fat and 3.9% fiber (16-18% total dietary fiber) [24]. Fecal samples collected from twenty-nine of the thirty dogs that completed the study contained sufficient quality for microbiota sequence analysis (Figure 1). One dog was withdrawn from the analysis due to inability to obtain a fecal sample after the 4-wk dietary intervention. No gastrointestinal discomfort or changes in flatulence or fecal consistency were reported by the owners. Pyrosequencing of 16S rRNA barcoded amplicons resulted in a total of 852,979 total sequences with a mean and standard deviation of 14,706 ± 7057 reads per sample. Sequences are available at the NCBI sequences read archive (http://www.ncbi.nlm.nih.gov/Traces/sra/) under the accession number SRP045271.

Multi-colored stacked bar graphs represent the relative abundance of bacterial genera of all dogs at baseline (Figure 2). Alpha diversity and species richness were not different among treatments (Figure 3). Based on 97% OTU composition, the PCoA of unweighted Unifrac distances (abundance of bacterial species was not accounted for; Figure 4A indicated that OTU composition was not more similar within diet*time categories than across categories (*t* = -3.089; *P* = 0.517, 2-tailed, 2-sample Monte Carlo *t* test with 999 iterations). Similarly, PCoA of weighted Unifrac distances between samples based on their 97% OTU composition and abundances (Figure 4B) indicated that gut microbial communities were not more similar within diet*time categories than across categories (*t* = -0.985; *P* = 1, 2-tailed, 2-sample Monte Carlo *t* test with 999 iterations). Predominant bacterial phyla present in all dogs at baseline included Firmicutes, Fusobacteria, Actinobacteria, Proteobacteria, and Bacteroidetes (data not shown). Firmicutes composed about 88-94% of bacterial sequences, Fusobacteria composed 0.9-9.5% of bacterial sequences, Actinobacteria composed 1.4-4.5% of bacterial sequences, and Proteobacteria and Bacteroidetes each contributed to only 0.2-0.5% and 0.06-0.3% of sequences, respectively (data not shown). Predominant bacterial genera present in all dogs at baseline included *Clostridium*, *Blautia*, undetermined *Lachnospiraceae*, undefined *Ruminococcus*, *Fusobacterium*, *Dorea*, and *Catenibacterium* (Figure 3).

Predominant bacterial phyla present in all dogs at wk. 4 included Firmicutes, Fusobacteria, Actinobacteria, Proteobacteria, and Bacteroidetes (Table 2). Firmicutes composed about 84-92% of bacterial

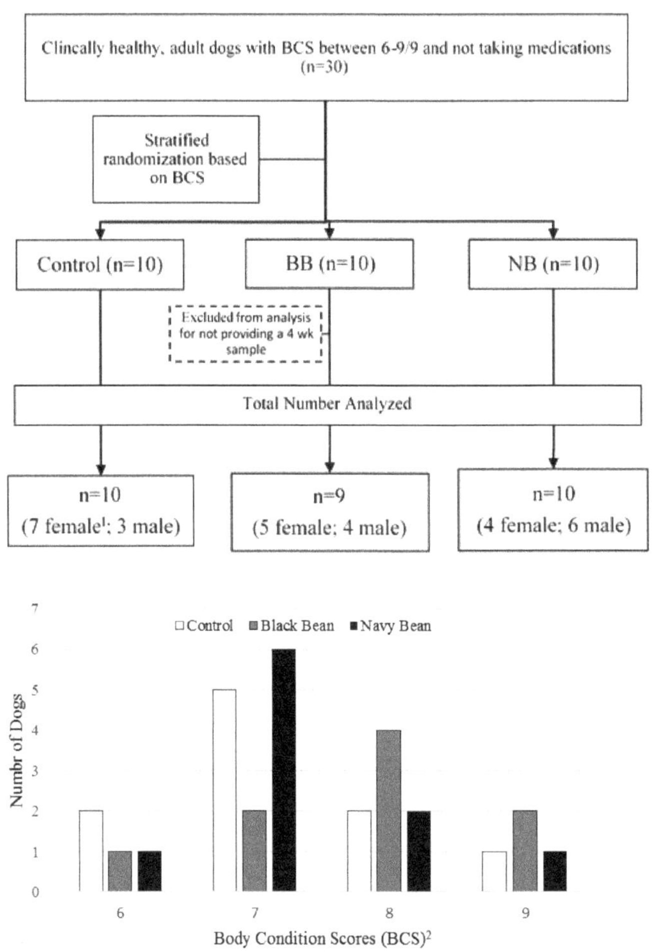

¹All but one female participant in the control group was spayed and all males were castrated.
²Body Condition Score (BCS): 9-point scale was used, where BCS 4 and 5 are ideal, 6 and 7 are overweight, and 8 and 9 are obese[27].

Figure 1: Study design with sex and body condition score distribution of overweight or obese dogs fed control or bean based weight loss diets.

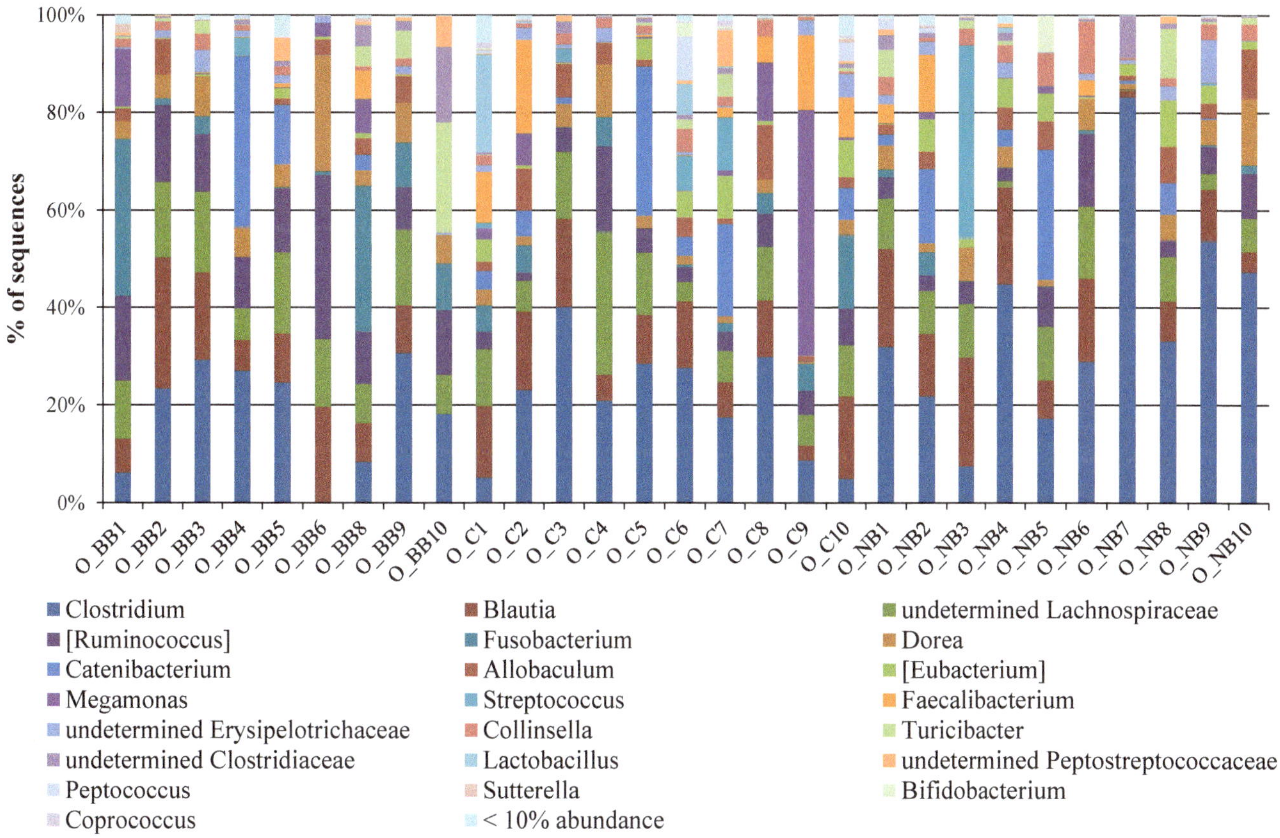

Figure 2: Multi-colored stacked bar graphs represents the relative abundance of bacterial genera (expressed as a percentage of sequences) in feces of overweight or obese dogs at baseline (wk. 0).

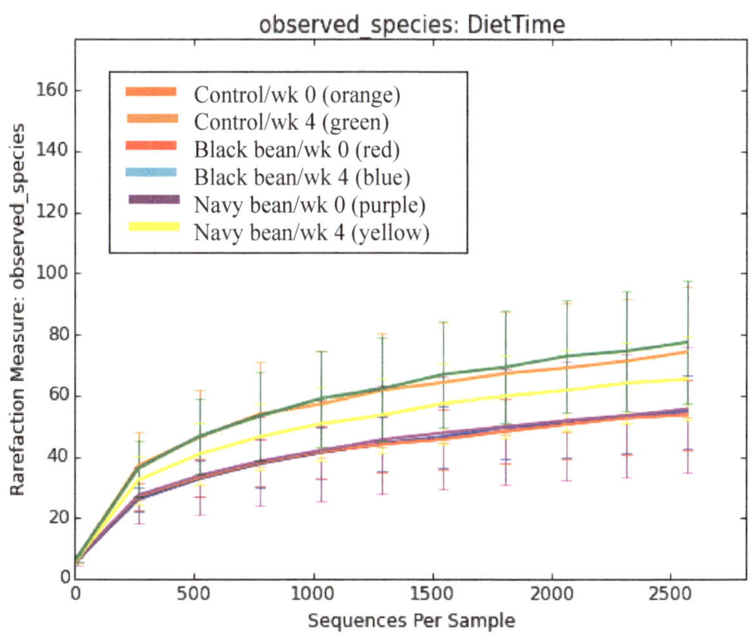

Figure 3: Rarefaction curve of 16S rRNA gene sequences from fecal bacterial samples among dogs fed bean powder-containing weight loss diets.

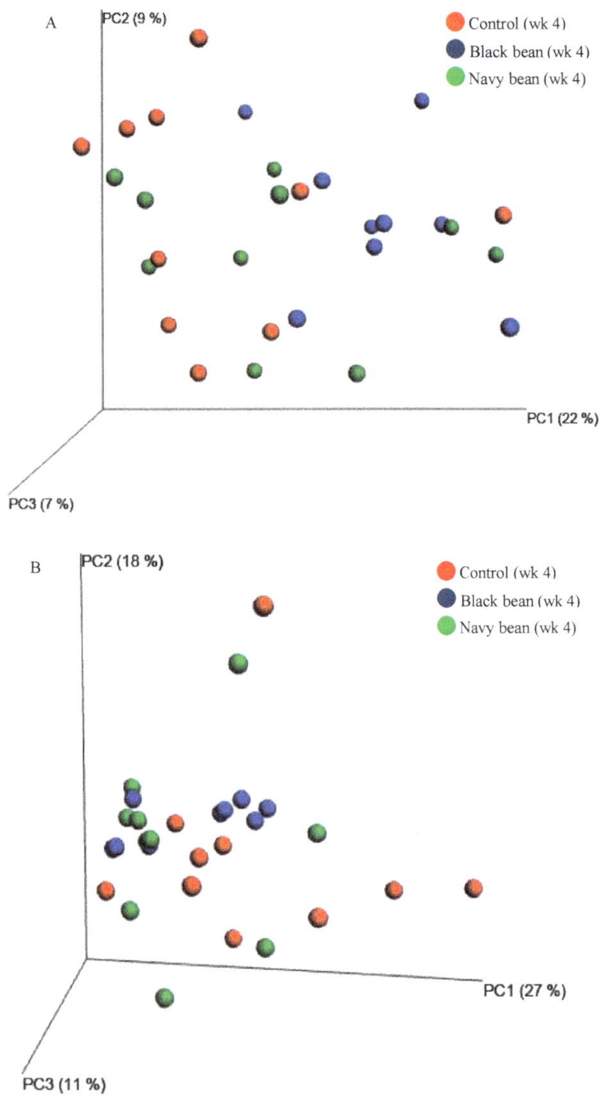

Figure 4: Principal coordinates analysis (PCoA) of unweighted UniFrac distances of fecal bacterial samples among dogs fed bean powder-containing weight loss diets after a 4-wk treatment period based on their 97% OTU composition (abundance of bacterial species was not accounted for; A). This plot indicates that OTU composition was not more similar within diet'time categories than across categories (t = -3.089; P = 0.517, 2-tailed, 2-sample Monte Carlo t test with 999 iterations). Similarly, PCoA of weighted Unifrac distances between samples based on their 97% OTU composition and abundances (B) indicates that gut microbial communities were not more similar within diet'time categories than across categories (t = -0.985; P = 1, 2-tailed, 2-sample Monte Carlo t test with 999 iterations).

sequences, Fusobacteria composed about 4-12% of bacterial sequences, Actinobacteria composed about 1-2% of bacterial sequences, and Proteobacteria, and Bacteroidetes each contributed to only 0.2-1.4% and 0.05-0.2% of bacterial sequences, respectively. No dramatic shifts related to treatment were observed in the unweighted PCoA plot, but dogs consuming BB appeared to cluster together in the weighted PCoA plot (Figures 4A and 4B).

Predominant fecal bacterial families present in all dogs at wk. 4 included *Lachnospiraceae*, *Clostridiaceae*, *Erysipelotrichaceae*, and *Fusobacteriaceae*. *Lachnospiraceae* composed about 27-43% of bacterial sequences, *Clostridiaceae* composed about 19-30% of bacterial sequences, *Erysipelotrichaceae* composed about 10-16% of bacterial sequences, and *Fusobacteriaceae* composed about 4-12% of bacterial sequences. Predominant fecal bacterial genera included *Clostridium*, *Blautia*, *Fusobacterium*, and undefined *Lachnospiraceae*. Baseline variation in the microbiota composition was significant between the control, NB, and BB groups, making differences at wk. 4 difficult to interpret (Figure 3). The relative abundance of fecal undefined *Ruminococcus* (phylum Firmicutes) was greater (P = 0.02) in dogs fed BB (8.50%) when compared to dogs fed the control diet (3.37%) at wk. 4. The relative abundance of Ruminococcaceae *Ruminococcus* tended to be higher (P = 0.05) in dogs fed the CON diet (0.10%) compared to dogs fed the BB diet (0.01%), but was similar at baseline. The relative abundance of fecal *Dorea* (phylum Firmicutes) tended to be lower (P = 0.05) in dogs fed the control or NB diet (3.53% and 3.23%, respectively) when compared to dogs fed BB (6.56%), this difference was not significant at baseline. The relative abundance of fecal *Faecalibacterium* (phylum Firmicutes) tended to be lower (P = 0.05) in dogs fed BB (0.42%) when compared to dogs fed the control diet (4.80%), and was significantly different at baseline. The relative abundance of fecal *Blautia* (phylum Firmicutes) was numerically greater (P = 0.18) in dogs fed BB or NB (18.77% and 16.03%, respectively) when compared to dogs fed the control diet (11.76%), but did not reach statistical significance.

Discussion

Black or navy bean consumption led to few changes in the fecal microbiota of this clinically healthy, diverse breed, overweight and obese companion dog population. No gastrointestinal discomfort or changes in flatulence or fecal consistency were reported by the owners, which supports both the safety and tolerability of adding 25% cooked bean powder to dog food. This finding is consistent with our previous report demonstrating that 25% NB intake did not disrupt the fecal microflora of healthy weight companion dogs [35]. The baseline compositions of these overweight or obese dogs varied significantly with relative abundances of Firmicutes, Fusobacteria, and Actinobacteria resembling previous reports [35,36]. As such, several of the changes observed may be attributed to the variation in baseline fecal microbiota (e.g. Firmicutes undefined *Ruminococcus* and *Faecalibacterium*), however Ruminococcaceae *Ruminococcus*, *Dorea* (phylum Firmicutes) and *Blautia* (phylum Firmicutes) differed in at least one of the diet groups at wk. 4, and can be considered diet-modifiable. Human consumption of beans or other fermentable fibers have shown similar observational changes. For example, increased fecal *Ruminococcus* was observed in human stool following the increased consumption of resistant starch [37,38]. In dogs, fecal *Ruminococcus* numerically increased when fed fermentable fibers [23]. The dogs in the current study followed a similar pattern, which may be partially due to the resistant starch content of beans. *Blautia* are also part of the butyrate-producing bacteria group in the gut, which proliferate in response to microbial fermentation of certain carbohydrate substrates [39-41]. Increased fecal *Blautia* was observed in response to resistant starch supplementation using an *in vitro* model [42], and in this case suggests increased content of plant polysaccharides from bean powders reaching the colon for fermentation. Furthermore, Suchodolski et al. [43], who evaluated the impact of diarrhea and inflammatory bowel disease on the fecal microbiome of dogs, observed a decrease in fecal *Blautia* in dogs with acute diarrhea. These findings suggest *Blautia* has roles in maintaining a healthy canine intestinal microbiome and may be supported by the prebiotics found in common beans.

End-products of microbial fermentation were not evaluated in

			Diet				
Phylum	Family	Genus	Control	Black Bean	Navy Bean	Pooled SEM	P-Value
Actinobacteria			**1.36**	**2.25**	**2.33**	**0.59**	**0.44**
	Bifidobacteriaceae	*Bifidobacterium*	0.05	0.01	0.04	0.03	0.63
	Coriobacteriaceae	*Collinsella*	1.24	2.14	2.23	0.57	0.40
		Slackia	0.06	0.04	0.06	0.03	0.90
Bacteroidetes			**0.27**	**0.05**	**0.33**	**0.13**	**0.32**
	Bacteroidaceae	*Bacteroides*	0.08	0.05	0.14	0.07	0.67
	Prevotellaceae	*Prevotella*	0.15	0.00	0.15	0.07	0.27
Firmicutes			**84.07**	**88.82**	**92.14**	**3.84**	**0.33**
	Clostridiaceae	Unclassified Clostridiaceae	0.90	0.58	0.53	0.14	0.13
		Clostridium	18.36	29.76	26.75	4.65	0.22
		Sarcina	0.01	0.00	0.00	0.01	0.66
	Enterococcaceae	*Enterococcus*	0.02	0.09	0.01	0.04	0.40
	Erysipelotrichaceae	Unclassified Erysipelotrichaceae	2.78	2.46	2.99	0.69	0.87
		Allobaculum	3.22	4.11	4.01	1.08	0.81
		Bulleidia	0.39	0.01	0.00	0.23	0.41
		Catenibacterium	3.80	2.48	4.01	1.63	0.78
		Coprobacillus	0.06	0.14	0.03	0.05	0.23
		[Eubacterium]	3.65	1.73	5.41	1.90	0.41
	Lachnospiraceae	Unclassified Lachnospiraceae	8.46	9.84	9.25	1.89	0.88
		Blautia	11.76	18.77	16.03	2.58	0.18
		Coprococcus	0.24	0.10	0.30	0.10	0.35
		Dorea	3.53[x]	6.56[y]	3.23[x]	1.00	0.05
		Epulopiscium	0.01	0.01	0.003	0.01	0.62
		Roseburia	0.020	0.001	0.003	0.01	0.28
		[Ruminococcus]	3.37[a]	8.50[b]	6.65[ab]	1.21	0.02
	Lactobacillaceae	*Lactobacillus*	0.73	0.03	0.01	0.43	0.41
	Peptococcaceae	*Peptococcus*	1.18	0.03	0.51	0.50	0.29
	Peptostreptococcaceae	Unclassified Peptostreptococcaceae	0.46	0.10	0.26	0.12	0.11
		Clostridium	0.00	0.01	0.03	0.01	0.32
	Ruminococcaceae	*Butyricicoccus*	0.10	0.02	0.08	0.03	0.21
		Faecalibacterium	4.80[y]	0.42[x]	2.51[xy]	1.17	0.05
		Ruminococcus	0.10[y]	0.01[x]	0.02[xy]	0.03	0.05
	Streptococcaceae	*Streptococcus*	6.37	0.35	3.55	3.98	0.58
	Turicibacteraceae	*Turicibacter*	1.63	0.34	0.67	0.53	0.22
	[unclassified]		2.24	2.23	2.82	0.66	0.77
	Veillonellaceae	*Megamonas*	4.95	0.12	2.02	1.65	0.13
		Megasphaera	0.13	0.00	0.00	0.05	0.15
		Phascolarctobacterium	0.38	0.00	0.28	0.19	0.37
Fusobacteria			**12.90**	**8.65**	**4.49**	**3.68**	**0.28**
	Fusobacteriaceae	*Cetobacterium*	0.80	0.00	0.00	0.48	0.40
		Fusobacterium	12.11	8.65	4.49	3.70	0.35
Proteobacteria			**1.40**	**0.24**	**0.71**	**0.37**	**0.11**
	Alcaligenaceae	*Sutterella*	0.51	0.06	0.36	0.24	0.42
	Campylobacteraceae	*Campylobacter*	0.04	0.00	0.05	0.03	0.45
	Helicobacteraceae	*Helicobacter*	0.10	0.12	0.02	0.07	0.60
	Succinivibrionaceae	*Anaerobiospirillum*	0.02	0.01	0.00	0.01	0.43
	Enterobacteriaceae	*Escherichia*	0.02	0.00	0.01	0.01	0.17

[a,b]Mean values within the same row not sharing common superscript letters differ ($P < 0.05$) due to diet

[x,y]Mean values within the same row not sharing common superscript letters differ ($P \leq 0.10$) due to diet

Table 2: Predominant bacterial phyla and genera (expressed as a percentage of sequences) in feces of overweight or obese dogs fed control or bean powder-containing weight loss diets after a 4-wk treatment period.

these dogs, yet the shifts in such bacterial populations suggest that there would be increased carbohydrate fermentation, namely for short-chain fatty acid production. Increased fecal short chain fatty acids are expected to have positive impacts on gut health in overweight dogs losing weight and merits continued evaluation. For instance, increased abundance of fecal *Lachnospiraceae* has been associated with increased butyrate production [44-46]. Furthermore, increased propionate production has been previously associated with decreased serum lipids [47], which were demonstrated in the overweight/obese dogs consuming beans in the current study [24].

It should be emphasized that the dogs in the current study not only received bean powder-dietary treatments, but also underwent a 4-wk weight loss phase. This combination of treatments may lead to differences in the microbiome not accounted for by dietary changes alone. In humans and rodent models, researchers have observed increased fecal Bacteroidetes and decreased Firmicutes during weight loss [48-51]; though shifts in these groups were not observed in the current short-term weight loss study. Interestingly, the predominant bacterial phyla observed herein at both baseline and wk. 4 was similar to those of the lean dog group observed by Park et al. [52]. However, as the primers utilized in this study have a bias against Bacteroidetes, further research is necessary to determine if bacteria in the Bacteroidetes phyla also increase in canine populations during weight loss in the long term.

Although several fecal microbiota shifts were observed in the current study, the overall gut microbial populations remained stable in all dogs consuming bean-based or control diets. This may be due, in part, to the matched macro- and micronutrient profiles of the diets. However, bean based canine diets were shown to differ in phytochemical diversity, despite the nutrient match [53], and differences in phenolic compounds have been reported between bean cultivars that may influence metabolism by microbiota when compared to microbial composition [2,54-56]. Lin et al. [56] evaluated the polyphenolic profile of several common dry beans from different commercial market classes, and concluded that black beans and navy beans had similar hydroxycinnaminic acid derivatives. However, the black bean group had 3 identified anthocyanins (flavonoids), whereas the navy bean group had no flavonoids detected [56]. Thus, more research is necessary to identify bioactive components of the beans that may be responsible for subtle shifts in the metabolic function of the gut microbiome, for resulting health implications.

In conclusion, although the PCoA plots do not demonstrate dramatic treatment-related shifts in the fecal microbiota, the shifts in relative abundance of some taxa were associated with the consumption of cooked bean powders. The interpretation of these data is subject to several limitations. First, the dogs studied were part of a free-living population, with the potential for different exposures to environmental factors, including foods other than the assigned treatment diets. Second, the dogs were not acclimated to a control diet prior to baseline measurements, potentially masking bean diet treatment-related shifts. Because of this, it is highly recommended that future studies aiming to investigate changes in gut microbiota over time with companion dogs should incorporate a run-in period with the same placebo-control diet for at least 10 days prior to collection or utilize a Latin square design and have higher animal number due to high variability. Despite these limitations and high individual variability, this study supports that a cooked bean based canine diet only modestly shifts a healthy microbiome, and thus provides rationale for continued investigation to enhance canine gut health. Future research is warranted to better understand the impact of cooked beans on clinical obesity and obesity-related comorbidities of a free-living canine population.

Acknowledgements

The authors declare no conflict of interest. One author (Ryan) is participating in efforts to commercialize novel dog food formulations. The current study and data analyses were completed prior to Ryan participating in commercialization and are, therefore, not biased though may be perceived as a potential conflict of interest. Supported in part by ADM Alliance Nutrition, Inc., Quincy, IL, USA.

References

1. Bennink MR, Rondini E (2008) Dry Beans and Human Health: An Overview of the Status of the Science on Dry Beans and Human Health. The Bean Institute.
2. Tiwari BK, Singh N (2012) Pulse Chemistry and Technology. The Royal Society of Chemistry, Cambridge, UK.
3. Rosa CO, Costa NM, Leal PF, Oliveira TT (1998) The cholesterol-lowering effect of black beans (*Phaseolus vulgaris*, L.) without hulls in hypercholesterolemic rats. Arch Latinoam Nutr 48: 299-305.
4. Anderson JW, Major AW (2002) Pulses and lipaemia, short- and long-term effect: potential in the prevention of cardiovascular disease. Br J Nutr 883: S263-S271.
5. Hangen L, Bennink MR (2002) Consumption of black beans and navy beans (*Phaseolus vulgaris*) reduced azoxymethane-induced colon cancer in rats. Nutr Cancer 44: 60-65.
6. Hu FB (2003) Plant-based foods and prevention of cardiovascular disease: an overview. Am J Clin Nutr 78: 544S-551S.
7. Finley JW, Burrell JB, Reeves PG (2007) Pinto bean consumption changes SCFA profiles in fecal fermentations, bacterial populations of the lower bowel, and lipid profiles in blood of humans. J Nutr 137: 2391-2398.
8. Winham DM, Hutchins AM (2007) Baked bean consumption reduces serum cholesterol in hypercholesterolemic adults. Nutr Res 27: 380-386.
9. Zhu Z, Jiang W, Thompson HJ (2012) Edible dry bean consumption (*Phaseolus vulgaris* L.) modulates cardiovascular risk factors and diet-induced obesity in rats and mice. Br J Nutr 108: S66-S73.
10. Campos-Vega R, Garcia-Gasca T, Guevara-Gonzalez R, Ramos-Gomez M, Oomah BD, et al. (2012) Human gut flora-fermented nondigestible fraction from cooked bean (*Phaseolus vulgaris* L.) modifies protein expression associated with apoptosis, cell cycle arrest, and proliferation in human adenocarcinoma colon cancer cells. J Agric Food Chem 60: 12443-12450.
11. Courcier EA, Thomson RM, Mellor DJ, Yam PS (2010) An epidemiological study of environmental factors associated with canine obesity. J Small Anim Pract 51: 362-367.
12. Samal L, Pattanaik A, Mishra C (2011) Application of molecular tools for gut health of pet animals: A review. J Adv Vet Res 1: 38-46.
13. Ouwehand AC, Derrien M, de Vos W, Tiihonen K, Rautonen N (2005) Prebiotics and other microbial substrates for gut functionality. Curr Opin Biotechnol 16: 212-217.
14. Vieira AT, Teixeira MM, Martins FS (2013) The role of probiotics and prebiotics in inducing gut immunity. Front Immunol 4: 445.
15. Moloney RD, Desbonnet L, Clarke G, Dinan TG, Cryan JF (2014) The microbiome: stress, health and disease. Mamm Genome 25: 49-74.
16. Zeng H, Lazarova DL, Bordonaro M (2014) Mechanisms linking dietary fiber, gut microbiota and colon cancer prevention. World J Gastrointest Oncol 6: 41-51.
17. Suchodolski JS (2011) Companion animals symposium: microbes and gastrointestinal health of dogs and cats. J Anim Sci 89: 1520-1530.
18. Suchodolski JS, Camacho J, Steiner JM (2008) Analysis of bacterial diversity in the canine duodenum, jejunum, ileum, and colon by comparative 16S rRNA gene analysis. FEMS Microbiol Ecol 66: 567-578.
19. Suchodolski JS, Dowd SE, Westermarck E, Steiner JM, Wolcott RD, et al. (2009) The effect of the macrolide antibiotic tylosin on microbial diversity in the canine small intestine as demonstrated by massive parallel 16S rRNA gene sequencing. BMC Microbiol 9: 210.
20. Middelbos IS, Vester Boler BM, Qu A, White BA, Swanson KS, et al. (2010) Phylogenetic characterization of fecal microbial communities of dogs fed diets with or without supplemental dietary fiber using 454 pyrosequencing. PLoS One 5: e9768.
21. Handl S, Dowd SE, Garcia-Mazcorro JF, Steiner JM, Suchodolski JS (2011) Massive parallel 16S rRNA gene pyrosequencing reveals highly diverse fecal bacterial and fungal communities in healthy dogs and cats. FEMS Microbiol Ecol 76: 301-310.
22. Swanson KS, Dowd SE, Suchodolski JS, Middelbos IS, Vester BM, et al. (2011) Phylogenetic and gene-centric metagenomics of the canine intestinal microbiome reveals similarities with humans and mice. ISME J 5: 639-649.
23. Beloshapka AN, Dowd SE, Suchodolski JS, Steiner JM, Duclos L, et al. (2013) Fecal microbial communities of healthy adult dogs fed raw meat-based diets with or without inulin or yeast cell wall extracts as assessed by 454 pyrosequencing. FEMS Microbiol Ecol 84: 532-541.
24. Forster GM, Ollila CA, Burton JH, Hill D, Bauer JE, et al. (2012) Nutritional weight loss therapy with cooked bean powders regulates serum lipids and biochemical analytes in overweight and obese dogs. J Obes Wt Loss Ther 2: 149.
25. Qin J, Li R, Raes J, Arumugam M, Burgdorf KS, et al. (2010) A human gut

microbial gene catalogue established by metagenomic sequencing. Nature 464: 59-65.

26. Bischoff SC (2011) 'Gut health': a new objective in medicine? BMC Med 9: 24.

27. Laflamme D (1997) Development and validation of a body condition score system for dogs. Canine Pract 22: 10-15.

28. AAFCO (2010) Official Publication. Association of American Feed Control Officials Inc., Oxford, (IN).

29. National Research Council (NRC) (2006) Nutrient requirements of dogs and cats. National Academic Press, Washington, D.C., USA.

30. Dowd SE, Sun Y, Wolcott RD, Domingo A, Carroll JA (2008) Bacterial tag-encoded FLX amplicon pyrosequencing (bTEFAP) for microbiome studies: bacterial diversity in the ileum of newly weaned Salmonella-infected pigs. Foodborne Pathog Dis 5: 459-472.

31. Hooda S, Boler BM, Serao MC, Brulc JM, Staeger MA, et al. (2012) 454 pyrosequencing reveals a shift in fecal microbiota of healthy adult men consuming polydextrose or soluble corn fiber. J Nutr 142: 1259-1265.

32. Caporaso JG, Kuczynski J, Stombaugh J, Bittinger K, Bushman FD, et al. (2010) QIIME allows analysis of high-throughput community sequencing data. Nat Methods 7: 335-336.

33. Holscher HD, Caporaso JG, Hooda S, Brulc JM, Fahey GC Jr, et al. (2015) Fiber supplementation influences phylogenetic structure and functional capacity of the human intestinal microbiome: Follow-up of a randomized controlled trial. Amer J Clin Nutr 101: 55-64.

34. Bokulich NA, Subramanian S, Faith JJ, Gevers D, Gordon JI, et al. (2013) Quality-filtering vastly improves diversity estimates from Illumina amplicon sequencing. Nat Methods 10: 57-59.

35. Kerr KR, Forster G, Dowd SE, Ryan EP, Swanson KS (2013) Effects of dietary cooked navy bean on the fecal microbiome of healthy companion dogs. PLoS One 8: e74998.

36. Handl S, German AJ, Holden SL, Dowd SE, Steiner JM, et al. (2013) Faecal microbiota in lean and obese dogs. FEMS Microbiol Ecol 84: 332-343.

37. Abell GC, Cooke CM, Bennett CN, Conlon MA, McOrist AL (2008) Phylotypes related to *Ruminococcus bromii* are abundant in the large bowel of humans and increase in response to a diet high in resistant starch. FEMS Microbiol Ecol 66: 505-515.

38. Martínez I, Kim J, Duffy PR, Schlegel VL, Walter J (2010) Resistant starches types 2 and 4 have differential effects on the composition of the fecal microbiota in human subjects. PLoS One 5: e15046.

39. Barcenilla A, Pryde SE, Martin JC, Duncan SH, Stewart CS, et al. (2000) Phylogenetic relationships of butyrate-producing bacteria from the human gut. Appl Environ Microbiol 66: 1654-1661.

40. Pryde SE, Duncan SH, Hold GL, Stewart CS, Flint HJ (2002) The microbiology of butyrate formation in the human colon. FEMS Microbiol Lett 217: 133-139.

41. Fukuda S, Toh H, Taylor TD, Ohno H, Hattori M (2012) Acetate-producing bifidobacteria protect the host from enteropathogenic infection via carbohydrate transporters. Gut Microbes 3: 449-454.

42. Yang J, Martínez I, Walter J, Keshavarzian A, Rose DJ (2013) *In vitro* characterization of the impact of selected dietary fibers on fecal microbiota composition and short chain fatty acid production. Anaerobe 23: 74-81.

43. Suchodolski JS, Markel ME, Garcia-Mazcorro JF, Unterer S, Heilmann RM, et al. (2012) The fecal microbiome in dogs with acute diarrhea and idiopathic inflammatory bowel disease. PLoS One 7: e51907.

44. Duncan SH, Lobley GE, Holtrop G, Ince J, Johnstone AM, et al. (2008) Human colonic microbiota associated with diet, obesity and weight loss. Int J Obes (Lond) 32: 1720-1724.

45. Louis P, Young P, Holtrop G, Flint HJ (2010) Diversity of human colonic butyrate-producing bacteria revealed by analysis of the butyryl-CoA:acetate CoA-transferase gene. Env Microbiol 12: 304-314.

46. Van den Abbeele P, Belzer C, Goossens M, Kleerebezem M, De Vos WM, et al. (2013) Butyrate-producing *Clostridium* cluster XIVa species specifically colonize mucins in an in vitro gut model. ISME J 7: 949-961.

47. den Besten G, van Eunen K, Groen AK, Venema K, Reijngoud DJ, et al. (2013) The role of short-chain fatty acids in the interplay between diet, gut microbiota, and host energy metabolism. J Lipid Res 54: 2325-2340.

48. Ley RE, Bäckhed F, Turnbaugh P, Lozupone CA, Knight RD, et al. (2005) Obesity alters gut microbial ecology. Proc Natl Acad Sci U S A 102: 11070-11075.

49. Kalliomäki M, Collado MC, Salminen S, Isolauri E (2008) Early differences in fecal microbiota composition in children may predict overweight. Am J Clin Nutr 87: 534-538.

50. Nadal I, Santacruz A, Marcos A, Warnberg J, Garagorri JM, et al. (2009) Shifts in clostridia, bacteroides and immunoglobulin-coating fecal bacteria associated with weight loss in obese adolescents. Int J Obes 33: 758-767.

51. Zhang H, DiBaise JK, Zuccolo A, Kudrna D, Braidotti M, et al. (2009) Human gut microbiota in obesity and after gastric bypass. Proc Natl Acad Sci U S A 106: 2365-2370.

52. Park HJ, Lee SE, Kim HB, Isaacson RE, Seo KW, et al. (2015) Association of obesity with serum leptin, adiponectin, and serotonin and gut microflora in beagle dogs. J Vet Intern Med 29: 43-50.

53. Forster GM, Heuberger AL, Broeclking CD, Bauer JE, Ryan EP (2015) Consumption of cooked navy bean powders modulate the canine fecal and urine metabolome. Curr Metabolomics 3: 90-101.

54. Campos-Vega R, Loarca-Piña G, Oomah BD (2010) Minor components of pulses and their potential impact on human health. Food Res Int 43: 461-482.

55. Zhang C, Monk JM, Lu JT, Zarepoor L, Wu W, et al. (2014) Cooked navy and black bean diets improve biomarkers of colon health and reduce inflammation during colitis. Br J Nutr 111: 1549-1563.

56. Lin LZ, Harnly JM, Pastor-Corrales MS, Luthria DL (2008) The polyphenolic profiles of common bean (*Phaseolus vulgaris* L.). Food Chem 107: 399-410.

Effect of Dietary on Live Weight and Testicular Development in Ouled Djellal Ram Lambs During the Prepubertal Period in Western Algeria

Zineddine Esma* and Bereksi Reguig Karima

Département de Biologie/Université UDL de Sidi-Bel-Abbès, Algéria

Abstract

The aim of our study was to investigate the effect of the feeding level on the testicular and body weight growth of Ouled Djellal ram lambs. The study lasted 3 months (15 March to 15 June 2015) from post-weaning until prepubertal period at the Technical Institute Farms (ITELV) Lamtar of Sidi-bel-Abbes (Western Algeria). Twenty Ouled Djellal lambs of 3-4 months of age were weighed and alloted into two equal groups of Low (n=10) or High (n=10) nutrition plane. Each group received, in addition to a basal diet, 200 g and 400 g head^{-1}day^{-1} respectively. Monthly measurements of live weight and testicular volume of lambs were recorded. During the trial, the High group showed a significant greater live weight compared to the low group. Whereas, the testicular growth was a gradual and linear increase according to the two groups (low and high) without significant differences. However, all measurements of testis, live weight and age were positively correlated with one another at both low and high groups during the trial. It was concluded that postweaning nutrition management had a strong influence on lamb live weight, which in turn was related to testicular growth and prepubertal period in Ouled Djellal ram lambs. The strategy foucussed feeding is necessary to optimise weight and tesicular growth of ram lambs replacements. Also, the nutrition management may be a useful tool to maximize productivity in flocks.

Keywords: Live weight; Ouled Djellal lambs; Nutrition; Prepubertal period; Testicular volume; Weaning

Introduction

In Algeria, sheep breeding represents 81.6% of the total domestic animal production (with 26.88 millions head) and mutton provides more than 56% of the national red meat production [1]. The Ouled Djellal is the main native sheep breed. It is adapted to steppe conditions and has exceptional qualities for red meat and wool production [1]. Recognition of the reproductive characteristics of a sheep breed is an essential starting point towards improving its productivity [2]. Characterization of puberty and early sexual development is a valuable tool for selection within the males of a breed [3]. In fertility studies in livestock there is a tendency to focus more on the female side with much less emphasis on the male side [2]. However, male fertility is as important as that of the female [4,5].

In general, sexual development of ram lamb appears to be more closely associated with body growth than with chronological age [6]. Dyrmundsson [7] concluded that body weight was a better criterion for the attainment of puberty than the chronological age alone. A review by Toe et al. suggested that measures of testicular size have received considerable attention as possible selection criteria for improving fertility in sheep, primarily because of their high heritable and their favourable to neutral association with female reproduction. The purpose of this investigation was to evaluate the effect of level of dietary on onset of prepubertal period and also to reseach its linkage with testicular and body weight growth of Ouled Djellal ram lambs.

Materials and Methods

The present study was conducted at the Technical Institute Farms (ITELV) Lamtar of Sidi-bel-Abbes (Western Algeria). This farm is located in Lamtar (25 km on the road to Tlemcen), at an altitude of 560 m (average minimum temperature 10.38°C, average maximum temperature 25.22°C, annual rainfall 372 mm). Twenty Ouled Djellal lambs of 3-4 months old were used. The lambs were weaned at 100 ± 10 days of age and then housed in a sheepfold under natural condition. They were weighed and allotted into two equal groups of Low (n=10) or High (n=10) nutrition plane. Each group received, in addition to a basal diet (good quality pasture) 200 g and 400 g of concentrate feed containing barley (50%), corn (10%), wheat bran (37.5%) and vitamin mineral compound (2.5%) by head^{-1}day^{-1} respectively. Lambs concentrate feed contained also 92.36% dry matter which it composed of: 72.68% carbohydrates, 15% proteins, 2% lipids, 1% calcium, 0.55% phosphorus and vitamins (A: 500000 UI, D3: 75000 UI, E: 1000 UI). Hay and water were provided *ad libitum*. At the date of 15th March the lambs were identified by numerated loops in the ear. Body weight and testicular volume of lambs were measured monthly for 3 months (15 April-15 June 2015). The volume of testis was calculated as reported by Marson et al. [8]. The length and wide of each testis were measured with a calliper after forcing it against the scrotum.

Volume Testicular (cm^3)=$W^2 \times L \times \pi/6$ (with W: testicular width and L: testicular length)

All statistical analyses were carried out using the Stat View program (version 5; 1998 France SAS Institute Inc.). Data were analyzed using the "Student t test" (with a 5% significance level). Correlations between measurements were obtained by means on the Pearson correlation test.

Results and Discussion

The average means and standard deviations of live weights for different age periods are shown in Table 1. Live weights increased continuously at different average ages respectively 20.22 ± 2.11 kg at 102 ± 11.86 days to 23.57 ± 1.95 kg at 133 ± 11.86 days and 26.55 ± 2.59 kg at 163 ± 11.86 days (significant difference : $p<0.0001$). Results in the present study indicated that the average lamb live weights of the two groups (Low and High) tend to increase throughout during

***Corresponding author:** Zineddine Esma, Médecin Vétérinaire and Maître Assistante A, Département de Biologie/Université UDL de Sidi-Bel-Abbès, Algéria
E-mail: zineddinevet@gmail.com

the trail. The means live weights of lambs on diet 1 were significantly higher than those for animals on the diet 2 (18.65 ± 1.02 vs 21.80 ± 1.70 kg : significant difference with p=0.001), (22.15 ± 0.94 vs 25.00 ± 1.63 kg : significant difference p=0.0018), and (24.30 ± 0.71 vs 28.80 ± 1.56 kg: very significant difference with p<0.0001). However, increasing the concentrate component of feed intake indicates an apparent influence on weight gain which it mentioned with the findings 3.15 kg, 2.85 kg and 4.5 kg respectively between the lambs of lower and higher groups.

Our values were superior to comparable compared with results reported by Titaouine [9] which has advanced average of 16.92 ± 1.22 kg, and 22.56 ± 1.50 kg respectively for 90 days and 120 days in Appearance lambs Ouled high Djellal the level the cradle region of this breed of sheep (Wilaya of Biskra) although Yilmaz and Altin [10] have advanced an average of 19.71 kg at 100 days of age in lambs from Chios cross breed Kıvırcık × F1 in Turkey.

Our results were also higher than those estimated by some Algerian authors who recorded 15.79 alive means weight of ± 2.15 kg and 18.85 ± 3.05 kg at 60 days and 120 days respectively in race lambs Rembi in Tiaret (western Algeria) [11] and by Dekhili and Mahnane [12] who found an average weight of lambs of 17.80 ± 0.42 kg at 90 days in the race Ouled Djellal in Setif (eastern Algeria). As for the level of the Mediterranean basin, for example, in Tunisia, averages 15 to 20 kg at the age of 3 months to 3.5 months at the Ghezala farm and 18-23 Kg at 3.5 months of age in farm Fretissa at the same breed of sheep called the Sicilo- Sarde [13] while Chafri and Mahouachi [14] found an average of 14.2 kg at 24 weeks or 6 months of age in lambs D'man race receiving a high diet. In Morocco, Elfadili [15] reported an average of 17.24 ± 0.35 kg at 90 days in the local race Beni Guil. However, our results were lower than those recorded by Boussena et al. [16] who obtained 22.07 average weight of ± 0.94 kg, and 25.82 ± 1.17 kg, respectively, at 90 days and 120 days in breed lambs Ouled Djellal late weaned at an average age of 122.65 ± 1.18 kg and housed at the demonstration farm of the technical institute farms Ain M'lila (North - East Algeria) while Lamrani et al. [17] who noted an average live weight of 31.09 ± 0.98 kg) at 6 months of age in lambs of the same race at the Guelma region (North - East Algeria).

In general, the significant increase in live weight may be explained by the dietary transition that suffered the lamb during the weaning period wich the milk food was replacing by the solid food and he received a high level of concentrate energy. It will allow to transform the monogastric to a ruminant (development of other gastric pouches and increasing the efficiency of the digestive tract).

Our results differ significantly more or less compared to those obtained by other authors because there are several factors influencing the weight of lambs in the post- weaning period (weaning age : early or late weaning), genotype (breeds) factors related to the mother (maternal age, parity, maternal qualities, level of milk production ... etc.), type of birth (single or double), diet (food transition, quantity and quality concentrated and distributed availability and forage type offered including individual intake capacity of the lamb) and the type of farming (intensive, semi- intensive or extensive depending on the type of production).

Table 2 summarize the development of testicular volumes of Ouled Djellal ram lambs during the present trial. Our results revealed that a gradual and linear increase in testicular volume from 3 to 6 months at different average age periods in the two groups (High and Low) wich it recorded the values : 34.76 ± 6.31 cm^3 to 102 ± 11.86 days and 41.38 ± 6.60 cm^3 133 ± 11.86 days while 53.12 ± 10.87 cm^3 is estimated at 163 ± 11.86 days (highly significant difference with p<0.0001). This finding is in agreement with that observed by Attal et al. who report that testicular growth is initially slow during the period of infancy, is accelerating between 3 and 12 months in the establishment of spermatogenesis in the Normande cattle breed males.

A gradual and linear increase in testicular volume was observed from two to six months of age for both of the lower and higher groups with the findings were 33.11 ± 4.56 vs 36.41 ± 7.56 cm^3: no significant difference with p=0.23), (39.04 ± 5.45 vs 43.71 ± 7.09 cm^3 : no significant difference with p=0.12) and (48.54 ± 12.00 vs 57.69 ± 7.67 cm^3 : no significant difference with p=0.06), although the beginning of the experiment, a slight gap was gradually observed 3.29 cm^3, 4.67 cm^3 to reach the threshold of 9.14 cm^3 until the end of the study period (6th month corresponding to the pre-pubertal age).

Lambs having larger testis produce more sperm later [18,19]. However, scrotal circumference is considered the best indicator of sexual development in males [20] and differs by breeds [21].

Our results were lower than those reported by Kahal [22] who advanced the following values : 37.62 ± 4.52 cm^3, 47.39 ± 5.01 cm^3,

Groups	Effective	(102 days)	(133 days)	(163 days)
Group Lower	n=10	18.65 ± 1.02^a	22.15 ± 0.94^a	24.30 ± 0.71^a
Group Higher	n=10	21.80 ± 1.70^b	25.00 ± 1.63^b	28.80 ± 1.56^b
AM ± SD*	n=20	20.22 ± 2.11$^\alpha$	23.57 ± 1.95$^\beta$	26.55 ± 2.59$^\omega$

Total average mean and standard deviation
a,b: Values with different letters in the same column are significantly different (p<0.05)
α,β,ω: Values with different superscripts in the same row are significantly different (p<0.0001)

Table 1: Changes in live weight (kg) in Ouled Djellalram lambs according to the average age.

Testicular Volume (cm^3)	Effective	(102 days)	(133 days)	(163 days)
Group Lower	n=10	33.11 ± 4.56	39.04 ± 5.45	48.54 ± 12.00
Group Higher	n=10	36.41 ± 7.56	43.71 ± 7.09	57.69 ± 7.67
AM ± SD*	n=20	34.76 ± 6.31$^\alpha$	41.38 ± 6.60$^\beta$	53.12 ± 10.87$^\omega$

*Total average mean and standard deviation
The values in the same column are not significantly different (p>0.05).
α, β, ω: values with different superscripts in the same row are significantly different (p<0.0001).

Table 2: Changes in testicular volume in Ouled Djellal ram lambs according to the average age.

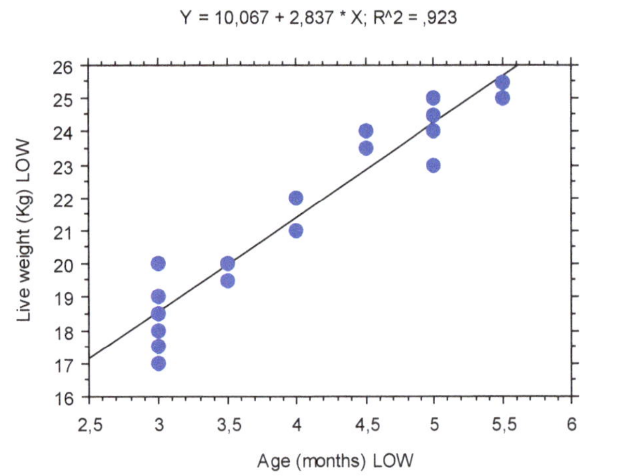

Figure 1: Development of live weight (Kg) in Ouled Djellal ram lambs from 3 to 6 months of age (Low group).

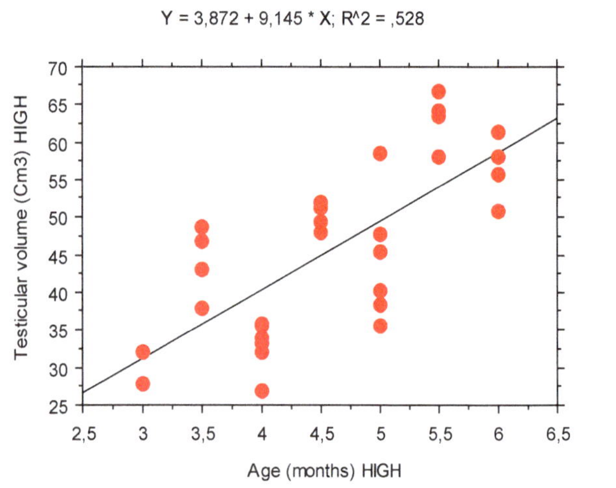

Figure 4: Development of testicular volume (cm³) in Ouled Djellal ram lambs from 3 to 6 months of age (High group).

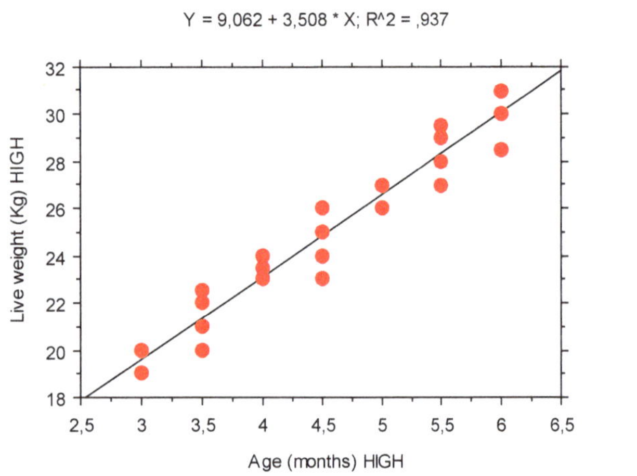

Figure 2: Development of live weight (Kg) in Ouled Djellal ram lambs from 3 to 6 months of age (High group).

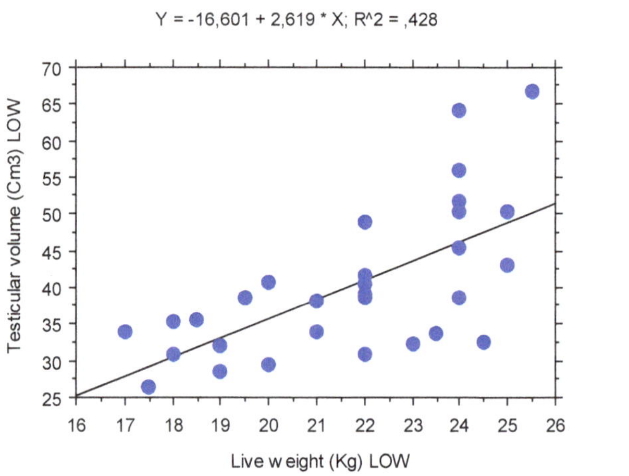

Figure 5: Development of testicular volume (cm³) and live weight (Kg) in Ouled Djellal ram lambs from 3 to 6 months of age (Low group).

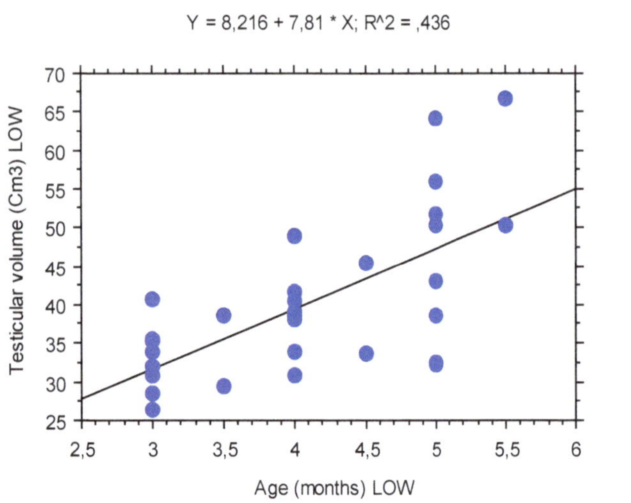

Figure 3: Development of testicular volume (Cm³) and live weight (Kg) in Ouled Djellal ram lambs from 3 to 6 months of age (Low group).

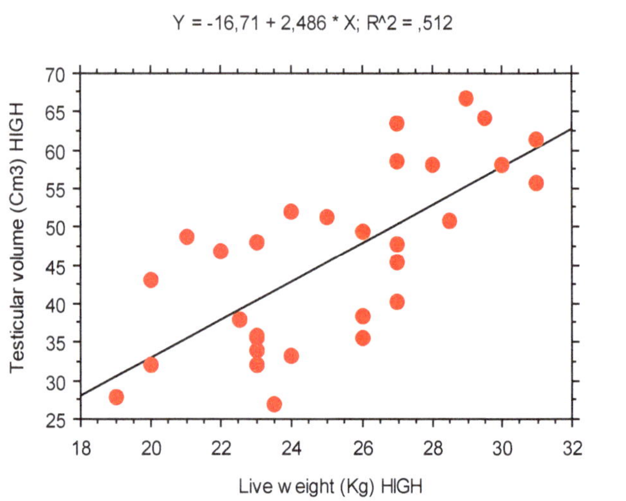

Figure 6: Development of testicular volume (cm³) and live weight (Kg) in Ouled Djellal ram lambs from 3 to 6 months of age (Higher group).

62.79 ± 6.98 cm^3 to 3 months, respectively, 4 months and 5 months of age in Ouled Djellal ram lambs keeping at the experimental station of EL- Meniaa and receiving two levels of dietary supplementation based on barley (250 g or 500 g/head/day). While Koyuncu et al. [23] reported an average testicular volume (measured by immersing the testicles in a graduated container of water) of 87.57 ± 5.92 cm^3, and 157.49 ± 5.98 cm^3 to 2 months and 6 months of age respectively in Turkey Kivircik ram lambs (farming system intensive and weaning at 60 days) [24,25].

Our results differ significantly from those reported by other authors as lambs in experiment were receiving different diets related to the types of forage offered and the quality and quantity of concentrate supplementation consumed. Furthermore, methods of measurement of testicular volume differs from one practitioner to another (calipers, orchidometer, graduated with water container .... etc.). The differences among all the studies in the literature may be due to breed, age, season and feeding strategies and other environmental/management practices [26-29].

Correlations between different parameters (age, live weight and testicular volume)

Live weight of Ouled Djellal ram lambs were positively correlated with the age according both of the two groups (High: R=0.96 and Low: R=0.96). Our results were similar to those reported by Elmaz et al. [2] which showed strong correlation between age and weight (R=0.89) [30,31] (Figures 1 and 2).

Testicular volume of Ouled Djellal ram lambs were positively correlated with the age according both of the two groups (Higher : R=0.72 and Lower : R=0.66) [32]. Our findings were in agreement with those reported by Elmaz et al. [2] which showed strong correlation between age and weight (R=0.83) [33,34] (Figures 3-6).

Regression equation presented in Figure 6 describe the relationship with body weight and testicular volume of ram lambs of both the two groups (High : R=0.65 and Low : R=0.71). In agreement with Chafri et al. [24] reported that scrotal circumference is strongly correlated with live weight of lambs D'man race with a coefficient of R=0.95) and Elmaz et al. [2] which showed strong correlation (R=0.86) between body weight and testicular volume. These results also corroborated those of Toure and Meyer [25]. The trend of testicular and body growth noticed in this study was similar also to that described by Mahouachi and et al. [26] in Dman lambs and Courot Richetin [27] in Ile-de-France ram lambs [35-38].

Conlusions

Depending on the results of the present study it was possibly to confirm the effect of a high level and adequate diet on weight and testicular growth in Ouled Djellal ram lambs from the early age just after weaning until the prepubertal age of six months. Moreover, a close relationship was found between the different parameters live weight, testicular volume and age of the animals throughout the period of the experiment. Therefore, the nutrition management during the crucial period of development may be a useful tool to maximize productivity in flocks and it can be considered to reduce the costs of keeping surplus ram lambs.

References

1. Nedjraoui N (2006) Appui à la mise en œuvre du NEPAD-PDDAA. Volume V. de V du NEPAD-PDDAA. Appui au développement de la filière ovine avec installation d'un abattoir aux normes internationales dans la wilaya de Djelfa (Algérie).
2. Elmaz Ö, Cirit U, Demir H (2007) Relationship of testicular development with age, body weight, semen characteristics and testosterone in Kivircik ram lambs. S Afr J Anim Sci 37: 269-274.
3. Benyoucef MT, Madani T, Abbas K (2000) Systèmes d'élevage et objectifs de sélection chez les ovins en situation semi-aride algérienne. In: Gabiña D (ed). Analysis and definition of the objectives in genetic improvement programmes in sheep and goats. An economic approach to increase their profitability. Zaragoza: CIHEAM. pp: 101-109.
4. Davidson, JN, Farver TB (1980) Conception rate of Holstein bulls for artificial insemination on a California dairy. J Dairy Sci 63: 621-626.
5. Syrstad O (1981) Selection for fertility on the basis of AI data. Livestock Prod Sci 8: 247-252.
6. Dýrmundsson ÓR, Lees JL (1972) Puberal development of Clun Forest ram lambs in relation to time of birth. J Agri Sci 79: 83-89.
7. Dyrmundsson OR (1973) Puberty and early reproductive performance in sheep rams lambs. Animal Breeding Abstracts 41: 419-430.
8. Marson J, Meuris S, Cooper RW, Jouannet P (1991) Puberty in the Male Chimpanzee: Progressive Maturation of Semen Characteristics. Biol Reprod 44: 448-455.
9. Titaouine M (2015) Approche de l'étude zootechnico-sanitaire des ovins de la race Ouled Djellal dans l'Est Algérien : Evolution des paramètres biochimiques et hématologiques en fonction de l'altitude. Université El- Hadj Lakhdar de Batna (Algérie). Thèse Doctorale ès Science, p: 45.
10. Yilmaz M, Altin T (2011) Growth characteristics in lambs of estrus synchronized ewes in grower conditions. Turk J Vet Anim Sci 35: 421-429.
11. Benchohra M, Boulkaboul A, Aggad H, Amara K, Hémida H (2014) Production laitière, croissance et comportement des agneaux chez le mouton Rembi en période d'allaitement. Algerian Journal of arid environment 4: 31-41.
12. Dekhili M, Mahnane S (2004) Facteurs de l'accroissement en poids des agneaux Ouled Djellal de la naissance au sevrage. Rencontres de la Recherche sur les Ruminants 11: 235.
13. Rouissi H, Ben Souissi N, Dridi S, Chaieb K, Tlili S, et al. (2001) Performances zootech niques de l a race ovine Si ci l o-Sarde en Tunisie. In: Productionsystems and product quality in sheep and goats. Rubino R, Moran d-Fehr P (eds.). Zaragoza: CIHEAM, pp: 231-236.
14. Chafri N, Mahouachi M (2011) Effet du niveau alimentaire intra-uterin sur le moment d'apparition de la puberté et la croissance testiculaire et corporelle chez les agneaux de la race D'man. Renc Rech Ruminants 18: 105.
15. El fadili M (2008) Performances en croisement et facteurs de variation des ovins Beni Guil au Maroc : Caractères de reproduction de la brebis et de viabilité et de croissance pré-sevrage des agneaux. Revue d'élevage et de médecine vétérinaire des pays tropicaux 61: 197-202.
16. Boussena S (2013) Performances de reproduction chez les ovins Ouled Djellal: Avènement de la puberté et évolution des caractéristiques séminales chez le mâle jusqu'à l'âge de 1 an (Algérie). Thèse Doctorale ès Sciences. Université de Constantine (Algérie) 1: 55.
17. Lamrani F, Benyounes A, Benyounes A (2015) Croissance d'agneaux Ouled Djellal élevés sur chaumes de céréales dans la région de Guelma, Algérie. Livestock Res Rural Develop, p: 27.
18. Courot M, Ortavant R (1980) Endocrine control of spermatogenesis in the ram. J Reprod Fertil 30: 47-60.
19. Oatley JM, Tibary A, de Avila DM, Wheaton JE, McLean DJ, et al. (2005) Changes in spermatogenesis and endocrine function in the ram testis due to irradiation and active immunization against luteinizing hormone-releasing hormone. J Anim Sci 83: 604-612.
20. Notter DR, Lucas JR, McClaugherty FS (1981) Accuracy of estimation of testis weight from *in situ* testis measures in ram lambs. Theriogenology 15: 227-234.
21. Belibasaki S, Kouimtzis S (2000) Sexual activity and body and testis growth in prepubertal ram lambs of Friesland, Chios, Karagouniki and Serres dairy sheep in Greece. Small Rumin Res 37: 109-113.
22. Kahal A (2010) Effet de l'alimentation sur la fonction sexuelle au cours de l'installation de la puberté chez les agneaux de race Oulad Djella. Mémoire de Magister en Sciences de la Nature. Université des Sciences de la Technologie Houari Boumediene (Algérie), p: 36.

23. Koyuncu M, Karauzun S, Ozis S, Duru S (2005) Development of testicular dimensions and size, and their relationship to age and body weight in growing Kivircik (Western Thrace) ram lambs. Czech J Anim Sci 50: 243-248.

24. Chafri N, Mahouachi M, Ben Hamouda M (2008) Effets du niveau alimentaire après mise bas sur le développement de la fonction reproductive chez l'agneau de race prolifique D'man : Développement testiculaire et déclenchement de la puberté. Renc Rech Ruminants 15: 394.

25. Toure G, Meyer C (1990) Evolutions corporelle, testiculaire et comportementale chez l'agneau Djallonké. Agronomie africaine 2: 45-51.

26. Mahouachi M, Chafri N, Hamouda MB, Rekik M, Lassoued N (2011) Effets de la nutrition sur les performances reproductives chez l'agneau et le bélier. In: Options Méditerranéennes. Séries A. Mediterranean Seminars. OEP, Office de l'Elevage et des Pâturages, Tunis Belvédère (Tunisia); IRESA, Institution de la Recherche et de l'Enseignement Supérieur Agricole, Tunis Belvédère (Tunisia); CIHEAM-IAMZ.

27. Courot M, Richetin C (1962) Dévelopment du testicule chez l'agneau. Etablissement de la spermatogenèse. Ann Biol Anim Biochim Biophys 2: 25-41.

28. Agabriel J (2007) Alimentation des bovins, ovins et caprins: besoins des animaux, valeurs des aliments: tables Inra 2007. Versailles, FRA: Editions Quae, Résumé du livre, p: 307.

29. Aissaoui C, Chibani J, Bouzebda Z (2004) Etudes des variations de la production spermatique du bélier de race Ouled Djellal soumis à un régime pauvre. 11 ème Renc. Rech. Rum 14: 380.

30. Benyoucef MT, Zahaf A, Boutebila S, Benaissa T, Kaidi R, et al. (1995) Aspects organisationnels et techniques d'un programme d'étude génétique de la race ovine Hamra dans la région de l'Ouest (Algérie). In: Strategies for sheep and goat breeding. Zaragoza : CIHEAM. pp: 215-224. (Cahiers Options Méditerranéennes; n. 11). Meeting of the joint FAO/CIHEAM Network on Sheep and Goats, Subnetwork on Animal Resources, 1995/03/26-28, Sidi-Thabet (Tunisia).

31. Boucif A, Azzi N, Tainturier D, Niar A (2007) Variations saisonnières des paramètres reproductifs chez les béliers de deux races locales algériennes. Renc Rech Ruminants 14: 380.

32. Boussena S, Bouazizi O, Zerrougui S, Derquaoui L, Tainturier D (2013) Performances de croissance corporelle et testiculaire avant le sevrage chez les agneaux de race Ouled Djellal. Revue Méd Vét 164: 191-199.

33. Buckrell BC (1987) Management of reproduction. Can Vet J 28: 374-377.

34. Chellig R (1992) Les races ovines Algériennes. Office des Publications Universitaires. Alger, p: 80.

35. Dekhili M, Benkhlif R (2005) Bilan portant sur les performances reproductives d'un troupeau de Brebis Ouled-Djellal. Rencontres de la Recherche sur les Ruminants 12: 162.

36. Dekhili M (2010) Fertilité des élevages ovins type Hodna menés en extensif dans la région de Sétif. Agronomie 1-7.

37. Ministère de l'Agriculture et du Développement Rural (MADR) (2013) Statistiques Agricoles Série B.

38. Villeneuve L (2008) Restriction alimentaire des agnelles pré-pubères et impact sur leurs performances de croissance, de reproduction et de lactation. Mémoire de Maîtrise ès Sciences. Université de Laval (Canada), p: 2.

12

Effect of Cuff Placement on Blood Pressure Measurement in Conscious Healthy Dogs

Carlos F Agudelo[1]*, Shachar Dvir[1], Zeki Yilmaz[2] and Meric Kocaturk[2]

[1]Small Animal Clinic, University of Veterinary and Pharmaceutical Sciences Brno, Czech Republic
[2]Uludag University, Veterinary Teaching Hospital, Internal Medicine Department, 16059, Gorukle, Bursa-Turkey

Abstract

Blood pressure determination is a very helpful aid in the diagnosis and monitoring of several diseases in small animal medicine. Non-invasive methods for blood pressure measurement are currently the most rapid and practical alternative in the clinical setting, however only few studies have dealt with selecting the best cuff position for its determination. The aim of the study was to determine the best site for cuff placement (limbs and tail) during non-invasive blood pressure in healthy subjects. Arterial blood pressure was measured by use of an oscilometric system in 22 clinically healthy dogs. Five consecutive measurements were obtained from five different sites: left and right median arteries, left and right tibial cranial arteries and coccygeal artery then were compared. Significant differences were found in systolic blood pressure measured from the right hind limb. Heart rate, age, and weight were not found to have a significant influence on arterial blood pressure. We suspect that the long duration of the procedure was the culprit, leading to stress, which as a result, led to higher blood pressure on the mentioned limb. Based on our results, we concluded that all limbs as well as the tail are suitable sites for routine blood pressure determination, as long as the procedure is completed within a rational time period.

Keywords: Cuff placement; Non-invasive arterial blood pressure; Dogs; Oscillometry

Introduction

Scientific advancements in modern medicine have helped prolong significantly human life length. In the veterinary field, these achievements have been just marginal; more of them due to adequate veterinary preventive care, among others. However, it is expected that in the next decades there will be also great progresses in the field of companion animal medicine due to the tendency to suffer from conditions related to ageing, as occurs in human beings [1]. Diseases like chronic renal disease, cancer or heart disease are very common in the geriatric dog or cat [2]. A very common complication from the above mentioned circumstances is systemic hypertension, and when properly diagnosed, warrant classification and management. Systemic hypertension is of concern, because can cause injury to tissues, commonly referred to as Target-Organ Damage (TOD), which is generally a strong indication for antihypertensive therapy [3,4].

Recent advancements in diagnostic techniques to determine Blood Pressure (BP) make possible to obtain rapid and accurate measurements in conscious animals. One priority for a busy practitioner and owners is to obtain quick and reliable results by using non-invasive methods. Due to the increasing accuracy, reliability, and promptness of Non-Invasive Blood Pressure (NIBP) measurement systems, as well as their reasonable cost, they are now becoming a significant diagnostic tool in daily clinical practice [5]. Clinical applications range from routine screening (preventive care) through diagnosis and monitoring the course of a disease [6]. Regular follow-ups have been to gained a long-term trend-line of individual measurements [3,6]. As patients age, changes in the trend line can be used as an indication of a possible underlying disease [3]. To regard, many factors make BP determination in dogs very challenging. Since small animals have relatively small blood vessels and they possess fur, which complicates repeated measurements, BP determination in dogs is very challenging [7]. However, other factors such as breed, age, gender, and degree of anxiety also influence BP. Furthermore, there is a minute-to-minute spontaneous physiological change in BP, as well as circadian changes [4]. Due to the aforementioned reasons, during the last years, there have been attempts to increase the accuracy and reliability of NIBP techniques. The efforts to standardise have been initiated by the veterinary blood pressure society, aimed by the ACVIM, which devised a consensus statement in the form of a diagnostic protocol to minimize bias including human and devised related [3]. Although effects of body position on indirect BP measurements [8,9] and relations between BP measurement techniques and selected cuff positions in dogs [10] were reported, different cuff placements and its relation with physiologic parameters using a single BP method in healthy conscious dogs are not studied yet.

The aims of the present study were to determine BP values in different body places using an Oscillometric System (OS) in conscious healthy dogs, and determine relationships between BP and heart rate (HR), body weight, age and total measurement time.

Materials and Methods

Patients

Twenty-two dogs (5 males, 17 females) between 10 months and 10 years of age (5.3 ± 0.98), weighing between 3.5-40 kg (19.3 ± 4.6) participated in the study (Table 1). The subjects belonged to faculty staff and students of the University of Veterinary and Pharmaceutical Sciences Brno. No requirements, other than being clinically normal were established.

***Corresponding author:** Carlos F Agudelo, Assistant Professor, University of Veterinary Medicine and Pharmaceutical Sciences Brno, Small Animal Clinic, Palackeho tr. 1946/1, 612 42 Brno, Brno, 61242, Czech Republic
E-mail: cagudelo@vfu.cz

Measurement of BP

The procedure was conducted without the presence of the owners. During the procedure, only two individuals were present in the room - the investigator, which operated the equipment, and one assistant (nurse or student). A not populated room was specifically chosen for this purpose, which offered a quite environment, without interference. In there, dogs were allowed several minutes to acclimatize. Measurements of BP were acquired from the right and left median and cranial tibial arteries and coccygeal artery in both right and left lateral recumbent positions. The examined limb was contralateral to a side in which the patient was laying in order to maintain the limb at the approximate with the cuff at or close to the level of the right atrium and reduce the effect of pressure on the arteries. Commercial washable BP cuffs were used. The cuff size was determined (~40% of the circumference of the limb) and first applied to the left forelimb (medioproximal to the carpus). The patient was minimally restrained, and once it was calm, a series of 5 measurements of BP (systolic, diastolic and mean arterial pressures) were obtained. Subsequent measurements were carried out in this order: left hind limb (above the hock), base of the tail, right forelimb and right hind limb. The sequence of measurements was maintained in all patients and the time recorded (Table 1). An automatic OS was used (Vetmon 2200, Czech Republic). Values of systolic, mean and diastolic blood pressure (SAP, MAP and DAP respectively) were displayed. The highest and lowest values were discarded, and an average of the remaining values was calculated.

Statistical analysis

Normality of all variables was confirmed using Shapiro-Wilk test. To determine differences of BP between cuff sites ANOVA test was used. A Tukey's Honestly Significant Difference (HSD) Post-Hoc tests for one-way ANOVA were used to evaluate differences between means. Pearson's correlation coefficient was used to assess associations of BP with HR, weight and age. The results in all tests were considered significant when $p<0.05$

Results

A total of 550 measurements were obtained from 22 clinically normal dogs at 5 sites using an OS (Table 1). Though unrecorded, total measurement time for all BP was assessed from 35 to 90 minutes. All values distributed normally. ANOVA tests found significant differences between cuff placements for SAP ($p=0.01$) and MAP ($p=0.03$) whereas DAP did not show significant differences ($p=0.12$). Tukey HSD Post-Hoc tests revealed that source of difference in SAP (consequently in MAP) among placements was due to the values obtained from the right hind limb (Figure 1).

SAP and MAP values were found to be the highest in the right cranial tibial artery (158 mm Hg and 120 mm Hg respectively) (Figure 2). There were no correlations between of BP with HR, weight and age.

Discussion

In this study, BP measurements and its relation with body weight, age and measurement time were discussed based on five different cuff placements in healthy conscious dogs. Our results showed that all limbs and tail might be used for routine BP determination in dogs. There is only a handful of information in the literature and the web concerning cuff placement in veterinary patients. In general, different sources coincided that the limb one uses should be at heart level. Anecdotally on dogs, the best site for cuff placement would be over the metacarpal area and alternately, either the metatarsal area. On cats, between the elbow and the carpus, however the tail is also an acceptable site to measure

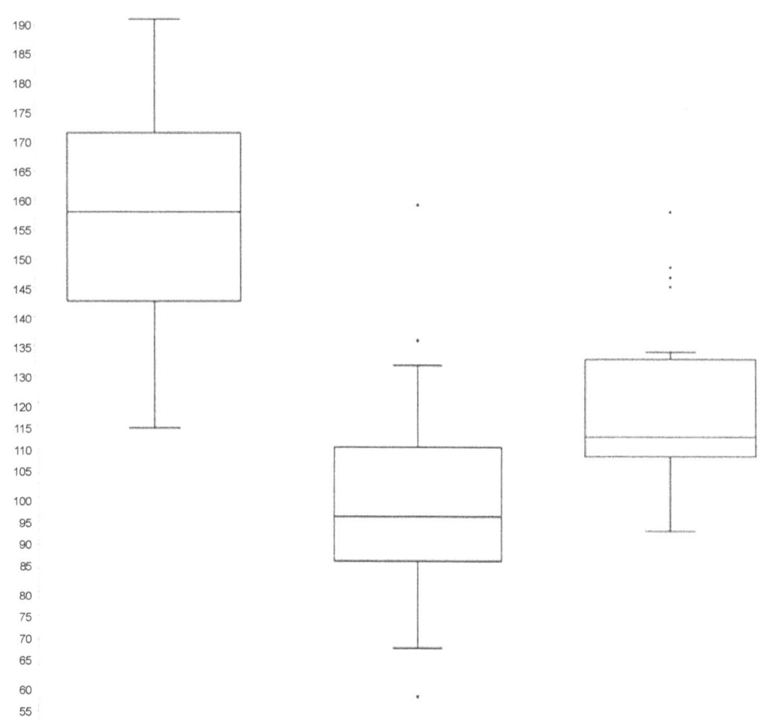

Figure 1: Results of average BP readings in 5 different cuff placements. The highest values were observed in the right hind limb at the end of whole procedure.

		Left									Right						
		Forelimb			Hind Limb			Tail			Forelimb			Hind Limb			
Breed	Weight	S	D	M	S	D	M	S	D	M	S	D	M	S	D	M	Duration
Golden retriever	34	131	80	105	155	71	90	127	69	92	148	86	101	138	96	113	60
manchester terrier	10	151	97	114	169	108	140	144	87	110	147	95	118	185	125	145	86
GSD (Ron)	40	165	102	121	172	104	119	153	88	108	156	128	123	162	108	127	80
Mixed	12	95	71	82	162	124	142	147	95	113	144	115	124	169	129	143	97
Golden retriever	25	121	59	79	121	40	83	97	53	68	126	73	92	149	57	103	37
Golden retriever	30	133	61	82	119	43	74	117	57	80	155	79	106	135	78	99	35
mixed	12	164	87	122	179	87	111	140	66	85	180	93	133	191	94	148	55
Visla	16	141	90	104	141	83	105	147	78	105	128	75	87	139	73	99	47
Wired-haired visla	20	145	92	107	126	70	88	151	101	116	127	94	105	176	95	108	122
WWT	6.5	190	96	142	155	121	133	167	100	131	193	152	167	159	113	131	60
mixed	32	147	78	90	160	78	112	134	61	99	131	74	95	140	89	110	60
mixed	28	119	73	85	136	93	109	126	66	83	138	64	92	152	92	113	82
mixed	16	132	78	96	168	72	105	145	81	102	142	88	109	178	92	114	45
Border Collie	15	156	100	131	142	81	96	121	64	85	137	85	103	148	97	114	95
Border Collie	15	117	71	86	129	64	83	134	84	105	135	72	96	142	87	112	79
Mini schnauzer	7	137	73	100	175	96	134	134	53	91	128	65	90	157	67	114	117
daschhound	8	190	121	133	203	104	161	123	57	93	145	66	89	162	88	114	42
Am. Staff Terrier	25	148	113	126	147	112	133	179	121	149	164	127	146	162	108	129	99
GS	25	121	62	77	144	103	117	113	73	99	119	66	96	121	79	95	30
mixed	13	132	74	101	184	100	141	136	74	99	147	69	98	170	94	117	80
Jack russel terrier	7	132	104	116	140	109	123	175	119	139	177	107	145	192	150	166	103
mixed	3.5	169	110	128	162	131	143	158	96	112	143	71	94	155	107	123	123

Table 1: Blood pressure measurements in 22 healthy dogs. Breed, weight, BP values (S: systolic; D: diastolic; M: mean), and duration of the protocol are engraved.

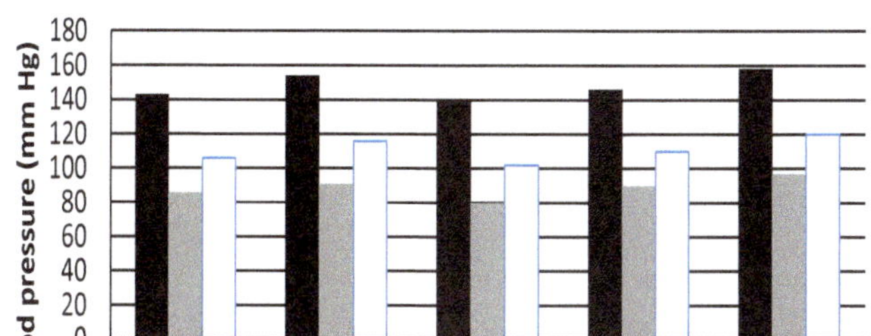

	Left forelimb	Left hindlimb	Tail	Right forelimb	Right hindlimb
SAP	143	154	139	146	158
DAP	86	91	80	90	97
MAP	106	116	102	110	120

Figure 2: Results of average BP readings in 5 different cuff placements. The highest values were observed in the right hind limb at the end of whole procedure.

BP in both species [11]. One study determined five measurement sites (coccygeal, metacarpal, metatarsal, tibial, and median arteries) by comparing OS and ultrasonic Doppler devices with a standardized invasive radio telemetric system [12]. OS showed that coccygeal and tibial sites were the most correlated whereas Doppler determined that metatarsal site provided the strongest correlation. Another study determined reference values of BP in unsedated Irish Wolfhounds by OS at the coccygeal artery and the effect of body position on BP showing that DAP was significantly lower when measured in a standing position compared to lateral recumbence [8]. Human studies have not shown uniformity in results, where both increases and decreases in BP were observed after changes in body position [13,14]. These findings certainly raise the question whether there is a relationship between hypertension and posture with regards to alterations in BP.

In our study, significant changes in SAP were observed which also probably affected by directly accurate changes in the MAP. Previous research comparing simultaneous direct and indirect BP measurements suggested that SAP varies the most, either due to greater liability or greater measurement error [15]. The same conducted work also found DAP to be the least variable, both within (moment-by-moment variability) and between occasions (day-to-day variability), therefore more accurately reflecting the *true* BP. The differences of SAP measurements due to cuff placements (limbs and tail) were higher than that of DAP and MAP measurements. This might be explained, at least in part, by the distal pulse wave amplification phenomenon. The pulse pressure increases from the central aorta to the peripheral muscular arteries in the extremities due to reflected pulse waves and distensibility (stiffness) differences between aorta and peripheral arteries [16]. However, one should interpret carefully any result due to measurement artefacts like stress or related with operator and used devices or to the fact that SAP between occasion's decreases as more measurements are obtained. Because the above reasons, we used healthy dogs belonging to students or staff because they are get used to manipulation and to the clinical environment. These findings support once more that more emphasis should be given to DAP rather than SAP when evaluating a patient's health status using OS.

One of the main problems encountered during the procedure was the length of the OS to obtain a measurement and in some instances when movements of the dog have caused to errors. As a result, instead of completing a series of 25 measurements within the allotted 30-45 minutes, in several cases it took up to 1.5 hours. Several studies have found that the traditional OS consistently underestimates BP in conscious dogs [12,17,18]. The use of high-definition oscilometric systems could refine accuracy of measurements, as it contains a 32 bit processor (compared to 8 bit processor in conventional OS) which is much less prone to errors. Undoubtedly, the length of the procedure had a significant effect on the accuracy of measurements (Table 1). First, it was difficult for some of the dogs to remain calm for such an extended period of time. Second, it was frustrating for the investigators, which could also have been sensed by the patients. Several studies have concluded that anxious dogs have higher SAP, DAP and MAP [4,17].

All measurements were done in lateral recumbence in order to maintain cuff places at roughly the level of the heart. When a measurement site that is much lower than the heart, will lead to falsely elevated values and vice versa [13]. This procedure was conducted in absence of the owners. White-coat effect might have increased in some patients due to the absence of the owners, however, several of the patients were owned by the clinic's staff and students, and therefore might have been less affected. This sequence might have influenced the results in some ways, since in most cases patients became calmer during the middle part of the procedure, and then more anxious towards the end. In humans, BP machines have become increasingly affordable, allowing individuals to measure their own BP at home, thus eliminating the potential white-coat effect. If this trend trickles into the veterinary community as HDO systems becomes more affordable like other diagnostics like urine glucose, etc.; remains to be seen.

Conclusion

Significant differences were found between SAP and consequently MAP obtained from and between the limbs and the tail, when measured in lateral recumbence. However, DAP showed to be the least variable then it could be used more truthfully in reproducing the *true* BP. There was no significant correlation between blood pressure, heart rate, weight, and age. Although there are many limitations to this kind of study, we achieved in to determine BP under "normal" clinical conditions; therefore the variations in the measurements, as presented throughout the study are an important reminder of the challenges faced daily by clinicians in obtaining accurate and reliable data. Although cuff placement is important, if it remains the same between occasions, its importance of the technique diminishes. Furthermore, it highlights the importance of regular monitoring of BP, in order to acquire trends, which are more correlated to patient's physical condition. Further study is may be required in order to reinforce our findings.

References

1. Docksai R (2014) Extending Pet Longevity: Our Companions in Sickness and in Health. The Futurist 48: 47-51.

2. Bush BM (1989) Pharmacy and Dispensing. In: Jones's Animal Nursing. 5th edn. Lane DR (Ed.). British Small Animal Veterinary, Pp: 351-378.

3. Brown S, Atkins C, Bagley R, Carr A, Cowgill L, et al. (2007) American College of Veterinary Internal Medicine consensus statement: Guidelines for the identification, evaluation, and management of systemic hypertension in dogs and cats. J Vet Intern Med 21: 542-558.

4. Egner B (2007) Blood pressure measurement-Basic principles and practical application. In: Essential facts of blood pressure in dogs and cats: a reference guide. 4th edn. Egner B, Carr A, Brown S (Eds.). Life learn, Inc., Pp: 1-14.

5. Erhardt W, Henke J, Carr A (2007) Techniques. In: Essential facts of blood pressure in dogs and cats: a reference guide. 4th edn. Egner B, Carr A, Brown S (Eds.). Life Learn Inc., Pp: 34-58.

6. Egner B, Erhardt W, Henke J, Carr A (2007) Indications for Blood Pressure Measurements. In: Essential facts of blood pressure in dogs and cats: a reference guide. 4th edn. Egner B, Carr A, Brown S (Eds.). Life Learn Inc., Pp: 15-31.

7. Remillard RL, Ross JN, Eddy JB (1991) Variance of indirect blood pressure measurements and prevalence of hypertension in clinically normal dogs. Am J Vet Res 52: 561-565.

8. Bright JM, Dentino M (2002) Indirect arterial blood pressure measurement in nonsedated Irish wolfhounds: reference values for the breed. J Am Anim Hosp Assoc 38: 521-526.

9. Rondeau DA, Mackalonis ME, Hess RS (2013) Effect of body position on indirect measurement of systolic arterial blood pressure in dogs. J Am Vet Med Assoc 242: 1523-1527.

10. Garofalo NA, Teixeira Neto FJ, Alvaides RK, de Oliveira FA, Pignaton W, et al. (2012) Agreement between direct, oscillometric and Doppler ultrasound blood pressures using three different cuff positions in anesthetized dogs. Vet Anaesth Analg 39: 324-334.

11. Turner SM (2005) Veterinary Ophthalmology: A Manual for Nurses and Technicians. Elsevier Health Sciences. 205 pages.

12. Haberman CE, Kang CW, Morgan JD, Brown SA (2006) Evaluation of oscillometric and Doppler ultrasonic methods of indirect blood pressure estimation in conscious dogs. Can J Vet Res 70: 211-217.

13. Netea RT, Smits P, Lenders JW, Thien T (1998) Does it matter whether blood pressure measurements are taken with subjects sitting or supine? J Hypertens 16: 263-268.

14. Lu LC, Wei TM, Li S, Ye XL, Zeng CL, et al. (2008) Differences in blood pressure readings between supine and sitting postions in hypertensive patients. Acta Cardiol 63: 707-711.

15. Bodey AR, Mitchel AR (1997) Longitudinal studies of reproducibility and variability of indirect (oscillometric) blood pressure measurements in dogs: evidence for tracking. Res Vet Sci 63: 15-21.

16. Avolio AP, Van Bortel LM, Boutouyrie P, Cockcroft JR, McEniery CM, et al. (2009) Role of pulse pressure amplification in arterial hypertension: experts' opinion and review of the data. Hypertension 54: 375-383.

17. Bodey AR, Michell AR, Bovee KC, Buranakurl C, Garg T (1996) Comparison of direct and indirect (oscillometric) measurement of arterial blood pressure in conscious dogs. Res Vet Sci 61: 17-21.

18. Chalifoux A, Dallaire A, Blais D, Lariviere N, Pelletier N (1985) Evaluation of the arterial blood pressure of dogs by two noninvasive methods. Can J Comp Med 49: 419-423.

Small Ruminant Brucellosis and Public Health Awareness in Two Districts of Afar Region, Ethiopia

Anteneh Hailu Tegegn[1], Aklilu Feleke[2], Wesinew Adugna[3] and Simenew Keskes Melaku[4*]

[1]*Semeral Veterinary Regional Laboratory, Afar, Ethiopia*
[2]*College of Veterinary Medicine and Agriculture, Addis Ababa University, PO Box 34, Bishoftu, Ethiopia*
[3]*VSF Suisse, Addis Ababa, Ethiopia*
[4]*College of Agriculture and Natural Resources, Dilla University, PO Box 419, Dilla, Ethiopia*

Abstract

Cross-sectional serological and questionnaire surveys were employed on small ruminants to determine the prevalence of brucellosis, identify risk factors and public health implications. Brucellosis is a bacterial disease with high economic and public health importance in the sub-Sahara countries in particular. A total of 1190 blood samples were collected from shoats (876 caprine and 314 ovine) in Chifra and Ewa districts. One hundred fifty five (13%) of the samples tested were positive using mRBPT. Further testing of the positive reactors for mRBPT with CFT revealed 147 (12.35%) seropositivity for brucella. The result showed that among the risk factors considered in the analysis, species, sex, age, parity number and flock size had statistically significant effect on seropositivity ($p<0.05$). Goats were more than 2 times (OR=2.34) at risk of getting infected with brucella than sheep. The seroprevalence was also significantly higher in female (13.8%) than in male (6.5%) animals. The odds of seropositivity in older animals are 2.36 times higher than that of younger ones. Individual animal seroprevalence was higher in larger flocks than in smaller ones (OR=0.68). The habit of drinking raw milk was practiced by almost all of the respondents. Poor awareness of the zoonotic importance of brucellosis and the practices of consuming raw milk and handling potentially infectious materials using bare hands pose a serious danger to small ruminant owners. There is a need for planning and implementation of joint programs by stakeholders in prevention and control of the disease as well as raising public awareness.

Keywords: Afar region; Brucellosis; CFT; Public health; RBPT; Small ruminants

Introduction

Brucellosis is a zoonotic bacterial disease caused by Brucella species and is primarily a disease of animals and humans are accidental hosts [1]. The disease is an important public health problem but neglected in many parts of the world [1-3]. The disease is more important in developing countries and has important economic and public health consequences [3]. Brucellosis has been virtually eradicated from majority of developed countries; but important disease among livestock and people in sub-Saharan Africa [4].

Infection in animals is strongly correlated with abortions in the last trimester of pregnancy and commonly affected animals include bovine, ovine, caprine, swine, and some other domestic animals including camels [3,5]. In animals, the primary sign of infection in females is abortion and in males epididymitis and orchitis and diagnosis can only be confirmed by laboratory tests that may even confirm latent infections [1]. Cross-transmission of brucellosis can occur among cattle, sheep, goats, camels and other species [6].

Brucellosis is a major cause of direct economic losses resulting from clinical disease, abortion, neonatal losses, reduced fertility, decreased milk production, emergency slaughtering of the infected animals and treatment costs. It also plays a significant role as a barrier for international trade of live animals by being used as an impediment to free animal movement and export [7]. Economic losses in small ruminants stem from breeding inefficiency, loss of lambs and kids, reduced wool, meat and milk production [8].

In Africa, little is known about its epidemiological status in animals and neither the factors contributing to its cross-species nor to human transmission [9]. The huge and diverse livestock species in Ethiopia are kept under different agro-ecological zones, management systems, migration and animal health care system. The predominant extensive husbandry practices of the country provide ample opportunities for mixing of different animal species at communal grazing areas and watering points [10].

More importantly, a close human-animal contact and tradition of raw animal product consumption make zoonosis among the major public health hazards, with particular implication to pastoral area. This requires a thorough epidemiological investigations including due consideration to identifying the major risk factors that predominantly influence the disease occurrence, and thus contribute to design appropriate and feasible national controlling strategies. Brucellosis in sheep and goats mainly caused by *Brucella melitensis* is characterized by abortion, stillbirths and reproductive failure. According to AU-IBAR [11], small ruminants' brucellosis was not reported from Ethiopia, although high prevalence rate of up to 13.6 by Wesinew et al. [5] in small ruminants. In Afar region very little attempts were done and there were no such studies yet in the current target districts. Therefore, this study is designed with the objectives to determine prevalence of brucellosis in small ruminants and its public health impact in Ewa and Chifra districts and to identify risk factors and sources of infection for livestock and humans.

***Corresponding author:** Simenew Keskes Melaku, College of Agriculture and Natural Resources, Dilla University, PO Box 419, Dilla, Ethiopia
E-mail: drsimenew@yahoo.com or simenew.keskes@aau.edu.et

Materials and Methods

Study area

The study was carried out in two districts namely Chifra and Ewa, located in Zone one and Zone four respectively of Afar National Regional State (ANRS). Chifra and Ewa districts are found 174 and 219 kilometer far from Semera town respectively. The districts are found adjacently and share boundary with Amhara region. Chifra district has 1 urban and 19 rural peasant associations while Ewa contains 1 urban and 9 rural peasant associations. May/June is the driest season of the year, 'hagay'. It is said to be unsuitable for browsing since bushes dry up. The main rainy season 'Karma', accounts for above 60% of the annual total rainfall are from July to September. This is followed by the best grazing season of 'Kayra' that occurs from September to November. Another minor rainy season is Sugum and appears during March and April. 'Gilal' is less severe dry season with relatively cool temperatures (November to March). Occasional rainfalls called dada may interrupt 'Gilal' [12].

Study animals

The study animals were indigenous Afar goat and sheep characterized by ILRI [13]. Ovine and caprine which were above 6 months of age with no history of vaccination against brucellosis were included in the study. Then individual animal age, species, sex, flock size and parity were recorded. The study animals consisted of 1190 traditionally managed small ruminants of which 146 ovine and 214 caprine were obtained from Ewa district while the remaining 168 ovine and 662 caprine were obtained from Chifra district.

Study design and sampling strategies

A cross-sectional study design was devised from November 2013 to April 2014 to determine the seroprevalence of brucellosis in sheep and goats from the two selected study districts. Two districts were selected purposively based on easier accessibility as well as ovine and caprine populations. At the present, there are 20 and 10 PAs in Chifra and Ewa districts, respectively. Peasant associations in the districts were selected simple randomly in the ratio of 2:1 (Chifra (6) and Ewa (3) districts, respectively). Peasant association is the lowest administrative unit within a district considered. A total of 1,190 sera samples were collected from 45 flocks of small ruminants.

Two districts from zone one and zone four of the existing five zones were selected purposively; and a multistage random sampling method were used to select the sampling units. Households were the sampling units and the principles of simple random sampling technique to select peasant associations and systematic random sampling to sample the households were followed at each stage of sampling. The numbers of animals included in the study were distributed proportionally over the PAs.

Sample size determination

The total number of animals to be sampled were calculated using Win Episcope 2.0, an improved epidemiological software for veterinary medicine developed for simple random sampling with the under mentioned assumption and an infinite population and inflated the estimated sample size to 1190 small ruminants [14]. A 5% absolute precision and 95% confidence interval were used for determining sample size. Since previous study in the region indicated that prevalence rate of 5.7% (Chifra) and 2.4% (Ewa), an expected prevalence of 20% were used to obtain the maximum sample size. Accordingly, 246 animals were the calculated sample size for each Chifra and Ewa district. In order to get representative sample for both districts inflated the sample size to 1190. Therefore; the appropriate sample sizes were 830 and 360 ovine and caprine for Chifra and Ewa district respectively. In general 1190 sera samples were collected from 45 flocks of small ruminants.

$$n = \frac{1.96^2 \times P_{exp}\ (1-P)}{d^2}$$

Where n=the total sample size

P=expected prevalence

d^2=absolute precision

Methodologies

Questionnaire survey: A structured questionnaire was administered to livestock owners/herders men after pretesting in the field properly and translated to the local language 'Afarigna'. Verbal consent was obtained from the respondents after the objective of the survey is explained to them before starting the interview. This questionnaire was designed for a survey of the potential risk factors associated with the disease in their flocks and to gather relevant information on the overall small ruminants' management practices, knowledge about zoonotic diseases, habit of consuming animal products, handling of aborted fetuses and other potentially contaminated materials.

Serological survey: Approximately 8 ml of blood from jugular vein of sheep and goats were collected aseptically using sterile plain vacutainer tubes. The samples were properly labelled and left for overnight at room temperature to allow clotting and the sera were decanted and stored in sterile Eppendorf tubes at -20°C in Samara Regional Veterinary Laboratory until tested for antibodies in National Veterinary Institute.

Modified Rose Bengal Plate Test (mRBPT): All sera samples collected were screened using the RBPT, according to the procedures described by Alton et al. [15] and the World Organisation for Animal Health [16,17]. This test was done at Semera Regional Veterinary Laboratory in order to screen positive samples by RBPT using RBPT antigen (Institue Pourquier 325, rue de la galèra 34097 Montpellier cedex 5, France). Positive sera were then retested using complement fixation test (CFT) at the National Veterinary Institute.

In brief, 75 µl of serum was mixed with 25 µl of antigen suspension on a glass plate and agitated. After four minutes of rocking, any visible agglutination was considered as positive [16]. Agglutinations were recorded as 0, +, ++ and +++, according to the degree of agglutination. A score of 0 indicates the absence of agglutination; + indicates barely visible agglutination; ++ indicates fine agglutination, and +++ indicates coarse clumping. Those samples with no agglutination (0) were recorded as negative while those with +, ++ and +++ were recorded as positive [17].

Complement Fixation Test (CFT): All the reagents required for CFT were evaluated by titration. Positive sera with RBPT were further tested with CFT for confirmation using standard *B. abortus* antigen (New Haw, Addleston, and Surrey KT15 3NB, UK). The CFT test proper and reagent preparation procedures were following the procedures outlined by Ref. [16]. Sera with strong reaction, more than 75% fixation of complement (3+) at a dilution of 1:5 or at least with 50% fixation of complement (2+) at a dilution of 1:10 and above were classified as positive [16].

Statistical analyses

Data obtained from both serological tests and questionnaire surveys were stored in Microsoft excel spreadsheet program. Descriptive and analytic statistics were computed using SPSS® Version 20.0. Logistic regression was employed to identify possible risk factors associated with seropositivity in sheep and goats. The degree of association was computed using odds ratio (OR) signified by 95% confidence intervals [14].

Results

Individual and flock level seroprevalence of brucellosis

The highest individual animal level seroprevalence was recorded in goat from species group in both Chifra and Ewa woredas. The overall flock level seroprevalence of brucellosis infection was 57.8% while it was 60% and 53.3% in Chifra and Ewa district respectively. The difference in seropositivity between species in both woredas was statistically significant ($p<0.05$) as presented in Table 1.

Risk factors affecting individual animal level seroprevalence of brucellosis

The results revealed that among the risk factors considered in the analysis, species, sex, age, parity number and flock size had statistically significant effect on seropositivity ($p<0.05$) as indicated in Table 2.

The risk factors with significant effect after univariate logistic regression test (species, sex, age, parity and flock size) were fitted in a multivariate model and the results showed that all the factors except districts had statistically significant effect on the seroprevalence of brucellosis in sheep and goat populations ($p<0.05$) (Table 3). Age was dropped from the multivariate model due to the likelihood of confounding the effects of parity. The results of univariate logistic regression analysis are presented in Table 4.

Zone	District	Species	No. Tested	CFT positive	p-value	Flock level	
						No tested	Positive (%)
	Chifra	Overall	830	104 (12.5%)	0.018	30	18 (60%)
1		Ovine	168	12 (7.14%)			
		Caprine	662	92 (13.8%)			
	Ewa	Overall	360	43(12.0%)	0.005	15	8 (53.3%)
4		Ovine	146	9 (6.16%)			
		Caprine	214	34 (15.89%)			

Table 1: Individual animal and flock level seroprevalence of brucellosis in sheep and goat populations in Chifra and Ewa woredas, Afar Region.

Risk factors	Category	Prevalence	OR	95% CI	p-value
Woreda	*1(Chifra)	12.5%		0.648-1.383	0.778
	4 (Ewa)	12%	0.947		
Species	*Ovine	6.7%		1.44-3.79	0.001
	Caprine	14.4%	2.34		
Sex	*Male	6.5%		0.24-0.75	0.003
	Female	13.8%	2.12		
Age/Years	*<2 years	2.8%			
	2-5 years	16.4%	5.86 7.1	1.84-3.02	0.000
	>5 years	20%			
Parity	*0	1.3%			
	1-2	10.2%	7.7 16.9	1.07-1.56	0.006
	3-4	22%			
Flock size	*≤ 25	36.8%		0.46-0.99	0.011
	>25	73%	1.93		

*Reference category; OR: Odds ratio; CI: Confidence interval

Table 2: Results of univariate logistic regression analysis of risk factors.

CFT	Odds Ratio	(95% CI)	p-value
Species	2.131	1.53-3.44	0.003
Sex	0.138	0.059-0.321	0.000
Parity	*2.038*	1.303-3.187	0.002
Flock size	*0.761*	0.684-1.523	0.011

Table 3: Multivariate logistic regression analysis of risk factors of brucellosis in small ruminants.

Risk factors	Category	Number of flocks	Infected flocks	(95% CI)	p-value	OR
Flock size	*≤ 25*	19	7	0.46-0.99	0.011	0.68
	>25	26	19			
Districts	*Chifra*	30	18	0.648-1.383	0.778	0.947
	Ewa	15	8			

OR: Odds ratio; CI: Confidence interval

Table 4: Risk factors associated with seroprevalence occurrence at flock level of small ruminants.

Risk factors affecting the flock level seroprevalence of brucellosis

Seroprevalence of brucellosis was statistically significant in larger sized flocks than in smaller ones and in Chifra than in Ewa ($p<0.05$) as stipulated in Table 4.

Public health importance of brucellosis

The results of the questionnaire survey on the perception and practices of livestock owners in the study areas are presented below. Most of the outcomes of the analysis of the questionnaire data showed that livestock owners in the studied areas are at high risk of contracting brucellosis from infected animals. Almost all the respondents in the studied areas were not aware of brucellosis as a disease affecting different species of livestock (91.1%) although all respondents (45 livestock owners) interviewed recognized the existence of abortion (locally called in Afarigna as "Feneg-dalay") among small ruminant flocks and most of them handle abortion materials with bare hand without protecting themselves (82.2%). The habit of drinking raw milk is practiced by all the 45 interviewed respondents (100%) while there is no habit of consuming raw meat.

Discussion

The flock level prevalence is higher than individual animal level and this characterizes the nature and importance of the disease in the large flock size. This signifies that brucellosis has significant economic implication in its ability to bring about morbidity at flock level. Above all the higher flock level prevalence can be considered as a serious public health concern. The study also demonstrated overall individual animal level seroprevalence of brucellosis in small ruminant was 12.35% (95% CI: 1.44-3.79). This is fairly comparable to the seroprevalence reported in Afar region by Ref. [5,18]. Since there is barely no vaccination or any other control mechanisms in the region increasing trend of prevalence is expected. Above all free movement and mixing of different herds and among species can also facilitate transmission and cross infection [19]. However, the current prevalence is lower than report by Al-Majali [20] (27.7%) and Hamidullah et al. [21] (34.88%) in Jordan. The reason for this discrepancy could be variation in management practices and level of frequent introduction of new animals. The prevalence in this study is higher than the findings by Tekleye and Kasali [22] in central highlands of Ethiopia. This could be due to the production system difference as mixed crop-livestock management is practiced in the latter.

There was statistical significant difference between ovine and caprine species. The higher seroprevalence of brucellosis in caprine 14.4% than in ovine 6.7% was comparable with Ref. [5]. This species prevalence difference might be due to the fact that ovine are more resistant than caprine and they do not shade the bacteria for long time and flocks with high numbers of ovine would have low prevalence [23]. Above all, caprine are the principal host of *B. melitensis*, whereas, ovine are not significantly infected even when kept in close contact with caprine [24]. In addition, infection in caprine can vary from acute to persistent occurrence for years whereas in ovine, the course of infection depends upon the dose of bacteria and they are resistant to re-infection.

There was statistical significant difference between male and female small ruminants in the current study. The higher seroprevalence of brucellosis in females (13.8%) than in male (6.5%) might be due to high concentration of erythritol, which is scarcely produced in male reproductive organs [25]. In addition, the Afar society supply male small ruminants to both the export and domestic markets while female small ruminants are used as replacement herd just like all pastoralists.

Animals with three or more parities showed significantly higher seroprevalence than animals with less than 3 parities. A statistically significant variation was also recorded between adults and young animals. It has been reported that brucellosis is essentially a disease of sexually mature animals [26]. Sexually mature and pregnant animals are more prone to Brucella infection and brucellosis than sexually immature animals of either sex [23]. On the other hand, it is also true that younger animals tend to be more resistant to infection and frequently clear an established infection, although latent infections can occur [27]. This may result from the hormone erythritol, which stimulate the growth and multiplication of Brucella organisms, tend to increase in concentration with age and sexual maturity [23]. No significant difference was seen between the two districts, since the similarity in agro-ecological conditions and livestock management system.

From the questionnaire survey, almost all small ruminant owners residing in the study area were able to recognize the occurrence of abortion in their flocks. More than 86% of the respondents had the habit of drinking raw milk and 82.2% of the respondents used to dispose of aborted fetuses barehanded. This may be due to lack of awareness about brucellosis together with existing habit of raw milk consumption and close contact between animals and humans.

Conclusions

Results of the present study show the importance of small ruminant brucellosis in Afar pastoral areas and identify the risk factors that contribute to the occurrence of the disease possible zoonotic implications. Critical assessment of the economic impact of the disease, which emanates from its effect on reproductive and production performance of animals, is worthy as the prevalence is high. Joint ventures among veterinary and public health professionals are of paramount importance to control this disease. Awareness creation among pastoralists on animal husbandry, disease prevention and risk of zoonotic diseases need to be undertaken. Large scale investigation level of infection in both animals and humans at risk should be done in Afar. Further studies focused on the isolation and molecular characterization of the circulating Brucella species is imperative.

References

1. Corbel MJ (2006) Brucellosis in humans and animals. World Health Organization, Geneva.
2. Hadush A, Pal M (2013) Brucellosis-An infectious re-emerging bacterial zoonosis of global importance. Int J Livest Res 3: 28-34.
3. Bekele WA, Tessema TS, Melaku SK (2013) *Camelus dromedarius* brucellosis and its public health associated risks in the Afar National Regional State in northeastern Ethiopia. Acta Vet Scand 55: 89.
4. Franco MP, Mulder M, Gilman RH, Smits HL (2007) Human brucellosis. Lancet Infect Dis 7: 775-786.
5. Adugna W, Tessema TS, Keskes S (2013) Sero-prevalence of small ruminants' brucellosis in four districts of Afar National Regional State, Northeast Ethiopia. Journal of Veterinary Medicine and Animal Health 5: 358-364.
6. Dawood HA (2008) Brucellosis in Camels (*Camelus dromedorius*) in the south province of Jordan. Am J Agri Biol Sci 3: 623-626.
7. Coelho AM, Coelho AC, Roboredo M, Rodrigues J (2007) A case-control study of risk factors for brucellosis seropositivity in Portuguese small ruminants herds. Prev Vet Med 82: 291-301.
8. Renukaradhya GJ, Isloor S, Rajasekhar M (2002) Epidemiology, zoonotic aspects, vaccination and control/eradication of brucellosis in India. Vet Microbiol 90: 183-195.
9. Megersa B, Biffa D, Niguse F, Rufael T, Asmare K, et al. (2011) Cattle brucellosis in traditional livestock husbandry practice in Southern and Eastern Ethiopia, and its zoonotic implication. Acta Vet Scand 53: 24.
10. Muma JB, Samui KL, Oloya J, Munyeme M, Skjerve E (2007) Risk factors for brucellosis in indigenous cattle reared in livestock-wildlife interface areas of Zambia. Prev Vet Med 80: 306-317.
11. AU-IBAR (2013) *Brucella melitensis* Infection. Know your animals' monthly series.
12. Afar Region Finance and Economy Bureau (ARFEB) (2007) Regional atlas of Afar region, Semera, Ethiopia.
13. International Livestock Research Institute (2006) Domestic animal genetic resources information system (DAGRIS) (Rege JEO, Ayalew W, Getahun E, Hanotte O, Dessie T), Addis Ababa, Ethiopia.
14. Thrusfield M (2007) Veterinary Epidemiology. Blackwell science Ltd., USA, pp: 228-242.
15. Alton GG (1990) *Brucella melitensis*. In: Animal Brucellosis. Nielsen K and Duncan R (eds). CRC Press, Boca Raton, Florida, USA, pp: 383-409.
16. Díez FG, León FC (2004) The Spanish translation of the Manual of Diagnostic Tests and Vaccines for Terrestrial Animals: current and future solutions. Rev Sci Tech 23: 1023-1031.
17. Nielsen K, Dunkan JR (1990) Animal Brucellosis. CRC Press Inc., USA, pp: 173-179.
18. Teshale S, Muhie Y, Dagne A, Kidanemariam A (2006) Seroprevalence of small ruminant brucellosis in selected districts of Afar and Somali pastoral areas of Eastern Ethiopia: the impact of husbandry practice. Revue Med Vet 157: 557-563.
19. Sharifi H, Mashayekhi K, Tavakoli MM (2015) Risk facts of small ruminant brucellosis: a crosssectional study in Southeast Iran 2012. Human & Veterinary Medicine. International Journal of the Bioflux Society 7: 42-45.
20. Al-Majali AM (2005) Seroepidemiology of caprine brucellosis in Jordan. Small Rumin Res 58: 13-18.
21. Hamidullah M, Khan R, Khan I (2009) Seroprevalence of brucellosis in animals in district Kohat NWFP and comparison of two serological tests. Pak Vet J 4: 242-243.
22. Bekele T, Kasali OB (1990) Brucellosis in sheep and goats in Central Ethiopia. Bull Anim Health Prod Afr 38: 23-25.
23. Radostits OM, Gay CC, Hinchcliff KW, Constable PD (2007) Veterinary Medicine: A textbook of the diseases of cattle, sheep, goats, pigs, and horses. 10th edn. Saunders Company, Philadelphia, USA, pp: 962-984.
24. Alton GG (1985) Epidemiology of *B. melitensis* in sheep and goats. In: *B.*

melitensis CEC seminar. Verger JM, Plommet M (eds.). Martinus Nijoff, Dordrecht-Bosten Lancaster, pp: 187-196.

25. Colmenero JD, Muñoz-Roca NL, Bermudez P, Plata A, Villalobos A, et al. (2007) Clinical findings, diagnostic approach, and outcome of *Brucella melitensis* epididymo-orchitis. Diagn Microbiol Infect Dis 57: 367-372.

26. Osman AY, Jesse FF, Abdulkadir A, Saharee AA (2016) The Epidemiology and Immunopathophysiology of Brucellosis in Small Ruminant. PJSRR 2: 11-21.

27. Walker R (1999) Brucella. In: Veterinary Microbiology and Immunology. Hirsh DC, Zee YC (Eds.). Blackwell Science, USA, pp: 196-202.

Evaluation of Amitraz and Diazinon against *Rhipicephalus decoloratus* and *Amblyomma variegatum* in Bako Agricultural Research Center

Temesgen Tesfaye[1], Chala Mohammed[1*], Lama Yimer[1], Misgana Duguma[1] and Mammo Mokonnen[2]

[1]*School of Veterinary Medicine, Wollega University, Nekemte, Ethiopia*
[2]*Bako Agricultural Research Center, Ethiopia*

Abstract

Ticks are blood feeding ectoparasites that induce huge production losses in livestock industry and creating serious public health problems in the world. Although the use of chemicals is still the most effective method of tick control, uncontrolled applications may have accelerated the emergence of tick resistance to several active ingredients available. This study was conducted to assess the efficacy of commonly used acaricides (amitraz and diazinon) against *Rhipicephalus decoloratus* and *Amblyomma variegatum* collected from cattle by using Adult immersion test method. The *in-vitro* test employed an adult immersion technique. For laboratory experiment, adult ticks collected were exposed to Amitraz or Diazinon. The *in-vitro* assay showed no statistically significant tickicidal difference (p>0.05) between these compounds, although amitraz proved a relatively better efficacy. For both acaricides, doubled concentration was more effective in tick killing. In conclusion, comparing the efficacy of the two acaricides, amitraz is the preferable one. Furthermore, right application and choice of acaricides, avoidance of uncontrolled utilization of commercial insecticides and Strategies involving the early detection of resistance needs to be pursued in order to avoid any resistance against ticks in cattle.

Keywords: *Amblyomma varigaieum*; *Rhipicephalus decoloratus* ticks; Amitraz; Diazinon; Efficacy; *In-vitro* testing; Cattle

Introduction

A wide range of internal and external parasitic diseases are found in domestic animals. Among external parasites, ticks are undoubtedly the most economically important ectoparasites of livestock on global scale [1]. The economic benefits of resolving questions about the epidemiology and control of tick-borne diseases in the vast cattle-producing areas of eastern and southern Africa, Latin America, Australia and the southern US motivated research by national and colonial governments in the affected countries plus efforts by international animal health companies to create and market products that provided a means for protecting cattle [2].

The infestation with ticks can cause vast losses in farm animal's production, due to tick borne diseases, tick paralysis and physical damage as well as to huge financial losses due to tick control [3]. The economic losses caused by the *Rhipicephalus microplus* tick are due to a reduction in meat and milk production, as well as a devaluation of leather due to skin lesions caused by high infestations and the possible installation of myiasis. This tick species is responsible for the transmission of Babesiosis (*Babesia bovis* and *B. bigemina*) and Anaplasmosis (*Anaplasma marginale*), hemoparasites that characterize the disease named Bovine Babesiosis and Anaplasmosis Complex. This tick also causes indirect economic harm due to the additional hours of work required, additional facility costs, acaricide acquisition and equipment used for its application [4].

The application of chemicals is still the most effective method of ticks' control. However, uncontrolled applications of commercial acaricides may have accelerated the emergence of tick resistance to several active ingredients available. Since acaricide introduction in Africa around 1890, tick treatment relying on different application methods have been the main method of tick control in Africa, leading to numerous problems; environmental pollution, development of resistant tick strains and escalating costs [5]. Likewise, in Ethiopia, over the past decade's ticks are mainly controlled by using variety of acaricides; including organochlorines, organophosphates, carbamates, amidines or synthetic pyrethroids. However, with the most widespread, under or over concentration and frequent use of organochlorines and organophosphates compounds; ticks are likely to develop resistance in many countries and in Ethiopia [6].

Repeated use of acaricides besides being the environmental hazard, it is exposed to be resisted by tick species through time, and this forces frequent application at high concentrations which is more critical to the environment. Tick acaricide resistance is reported in various parts of the countries where tick and tick borne diseases are of major problem. Since tick infestation is one of the major reported problems in the area, repeated use of acaricides is the only option in high tick seasons [6].

The most common method to control ticks is use of different types of chemical acaricides which are used in different method of applications such as dressing, spraying, systemic and dipping. The prolonged incorrect use of acaricides may cause resistance in ticks against acaricides. The resistance can be caused by numbers of mechanisms [7], and when resistant ticks survive, they pass this ability by genetic to their offspring, the higher reproductive rate of ticks that have heritable resistance factors well resulting to increase in proportion of population of tick that carry genes of acaricides resistance [8].

Ticks are of importance to veterinary medicine because they can be an annoyance, cause harm due to their blood feeding and they

***Corresponding author:** Chala Mohammed, School of Veterinary Medicine, Wollega University, PO Box 395, Nekemte, Ethiopia
E-mail: chalamohammed@wollegauniversity.edu.et

can transmit many pathologic organisms. Tick infestation and tick borne disease control is based mainly on the use of acaricides. Thus, the most widely used method for effective control of ticks is the direct application of acaricides to host animals. Tick acaricide resistance is reported in various parts of the countries where tick and tick borne diseases are of major problem. Since tick infestation and resistance to acaricides were one of the major problems in the area, repeated use of acaricides and inadequate application throughout an extended period may promote population selection of acaricide resistant of ticks in high tick seasons and increasing the resistance problem.

Therefore, the main Objective of this study was: To assess the efficacy of most frequently used acaricides for the control of ticks at Bako Agricultural Research Centre, Oromia Regional State, Ethiopia.

Materials and Methods

Description of study area

The study was conducted at Bako Agricultural Research Center from November 2015 to March 2016. It is situated at 258 Km west of Addis Ababa, in Gobu Sayo District, East Wollega Zone of Oromia regional state, Western Ethiopia and some 4 km away from the main high way that gains Addis Ababa to Nekemte. It is located at Latitude of 090 06'N and Longitude of 370 09'E, and an Altitude of 1650 meters above sea level. The district has an average rain fall of 886.5 mm and an average temperature of 21.2°C. The area was generally concluded as "Woina Dega" even though some of it was kola. The main rainfall season was from May to September, dry season being from December to April and their humidity was 57.83% [9].

The total area of the Bako Tibe District is about 64,469 hectares of land with animal population of 141,393 Cattle, 12,880 Sheep, 14,641 Goats, 3,795 Horses, 8,668 Donkeys, 1,054 Mules, 97,709 Poultry, 5,237 Feline and 4,894 Canine [10]. The vegetation type of the area is characterized by common savannah vegetation's like mango tree, *stetrespermum kunthiamum* (botoro), Dokma (locally), pilio stigma thonningii (wanza) acashia absinica(grar), *Carissa idylis* (agamsa) and others. The area is reach with wild game animals in main river systems and in savannah. Some of these wild animals are Apes, pigs, antelopes, Columbus monkey, baboons and others. According to the settlers and people, there are bushbucks, hyenas and others [9].

Study population

The study was conducted on different cattle breeds of Dairy Farm at Bako Agricultural Research Centre. It was carried out by collecting ticks from the animals for *in-vitro* efficacy evaluation of Amitraz 12.5% and Diazinon 60% EC. None of the cattle received acaricidal treatment one month before the start of tick collection for the experiments.

Tick collection

The Farm was selected on the history basis of complaints on acaricides failure. From the Farm, the engorged adult of *Rhipicephalus decoloratus* and *Amblyomma variegatum* were collected for *in-vitro* efficacy evaluation of Amitraz 12.5% and Diazinon 60% EC. At each collecting site, the entire body surfaces of the animals were examined thoroughly and adult ticks were collected from neck/dewlap, udder, perineum/anus and legs/belly in combination from the sampled cattle. The bottles were labeled by considering the predilection sites and sampled animals. All collected ticks were examined under stereomicroscope and identified to the Genus/species level using the taxonomic key described by [11].

Study methodology and procedures

For laboratory experiment, the engorged adult ticks were collected from Dairy Farm at Bako Agricultural Research Centre. The *in vitro* acaricidal efficacy study was conducted on two dominant tick species infesting Cattle in the area. Accordingly, *Ambylomma variegatum* and *Rhipicephalus (R.) decoloratus* were collected and exposed to Diazinon and Amitraz according to Holdsworth et al. [12] immersion technique.

The recommended (1:1000 for diazinon, 1:625 for amitraz), double (2:1000 for diazinon, 2:625 for amitraz) and half doses were prepared. 1 ml of each liquor was added on Petri dish with a filter paper fit at its bottom. Then, the acaricide was evenly distributed and 10 ticks of equal size were placed on each Petri dish and it was closed. This was done separately for each species of tick. Distilled water was used as a control. The number of ticks alive or dead was counted after 24 hours of exposure. The experiment was repeated three times for precision and mean value was taken for the analysis.

Data analysis

The Collected data were recorded, organized, edited and analyzed using statistical package for social sciences (SPSS) Version 20. The results generated from the investigation were expressed using descriptive statistics (mean ± standard error of mean, percentage and graphs).

Results

The present study revealed that a number of ticks died after exposure with acaricides in laboratory at recommended, half and double doses. There was no significant difference ($p>0.05$) between two acaricides on the killing effect at any of the three different concentrations tested against both species of ticks (Table 1). Although not statistically significant, amitraz seemed to be superior to diazinon as measured by antiparasitic efficacy (%) estimation against both *Amblyomma variegatum* and *R. decoloratus*. However, both compounds appeared to have a comparable and relatively better efficacy (>90% at recommended dose) against both *Amblyomma variegatum* and *R. decoloratus*. Both compounds produced maximum efficacy only at their double recommended dose. The mean number of ticks died after distilled water exposure was not more than one (Figures 1 and 2). For the *in vitro* experiments, antiparasitic efficacy (AE) of each treatment was calculated using the following equation [13]:

$$AE=[B-T/B]/B$$

Where AE is the antiparasitic efficacy, B is the mean number of surviving ticks in the control, and T is the mean number of surviving ticks in treatment (Table 1).

The sensitivity of *Amblyomma variegatum* to acaricides was compared based up on the result obtained. Even though, *Amblyomma variegatum* is sensitive to both acaricides at different concentration, it is relatively more sensitive to Amitraz as shown in Figure 1 above.

The study indicated that the sensitivity of. *R. decoloratus* to both acaricides was compared based up on the result obtained. *R. decoloratus* is moderately resistant to Diazinon when compared with amitraz as shown in Figure 2 above.

Discussion

The present study revealed that a number of ticks died after exposure with acaricides in laboratory at recommended, half and double doses. Even though, there was no significant difference ($p>0.05$)

Treated tick	Treatment	NE	MNS	MND	AE (%)
	Amitraz RD	10	1.33 ± 0.577	8.67 ± 0.577	98.52
	Amitraz HRD	10	4.00 ± 1.000	6.00 ± 1.000	95.56
	Amitraz DRD	10	0.67 ± 0.577	9.33 ± 0.577	99.25
Amblyomma variegatum	Diazinon RD	10	3.00 ± 1.000	7.00 ± 1.000	96.67
	Diazinon HRD	10	5.00 ± 1.000	5.00 ± 1.000	94.45
	Diazinon DRD	10	3.33 ± 0.577	6.67 ± 0.577	96.31
	Distilled Water	10	9.50 ± 0.548	0.50 ± 0.548	0
	Amitraz RD	10	3.00 ± 1.000	7.00 ± 1.000	96.89
	Amitraz HRD	10	5.00 ± 1.000	5.00 ± 1.000	94.82
	Amitraz DRD	10	1.67 ± 0.577	8.33 ± 0.577	98.27
R. decoloratus	Diazinon RD	10	5.00 ± 1.000	5.00 ± 1.000	94.82
	Diazinon HRD	10	6.00 ± 1.000	4.00 ± 1.000	93.79
	Diazinon DRD	10	3.33 ± 0.577	6.67 ± 0.577	96.55
	Distilled Water	10	9.83 ± 0.408	0.17 ± 0.408	0

Values are mean ± SD; RD=Recommended Dose; DRD=Double Recommended Dose; HRD=Half Recommended Dose; NE=Number of Ticks Exposed; MNS=Mean Number of Ticks Survived; MND=Mean Number of Ticks Died; AE=Antiparasitic Efficacy

Table 1: *In vitro* ticks killing effect of Diazinon and Amitraz at recommended, Half and double doses of 24 hours post exposure of Amblyomma *variegatum and* R. *decoloratus*.

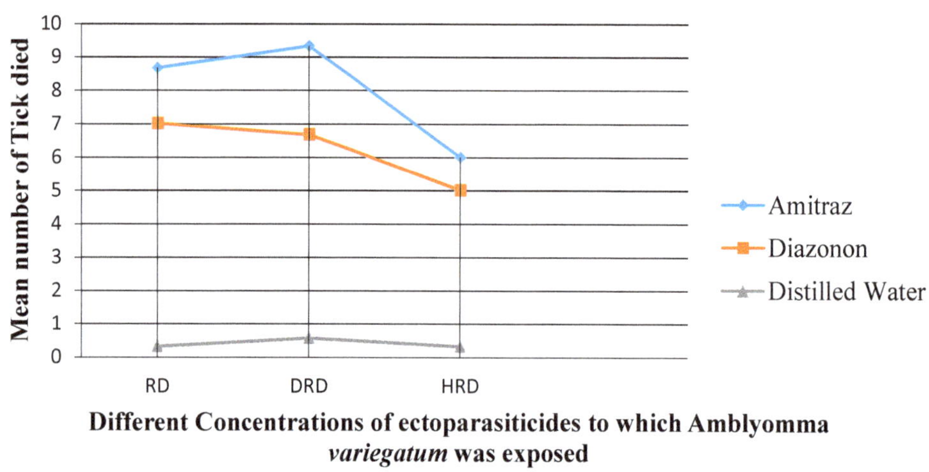

Figure 1: Relative comparison of *in vitro* killing effect of amitraz and diazinon at recommended, double and half concentrations against *Amblyomma variegatum*. RD=Recommended Dose; DRD=Double Recommended Dose; HRD=Half Recommended Dose.

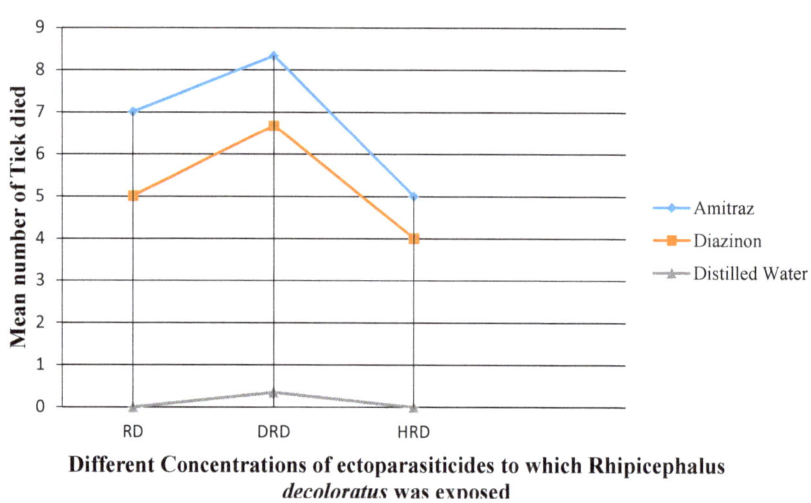

Figure 2: Relative comparison of *in vitro* killing effect of amitraz and diazinon at double, recommended and half concentrations against *R. decoloratus*. RD=Recommended Dose; DRD=Double Recommended Dose; HRD=Half Recommended Dose.

between two acaricides on the killing effect at any of the three different concentrations tested against both species of ticks, amitraz seemed to be effective than diazinon as measured by antiparasitic efficacy estimation against both *Amblyomma variegatum* and *R. decoloratus*. However, both compounds appeared to have a comparable and relatively better efficacy (>90% at recommended dose) against both *Amblyomma variegatum* and *R. decoloratus* and produced maximum efficacy only at their double recommended dose.

The present result showed that Amitraz (98.52) is more effective than Diazinon (96.67) at a recommended dose to *Amblyomma variegatum*. Present study agrees with Eshetu et al. [14] who reported that Amitraz at recommended concentration provides better efficient oviposition inhibition than Diazinon on Amblyomma and other ticks. However, the present study disagrees with the report of Furlong et al. [15] who found mean efficacy of 47.9% for amitraz, Santana [16] who reported a low efficacy of amitraz 40.5%, Campos and Oliveira [17] of 30.95% and Camillo et al. [18] also observed low efficacy of Amitraz in some tick populations, in Northeast region of Brazil. This difference might be associated with the method of application of acaricides.

The present finding shows that, Amitraz is the most preferable than Diazinon to control *R. decoloratus* ticks with the antiparasitic efficacy of 96.89% whereas that of diazinon is 94.82%. This finding was nearly similar with the finding of Dinka et al. [19] who worked at Borana and reported 100% efficacy of Amitraz and Souza et al. [20], in Southeast Brazil obtained mean Amitraz efficacy of 95%. The result also in consistent with the report of different authors from different areas at different time reported that the effectiveness of Amitraz over Diazinon [21]. Current study reveals that the sensitivity of *Amblyomma variegatum* to acaricides was compared based up on the result obtained. Even though, *Amblyomma variegatum* is sensitive to both acaricides at recommended and double dose, it is relatively more sensitive to Amitraz, but with no great variation on number of tick died due to the application of both drugs. Both compounds seemed to have a comparable and relatively better *in-vitro* efficacy (>90% at recommended dose) against *Amblyomma variegatum* with Antiparasitic Efficacy 98.52 of Amitraz and 96.67 Diazinon Recommended dose, after 24 hours post exposure. This finding is consistent with the report of similar result indicated by Turkson and Botchey [22] at Ghana, who reported that field strain of *Amblyomma variegatum* is resistant to organophosphates like Diazinon.

Generally, the species of ticks used in the study were compared based on their susceptibility to the acaricides used. Even though, both *Amblyomma variegatum* and *Rhipicephalus decoloratus* were sensitive to both acaricides at different concentration; they were relatively more sensitive to Amitraz than Diazinon The present study illustrated that the superiority of Amitraz over Diazinon in each concentration against both *Amblyomma variegatum* and *R. decoloratus*. The result also revealed that Rhipicephalus was relatively resistant to both acaricides than amblyomma. This resistance might be due to regular use of limited acaricide in the area since there is high infestation of ticks. The observation of the result was after 24 hours, which could be resulted by making rhipicephalus was seemed resistant to the drug.

Conclusion and Recommendations

The present research work demonstrated that amitraz has relatively conserved its tickicidal efficacy in vitro, on both tested tick species than diazinon. A clue of tick insusceptibility to diazinon was noted suggesting a need to consider correct application and choice of acaricides in order to avoid any resistance against ticks. The differences in the efficacy of the two evaluated acaricides (Amitraz and Diazinon) were most likely attributed from one of widespread, frequency, irregular application, inadequate spraying, and improper mixing of acaricides and on the use of acaricides stored for a long time after dilution.

Therefore, the following some basic management were forwarded as the recommendation to reduce the chances of developing acaricides resistance:

- Avoidance of uncontrolled utilization of commercial insecticides and dependence on limited type of acaricides and appropriate and good application of acaricides as prescribed by manufacturer.
- Use of appropriate dose of acaricides during treatment.
- Strategies involving the early detection of resistance and the use of integrated tick control are recommended.

Acknowledgements

The research was funded by Wollega University Research Ethiopia to which we are grateful. We would like to express our thanks to Bako Woreda Agricultural research center for their assistance during data collection. The research team is also grateful to study participants for their collaboration, enthusiasm and willingness to share us information.

Competing Interest

We declare that we have no any personal interest that inappropriately influences writing this article.

References

1. Zenebe S (2005) Ethiopian veterinary association (EVA). Addis Ababa, Ethiopia.
2. Taylor MA (2001) Recent developments in ectoparasiticides. The Vet J 161: 253-268.
3. Koney M (2004) Livestock production and health in Ghana. 2nd edn. Advent Press, Accra, pp: 4-21.
4. Gomes A (1998) O carrapato-do-boi Boophilus microplus: ciclo, biologia, epidemiologia, patogenia e controle. In: Carrapato, tristeza parasitária e tripanossomose dos bovinos. Kessler RH, Schenk MAM (eds.). Embrapa Gado de Corte.
5. Brito LG, Barbieri FS, Rocha RB, Oliveira M, Ribeiro ES (2011) Evaluation of the efficacy of acaricides used to control the cattle tick, *Rhipicephalus microplus*, in dairy herds raised in the Brazilian southwestern amazon. Vet Med Int 2011: 806093.
6. Yilma J, Adamu G, Zerbini E (2001) Biossay of acaricide resistance on three common cattle tick species at Holotta, Central Ethiopia. Rev Med Vet 152: 385-390.
7. Li AY, Chen AC, Miller RJ, Davey RB, George JE (2007) Acaricide resistance and synergism between permethrin and amitraz against susceptible and resistant strains of *Boophilus microplus* (Acari: Ixodidae). Pest Manag Sci 63: 882-889.
8. Kaljouw M (2009) Resistance to acaricides of Boophilus ticks from cattle in Ghana. MSc Thesis. Veterinary Medicine, Utrecht University, Netherlands.
9. Bako Agricultural Research Center (2014) Weather and climate desks. Bako, Ethiopia.
10. Bako Tibe Woreda Office of Agriculture and Rural Development (BTWOARD) (2015/16) Animal population information desks.
11. Kaiser N (1987) Tick survey, Ethiopia. Report on tick taxonomy and biology. Consultant report. Food and Agricultural Organization of the United Nations, p: 92.
12. Holdsworth PA, Kemp D, Green P, Peter RJ, De Bruin C, et al. (2006) World Association for the Advancement of Veterinary Parasitology (WAAVP) guidelines for evaluating the efficacy of acaricides against ticks (Ixodidae) on ruminants. Vet Parasitol 136: 29-43.
13. Wang GX, Han J, Feng TT, Li FY, Zhu B (2009) Bioassay-guided isolation

and identification of active compounds from *Fructus Arctii* against *Dactylogyrus intermedius* (Monogenea) in goldfish (*Carassius auratus*). Parasitol Res 106: 247-255.

14. Eshetu E, Dinede G, Lakew M, Tolosa T (2013) *In-vitro* efficacy evaluation of amitraz 0.025% and diazinon 0.06% against *Rhipicephalus pulchellus* and *Amblyomma gemma* in Borena pastoral area, Southern rangeland of Ethiopia. J Parasitol Vector Biol 5: 72-76.
15. Furlong J, Martins JR, Prata MCA (2007) The tick of cattle and resistance: we have to celebrate? A Hora Vet 27: 1-7.
16. Santana VLA (2000) Situation of chemical control of *Boophilus microplus* the sub-regions in the area of forest and wasteland in the state of Pernambuco, based on *in vitro* efficacy of acaricides in engorged females (Doctoral dissertation, Dissertation in Veterinary Science, Federal Rural University of Pernambuco, Recife, Pernambuco, Brazil).
17. Campos Júnior DA, Oliveira PRD (2005) *In vitro* valuation of acaricides efficiency to *Boophilus microplus* (Canestrini, 1887) (Acari: Ixodidae) from bovines at the region of Ilhéus, Bahia, Brazil. Ciênc Rural 35: 1386-1392.
18. Camillo G, Vogel FF, Sangioni LA, Cadore GC, Ferrari R (2009) *In vitro* evaluation of acaricides efficiency to bovine's ticks of Rio Grande do Sul State, Brazil. Ciênc Rural 39: 490-495.
19. Ayana D, Eshetu E, Waketole H, Abunna F (2013) *In vitro* Acaricidal efficacy evaluation trial of Ixodid ticks at Borana, Ethiopia. Ethiopian Vet J 17: 85-99.
20. de Souza AP, Sartor AA, Bellato V, Perussolo S (2003) Efficacy of acaricides in dairy cattle herds in southern region of Parana state, Brazil. Revista de Ciências Agroveterinárias (Journal of Agroveterinary Sciences) 2: 131-135.
21. Mekonnen S, Bryson NR, Fourie LJ, Peter RJ (2002) Acaricide resistance profiles of single-and multi-host ticks from communal and commercial farming areas in the Eastern Cape and North-West Provinces of South Africa. The Onderstepoort J Vet Res 69: 99-105.
22. Turkson PK, Botchey M (1999) Acaricide resistance in the cattle tick, *Amblyomma variegatum*, in the coastal savanna zone of Ghana. Ghana J Agric Sci 32: 199-204.

Effect of Imidacloprid on Reproduction of Female Albino Rats in Three Generation Study

Prerna Vohra* **and Kuldeep Singh Khera**

Department of Zoology, College of Basic Sciences and Humanities, Punjab Agricultural University, Ludhiana, Punjab, India

Abstract

In the present study, the effect of oral administration of imidacloprid over three generations on biochemical, histological and physiological alterations in female rats was assessed. Female rats were divided into three groups. Group 1 was control and was given corn oil, group 2 was administered imidacloprid at the rate of 10 mg/kg bw/day, group 3 was administered imidacloprid at the rate of 20 mg/kg bw/day. F0 and F1 generation female albino rats were dissected for this study. Weight of ovary decreased significantly at higher dose of treated female rats of F0 and F1 generation. Histopathology of ovary of group 2 and group 3 revealed different stages of follicles. The level of acid phosphatase (ACP) and alkaline phosphatase (ALP) increased significantly at higher dose in the ovary of females of both the generations. In either generation, non-significant changes were observed in fertility index, live birth index, gestation lengths and sex ratio. Female F1 pups in the 20 mg/kg/day group showed a significant decreased body weight on postnatal day 21 as compared to F0 pups on day 21.

Conclusion: The lower dose of imidacloprid (10 mg/kg/day T1) had no effect on various reproductive parameters of female rats and higher dose (20 mg/kg/day T2) of imidacloprid had some significant effects on feed consumption and reproductive parameters for three generation reproductive study.

Keywords: Imidacloprid; Female albino rats; Fertility index; Sex ratio; Reproductive parameters; Lower dose; Higher dose; Three generations

Introduction

Imidacloprid, a neonicotinoid the newest class of major insecticide has outstanding potency and systemic action for crop protection against piercing and sucking insect pests and also highly effective for control of flea on cats and dogs [1]. Few cases of acute human poisoning have been reported following ingestion of imidacloprid formulations [2,3]. There are some reports that show imidacloprid has an adverse effect on the reproductive tract [4], also this compound has been identified as having teratogenic [5], mutagenic [6] and carcinogenic [7] effects in animals and humans. Many pesticides having endocrine disruptor properties are also known to adversely impair the reproductive competence of males. Imidacloprid may adversely affect reproduction and cause developmental delays as a result of maternal toxicity. The effects of imidacloprid on reproduction and development were examined in a two generation, two-litter study in Wistar rats (30/sex/dose in the parental generation, P1). The dietary doses were 100, 250 and 700 ppm [8]. Maternal toxicity at 700 ppm included decreased body weight gain and food consumption with a marked reduction during lactation. In one study, pregnant rats fed technical grade imidacloprid throughout pregnancy and lactation at doses of 0, 100, 250 and 750 ppm revealed no effects other than significantly reduced food consumption (14% relative to controls) in the mother rats [9]. Imidacloprid was not found to affect reproductive variables or cause birth defects. However, reduced mean body weight and body weight gain relative to controls was observed in the males and females of all generations at the highest dietary concentration tested (700 ppm). At this concentration, parental animals also had reduced body weights, relative to controls, in association with reduced food consumption [10]. In spite of a number of studies on the effects of imidacloprid on reproductive behavior of animals, no information is available on the effect of imidacloprid on the two generation reproduction of rats when females were treated with imidacloprid. Aminotransferases and phosphatases are important and critical enzymes in the liver metabolic activity and are responsible for detoxification processes. So any interference in various enzyme levels lead to biochemical impairment and lesions of the tissue. The liver is the principal target of imidacloprid toxicity, as demonstrated by its elevated serum transaminase, alkaline phosphatase and/or glutamate dehydrogenase activities; and alterations of other clinical parameters. Therefore, this study was designed to investigate the effects of imidacloprid on three generation reproduction of rats (when only females were treated with imidacloprid).

Materials and Methods

Chemical

Commercial product of imidacloprid (Confidor, 17.8%, w/w imidacloprid as active ingredient) used in this study was purchased from the local market in Ludhiana, India.

Animals and experimental design

The study was conducted on sexually mature female albino rats, 3 months of age, weighing 100-150 g obtained from Guru Angad Dev Veterinary and Animal Sciences University (GADVASU), Ludhiana. The animals were housed in groups of two rats per cage. The rats were acclimatized for one week before using them for experimentation. The rats were maintained under controlled conditions of temperature (22 ± 2°C) and humidity (30-70%) with 12 h light and dark cycle. After acclimatization for one week, healthy rats were subjected to this study,

***Corresponding author:** Prerna Vohra, Department of Zoology, College of Basic Sciences and Humanities, Punjab Agricultural University, Ludhiana-141 004, Punjab, India, E-mail: vohra.prerna123@gmail.com

with 6 female rats constituting each group. Animals were divided into three groups. Group I served as control and given corn oil orally. Group II rats were given 10 mg/kg bw/day dose of imidacloprid. Group III rats were given 20 mg/kg bw/day dose of imidacloprid. The animals were given standard diet containing pelleted food and water *ad libitum*. The experimental protocol met the National guidelines on the proper care and use of animals in the laboratory research. The Institutional Animal Ethics Committee (IAEC) approved this experimental protocol. The study began with 6 female rats/group (F0 generation), and they were exposed to imidacloprid orally at 10 and 20 mg/kg bw/day. After 8-week administration of imidacloprid, each treated female was mated with a normal male having no dosage group and pregnant females were allowed to deliver and nurse their pups. F0 females were necropsied after weaning of their pups. Administration of imidacloprid was continued throughout the mating, gestation and lactation periods until necropsy. For the second generation, 6 female weanlings in each group of F0 generation were selected as F1 parents on post natal days 21-25 to equalize the mean body weights among groups as much as possible. The day on which F1 parental animals were selected was designated as day 0 of dosing for the F1 generation. F1 selected rats were given imidacloprid orally dissolved in corn oil mated after 8-week administration. They were allowed to deliver and nurse their F2 pups.

Dosing

Imidacloprid was dissolved in corn oil to obtain the desired test concentrations and given orally to female rats for two generations. Two doses of imidacloprid 10 and 20 mg/kg bw/day were given to females of F0 and F1 generation, and control rats of each generation were given corn oil. F0 females mated with normal males to get F1 generation and F1 females mated with normal rats to get F2 generation. 10 mg/kg/day dose was reported as NOEL (No Observed Effect Level Dose) by Bhardwaj et al. and Kapoor et al. [11,12] and other higher than NOEL was taken in the present study. Administration to F0 parental female animals was started at 3 months of age. Administration to F0 females lasted until necropsy through 10 weeks or more of the pre-mating, mating, gestational, lactational periods and during weaning of the F1 offspring. Administration to F1 parental animals was started from age of 6 weeks old, until necropsy through 8 weeks or more of the pre-mating, mating, gestational, lactational periods and during weaning of the F2 offspring.

Parental data (F0 and F1)

Clinical observations: Throughout the study, all F0 and F1 parental female rats were observed at least twice daily and cages were inspected daily for evidence of ill health or reaction to the treatment. F0 females underwent physical examinations beginning on the day treatment commenced, and weekly until mating. After mating, the physical examinations occurred on days 1, 7, 14, 21 and 28. The same schedule of examinations was used for the selected F1 rats. F0 females were weighed on the day treatment commenced, at weekly intervals until mating was detected, on days 0, 6, 13 and 20 after mating, on days 0, 4, 7, 14 and 21 of lactation and prior to necropsy. After selection, the F1 animals were weighed following the same schedule as the F0 animals.

Body weight and food consumption: All adult rats were observed daily for clinical signs of toxicity; food consumption and body weight were recorded weekly during mating, gestation and lactation period. For F0 females mean weekly food consumption was calculated for individual animals prior to mating. Mean daily food consumption was calculated for each F0 female based on the data recorded for the period days 0-5, 6-12 and 13-21 post-mating, and days 1-3, 4-6, 7-13 and 14-20 of lactation. Food consumption for the F1 animals was recorded at the same frequency following selection.

Mating procedures: At the age of 12 weeks after the 8 week administration period starting from six week old in the F0 animals, and at the age of 14-15 weeks after 8 week oral administration period from six weeks of age in the F1 animals, females were moved to the cages of male partners in the evening, and the males and females cohabited at a sex ratio of 1:1 through the mating period. Existence of a vaginal plug or sperm in the vaginal smear was examined every morning from the following day. When either was detected, it was judged that copulation had occurred and the day was defined as gestation day (GD) 0. The mating period was limited to two weeks. Pregnancy was confirmed by existence/absence of delivery and/or by investigating implantation sites at the time of necropsy. Beginning on day 20 after mating, females were inspected 3 times daily for evidence of parturition. The progress and completion of parturition was monitored, the numbers of live and dead offspring were recorded. Individual F1 offspring's were numbered; within each litter day 1-postpartum. The selected F1 generation was allocated to its specific treatment group when they were 6 weeks old.

Vaginal smears were obtained from the female animals everyday in the morning to examine the estrous cycle during four weeks before mating; starting from 12 weeks of age for the F0 parents and from 11 weeks old for the F1 parents, and the mean days of estrous cycle were calculated. Cases with estrous cycle other than 4 to 6 days were regarded as abnormal. F0 and F1 parental females were anaesthetized by chloroform. The following organs were weighed in all the F0 and F1 females: the liver, ovaries and uterus.

Biochemical analysis

After sacrification, the tissue sample of liver was homogenized in the phosphate buffer saline. The activities of aspartate aminotransferase (AST), alanine aminotransferase (ALT) were estimated by the method of Reitman and Frankel as described by Bergmeyer and acid phosphatase (ACP), alkaline phosphatase (ALP) was estimated by method of Bessey et al.

Processing of tissues for histopathology

All F1 and F2 rats were weighed and sacrificed by chloroform anesthesia. For histopathological studies, ovaries of treated and control rats were fixed in 10% formalin. After routine processing and dehydration of each tissue, paraffin sections were cut at 5 um and stained with hematoxylin-eosin for microscopic examination. Serial sections of ovary were studied for various observations like total number of follicles, number of normal and atretic follicles, oocyte and nucleus as described by Kaur and Guraya.

Offspring evaluation (F1 and F2)

All pups derived from F0 and F1 parents (F1 and F2 litters, respectively) were examined as soon as possible on the day of birth to determine the number and sex of pups, the number of live born and stillborn members of each litter and gross abnormalities. All individual offspring's were examined approximately 24 h after birth (day 1) and daily thereafter for any evidence of ill health. Litter size and mortality were recorded daily from days 1 to 21. The sex ratios of each litter were recorded. Individual body weights were recorded on days 0,4,7,14,21. The dams were removed and offspring weaned on day 21 of age, and the selection of the F1 generation was made on day 25. For the selected F1 females, sexual maturation was assessed daily from day 25 of age until vaginal opening occurred. Females that littered and reared offspring to weaning were euthanized on day 28 post-partum (after weaning). For all F0 and the selected F1 adult females, detailed necropsies involving full macroscopic examinations weighing of the liver, ovary and uterus was carried out.

Reproductive performance of F0 and F1 rats: The reproductive parameters from this study were expressed in terms of indices, weights and ratios that considered all stages from conception to weaning [13]. These parameters were defined below:

Fertility index (%)=(Number of females delivering /number of females cohabited) × 100

Live birth index (%)=(Number of live pups at day 0/number of pups born) × 100

4-day survival index (%)=(Number of live pups on day 4/ number of pups alive on day 0) × 100

21-day (weaning) survival index (%)=(Number of pups alive on day 21/ number of pups alive on day 4) × 100

Litter size=Number of pups/number of pregnant females

Body weights of pups=The body weight of pups were recorded on days 0, 4, 7, 14 and 21

Statistical analysis

All values were presented as the mean ± standard error of means (S.E.M). Comparisons were made between control and treated groups using "Analysis of Variance (ANOVA)" as a statgraphics statistical package. The body weight of parental animals, food consumption, length of estrous cycle, organ weight was evaluated by student t test for pairwise comparisons between control and individual treatment groups.

Results

Data for parental animals

Clinical signs and body weight: The most consistent finding was aggression/hyperactivity which was observed throughout the study in both F0 and F1 females of imidacloprid treated groups. Some females of the low and high dose groups had vaginal discharges. Mean estrous cycle days were significantly reduced in higher dose (T2) treated group of F0 females (4.06 ± 0.03, P<0.01) as compared to control (5 ± 0.21). In F1 females there was non-significant change in mean estrous cycle days. Body weight data of F0 and F1 females are shown in Table 1. The imidacloprid treated F0 and F1 females experienced reduction in body weight. The total weight gain of females reduced non significantly in T1 and T2 group (Table 2).

Organ weights of F0 and F1 parental rats: Organ weights of ovary and uterus for F0 and F1 parental animals are summarized in Table 3. The relative ovarian weight was significantly reduced in higher dose (T2) group in F0 and F1 generation. Weight of uterus increased in both F0 and F1 females.

Food consumption: During the pre-pairing phase, compared to controls, food consumption was significantly decreased in imidacloprid treated females as compared to control of both the generations (Table 4). Decreased food consumption in F1 generation was significant as compared to F0 generation. During most of gestation and lactation, feed intakes were significantly increased in higher dose (20 mg/kg/d) and non-significant increase was also seen in the 10 mg/kg/day dose group females (Tables 5 and 6). Average gestation length was slightly increased by 1-2 days in the higher dose group (23 days); all gestation lengths were within the expected range of 22-23.5 days. There was non-significant increase in length of gestation days in treated groups as compared to control in both the generations.

Biochemical analysis

There was significant increase in activity of liver ALT in F1 and F2 females. AST, ACP and AKP enzyme activity increased non-significantly in F1 and F2 females (Tables 7 and 8).

Offspring evaluation (F1 and F2)

Reproductive performance of F0 and F1: The reproductive performance of F0 and F1 rats were evaluated by looking at various parameters that included fertility index, live birth index, weaning index, litter size, body weight of pups and sex ratio. In F0 rats, imidacloprid treatment caused a non-significant change on the gestation length, litter size and the viability indices at the higher dose group compared to control (Table 9). Fertility index decreased in imidacloprid treated groups as compared to control in F0 and F1 generation.

Similarly, in F1 generation rats, no imidacloprid treatment related effect on gestation, viability and sex ratio was observed in the higher dose group compared to control. The body weight of F0 pups increased significantly, and at day 21 body weight of F1 pups was significantly lowered in high dose group as compared to control (Table 10).

Hormone levels

Progesterone and estrogen levels were estimated in plasma of control and treated rats of F1 and F2 generation (Table 5). In higher dose treated group there is non-significant decrease in progesterone level in F1 and F2 generation. Estrogen level showed non-significant increase in treated groups in both the generations (Table 11).

Histology

Histologically, sections of ovary of control rats showed different stages of follicles and sections of higher dose of treated rats showed more number of atreric follicles as compared to control rats. All the stages of follicular development viz. primary, secondary, tertiary, early

Weeks	F0			F1		
	Control	T 1	T 2	Control	T 1	T 2
I	101.67 ± 1.05	103.3 ± 1.52	103.33 ± 1.66	103.33 ± 1.67	105 ± 1.82	102.5 ± 2.14
II	107.5 ± 1.12	109.16 ± 1.40	110 ± 3.16	110 ± 1.29	110 ± 1.82	110 ± 1.82
III	117.5 ± 2.14	115 ± 1.17	115 ± 1.17	120.83 ± 2.38	120 ± 1.29	120 ± 1.82
IV	129.17 ± 2.00	136.67 ± 4.95	129.17 ± 3.98	139.17 ± 1.53	130 ± 1.29	130.83 ± 2.00
V	144.16 ± 3.33	141.6 ± 3.33	136.6 ± 4.95	149.1 ± 5.54	140.83±1.53	141.6 ± 6.54

Values are Mean ± SE of 6 animals in each group

Table 1: Effect of imidacloprid on weekly body weight of female albino rats before pairing of F0 and F1 generation as compared to control.

Traits	F0			F1		
	Control	T 1	T 2	Control	T 1	T 2
Mating	141.6 ± 3.06	152.5 ± 3.81	156.66 ± 3.07	158.33 ± 3.33	152.5 ± 6.02	152.5 ± 1.11
Gestation	152.5 ± 4.95	156.6 ± 4.21	173.33 ± 3.57*	169.16 ± 1.53	167.5 ± 2.50	166.6 ± 3.80
After delivery	146.6 ± 1.67	155 ± 3.65*	166.6 ± 2.47	158.33 ± 3.33	159.16 ± 4.36	145.8 ± 7.12
During lactation	165.8± 2.38	173.3 ± 8.33	186.6 ± 4.59**	185 ± 2.88	181.66 ± 3.07	176.6 ± 4.94

Values are Mean ± SE of 6 animals in each group
*Significantly different from control at P<0.05
**Significantly different at P<0.01

Table 2: Effect of imidacloprid on body weight of female albino rats after pairing of F0 and F1 generation as compared to control.

	Control	T 1	T 2
F 0 females			
No. of females examined	6	6	6
Final body weight (g)	129.16 ± 3.982	141.7 ± 3.333	156.7 ± 3.073
Ovary (g)	0.030 ± 0.002	0.029 ± 0.001	0.020 ± 0.001**
Uterus (g)	0.135 ± 0.021	0.172 ± 0.036	0.182 ± 0.031
F 1 females			
No. of females examined	6	6	6
Final body weight (g)	131.7 ± 4.013	140.8 ± 3.515	153.3 ± 7.490**
Ovary (g)	0.037 ± 0.001	0.036 ± 0.004	0.031 ± 0.001*
Uterus (g)	0.137 ± 0.020	0.206 ± 0.043	0.191 ± 0.015

Values represent the mean ± SE of 6 animals in each group
*Significantly different from control at P<0.05
**Significantly different from control at P<0.01

Table 3: Relative organ weights for F0 and F1 females.

antral and antral were observed in control and imidacloprid treated rats in F1 and F2 generation (Figures 1 and 2).

Discussion

The present three generation reproductive study was performed to provide general information concerning the effects of imidacloprid on the performance of female reproductive system, and on the growth and development of the offspring. Mean estrous cycle days were significantly reduced in T2 treated group of F0 females (4.06 ± 0.03, P<0.01) as compared to control (5 ± 0.21). Studies of Borgeest et al. [14] experienced a significant increase in the percentage of days in estrous phase compared with control and methoxychlor treated mice. It is obvious that monitoring of body weight provides information on health level of animals which can also be important interpretation of reproductive effects [15]. Body weight of females increased significantly during gestation and lactation period of F0 and F1 generation.

The relative ovarian weight was significantly reduced in higher dose (T2) group in F0 and F1 generation. Reduction in body weight at 20 mg/kg/day dose level as observed in the present study may be correlated with decreased sex organ weight (ovary weight) in both the generations, which reflects the effect of imidacloprid on the reproductive system. Organophosphates like methyl parathion, dimethioate and monocrotophos given to female albino rats have also resulted in significant decrease in the ovarian weights [16].

Food consumption of females before pairing for the F0 and F1 generation decreased significantly in treated females of both the generations. The decrease in feed consumption is correlated with decrease in body weight gain in all the treated groups [17] in the two generations. There was significant increase in food consumption of females during gestation and lactation in F0 and F1 generation. Significant increase in food consumption was observed on 13-21 days of gestation in both the generations. During the period of gestation and lactation metabolism increases by 82.5% on average and the female assimilates additionally 304 kcal (including 60.5 kcal for gestation and 243.5 kcal for lactation) [18]. Lactation makes considerably greater demands on the mother's body than pregnancy does in species where the young are helpless at birth and depend on mother's milk for a comparatively long time. The requirements for the production of milk are met partly from within, by the mobilization of the mother's body tissues, and partly from without, by an increased food intake [19]. Similar results were found by Margaret et al. [20] that at different intervals throughout the gestation and lactation periods, increased food consumption was observed in F0 generation females of the mid- and high-dose groups of stanol esters,

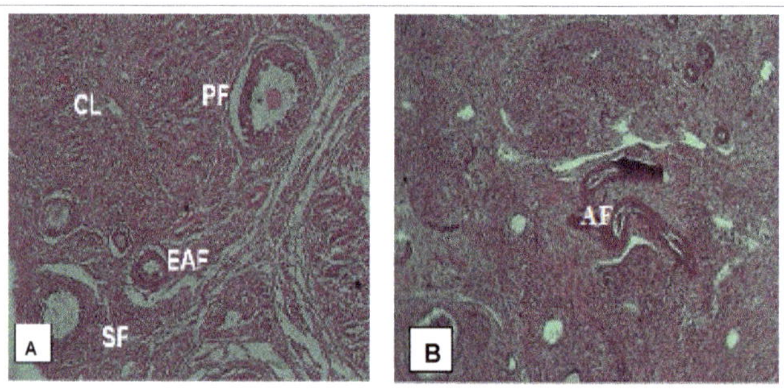

Figure 1: A. T.S of ovary of control rat of F1 generation showing different stages of follicles i.e., primary follicles (PF), secondary follicles (SF), tertiary follicles (TF), early antral follicles (EAF), antral follicle (AF) and corpus luteum (CL) (HE X100); **B.** T.S of ovary of T2 rat showing atretic primary, secondary and tertairy follicles..

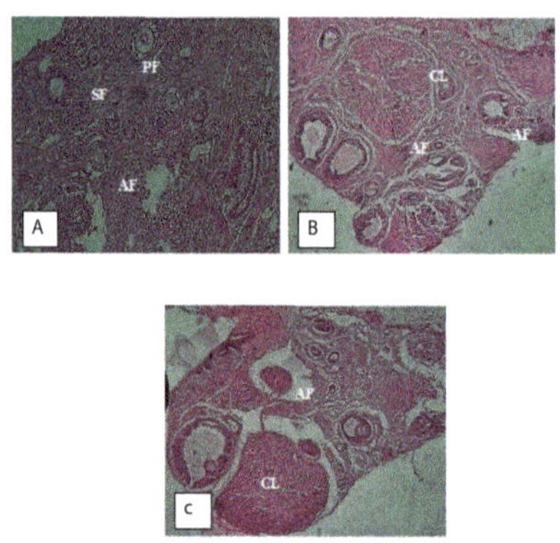

Figure 2: A. T.S of ovary of control rat of F2 generation showing different stages of follicles i.e., primary follicles (PF), secondary follicles (SF), tertiary follicles (TF), early antral follicles (EAF), antral follicle (AF) and corpus luteum (CL) (HE X100); **B.** T.S of ovary of T1 rat showing tertiaty, early antral and antral atretic follicles; **C.** T.S of ovary of T2 rat showing atretic primary, secondary and tertairy follicles and corpus luteum.

Week	Control	T 1	T 2
F0 generation			
1	18 ± 0.090	17 ± 0.271*	16.76 ± 0.391*
2	25 ± 0.000	22.95 ± 0.66	17.23 ± 0.030
3	30.5 ± 1.295	23.43 ± 0.632	19.14 ± 1.351
4	30.5 ± 2.108	29.29 ± 1.355	20.43 ± 0.271
F 1 Generation			
1	13.56 ± 2.306	12.89 ± 0.548[a]	12.28 ± 0.456
2	26.24 ± 2.741	24.76 ± 1.029	23.71 ± 1.355
3	33.86 ± 1.078	32.67 ± 1.046[a]	30.33 ± 0.475
4	34.42 ± 0.579	31.15 ± 0.811	30.65 ± 0.968

Values represent the mean ± SE of 6 animals in each group
*Significantly different from control at P<0.05
[a]Significantly different from T1 of F0 at P<0.01

Table 4: Food consumption of females before pairing for the F0 and F1 generation (g/animal/week).

F0 generation	Control	T 1	T 2
Gestation			
0-5 days	26.80 ± 0.000	26.80 ± 0.000	30.93 ± 1.307*
6-12	20.62 ± 0.688	24.15 ± 0.200	26.87 ± 0.295
13-21	24.09 ± 0.482	27.10 ± 0.662	27.97 ± 0.191**
Lactation			
1-3 days	28.54 ± 0.940	31.36 ± 1.574	33.19 ± 2.79*
4-6	29.30 ± 0.953	31.90 ± 1.364	33.62 ± 2.330
7-13	28.90 ± 1.079	31.55 ± 1.547	33.06 ± 2.551
14-20	28.75 ± 0.857	31.33 ± 1.526	32.96 ± 2.380

Values represent the mean ± SE of 6 animals in each group
*Significantly different from control at P<0.05
** Significantly different from control at P<0.01

Table 5: Food consumption of females during gestation and lactation for the F0 generation (g/animal/day).

F1 generation	Control	T 1	T 2
Gestation			
0-5 days	43.13 ± 1.499	38.93 ± 1.850	39.00 ± 1.820
6-12	43.52 ± 0.740	39.48 ± 0.314*	43.57 ± 1.065
13-21	33.87 ± 1.114	43.74 ± 0.625**	44.63 ± 1.042**
Lactation			
1-3 days	42.22 ± 1.921	42.06 ±1.471	43.44 ± 1.240
4-6	38.89 ± 1.890	43.78 ± 1.210	45.94 ± 1.381*
7-13	43.55 ± 1.164	45.79 ± 0.375	46.62 ± 0.792
14-20	43.57 ± 0.620	42.55 ± 1.221	44.31 ± 1.240

Values represent the mean± SE of 6 animals in each group
*Significantly different from control at P<0.05
**Significantly different from control at P<0.01

Table 6: Food consumption of females during gestation and lactation for the F1 generation (g/animal/day).

Parameters (µmole/g)	Dosage/mg/kg/d		
	0 (Control)	10	20
ALT	27.362 ± 3.34	57.85 ± 2.84***	66.27 ± 7.72***
AST	53.15 ± 8.90	59.88 ± 4.38	69.34 ± 4.13
AKP	51.85 ± 21.16	61.00 ± 0.93	65.33 ± 9.21
ACP	27.29 ± 4.06	33.12 ± 1.19	34.23 ± 2.78

Values represent the mean ± SE of 6 animals in each group
***Significantly different from control at P<0.001

Table 7: Liver biochemical data of female rats of F1 generation orally administered imidacloprid.

while increased food consumption was noted in F1 generation females of the mid- and high-dose groups during gestation. Such increases in food consumption are expected as a result of the animals' attempt to compensate for the reduced caloric value of the test diet compared to controls. Cripps and Williams [21] measured feed consumption during lactation in Sprague-Dawley rats and found an approximately 3- to 5-fold increase in daily feed consumption between post natal day 1 and post natal day 21. Similar increased food consumption during lactation in rats was reported by Shirley [22] and Arnold et al. [23].

Parameters (µmole/g)	Dosage/mg/kg/d		
	0 (Control)	10	20
ALT	26.80 ± 3.59	53.54 ± 5.71	63.73 ± 9.59**
AST	68.00 ± 9.89	61.08 ± 4.28	70.30 ± 3.35
AKP	50.70 ± 24.35	63.06 ± 2.50	69.00 ± 8.94
ACP	28.70 ± 3.96	35.23 ± 1.17	39.43 ± 2.10

Values represent the mean ± SE of 6 animals in each group
**Significantly different from control at P<0.01

Table 8: Liver biochemical data of female rats of F2 generation orally administered imidacloprid.

F 0 parents/F1 offspring	Control	T 1	T 2
Number of pairs at the start	6	6	6
Number of pregnant	6	5	5
Litter size	6	5	6.6
Fertility index of F0 female	100	83.33	83.33
Live birth index (%)	100	100	96.96
4-day survival index (%)	100	100	93.75
21-day survival index (%)	100	100	100
F 1 parents/F2 offspring	**Control**	**T 1**	**T 2**
Number of pairs at the start	6	6	6
Number of pregnant	6	5	5
Litter size	7	7.2	6.1
Fertility index of F0 female	100	83.33	83.33
Live birth index (%)	100	83.33	81.08
4-day survival index (%)	100	93.33	90
21-day survival index (%)	100	92.85	96.29

Table 9: Developmental findings for F1 and F2 pups.

There was non-significant increase in length of gestation days in treated groups as compared to control in both the generations. A slight increase in gestation length was observed in two generation study by Tyl et al. [24]. In F0 rats, no imidacloprid treatment related effect on the litter size and the viability indices (day 0 and 4) was observed at the higher dose group compared to control. Fertility index was slightly decreased in treated groups of both the generations. Similarly, in F1 generation rats, imidacloprid treatment caused non-significant change on fertility, survival index and litter size in the higher dose group compared to control. Suter et al. [8] also reported a mild effect or no effect on reproductive performance after exposure to imidacloprid. There were no effects on mating indices, fertility, gestation, litter size, mortality and no evidence of pathology at any dose level [25].

There was significant increase in ALT and AST activity in the liver. Bhardwaj et al. [11] also observed that oral administration of imidacloprid in female rats at the rate of 5, 10 and 20 mg/kg bw/day

Live pup weight (g)	Control	T 1	T 2
F 0 parents/F1 pups			
Day 0	3.90 ± 0.59	4.13 ± 0.24	6.08 ± 1.32**
Day 4	9.06 ± 0.59	9.05 ± 1.00	10.5 ± 2.27
Day 7	16.38 ± 0.50	16.01 ± 0.95	18.94 ± 4.01
Day 14	23.9 ± 1.19	22.83 ± 1.35	25.29 ± 5.38
Day 21	31.95 ± 6.78	30.44 ± 1.48	29.24 ± 1.48
F1 parents/F2 pups			
Day 0	2.73 ± 0.22	2.64 ± 0.19	2.81 ± 3.05
Day 4	6.38 ± 0.42	6.31 ± 0.10	6.62 ± 0.43
Day 7	13.09 ± 0.73	12.1 ± 0.93	12.67 ± 0.94
Day 14	17.29 ± 0.74	18.30 ± 0.86	17.60 ± 1.41
Day 21	29.93 ± 0.86	23.08 ± 2.46	20.74 ± 2.20**

Values represent the mean ± SE of 6 animals in each group
** Significantly different from control at P<0.01

Table 10: Effect of imidacloprid on the body weight gain of F1 and F2 pups.

Hormones	F1		
	Control	T 1	T 2
Progesterone (ng/ml)	19.8 ± 7.29	19.4 ± 7.46	7.3 ± 1.82
Estrogen (pg/ml)	253.3 ± 47.23	256.6 ± 34.02	256.6 ± 28.007
	F2		
Progesterone (ng/ml)	10.6 ±6.90	8.6 ± 2.71	8.5 ± 2.44
Estrogen(pg/ml)	201.6 ± 11.66	218.3 ± 19.73	235.0 ± 16.48

Table 11: Effect of imidacloprid on hormones of F1 and F2 generation.

for 90 days resulted in elevation of serum ALT, AST, glucose, Blood Urea Nitrogen (BUN). It has been suggested that an increase in alkaline phosphatase (ALP) level occurs due to the damage of the cells of liver, kidney, small intestine, and bone resulting in the liberation of this enzyme in the blood systems [26].

The body weight of F0 pups increased significantly on day 0, and at day 21 body weight of F1 pups was significantly lowered in higher dose group as compared to control. The body weight of F1 pups at day 21 in high dose group was significantly lowered compared to control. Svetlana [25] reported a decrease in body weight gain of offspring's up to 13% compared to control until weaning at postnatal day 21. Similar results were found by Leslie et al. that body weight gain of offspring was significantly decreased from days 21-25 for Han Wistar rat females receiving 7500 ppm and 25,000 ppm rebaudioside A. Pup body weight and weight gains were reduced throughout lactation, with statistically identified lower weights on post natal day 21 in all generations at 100 mg/kg/day [27].

Oral administration of cypermethrin to female rats has resulted in significant decrease in plasma progesterone levels [28]. Earlier studies of Mani et al. also observed significant reduction in testicular enzyme 17 β-hydroxysteroid dehydrogenase, responsible for testosterone biosynthesis in male rats exposed to fenevalerate which may ultimately be leading to net decrease in testosterone concentration in group of rats [29].

Two doses of imidacloprid to female rats over two successive generations resulted in some effects on weight gain, food consumption, fertility index and showed no effects on gestation index, weaning index, sex ratio, live birth index of F1 and F2 pups [30,31]. Higher dose of imidacloprid (20 mg/kg bw/day) in both the generations showed a reduction in their body weight and food consumption and some effects on reproduction. Lower dose of imidacloprid (10 mg/kg bw/day) showed non-significant effects. Thus 10 mg/kg/day dose of imidacloprid which has been reported as NOEL (No Observed Effect Level) dose has no adverse effects on either generation. Studies on imidacloprid have indicated 10 mg/kg/day as No Observed Effect Level (NOEL) as evidenced by various biochemical, hematological, neurobehavioral and oxidative stress parameters and produced significant changes at high dose levels (20 mg/kg/day) [11,12]. There have been no studies reported in the literature concerning the effects of imidacloprid on multigenerational reproduction after oral exposure to imidacloprid in female rats [32]. In our multigenerational experiment, the results indicated only minimal effects upon reproductive performance of rats. Imidacloprid exposure caused reduction in fertility index of both the generations. Suter et al. [8] also reported a mild effect or no effect on reproductive performance after exposure to imidacloprid.

Conflict of Interest Statement

The authors declare that there are no conflicts of interest.

Acknowledgements

We are thankful to Department of Zoology, PAU Ludhiana for providing facilities for conducting research.

References

1. Yamamoto I, Tomizawa M, Saito T, Miyamoto T, Walcott EC, et al. (1998) Structural factors contributing to insecticidal and selective actions of neonicotinoids. Arch Insect Biochem Physiol 37: 24-32.
2. Wu IW, Lin JL, Cheng ET (2001) Acute poisoning with the neonicotinoid insecticide imidacloprid in N-methyl pyrrolidone. Clin Toxicol 39: 617-621.
3. Proença P, Teixeira H, Castanheira F, Pinheiro J, Monsanto PV, et al. (2005) Two fatal intoxication cases with imidacloprid: LC/MS analysis. Forensic Sci Int 153: 75-80.
4. Rouchard J, Gustinm F, Wauters A (1994) Soil organic matter aging and its effect on insecticide imidacloprid soil biodegradation in sugar beet crop. Toxicol Environ Chem 45: 149-155.
5. Pike KS, Reed GL, Graf GT, Allison D (1993) Compatibility of imidacloprid with fungicides as a seed-treatment control of russian wheat aphid (Homoptera: Aphidae) and effect on germination, growth, and Yield of Wheat Barley. J Econ Entomol 86: 586-593.
6. Placke FJ, Weber E (1993) Method of determining imidacloprid residues in plant materials. Pflanzenschutz-Nachrichten Bayer 46: 109-182.
7. Scholz K, Spiteller M (1992) Influence of groundcover on the degradation of 14C-imidacloprid in soil. Proceeding of the Brighton Crop Protection Conference, pp: 883-888.
8. Suter P, Biedermann K, Luetkemeier H, Wilson J, Terrier C (1990) NTN 33893 Technical. Multiple Generation Study in Rats. RCC, Research and Consulting Company AG. Itingen, Switzerland. Study No. 100647. DPR Vol. 51950-0019 # 119496.
9. Sheets L (2001) A Developmental Neurotoxicity Screening Study with Technical Grade Imidacloprid in Wistar Rats: Lab Project Number: 99-D72-DV: 110245.
10. Solecki R (2001) Toxicological evaluations, pesticide residues in food. Pest Bio div Federal institute for health protection of consumers and veterinary medicine, Berlin, Germany.
11. Bhardwaj S, Srivastava MK, Kapoor U, Srivastava LP (2010) A 90 days oral toxicity of imidacloprid in female rats: morphological, biochemical and histopathological evaluations. Food Chem Toxicol 48: 1185-1190.
12. Kapoor U, Srivastava MK, Srivastava LP (2011) Toxicological impact of technical imidacloprid on ovarian morphology, hormones and antioxidant enzymes in female rats. Food Chem Toxicol 49: 3086-3089.
13. Oser BL, Oser M (1956) Nutritional studies on rats of diets containing high levels of partial ester emulsifiers. II. Reproduction and lactation. J Nutr 60: 489-505.
14. Borgeest C, Symonds D, Mayer LP, Hoyer PB, Flaws JA (2002) Methoxychlor may cause ovarian follicular atresia and proliferation of the ovarian epithelium in the mouse. Toxicol Sci 68: 473-478.

15. Aly HA, Domènech O, Abdel-Naim AB (2009) Aroclor 1254 impairs spermatogenesis and induces oxidative stress in rat testicular mitochondria. Food Chem Toxicol 163: 1733-1738.

16. Kaur S, Dhanju CK (2005) Biochemical effects of some organophosphorus pesticides on the ovaries of albino rats. Indian J Physiol Pharmacol 49: 148-152.

17. Bhadaniya AR, Joshi DV, Patel BJ, Kalaria VA, Padodara RJ, et al. (2012) Toxico-pathological studies on experimentally induced acephate toxicity in wistar rats (Rattus norvegicus). Wayamba J Animal Sci 4: 451 -458.

18. Migula P (1969) Bioenergetics of pregnancy and lactation in European Common Vole. Acta theriologica 14: 169-179.

19. Widdowson EM (1976) Changes in the body and its organs during lactation: nutritional implications. Ciba Found Symp 45: 103-118.

20. Whittaker MH, Frankos VH, Wolterbeek AP, Waalkens-Berendsen DH (1999) Two-generation reproductive toxicity study of plant stanol esters in rats. Regul Toxicol Pharmacol 29: 196-204.

21. Cripps AW, Williams VJ (1975) The effect of pregnancy and lactation on food intake, gastrointestinal anatomy and the absorptive capacity of the small intestine in the albino rat. Br J Nutr 33: 17-32.

22. Shirley B (1984) The food intake of rats during pregnancy and lactation. Lab Anim Sci 34: 169-172.

23. Arnold DL, Bryce FR, Clegg DJ, Cherry W, Tanner JR, et al. (2000) Dosing via gavage or diet for reproduction studies: a pilot study using two fat-soluble compounds-hexachlorobenzene and aroclor 1254. Food Chem Toxicol 38: 697-706.

24. Tyl RW, Myers CB, Marr MC, Sloan CS, Castillo NP, et al. (2008) Two-generation reproductive toxicity study of dietary bisphenol A in CD-1 (Swiss) mice. Toxicol Sci 104: 362-384.

25. Svetlana EK, Numay RR, Thomas BM (2006) Imidacloprid. Risk Characterization Document. Dietary and Drinking Water Exposure. California EPA (Environmental Protection Agency).

26. Zimmerman HJ (1969) Serum enzymes determination as an aid to diagonosis. In: Clinical diagnosis by Laboratory methods. Dawidson I, Henry JB (eds). WB Saunders Company, Philadelphia, USA, p: 719.

27. Hanley TR Jr, Breslin WJ, Quast JF, Carney EW (2002) Evaluation of spinosad in a two-generation dietary reproduction study using Sprague-Dawley rats. Toxicol Sci 67: 144-152.

28. Saleem FM, Elmonsoury EGA, Yousef AE (1996) Reproductive performance in rats and ewes treated with pyrethroid (ectomin). Assiut Vet Med J 34: 103-123

29. Chao S, Casida JE (1997) Interaction of imidacloprid metabolites and analogs with the nicotinic acetylcholine receptor of mouse brain in relation to toxicity. Pestic Biochem Physiol 58: 77-88.

30. Curry LL, Roberts A, Brown N (2008) Rebaudioside A: two-generation reproductive toxicity study in rats. Food Chem Toxicol 46 Suppl 7: S21-30.

31. Baligar PN, Kaliwal BB (2002) Reproductive toxicity of carbofuran to the female mice: effects on estrous cycle and follicles. Ind Health 40: 345-352.

32. Wilen R, Bastomsky CH, Naftolin F (1981) Control of puberty in female rats: the effect of PTU-induced hypothyroidism and systematic undernutrition. Pediatr Res 5: 169-171.

Staphylococcus: Isolation, Identification and Antimicrobial Resistance in Dairy Cattle Farms, Municipal Abattoir and Personnel in and Around Asella, Ethiopia

Fufa Abunna[1]*, Tekeste Abriham[1], Fikru Gizaw[2], Takele Beyene[1], Ashenafi Feyisa[1], Dinka Ayana[1], Bedaso Mamo[1] and Reta Duguma[1]

[1]*College of Veterinary Medicine and Agriculture, Addis Ababa University, PO Box 34, Bishoftu, Oromia, Ethiopia*
[2]*College of Veterinary Medicine, Semera University, PO Box 132, Samara, Ethiopia*

Abstract

A cross sectional study was conducted between February, 2014 and April, 2014 to isolate and identify *Staphylococcus* from dairy cattle farms and municipal abattoir; and to evaluate antimicrobial sensitivity for isolates in and around Asella, Ethiopia. An over all of 181 samples were collected and processed from nine dairy cattle farms (87) and seven municipal abattoir visits (94). Accordingly, 42 (23.2%) udder milk, 9 (5.0%) tank milk, 9 (5.0%) polled bucket swab, 9 (5.0%) tank swab, 9 (5.0%) polled hand swab, 9 (5.0%) polled nasal swab, from dairy cattle farms; and 66 (36.5%) meat swab, 7 (3.9%) polled knife swab, 7 (3.9%) polled slaughter line swab, 7 (3.9%) polled hand swab and 7 (3.9%) polled nasal swab from municipal abattoir visits were collected. The result showed the overall proportion of *Staphylococcus* was 89 (49.2%). Staphylococcal species were more predominant in abattoir 50/94 (53.2%) than farms 39/87 (44.8%), but there was no significant difference between them because $p>0.05$ at 95% confidence interval. Also high proportion of *Staphylococcus* was isolated from polled farm nasal swab 8/9 (88.9%), but this difference between sample type and the presence of *Staphylococcus* is not significant, because p-value (0.303) is greater than 0.05 at 0.05 level. Up on isolation and identification 35 (19.3%), 6 (3.3%), 24 (13.3%), 24 (13.3%) were *S. aureus*, *S. intermedius*, *S. hyicus* and Coagulase Negative Staphylococci (CNS), respectively. From total positive samples, 55 isolates were tested for antimicrobial susceptibility to different 15 antimicrobial discs. The comparative efficacies of antimicrobials used indicates Gentamycin, Kanamycin, Chloramphenicol, Ciprofloxacillin, and Sulphamethoxazole trimethoprim, were the most effective antibiotics where by 94.5%, 89.1%, 81.8%, 81.8%, and 81.8% respectively. Good hygienic practices should be followed both in dairy cattle farms and municipal abattoir including working personnel and equipment's used; and antimicrobials susceptibility test should be carried out at regular intervals to find out the development of resistance against the most commonly applied antibiotics.

Keywords: Abattoir; Antimicrobial susceptibility; Asella; Farm; Identification; Isolation; *Staphylococcus*

Introduction

Globally, millions of people suffer from communicable and non-communicable diseases caused by contaminated foods [1,2]. There are three ways people are exposed to Food Borne Diseases (FBD) due to pathogenic bacteria in foods of animal origin meat (beef, mutton, pork), dairy (milk, cheese, yoghurt, ice cream) and eggs [3,4]. Food borne diseases are universal public health problems and the implications are great including health and economic losses [5,6].

Food borne diseases or food poisonings are defined by the World Health Organization (WHO) as an illness or diseases of infectious or toxic nature caused by the consumption of foods or water contaminated with bacteria and/or their toxins, parasites, viruses, or chemicals [7,8]. Food borne diseases are major health problems in developed and developing countries. The World Health Organization (WHO) estimated that in developed countries, up to 30% of the population suffers from food borne diseases each year, whereas in developing countries up to 2 million deaths are estimated per year [9]. Many diseases are communicable and caused by micro-organisms that enter into the body via food [10]. Numerous outbreaks of gastroenteritis have been associated with ingestion of raw foods, foods incorporating raw ingredients or foods obtained from unsafe sources [11,12].

In the last few decades, staphylococcal food poisoning has been reported as third cause of food-borne illnesses in the world. Among the foods implicated in staphylococcal food poisoning, milk, dairy products and meats, particularly handled foods, play a vital role since entero-toxigenic strains of *S. aureus* have been commonly isolated in them [13]. *S. aureus* is present in a variety of locations on the dairy farms, and several studies suggested that transfer of *S. aureus* between humans and cows is possible [14]. Multidrug-resistant staphylococcal isolates such as Methicillin-Resistant *S. aureus* (MRSA) were isolated primarily from human samples, but such isolates were detected in animal samples [15,16]. Thus, the transfer of *S. aureus* between humans and cows may result in serious problems.

Milk, dairy products and meat, especially handled foods, are common vehicles that are frequently implicated in Staphylococcal Food Poisoning (SFP) [17,18]. Milk can be contaminated for example by *Staphylococcus aureus* when there is infection of the mammary gland or by bad hygiene habits, such as coughing or sneezing and not washing hands when handling milk storage equipment, during or after milking, and in this case, human activity is responsible for the contamination, as these bacteria colonizes the nasal pathways in human beings [19]. With regards to meat, it is a good material for bacterial growth; its quality

***Corresponding author:** Fufa Abunna, College of Veterinary Medicine and Agriculture, Addis Ababa University, PO Box 34, Bishoftu, Oromia, Ethiopia
E-mail: fufa.abunna@aau.edu.et

depends on the initial bacterial contamination. This contamination causes meat deterioration, lowers quality and sometimes illness may be caused by bacterial pathogens or their toxins through meat and meat products [20]. External contamination of meat is a constant possibility from the moment of bleeding until consumption [21]. The possible sources of these bacteria are likely resulted from the skin of the animal from which the meat was obtained. Other potential sources of microbial contaminations are the equipment used for each operation that is performed until the final product is eaten; the clothing and hands of personnel and the physical facilities themselves are all implicated [22].

Poor personal hygiene, improper cleaning of storage and preparation areas and unclean utensils cause contamination of raw and cooked foods. Mishandling of raw and cooked foods allows bacteria to grow. Man's respiratory passages, skin and superficial wounds are common sources of *S. aureus*. When *S. aureus* is allowed to grow in foods, it can produce a toxin that causes illness. Although cooking destroys the bacteria, the toxin produced is heat stable and may not be destroyed. Many foods will support growth of staphylococci and toxin production. Good personal hygiene while handling foods will help keep *S. aureus* out of foods, and refrigeration of raw and cooked foods will prevent the growth of these bacteria if any are present [23].

In developing countries, the surveillance system of FBD hardly exists and it is therefore, difficult to estimate the real magnitude of the problem. Even in countries where surveillance services are very efficient, the precise incidence of food poisoning is not known, as outbreaks are often not reported to public health authorities. Hence, the incidence of FBD caused by staphylococci is thought to be much higher than reported since many cases remain undeclared [17,24]. Therefore, the objectives of this study were to isolate, and identify *Staphylococcus* species and evaluate antimicrobial susceptibility patterns in dairy cattle farms, abattoir and human in and around Asella town.

Materials and Methods

Study area

The study was conducted in Asella town dairy farms and municipal abattoir from February to April 2014. Asella town is located in Oromia region. The town, which is the capital of Arsi zone, is located at about 175 km Southeast of Addis Ababa at 6°59' to 8°49' N latitudes and 38°41' to 40°44' E longitudes with an altitude of the area ranges from 2500 to 3000 metre above sea level. Agricultural production system of the study area is of mixed crop and livestock production. Dairy farming using improved breeds is a common practice in urban and peri-urban areas. The area is characterized by mid subtropical temperature ranging from 5°C-28°C and with relative humidity ranging from 43 to 60%. The annual average rainfall is 1200 mm and mostly with clay type of soil and in rare case black soil. The area has a bimodal rainfall occurring from March to April (short rainy season) and July to October (long rainy season). The area covers 23674.72 km square and topographically has highland escapement and lowland areas. The area is densely populated, with livestock population of 85,893 cattle, 57,118 sheep, 10,725 goats, 7841 horses, 15,642 donkeys, 517 mules and 35,489 poultry. The farmers in the area practice mixed crop-livestock farming system. The high land areas are found centrally and the low lands dominate the periphery of the area [25].

Study population

The study population were dairy cows, dairy cow milkers, slaughtered cattle's and abattoir personnel. In addition, samples were taken from materials used in milking process (farm) and slaughtering process (abattoir).

Sampling method

A total of 181 samples were collected from dairy cattle farms (87) and municipal abattoir (94). The sample size was fixed based on the representative samples taken from selected dairy cattle farms and municipal abattoir. Probability sampling (simple random) was used to select the population to be sampled. Samples were taken from nine dairy cattle farms including small scale farms and seven municipal abattoir visits. Accordingly, 42 (23.2%) udder milk, 9 (5.0%) tank milk, 9 (5.0%), 9 (5.0%) polled bucket swab tank swab, 9 (5.0%) polled farm hand swab, 9 (5.0%) polled nasal swab, 66 (36.5%) meat swab, 7 (3.9%) polled knife swab, 7 (3.9%) polled slaughter line swab, 7 (3.9%) polled abattoir hand swab and 7 (3.9%) polled abattoir nasal swab was collected from representative dairy cattle farms and municipal abattoir visits in and around Asella.

Study design

A cross sectional study was carried out to isolate and identify *Staphylococcus* from selected dairy cattle farms and a municipal abattoir visit from February, 2014 to April, 2014. In addition, *in vitro* antibiotic susceptibility test was undertaken using fifteen antimicrobial discs via disc diffusion test.

Study methodology

Sample type: A total of 181 samples containing eleven sample types were collected from selected dairy cattle farms and municipal abattoir in Asella town and its surroundings. These sample types include udder milk from cows, tank milk from total collected milk in the farm, bucket swab from bucket (polled), hand (polled) and nasal swabs (polled) from milkers' hand from selected dairy farms; and meat swab from slaughtered cattle, slaughter line swab from hanging materials (polled), knife swab from knives (polled), hand (polled) and nasal swab (polled) from slaughterers from municipal abattoir was taken.

Sampling procedure transportation and storage

Meat, polled slaughter line, polled knives, polled abattoir hand and nasal swabs from municipal abattoir; and polled bucket, polled farm hand and nasal swabs from selected representative dairy cattle farms were collected using 10 milliliter of buffered peptone water containing sterile test tubes and transported inside ice containing ice box. And udder milk and tank milk was collected using sterile test tube and transported with ice containing ice box. For good collection of milk sample the teat were wiped thoroughly with 75% ethyl alcohol. The sterile collection of bottle was used and the first stream of milk from each quarter was discarded. The milk sample then held in an ice box for transportation to the laboratory. In the laboratory samples was cultured immediately or stored at +4°C. Swabs samples were collected using sterile cotton swabs from abattoir (meat, slaughter line, knives, hand and nasal swab), and farm (bucket, tank, hand and nasal swab). Each sterile cotton swab was dipped into sterile distilled water prior to collection.

Meat swab was taken from slaughtered carcass after flaying process was undertaken from neck and front leg, thoracic wall, abdominal wall and thigh region to make a representative sample of the carcass. This was undertaken by rotating the sterile applicator swab on those regions. Swabs from materials from abattoir (slaughter line and knives) and farm (bucket and tank) were collected by using sterile applicator swab through rotating on the body (inside) of the materials. Swab from slaughter house personnel from abattoir and milkers' hand from farm was taken by wiping both hands with sterile applicator swab. Nasal swab for culture was obtained by firmly rotating new pre-moistened cotton-tipped swabs on both nares of volunteer dairy farm milkers' hand and slaughterers. After swab was taken, subsequently, it is put into a single screw capped test tube containing 10 ml of buffered peptone water as transporting media. Then, samples for culture were placed in racks for easy handling and held in an icebox, properly packed and kept cold. Finally, it was transported to the microbiology department of Asella regional laboratory to be processed.

Antimicrobial susceptibility test was performed on selected *Staphylococcus* isolates according to the criteria of the Clinical and Laboratory Standards Institute [26]. For susceptibility test, one antimicrobial from each subclass of antimicrobials which were commonly used for treatment of bovines or considered as important antimicrobial agents for human were selected for antibiogram based on the criteria of Clinical and Laboratory Standards Institute [26]. Thus, antimicrobials included in this study were Erythromycin (E/15 μg), Ciproflocaxin (CIP/5 μg), Penicillin G (P/10 Units), Sulphamethoxazole trimethoprim (SXT/25 μg), Amoxacillin (AML/25 μg), Chloramphenicol (C/30 μg), (Oxoid), Tetracycline (TE/30 μg), Cefoxitin (FOX/30 μg), Cloxacillin (OB/5 μg), Kanamycin (K/30 μg), Nalidixic acid (NA/30 μg), Nitrofurantion (F/50 μg), Streptomycin (S/10 μg), Vancomycin (VA/30 μg) and Gentamycin (CN/10 μg) (Biomerioux). Finally, the diameters of the zone of inhibition around the disks were measured to the nearest millimeter using rulers, and the isolates were classified as susceptible, intermediate and resistant according to the interpretative standards of Clinical and Laboratory Standards Institute [26]. Moreover, isolates showing resistance to three or more antimicrobial subclass were considered as multidrug resistant.

Data management and analysis

After the data was collected using different formats, Microsoft Excel was used for data management, computation of descriptive statistics and drawing graphs. Computation of descriptive statistics was conducted using SPSS version 20.0, 2011 software. Descriptive statistics such as percentages, proportions and frequency distributions were applied to compute some of the data. The Pearson's chi-square (χ^2) test at a significance level of 5% and 95% Confidence Interval was used to determine the differences of prevalence of *Staphylococcus*, *Staphylococcus* species and *Staphylococcus* and staphylococcal species between samples examined, sample source and sample types. The difference was statistically significant if the p- value was less than 0.05, but in significant if p- value is greater than 0.05.

Results

An overall of 181 examined samples, 89 (49.2%) were positive for *Staphylococcus* species, and after isolation and identification of *Staphylococcus* species from the total sample 35 (19.3%), 6 (3.3%), 24 (13.3%), 24 (13.3%) were *S. aureus*, *S. intermedius*, *S. hyicus* and coagulase negative Staphylococci (CNS), respectively. As the result shows *S. aureus* is the most prevalent staphylococcal species followed by *S. hyicus* and CNS; and lastly *S. intermedius.* From 181 samples, 94 (51.9%) and 87 (48.1%) were collected and examined from abattoir and farms, respectively. Staphylococcal species were more predominant in abattoir 50/94 (53.2%) than farms 39/84 (44.8%), but there was no significant difference between them because p-value (0.261)>0.05 at 95% confidence interval (Table 1).

Also high proportion of *Staphylococcus* was isolated from polled farm nasal swab 8/9 (88.9%), consequently followed by polled knives swab 5/7 (71.4%), polled abattoir nasal swab 4/7 (57.1%), meat swab 35/66 (53.0%), 3/7 (42.9%) (for each polled slaughter line swab and polled abattoir hand swab), udder milk 19/42 (45.2%) and 3/9 (33.3%) (for each tank milk, polled bucket swab, polled farm hand swab and tank swab). But this difference between sample type and the presence of *Staphylococcus* is not significant, because p-value (0.303) is greater than 0.05 at 0.05 level (Table 2).

From abattoir visits 94 samples were cultured for isolation and identification of *Staphylococcus*. The isolation result showed 50 (53.2%) were positive for *Staphylococcus* species. Upon identification *S. aureus* 22 (23.4%) was most predominant followed by *S. hyicus* 15 (16.0%), CNS 11(11.7%) and *S. intermedius* 2 (2.1%). In the abattoir visit five types of samples were examined including 66 (70.2%) meat swab, 7 (7.4%) slaughter line swab, 7 (7.4%) polled knife swab, 7 (7.4%) polled hand swab, and 7 (7.4%) polled nasal swab. Out of these 4 (57.1%), 4 (57.1%), 35 (53.0%), 3 (42.9%), and 3 (42.9%); polled nasal swab, polled knives swab, meat swab, polled hand and slaughter line swab, respectively were positive for staphylococcal species.

Out of nine farms 87 representative samples were taken and examined that 39 (44.8%) were positive for staphylococcal species. From these 13 (14.9%), 4 (4.6%), 9 (10.3%) and 13 (14.9) were *S. aureus*, *S. intermedius*, *S. hyicus*, and CNS, respectively.

In each farm six sample types including udder milk 42 (48.3%), tank milk 9 (10.3%), polled bucket swab 9 (10.3%), tank swab 9 (10.3%), polled hand swab 9 (10.3%), and polled nasal swabs 9 (10.3%) were processed. The status of *Staphylococcus* was high in polled nasal swab 8 (88.9%) followed by udder milk 19 (45.2%), tank milk 3 (33.9%), tank swab 3 (33.9%), polled bucket swab 3 (33.9%) and polled hand swab 3 (33.9%). But there is no significance difference between sample types, because p value 0.109 is greater than 0.05 at the 0.05 level.

A total of 32 samples, of which 16 (50.0%) polled hand swab and 16 (50.0%) polled nasal swab was taken and examined both from selected representative dairy cattle farms milkers' hand 14 (43.75%) and municipal abattoir slaughterers 18 (56.25%). From these 32 samples 18 (56.25%) were found to be positive for *Staphylococcus* species, and upon identification 7 (21.9%), 6 (18.8%), 5 (15.6%), and 0 (0%) were *S. aureus*, CNS, *S. hyicus* and *S. intermedius*, respectively.

As the result shows the status of *Staphylococcus* species was higher in dairy cattle farm milkers' hand 11/18 (61.1%) than municipal abattoir slaughterers 7/14 (50%). But the difference was not significant because p-value (0.53) is greater than 0.05 at 0.05 levels.

Sample source	*Staphylococcus* species								Total	
	S. aureus		*S. intermedius*		*S. hyicus*		CNS			
	n	%	n	%	n	%	n	%	n	%
Abattoir(n=94)	22	23.4	2	2.1	15	16	11	11.7	50	53.2
Farm (n=87)	13	14.9	4	4.6	9	10.3	13	14.9	39	44.8
Total (N=181)	35	19.3	6	3.31	24	13.3	24	13.3	89	49.2
X^2 (P- value)	2.071(0.15)		0.860 (0.35)		1.238(0.266)		1.238(0.412)		1.265(0.261)	

Table 1: Proportion or percentage of staphylococcal isolates from municipal abattoir and dairy cattle farms in and around Asella.

From total positive samples, 55 (22 (40.0%) *S. aureus*, 4 (7.3%) *S. intermedius*, 18 (32.7%) *S. hyicus*, 11 (20.0%) CNS) was tested for susceptibility to different 15 antimicrobial discs. The comparative efficacies of antimicrobials used indicate Gentamycin, Kanamycin, Chloramphenicol, Ciprofloxacillin, and Sulphamethoxazole trimethoprim, were the most effective antibiotics where by 94.5%, 89.1%, 81.8%, 81.8%, and 81.8% respectively. Penicillin G (14.5%), Nalidixic acid (25.5%), have shown the poorest in efficacy against staphylococcal isolates. The number and percentage of susceptibility pattern of 55 staphylococcal isolates with fifteen antimicrobials are listed on Table 3.

As the result shows staphylococcal species have showed a slightly variable susceptibility pattern toward antimicrobials (Table 4). *S. aureus* is highly susceptible (90.9%) to both Gentamycin and Kanamycin; and highly resistant to Penicillin G (95.5%). *S. intermedius* also showed greater susceptibility (100.0%) towards Gentamicin, Amoxicillin, Chloramphenicol, Sulphamethoxazole trimethoprim, Tetracycline, Vancomycin and Kanamycin; but is resistant to Penicillin G (75.0%). Similarly, *S. hyicus* was highly susceptible to Gentamycin (94.4%), but resistant to Penicillin G (94.4%). More over coagulase negative staphylococci (CNS) have showed high susceptibility (100.0%) to Gentamycin, Kanamycin and Chloramphenicol; but they were slightly resistant to Cloxacillin (63.6%).

In respect to resistance 40/55 (72.7%) (Table 5) staphylococcal species have developed a multi drug resistance. The result also shows 20/22 (90.4%), 1/4 (25.0%), 13/18 (72.2%), and 6/11 (54.5%) of multi drug resistance was developed in *S. aureus*, *S. intermedius*, *S. hyicus* and CNS, respectively. And generally only 2/55 (3.6%) staphylococcal isolates have shown no resistance against the previously mentioned fifteen antimicrobials (Table 5).

Discussion

Staphylococcus species are prevalent food-borne bacterial pathogens that cause food poisoning in humans when ingested in contaminated foods, including dairy products. They cause SFP by toxin production [27]. *Staphylococcus* species can indeed be easily eliminated from foods by heat treatment (in pasteurized foods) or by competition with other flora (in fermented foods), whereas SEs resist most of the treatments used during food processing. Hence, the surveillance of food for microbial contamination is vital for the protection of public health and consumer interests. Production of safe food also has important economic implications in an increasingly competitive global market. The organisms can gain access to raw milk and milk products either by direct excretion from udders having clinical and subclinical staphylococcal mastitis or by contamination from food handlers [28,29].

	Staphylococcal species (n %)				
Sample type	*S. aureus*	*S. intermedius*	*S. hyicus*	CNS	Total (n%)
MS (n=66)	13 (19.7)	2 (3)	13 (19.7)	7 (10.6)	35 (53.0)
KS (n=7)	3 (42.9)	0 (0.0)	1 (14.3)	1 (14.3)	5 (71.4)
SLS (n=7)	3 (42.9)	0 (0.0)	0 (0.0)	0 (0.0)	3 (42.9)
AHS (n=7)	3 (42.9)	0 (0.0)	0 (0.0)	0 (0.0)	3 (42.9)
ANS (n=7)	0 (0.0)	0 (0.0)	1 (14.3)	3 (42.9)	4 (51.7)
UM (n=42)	5 (11.9)	2(4.8)	4 (9.5)	8 (19.0)	19 (45.2)
TM (n=9)	1 (11.1)	1 (11.1)	1 (11.1)	0 (0.0)	3 (33.3)
BS (n=9)	0 (0.0)	1 (11.1)	0 (0.0)	2 (22.22)	3 (33.3)
TS (n=9)	3 (33.3)	0 (0.0)	0 (0.0)	0 (0.0)	3 (33.3)
FHS (n=9)	1 (11.1)	0 (0.0)	2 (22.2)	0 (0.0)	3 (33.3)
FNS (n=9)	3 (33.3)	0 (0.0)	2 (22.2)	3 (33.3)	8 (88.9)
Total (N%)	35 (19.3)	6 (3.3)	24 (13.3)	24 (13.3)	89 (49.2)
X^2 (P Value)	15.82 (0.11)	5.59 (0.85)	9.01 (0.52)	17.02 (0.07)	11.76 (0.30)

Key: MS: Meat Swab; KS: Knive Swab; SLS: Slaughter Line Swab; AHS: Abattoir Hand Swab; ANS: Abattoir Nasal Swab; UM: Udder Milk; TM: Tank Milk; BS: Bucket Swab; TS: Tank Swab; FHS: Farm Nasal Swab; FNS: Farm Nasal Swab; CNS: Coagulase Negative Staphylococci.

Table 2: Number and percentage of *Staphylococcus* species with samples type taken in and around Asella municipal abattoir and selected dairy cattle farms.

S. No	Name of antimicrobial	Susceptibility pattern		
		Susceptible (n %)	Intermediate (n %)	Resistant (n %)
1	Amoxicillin (AML)	32 (58.2)	0 (0.0)	23 (41.8)
2	Cefoxitin (FOX)	37 (67.3)	0 (0.0)	18 (32.7)
3	Chloramphenicol (C)	45 (81.8)	0 (0.0)	10 (18.2)
4	Ciprofloxacin (CIP)	45 (81.8)	7 (12.7)	3 (5.5)
5	Cloxacillin (OB)	26 (47.3)	0 (0.0)	29 (52.7)
6	Erythromycin (E)	34 (61.8)	10 (18.2)	11 (20.0)
7	Gentamicin (CN)	52 (94.5)	2 (3.6)	1 (1.8)
8	Kanamycin (K)	49 (89.1)	2 (3.6)	4 (7.3)
9	Nalidixic acid (NA)	14 (25.5)	9 (16.4)	32 (58.2)
10	Nitrofurantion (F)	25 (45.5)	7 (12.7)	23 (41.8)
11	Penicillin G (P)	8 (14.5)	0 (0.0)	47 (85.5)
12	Streptomycin (S)	36 (65.5)	10 (18.2)	9 (16.4)
13	Sulphamethoxazole trimethoprim (SXT)	45 (81.8)	4 (7.3)	6 (10.9)
14	Tetracycline (TE)	34 (61.8)	8 (14.5)	13 (23.6)
15	Vancomycin (VA)	38 (69.1)	0 (0.0)	17 (30.9)

Table 3: Antimicrobial susceptibility of staphylococcal isolates (n=55).

Drug name	Antimicrobial susceptibility pattern of *Staphylococcus* species											
	S. aureus			*S. intermedius*			*S. hyicus*			CNS		
	S n%	I n%	R n%	S n%	I n%	R n%	S n%	I n%	R n%	S n%	I n%	R n%
AML	13(59.1)	0(0.0)	9(40.9)	4(100)	0(0.0)	0(0.0)	7(38.9)	0(0.0)	11(61.1)	8(72.7)	0(0.0)	3(27.3)
FOX	19(86.4)	0(0.0)	3(13.6)	2(50.0)	0(0.0)	2(50.0)	8(44.4)	0(0.0)	10(55.6)	8(72.7)	0(0.0)	3(27.3)
C	15(68.2)	0(0.0)	7(31.8)	4(100)	0(0.0)	0(0.0)	15(83.3)	0(0.0)	3(16.7)	11(100)	0(0.0)	0(0.0)
CIP	18(81.8)	3(13.6)	1(4.5)	3(75.0)	1(25.0)	0(0.0)	14(77.8)	2(11.1)	2(11.1)	10(90.9)	1(9.1)	0(0.0)
OB	13(59.1)	0(0.0)	9(40.9)	3(75.0)	0(0.0)	1(25.0)	6(33.3)	0(0.0)	12(66.7)	4(36.4)	0(0.0)	7(63.6)
E	14(63.6)	4(18.2)	49(18.2)	3(75.0)	1(25.0)	0(0.0)	9(50.0)	5(27.8)	4(22.2)	8(72.7)	0(0.0)	3(27.3)
CN	20(90.9)	2(9.1)	0(0.0)	4(100)	0(0.0)	0(0.0)	17(94.4)	0(0.0)	1(5.6)	11(100)	0(0.0)	0(0.0)
K	20(90.9)	1(4.5)	1(4.5)	4(100)	0(0.0)	0(0.0)	14(77.8)	1(5.6)	3(16.7)	11(100)	0(0.0)	0(0.0)
NA	3(13.6)	5(22.7)	14(63.6)	1(25.0)	1(25.0)	2(50.0)	6(33.3)	2(11.1)	10(55.6)	4(36.4)	1(9.1)	6(54.5)
F	9(40.9)	5(22.7)	8(36.4)	2(50.0)	0(0.0)	2(50.0)	6(33.3)	2(11.1)	10(55.6)	8(72.7)	0(0.0)	3(27.3)
P	1(4.5)	0(0.0)	21(95.5)	1(25.0)	0(0.0)	3(75.0)	1(5.6)	0(0.0)	17(94.4)	5(45.5)	0(0.0)	6(54.5)
S	15(68.2)	3(13.6)	4(18.2)	3(75)	1(25.0)	0(0.0)	11(61.1)	3(16.7)	4(22.2)	7(63.6)	3(27.3)	1(9.1)
SXT	19(86.4)	0(0.0)	3(13.6)	4(100)	0(0.0)	0(0.0)	12(66.7)	4(22.2)	2(11.1)	10(90.9)	0(0.0)	1(9.1)
TE	13(59.1)	2(9.1)	7(31.8)	4(100)	0(0.0)	0(0.0)	9(50.0)	4(22.2)	5(27.8)	8(72.7)	2(18.2)	1(9.1)
VA	18(81.8)	0(0.0)	4(18.2)	4(100)	0(0.0)	0(0.0)	8(44.4)	0(0.0)	10(55.6)	8(72.7)	0(0.0)	3(27.3)

Key: S: Susceptible; I: Intermediate; R: Resistant; n: Number; CNS: Coagulase Negative *Staphylococcus* AML: Amoxicillin (25 µg); FOX: Cefoxitin (30 µg); C: Chloroamphenicol (30 µg); (Oxoid); CIP: Ciproflocaxin (5 µg); OB: Cloxacillin (5 µg); E: Erythromycin (15 µg); CN: Gentamicin (10 µg); K: Kanamycin (30 µg); NA: Nalidixic acid (30 µg); F: Nitrofurantion (50 µg); P: Penicillin G (10 units); S: Streptomycin (10 µg); SXT: Sulphamethoxazole trimethoprim (25 µg); TE: Tetracycline (30 µg); VA: Vancomycin (30 µg).

Table 4: Antimicrobial susceptibility patterns of each *Staphylococcus* species.

Number of antimicrobials	Resistance (number and percentage)
Zero	2 (3.6)
One	4 (7.3)
Two	9 (16.4)
Three	6 (10.9)
Four	9 (16.4)
Five	8 (14.5)
Six	5 (9.1)
Seven	2 (3.6)
Eight	5 (9.1)
Nine	1 (1.8)
Ten	1 (1.8)
Eleven	2 (3.6)
Thirteen	1 (1.8)
Total	**55 (100.0)**
MDR	40 (72.7)

MDR: Multi Drug Resistant

Table 5: Number and percentages of resistant staphylococcal isolates to antimicrobials.

In fact, tissues from healthy animal are sterile however, it has been pointed that during slaughter, dressing and cutting, microorganisms are introduced chiefly from the exterior of the animal and its intestinal tract but in general more microorganisms are added from knives, cloths, air, carts and equipment's. External contamination of meat will occur possibility from the moment of bleeding until consumption [21]. Among the factors that affect microbial growth in meat are intrinsic properties (physical and chemical properties of meat) and extrinsic (environmental factors), however the factors having the greatest influence on the growth of microorganisms in meat and meat products are the storage temperature, moisture and oxygen availability [30]. The possible sources of these bacteria are likely resulted from the skin of the animal from which the meat was obtained. Other potential sources of microbial contaminations are the equipment used for each operation until the final product is eaten; the clothing and hands of personnel and the physical facilities themselves are all implicated [22].

In the present study, 181 samples consisting of 94 municipal abattoirs, 87 dairy cattle farm originated samples were examined. The isolation and identification results proved the presence of the *Staphylococcus* in abattoir and farm originated samples examined in the study area. As the result, the proportion of *Staphylococcus* was found to be 53.2% (50/94), and 44.8% (39/87) from abattoir, and farm samples respectively. The overall proportion of *Staphylococcus* was 49.2% (89/181). A high proportion of *Staphylococcus* was recorded in municipal abattoir than dairy cattle farm samples. The reason for these could be hypothesized to be the poor hygienic status of the municipal abattoir. The proportional distribution of *Staphylococcus* among sample types is 35/66 (53.0%) in meat swab, 5/7 (71.4%) in polled knives swab, 3/7 (42.9%) in slaughter line swab, 3/7 (42.9%) in polled abattoir hand swab, 4/7 (57.1%) in polled abattoir nasal swab, 19/42 (45.2%) in udder milk, 3/9 (33.3%) in tank milk, 3/9 (33.3%)in polled bucket swab, 3/9 (33.3) tank swab, 3/9 (33.3%) polled farm hand swab and 8/9 (88.9%) polled farm nasal swab. From the samples containing staphylococci, *S. aureus* was detected 19.3% (35/181) of which 23.4% (22/50) abattoir and 14.9% (13/39) from farm samples. The farm result was slightly lower than 15.5% (51/328), [31] in around Addis Ababa; 17.2%, [32] in Egypt and 19.5%, [33] who isolated *S. aureus* strains from human and animal sources. Of the farm sample 5/42 (11.9%), 1/9 (11.1%), 0 (0.0%), 3/9 (33.3%), 1/9 (11.1%), and 3/9 (33.3%); udder milk, tank milk, polled bucket swab, tank swab, polled hand and nasal swab, respectively, were positive for *S. aureus* The findings of the present study revealed a lower proportional rate than 75% in 220 bovine bulk milk reported in [34], 68% (15/22) in [5], 61.3% (49/80) in [35], and 40% (32/81) in [36], but higher than [37] which was 8% (8/100) in udder milk and 10% (10/100) in tank milk. Also the present result shows the proportion of *S. aureus* in polled farm nasal swab 3/9 (33.3%) was higher than [38], 4/31(13%) and [33] who reported 20% from nasal swabs of diseased human. The difference in percentage of *S. aureus* in these reports could be explained either by the different microbiological techniques used in these studies, differences in the origin of the samples or by geographical differences. The *S. aureus* incidence at a considerable high percentage indicates the alarming situation both for dairy farms and for public health as well.

As the result shows *S. intermedius* have an overall proportion of 6/181 (3.3%), of which 2/94 (2.1%) and 4/87 (4.6%) are from abattoir and farm respectively. In addition, the proportion of *S. intermedius* was 2/66 (3%), 2/42 (4.8%), 1/9 (11.1%), 1(11.1%) in meat swab, udder milk, tank milk and bucket swab respectively, which was lower than [37] of 6/100 (6%) bucket milk and in agreement with 11/100 (11%) tank milk, but higher than 2% of 81 milk and milk product samples by [36]. The difference may be due to different procedures followed, geographical differences and origin of sample.

From 181 samples 24 (13.3%) was isolated to be *S. hyicus*, of these 13/66 (19.7%), 1/7 (14.3%), 1/7 (14.3%), 4/42 (9.5%), 1/9 (11.1%), 2/9 (22.2%), and 2/9 (22.9%); meat swab, polled knives swab, polled abattoir nasal swab, udder milk, tank milk, polled hand swab and polled farm nasal swabs respectively were distinguished. This result was higher than [37] who reported 6/100 (6%) bucket milk and 6/100 (6%) tank milk in Bishoftu town. This was may be due to poor hygienic status of the area.

In the past, CNS was often regarded as skin flora opportunists but recent data now indicate that they are associated with several subclinical and clinical infections [39]. In the current study 7/66 (10.6%) meat swab, 1/7 (14.3%) polled knives swab, 3/7 (42.9%) polled abattoir nasal swab, 8/42 (19.0%) udder milk, 2/9 (22.2%) polled bucket swab, 3/9 (33.3%) polled farm nasal swab was obtained with overall proportion of 24/181 (13.3%). It was lower than the investigation of [40] who reported CNS 54% in raw milk of cattle in Mongolia and [41] of 29% in 1036 samples.

In the current study 55 staphylococcal isolates were tested using fifteen antimicrobials. From these isolates Gentamycin, Kanamycin, Sulphamethoxazole trimethoprim, Chloramphenicol, and Ciprofloxacin were the most effective antimicrobials showing 94.5% to 81.1% susceptibility (Table 3). Because these drugs were the least frequently used in the study area in Veterinary services, thus no such more resistance was developed [42]. As [43] suggestion the development of antibiotic resistance is nearly always as a result of repeated therapeutic use and/or indiscriminate usage of them. The current study has showed very high level of resistance (85.5%) of *Staphylococcus* species isolates against Penicillin G. Moreover *S. aureus* have shown the resistance of Penicillin G was found to be 95.5% (Table 5), which is similar to [31] 96.7% and [44] 87.2%. This high level of resistance was due to isolate produced a penicillinase enzyme (a type of β-lactamase) that hydrolysed the beta-lactam ring of penicillin [45].

From 55 *Staphylococcus* species isolates tested 40/55 (72.9%) have developed multi drug resistance, which means those isolates are resistant to more than three antimicrobials. *Staphylococcus aureus* have developed higher degree of multi drug resistance 20/22 (90.9%) which was slightly higher than [46] report (79%). This was due to *S. aureus* strains have developed multidrug resistance worldwide with broad diversity in prevalence rate in different regions.

Conclusion

Staphylococcus species were prevalent in municipal abattoir and selected dairy cattle farms in Asella, South-eastern Ethiopia. *Staphylococcus aureus* was proportionally higher when compared to another Staphylococcal species. Over all, the presence of pathogenic *Staphylococcus* poses a health hazard and rise concerns about the safety of these food products. In addition, antimicrobial susceptibility showed that *Staphylococcus* species are highly sensitive to Gentamicin, Kanamycin, Chloramphenicol, Ciprofloxacillin, and Sulphamethoxazole trimethoprim; and also are more resistant Penicillin and Nalidixic acid. Moreover, most of *Staphylococcus* species isolates have developed multi drug resistance.

Conflict of Interests

The authors have not declared any conflict of interests.

Authors' Contributions

TB participated in research coordination, study design, data analysis, Antimicrobial susceptibility tests, and manuscript drafting and final revision. TA participated in sample collection, bacterial culture and identification Antimicrobial susceptibility tests and drafting manuscript. FG participated in study supervision, bacterial identification and Antimicrobial susceptibility tests. RD conceived the research idea and participated in its design, coordination and data analysis. TB, AF, DA, BM coordinated and supervised the study, provided valuable information and the design of the study. All authors agreed with the results and conclusions; and read and approved the final manuscript.

Acknowledgements

The authors greatly appreciate Addis Ababa University for funding this research.

References

1. Baron F (2007) Review on *Staphylococcus aureus* and food poisoning. Genet Mol Res 2: 163-176.
2. Pal M (2007) Zoonoses. 2nd edn. Satyam Publishers, Jaipur, India, pp: 138-139.
3. Hobbs BC, Roberts D (1981) Food Poisoning and Food Hygiene. 4th edn. Edward Arnold, London, Great Britain, p: 27.
4. Ash M (2008) Staphylococcus aureus and Staphylococcal Enterotoxins. In: Foodborne microorganisms of public health importance. 5th edn. AIFST (NSW Branch), Sydney, Australia, pp: 313-332.
5. Loir Y, Baron F, Gautier M (2003) Staphylococcus aureus and food poisoning. Genet Mol Res 2: 63-76.
6. Kerouanton A, Hennekinne J, Letertre C, Petit L, Chesneau O, et al. (2007) Characterization of Staphylococcus aureus strains associated with food poisoning outbreaks in France. Int J Food Microbiol 115: 369-375.
7. Aycicek H, Cakiroglu S, Stevenson T (2005) Incidence of Staphylococcus aureus in ready to eat meals from military cafeterias in Ankara, Turkey. Food Control 16: 531-534.
8. Bania J, Dabrowska A, Bystron J, Korzekwa K, Chrzanowska J, et al. (2006) Distribution of newly described enterotoxin-like genes in Staphylococcus aureus from food. Int J Food Microbiol 108: 36-41.
9. World Health Organization (2007) Food Safety - Food borne diseases and value chain management for food safety. "Forging links between Agriculture and Health" CGIAR on Agriculture and Health Meeting in WHO/HQ.
10. Essex-caster A (1987) A synopsis of public health and social medicine. 2nd edn. Sons Ltd., Bristol: Sohn Wright.
11. Hopkins RS, Juranek DD (1991) Acute giardiasis: an improved clinical case definition for epidemiologic studies. Am J Epidemiol 133: 402-407.
12. Ateba CN, Mbewe M, Moneoang MS, Bezuidenhout CC (2010) Antibiotic-resistant Staphylococcus aureus isolated from milk in the Mafikeng Area, North West province, South Africa. S Afr J Sci 106: 1-6.
13. Zadoks R, van Leeuwen W, Barkema H, Sampimon O, Verbrugh H, et al. (2000) Application of pulsed-field gel electrophoresis and binary typing as tools in veterinary clinical microbiology and molecular epidemiologic analysis of bovine and human Staphylococcus aureus isolates. J Clin Microbiol 38: 1931-1939.
14. Asao T, Kumeda Y, Kawai T, Shibata T, Oda H, et al. (2003) An extensive outbreak of staphylococcal food poisoning due to low-fat milk in Japan: estimation of enterotoxin A in the incriminated milk and powdered skim milk. Epidemiol Infect 130: 33-40.
15. Lee JH, Jeong JM, Park YH, Choi SS, Kim YH, et al. (2004) Evaluation of the methicillin-resistant Staphylococcus aureus (MRSA)-screen latex agglutination test for detection of MRSA of animal origin. J Clin Microbiol 42: 2780-2782.
16. Jay J (2000) Modern Food Microbiology. 6th edn., Aspen Food Science Text Series, Aspen Publishers Inc., Gaithersburg, Maryland, pp: 441-456.
17. Smith K (2007) Handbook of Foodborne pathogenic microorganisms and natural toxins. Food and Drug Administration, Center for Food Safety and Appl Nutr 10: 119-150.
18. Murray P, Rosenthal KS, Pfaller MA (2015) Microbiología médica. Elsevier, Brasil.
19. Yousuf A, Ahmed M, Yeasmin S, Ahsan N, Rahman M, et al. (2008) Prevalence of Microbial Load in Shrimp, Penaeus monodon and Prawn, Macrobrachium rosenbergii from Bangladesh. World J Agric Sci 4: 852-855.

20. Lawrie RA (1984) The preservation effect of smoke on meat. Meat Science Pergaman Press Inc., Maxwell House Fair View Park-Elmford, New York, pp: 49-52.

21. Rombouts F, Nouts R (1994) Food Microbiology and Hygiene. Encyclopedia Hum Biol Acad Press 3: 661-665.

22. Wagner AB Jr (2008) Bacterial Food Poisoning. Texas Agri Life Extension.

23. Walderhaug M (2007) Food borne pathogenic microorganisms and natural toxins. Food and Drug Administration, Centre for Food Safety and Applied Nutrition 28: 48-65.

24. Plan A (2007) Economic Development Office (APEDO) Socio Economic on Arsi Zone.

25. CLSI (2008) Performance Standards for Antimicrobial Disk and Dilution Susceptibility Tests for Bacteria Isolated from Animals. Clinical and Laboratory Standards Institute 28: M31-A3.

26. Salandra G, Goffredo E, Pedarra C, Nardella M, Parisi A, et al. (2008) Occurrence, characterization and antimicrobial resistance pattern of Staphylococcus species isolated from dairy products in southern Italy. Int J Food Microbiol 9: 327-360.

27. Soomro A, Arain M, Khashkeli M, Bhutto B, Memon A (2003) Isolation of Staphylococcus aureus from milk products sold at sweet-meat shops of Hyderabad, Pakistan. Online J Biol Sci 3: 91-94.

28. Kalorey DR, Shanmugam Y, Kurkure NV, Chousalkar KK, Barbuddhe SB (2007) PCR-based detection of genes encoding virulence determinants in Staphylococcus aureus from bovine subclinical mastitis cases. J Vet Sci 8: 151-154.

29. Forest DC, Harold DA, Judge BA, Robert EA (1985) Different Types of Meat and Meat product consumed by Nigerian. Principle of meat science. Pub WA. Freeman and Co., pp: 4-178.

30. Mekuria A, Asrat D, Woldeamanuel Y, Tefera G (2013) Identification and antimicrobial susceptibility of Staphylococcus aureus isolated from milk samples of dairy cows and nasal swabs of farm workers in selected dairy farms around Addis Ababa, Ethiopia. Afr J Microbial Res 7: 3501-3510.

31. El-Seedy FR, El-Shabrawy M, Hakim AS, Dorgham SM, Ata S, et al. (2010) Recent Techniques used for isolation and characterization of Staphylococcus aureus from mastitic cows. Am J Sci 6: 1-8.

32. Jakee J, Nagwa S, Bakry M, Sahar A, Zouelfakar E, et al. (2008) Characteristics of Staphylococcus aureus strains isolated from human and animal sources. J Agric Environ Sci 4: 221-229.

33. Jorgensen H, Mork T, Rorvik L (2005) The occurrence of Staphylococcus aureus on a farm with small-scale production of raw milk cheese. J Dairy Sci 88: 3810-3817.

34. Hein I, Jorgensen H, Loncarevic S, Wagner M (2005) Quantification of Staphylococcus aureus in unpasteurised bovine and caprine milk by real-time PCR. Res Microbiol 156: 554-563.

35. Bendahou A, Lebbadi M, Ennanei L, Essadqui F, Abid M (2008) Characterization of Staphylococcus species isolated from raw milk and milk products (lben and jben) in North Morocco. J Infect Dev Ctries 2: 218-225.

36. Tegegne MA (2009) Isolation and identification of Staphylococcus species from cottage cheese and raw bovine milk in Debre zeit, Ethiopia. MSc Thesis, Faculty of Veterinary Medicine, Addis Ababa University, Debreziet, Ethiopia.

37. Kateete D, Kabugo U, Baluku H, Nyakarahuka L, Kyobe S, et al. (2013) Prevalence and Antimicrobial Susceptibility Patterns of Bacteria from Milkmen and Cows with Clinical Mastitis in and around Kampala, Uganda. PLoS ONE 8: e63413.

38. Shah M (2003) Molecular pathogenesis of Staphylococcus aureus and other staphylococci. J Appl Bacteriol 59: 207-221.

39. Tsegmed U (2006) Staphylococci isolated from raw milk of yak and cattle in Mongolia. Studies on the occurrence, characterization, detection of enterotoxin and antimicrobial susceptibility profile of the isolates. Swedish University of Agricultural Sciences, Uppsala, Sweden.

40. Lamprell H, Villard L, Chamba JF, Beuvier E, Borges E, et al. (2004) Identification and biotyping of coagulase-positive staphylococci (CPS) in ripened French raw milk cheeses and their in vitro ability to produce enterotoxins. Rev Med Vet 155: 92-96.

41. Birhanu A, Diriba L, Iyob I (2013) Study of bovine mastitis in Asella government dairy farm of Oromia Regional state, South Eastern Ethiopia. Int J Curr Res Acca Rev 1: 134-145.

42. Jaimes EC, de los Monteros LEE, Renata D (2002) Epidemiology of drug resistance; the case of Staphylococcus aureus and coagulase negative staphylococci infections. Salud pública Méx 44: 108-112.

43. Sori T, Hussien J, Bitew M (2011) Prevalence and susceptibility assay of Staphylococcus aureus isolated from bovine mastitis in dairy farms of Jimma town, South West Ethiopia. J Anim Vet Adv 10: 745-749.

44. Cavalieri SJ, Harbeck RJ, McCarter YS, Ortez JH, Rankin ID, et al. (2005) Manual of antimicrobial susceptibility testing. American Society for Microbiology. Library of Congress Cataloging-in-Publication Data, USA, p: 102.

45. Chao G, Zhou X, Jiao X (2007) Prevalence and antimicrobial resistance of food borne pathogens isolated from food products in China. Foodborne Pathog Dis 4: 277-284.

46. Normanno G, La Salandra G, Dambrosio A, Quaglia NC, Corrente M, et al. (2007) Occurrence, characterization and antimicrobial resistance of enterotoxigenic Staphylococcus aureus isolated from meat and dairy products. Int J Food Microbiol 115: 290-296.

Major Health Challenges of Dairy Cattle in Hawassa Town SNNPRS, Ethiopia

Nigussu Fasil[2]*, Terefe Simon Juta[1] and Dessie Sheferaw[2]

[1]*Department of Parasitology and Pathology, Jigjiga University, Jigjiga, Ethiopia*
[2]*School of Veterinary Medicine, Hawassa University, Ethiopia*

Abstract

The aim of this study was to assess major health challenges of dairy cattle in Hawassa town, Ethiopia, which occurred on November 2014 up to April 2015. A single visit-multiple subject formal survey technique was used to collect data from 20 dairy farming which were selected at random and were interviewed using pre-tested, structured questionnaire which indicated that over all prevalence in this study was 33.6% (n=269) cattle were found affected by either one or more of health challenges. It appeared from the study that LSD (30.1%), mastitis (20.4%), hypocalcaemia (17.5%), repeated breeding (13%), RFM (10%) and parturient paresis (6.7%) were identified as the most frequently occurring diseases. Results of the major dairy cattle disease in the study area ranked LSD as number one disease occurred in different dairy farms, followed by mastitis (20.4%) and hypocalcaemia (17.5%). The degree of association of risk factors was assessed and parity, age, farm scale, and management system found to be directly associated. As the result shows age with dystocia directly associated and have good significances with the x^2=12.479 and p-value =0.002, and LSD associated with farm scale but not significant, with the x^2=4.705 and ($p>0.05$) and also abortion associated with management system but have no significance ($p>0.05$). This particular study indicated major health challenges which included hypocalcaemia, ketosis, abortion, RFM, parturient paresis, repeated breeding, diarrhea, bloat, and anestrous, uterine prolapsed, vaginal prolapsed, dystocia and LSD were one of the major reproductive and metabolic disorders responsible for the low reproductive performance of dairy cows.

Keywords: Age; Breed; Cattle; Dairy farm; Hawassa; Health

Abbreviations: DVM: Doctor of Veterinary Medicine; P-Value: Expected Prevalence; RFM: Retained Fetal Membrane; SPSS: Stastical Package for Social Science; LSD: Lumpy Skin Disease; χ^2: Chi-square test.

Introduction

Ethiopia has the largest livestock population being the first in Africa countries and the 10th in the world and holds large potential for dairy development due to its large livestock population and Urban and peri-urban livestock production constitutes an important sub-sector of the agricultural production system [1]. In Ethiopia, livestock represents a major national resource and form an integral part of the agricultural production system [2]. The livestock sector in general and the dairy industry in particular do not provide the expected contribution to the national income despite their large numbers due to several factors. The development of the dairy sector in the country is hindered by a number of technical, institutional and socio-economic constraints. The growth in milk production has been slow and the annual milk production is estimated to be 1,089,488,251 liters [3] which doesn't meet even the domestic demand for dairy products. As a result the country imports large volumes of dairy products per annum to meet the domestic demand. In 2005, for instance, the country imported 457,260 kg of milk (liquid and powder) which is equivalent to 3,026,724 Birr [3].

Despite the huge number of cattle and their dairy industry the productivity is low due to the constraints of disease, scarcity of feed, inefficient and insufficient AI, veterinary services nutrition, poor management, lack of marketing facilities and opportunity, inadequate animal health services, uncoordinated development programs between various levels of government institutions and /or non-government organizations and poor performance of indigenous breeds. These constraints result in health challenges of dairy cattle [4].

Major health challenges of dairy cattle were consists of ketosis, hypocalcaemia, metritis, retained fetal membranes, LSD, bloating, mastitis and uterine prolapsed. All of these diseases are related to one another, with complicated cause and effect mechanisms in place. Numerous studies [5-10] had shown that postpartum diseases can affect the length of calving interval, the number of days open, and the reproductive efficiency in general. These diseases can also affect the overall productivity of dairy cows by reducing milk yield. Studies conducted so far in Ethiopia [11-15] revealed poor reproductive performance of dairy cows in the tropics. For feasible intervention, the poor reproductive performance of dairy cows should warrant investigation on the types and magnitudes of the existing postpartum problems. These constraints also result in poor reproductive performance of dairy cattle. Among the major problems that have a direct impact on reproductive performance of dairy cows are: abortion, retention of the fetal membrane (RFM) and metritis. These results in considerable economic losses to the dairy industry due to slower uterine involution, reduced reproductive rate, prolonged inter conception and calving interval, cost of medication, drop in milk production, reduced calf drop, and early depreciation of potentially useful cows [16,17].

Although, the major health problems are greatly responsible for high economic loss in the dairy industry, there is scarcity of reliable information regarding the reproductive performances of dairy cows in subsistence dairy farms in the tropics, particularly in Ethiopia. Information pertaining to reproductive performance and interacting factors is of paramount importance primarily to the livestock owners and also to the extension agents, veterinarians and researchers. Moreover, it

***Corresponding author:** Nigussu Fasil, Assistant Professor, School of Veterinary Medicine, Hawassa University, Ethiopia
E-mail: fasilkedesegne@yahoo.com

can assist in the development of strategies and prioritization of possible intervention options for performance improvement [18]. Dairy cattle require minerals in their diet for optimal productivity. These are derived from the feed and fodder. The input of minerals through feed and water must balance their output through faces, urine and milk to maintain the animal's health. If the output exceeds input, the animals meet out their normal requirements by mobilization from its body reserves for a shorter period. But continuous imbalances develop into productivity related problems.

Nutritional imbalances, deficiencies, or erratic management of feeding programs for dairy cows can create large numbers and various types of health problems generally categorized as metabolic diseases. Most periparturient abnormalities have some metabolic element as a component of the cause of clinical disease. The metabolic disturbance of milk fever can be measured through low serum calcium concentrations. Negative energy balance, fat mobilization and subsequent elevations in ketone body concentrations play a contributing role in the expression of fatty liver syndrome, clinical ketosis, and abomasal displacement. A negative energy balance may also increase the risk of retained placenta, metritis, and mastitis through impaired immune function.

Therefore, the objectives of present study were;

- To identify major health challenges of dairy cattle found in different dairy farms.
- To assess risk factors that cause to occurrence of health challenges in dairy cow.

Materials and Methods

Description of the study area

The cross sectional study was conducted from November, 2014 up to April, 2015, in Hawassa, capital city of the Southern Nations Nationalities and Peoples Regional State (SNNPRS), which is one of the high potential areas for milk production in Southern Ethiopia. It is located 275 km south of Addis Ababa along the Addis Ababa - Moyale highway. Hawassa is situated at an altitude of 1750 m above sea level and according to an estimate, it lies between 6°83' to 7°17' N and 38°24' to 38°72' E. Hawassa receives an average annual rainfall of 955 mm with mean annual temperature of 20°C [3] (Figure 1).

Study design and method of sampling

The cross-sectional study design was needed to determine the prevalence of hypocalcaemia, parturient paresis, ketosis, bloat, mastitis, uterine prolapsed, vaginal prolapsed, dystocia, abortion, anestrous, diahorrea, payometra, retained fetal membrane, LSD and its risk factors that predisposes to this major health challenges. The study was a questionnaire data collection and analysis to establish the prevalence and to identify the major health challenges in the selected

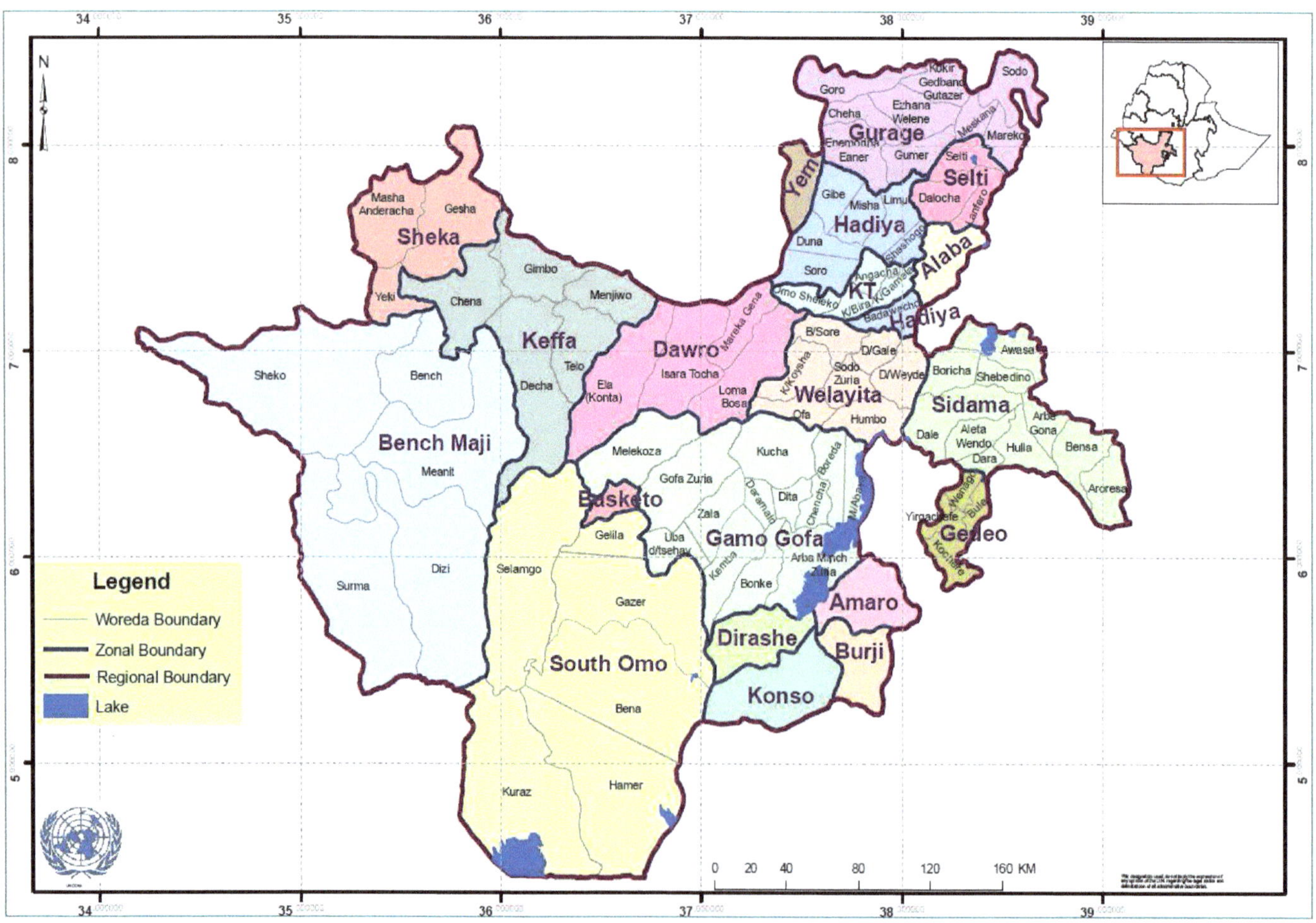

Figure 1: The regional map of SNNPRS.

farms. Farms purposively selected based their accessibility number of dairy populations in the area. Animals were selected by using simple random methods.

Study animals

The exotic, local and cross breeds of cows were used in this study. Addition to this extensively managed cross breeds that high grade Holstein Fresian, predominantly Holstein-indigenous zebu cross breeds and indigenous local zebu lactating cows in dairy farms were taken to this study. The history of the animals like age, parity, farm scale, stage of lactation, lactation number, milk yield, body condition, nutritional condition, symptoms observed by the owner, past and present history regarding other illness, and have different production system (extensive, semi-intensive and intensive type of management) were recorded in selected farms in Hawassa town.

Data collection

Questionnaires survey method: Structured questionnaire was prepared and used to collect information from 20 dairy farm owners by regular farm visit interview and recorded lists about major health challenges of their dairy cattle on individual level were studied. The questionnaires were checked for clarity of the questions prior the interview. Prior the interview, respondents were briefed to the objective of the study. Following that, the actual questions and questionnaires were presented. Accordingly, information about the parity, breed, feeding system, production system, and type of feed, health care and major health challenges such as hypocalcaemia, ketosis, abortion, mastitis, parturient paresis, anoestrus, uterine and vaginal prolapse, bloat, repeat breeding and LSD were collected on individual cattle level. From 20 selected dairy farms five farms have well recorded data list was needed to this study. In order to identify dairy farms considered in the current study, an initial list of dairy farms in the city was obtained from Hawassa City Administration Agricultural and Rural Development Office.

Data analysis

The data was presented using the descriptive statistics, the retrospective data results was entered to a Microsoft Excel sheet 2007 and analyzed using a software SPSS' version 20. Different factors include age, breed, productivity, parity, management, farm scale and body condition score that were considered during the study period were analyzed using the Chi-square technique. The possible association of dystocia, abortion, and LSD with age, management, and farm scale respectively was also tested using these techniques. In all chi-square test application, probability of $p<0.05$ was considered statistically significant.

Results

In the cross sectional study of questionnaire LSD, mastitis, hypocalcaemia, and repeated breeding were found to be the major health challenges occur in Hawassa town dairy farm, containing (30.1%), (20.4%), (17.5%) and (13%), respectively. Other health problems observed with lower prevalence include retain fetal membrane (10%), parturient paresis (6.7%), diarrhea (6.3%), dystocia (5.6%), anestrous (5.6%), ketosis (5.2%), abortion (5.2%), bloat (4.5%), payometra (3.7%), uterine prolapse (3.7%) and vaginal prolapse (2.2%) accounting were obtained from study.

From the total of 269 dairy cattle, 129 (47.9%) were managed semi-intensive, 38 (14.1%) were intensively and 102 (37.9%) were extensively and of which 250 (92.9%) were cross breed and the rest 19 (7.1%) were local breed. Most of the animal were adult age group encountered, 222 (82.5%), the rest of them were 23 (8.6%) young and 24 (8.9%) old age group. The parity of the animal is few, moderate, and high, which was in number showed 194 (72.1%), 62 (23.0%) and 13 (4.8%) respectively.

Major health challenges identified in dairy farms

The major health challenges identified were LSD (30.1%), mastitis (20.4%) and hypocalcaemia (17.5%), as summarized on Table 1, bellow. In this study 33.6% (n=269) cattle were found affected by either one or more of health challenges.

Association of risk factors with health challenges of dairy cattle

In this study among risk factors age, farm scale, parity and management system were considered to assess its association with the occurrence of the health challenges as shown on the tables below (Table 2).

Table 3 showed that there is statistically significant ($p<0.05$) variation with regard to age and dystocia. Highest prevalence was found in cattle with age group adult and followed by age group young while the least in cows with age group old. The prevalence rate of LSD at farm scale level is higher in small farm scale (46.1%) than in medium (26.3%) and large (33.3%) farm scale.

As shown on the Tables 4 and 5 above, statistically no significant difference ($P>0.05$) was found in the prevalence of health challenges with respect to management system.

Discussion

In the present study (33.6%) of dairy cattle in the study areas were affected by either one or major health challenges based on questionnaires to the owners. Major health challenges are LSD, mastitis, hypocalcaemia, and repeated breeding were found to be the major health challenges occur in Hawassa town dairy farm, containing (30.1%), (20.4%), (17.5%) and (13%), respectively. Recent survey which assesses the risk factors and financial impacts of LSD in selected districts of North-eastern Ethiopia (Tigray and Afar Regional States) conducted by Birhanu [19] reported a higher herd prevalence of (51%) and (37%) was recorded in Afar and Tigray Region respectively which is higher result from present study (30.1%), this variation might be due to environment, breed of animal and management system. The prevalence rate of mastitis (20.4%) recorded in this study is higher than to the reports done in different dairy farms in Hawassa town (4.9%) by

Challenges	Frequency	Percentage (%)
Hypocalcaemia	47	17.5
Payometra	10	3.7
Parturient paresis	18	6.7
Diahorrea	17	6.3
Ketosis	14	5.2
Bloat	12	4.5
Mastitis	55	20.4
Dystocia	15	5.6
Abortion	14	5.2
RFM	27	10
Uterine prolapsed	10	3.7
Vaginal prolapsed	6	2.2
Anestrous	15	5.6
Repeated breeding	35	13
LSD	81	30.1

Table 1: Frequency and Prevalence rate of major health problems of dairy Cattle in Hawassa town.

Risk factors	No. of cattle	Percentage
Age		
Young (<4 years)	23	8.6
Adult (4-8 years)	222	82.5
Old (>9 years)	24	8.9
Parity		
Few (<3 birth)	194	72.1
Moderate (3-5 birth)	62	23.0
High (>5 birth)	13	4.8
Productivity		
No	1	4
Low	157	58.4
Medium	94	34.9
High	17	6.3
Breed		
Local	19	7.1
Cross	250	92.9
Body condition		
Poor	78	29.0
Medium	138	51.3
Good	53	19.7
Management system		
Extensive	103	38.3
Semi-intensive	128	47.6
Intensive	38	14.1
Farm scale		
Small	26	9.7
Medium	171	63.6
Large	72	26.8

Table 2: Association of risk factors with health challenges of dairy cattle.

Challenge	Age				χ^2	P- value
Dystocia	Young	adult	Old	Total		
-ve	18	213	23	254	12.479	0.002
+ve	5	9	1	15		
Total	23	222	24	269		

Table 3: Association of age group with health challenge.

Challenges	Farm scale				χ^2	P- value
LSD	Small	Medium	Large	Total		
-ve	14	126	48	188	4.705	0.095
+ve	12	45	24	81		
Total	26	171	72	269		

Table 4: Association of farm scale with health challenge.

Challenges	Management system				χ^2	P-value
Abortion	Extensive	Semi-intensive	intensive	Total		
-ve	99	122	34	255	2.615	0.270
+ve	4	6	4	14		
Total	103	128	38	269		

Table 5: Association of management system with health challenge.

Nibret et al. [20]; in and around Mekelle (6.55%) by Wudu [21] and in central high lands of Ethiopia (6.6%) by Mungube et al. [22]. While it was comparable in the reports done in and around Sebeta (16.1%) by Hunderra et al. [23]; in Dire Dawa Administrative Council and Eastern Hararghe Zone (19.8%) by Birhanu [24]; in two major state owned dairy farms at Rapi and Debre Zeit, Ethiopia (21%) by Workineh et al. [25]; but it was lower in the research finding in selected areas of southern Ethiopia (37%) by Kerro and Tareke [26].

The prevalence rate of hypocalcaemia (17.5%) recorded in this study is lower than the result (30.2%) reported by Samuel et al. [27] this difference may be management, type of breed and study population. Most of the literatures suggest that when the incidence of milk fevers increases above (10%) in their third or latter lactation, considerations should be given to a specific control program [28]. Therefore, these results indicated that control methods are required to avoid loss due to milk fever. Milk fever is caused by a severe deficiency of metabolizable calcium ion in the circulation. This could be attributed due to several risk factors [29]. The risk factors identified in this study include milk yield, parity and breed of the cows.

The higher prevalence of repeated breeding (13%) found in the present study is in close agreement with (13%) reported by Micheal [30] in and around Hawassa and (13.08%) by Adane et al. [31] but higher than (11.4%) reported by Hadush et al. [32] from central Ethiopia. Repeated breeding can be caused by a number of factors, including sub-fertile bulls, endocrine imbalance, malnutrition, reproductive tract infections and poor management practices such as wrong time of insemination or faulty heat detection, inappropriate semen handling and insemination techniques [33]. In addition to these, communal use of bull for natural services also considered as contributing factor. Hence the difference between the findings of the current study and previous reports may be attributed to the above-mentioned factors.

Other health problems observed with lower prevalence include retain fetal membrane (10%), parturient paresis (6.7%), diarrhea (6.3%), dystocia (5.6%), anestrous (5.6%), ketosis (5.2%), abortion (5.2%), bloat (4.5%), payometra (3.7%), uterine prolapse (3.7%) and vaginal prolapse (2.2%) were obtained.

The prevalence rate of RFM (10%) in recent study is similar with the (8.6%) reported by Molalegn and Shiv [34] and lower than (14.2%) reported by Mamo [35] and 19.2% by Gashaw et al. [36]. The variation in the incidence of RFM attributed to variations in predisposing factors to which the animals are subjected to nutritional status and management problems such as lack of exercise. Dystocia that accounted (5.9%) of the problems is an important predisposing factor for occurrence of RFM. Previous report (5.79%) on the prevalence of dystocia by Mamo [35] in small holder dairy cows in and around Debre Zeiet fairly agrees to the prevalence of (5.6%) obtained in this study. However, the current finding is lower than the prevalence of (7.7%) reported by Dawit and Ahmed [37], and higher than those (3.8%) of Gashaw et al. [36]. This variation in the occurrence of dystocia due to the fact that it is influenced by the factors such as, age and parity of the dam as well as breed of the sire. Inseminating cows with semen collected from large sized bulls without taking into account the size and age of cows is an important factor in precipitating dystocia [38].

The prevalence of anestrous observed in this study (5.6%) was lower than the results of Hadush et al. [32], who reported (12.9%) in dairy cattle in Debre Zeit and Befekadu [39], who reported (24%) in cross breed dairy cows in central high lands of Ethiopia. This variation might be due to the age, faulty heat detection, and breed and management system differences.

The prevalence rate of abortion (5.2%) recorded in this study was higher than the result (2.2%) reported by Bekana et al. [34] in Nazret, but is lower than the (9.0%), (13.9%) and (14.6%) reported by Dawite and Ahmed [37], Molalegn and Shiv [34] and Hunduma [40] respectively. The lower prevalence rate of abortion may be attributed to the increasing practice of AI in the study area where the semen is collected from bulls free from brucellosis, in addition breed, management system specially feeding and sanitation. Study methodology and geographical location differences are all sources of differences in prevalence of abortion [36].

The prevalence rate of vaginal prolapse (2.2%) recorded in this study is lower than the result (5.2%) reported by Kidusan [41] but is higher than the (1.2%) reported by Dawite and Ahmed [37]. This variation might be due to management system (feeding), abortion, RFM, dystocia and breed of animals.

The prevalence rate of ketosis (5.2%) recorded in this study is lower than the result (11.2%) reported by Mulat et al. [42] in and around Addis Ababa. The highest prevalence of ketosis was recorded in the month of January. This indicates that ketosis occurred mostly during the winter season as the animals are usually housed and there is scarce of pasture [43].

There was both reproductive and metabolic problems (49%) and (29.4%) respectively. This result indicates that it is higher value than the prevalence (43.3%) reported by Adane et al. [31] in urban and per urban area of Hossana, (44.3%) by Hadush et al. [32] in central Ethiopia and (40.3%) by Dawite and Ahmed [37] in Northeast Ethiopia. This difference might be due to sample size, production system, study methodology and breed of animals as well as environmental factors.

The higher prevalence rate of health challenges in cross breed animals 92.9% (n=250) than local breed 7.1% (n=19) may be due to the fact that cross breeds are less adapted to tropical conditions of high temperature and humidity, disease and low feed quality than zebu cattle [44-46] making them more susceptible than indigenous zebu. In addition to this the risk factors like age group, parity, management system; farm scale, body condition and productivity are great effect up on major health challenges of dairy cattle.

Conclusion and Recommendation

The result found in the current study was an agreement with the other studies those metabolic and reproductive problems which have adverse effects on the health, production and reproduction indices of the dairy cow. Hypocalcaemia, ketosis, bloat, mastitis, uterine and vaginal prolapse, LSD, abortion, dystocia, RFM, anestrous and diahorrea were major health challenge in the dairy farm. Age, breed, parity, and management systems were the most important predisposing risk factor for the various health challenges. Development of practical management strategies to cope with the negative effects associated with reproductive and health problems on dairy cattle is critical in this study area. Therefore, the following recommendation will be forwarded:

- Providing an adequate amount of a properly formulated and delivered ration,
- Providing a clean, comfortable and minimal-stress environment.
- There should be proper animal management, cleanliness and good hygiene on dairy farms.
- Improving veterinary services with respect to adequate vaccination.
- There should be Routine and periodical examination of cows during postpartum period.
- Screening, sanitation, serious follow up and health care are very important.

Acknowledgements

To begin with, I would like to express my thanks to my academic advisor, Dr. Nigussu Fasil, who had made professional advices and critical comments, without which my study would have not reached to this stage of completion. My thanks also extend to my co-advisors, Dr. Desse Shiferaw. They all contributed invaluable advices and comments to my study from the step of inception up to the completion of this DVM, Thesis research work. My family, particularly my dad Simon Juta, wishes long life, additionally my golden sisters Minitiwab Simon, Tsedal Simon and my diamond brother Abebayehu Simon, I'm very much grateful to your ever supports to all my educational works. Prior to all, "GOD IS GREAT!!" is my ever saying to all great deeds he did to me.

References

1. Tegegne A, Tadesse M, Yami A, Mekasha Y (2000) Market-oriented urban and peri-urban dairy systems. Urban Agriculture Magazine 1: 23-24.
2. IFPRI (2006) Atlas of the Ethiopian Rural Economy. International Food Policy Research Institute (Washington, DC), Central Statistical Agency (Addis Ababa), Ethiopian Development Research Institute (Addis Ababa).
3. BoFED (2007) Bureau of Finance and Economic Development, Southern Nations, Nationalities and People's Regional State (SNNPR).
4. Drug Administration and Control Authority (2006) Standard veterinary treatment guide lines for Veterinary Clinics. 1st edition. Pp: 3-13.
5. Borsberry S, Dobson H (1989) Periparturient diseases and their effect on reproductive performance in five dairy herds. Vet Rec 138: 217-219.
6. Gröhn Y, McCulloch C, Saloniemi H (1990) Epidemiology of mammary gland disorders in multiparous Finnish Ayrshire cows. Prev Vet Med 8: 241-252.
7. Rajala PJ, Gröhn YT (1998) Effects of dystocia, retained placenta, and metritis on milk yield in dairy cows. J Dairy Sci 81: 3172-3181.
8. Ferguson J, Galligan D (2000) Assessment of Reproductive Efficiency in Dairy Herds. Educ Proc Vet 22: 150-158.
9. LeBlanc SJ, Duffield TF, Leslie KE, Bateman KG, Keefe GP, et al. (2002) Defining and diagnosing postpartum clinical endometritis and its impact on reproductive performance in dairy cows. J Dairy Sci 85: 2223-2236.
10. LeBlanc SJ (2008) Postpartum uterine disease and dairy herd reproductive performance: a review. Vet J 176: 102-114.
11. Negussie E, Brannang E, Banjaw K, Rottmann O (1998) Reproductive performance of dairy cattle at Asella livestock farm, Arsi, Ethiopia. I: Indigenous cows versus their F1 crosses. J Anim Breed Genet 115: 267-280.
12. Shiferaw Y, Tenhagen BA, Bekana M, Kassa T (2003 Reproductive Disorders of Crossbred Dairy Cows in the Central Highlands of Ethiopia and Their Effect on Reproductive Performance. Trop Anim Health Prod 37: 427-441.
13. Asseged B, Birhanu M (2004) Survival analysis of calves and reproductive performance of cows in commercial dairy farms in and around Addis Ababa, Ethiopia. Trop Anim Health Prod 36: 663-672.
14. Ibrahim N, Abraha A, Mulugeta S (2011) Assessment of reproductive performances of crossbred dairy cattle (Holstein Friesian× Zebu) in Gondar town. Global Vet 6: 561-566.
15. Dinka H (2012) Reproductive performance of crossbred dairy cows under smallholder condition in Ethiopia. Int J Livestock Prod 3: 25-28.
16. Thomas C (1989) A preliminary survey on infertility aspects of selected dairy farms around Addis Ababa. A seminar presented to the orientation course in Tropical Animal and Health Production, Addis Ababa University, Faculty of Veterinary Medicine, Debre Zeit, Ethiopia.
17. Barnouin J, Chacronac J (1992) A nutritional risk factor for early metritis in dairy farms in France. Pre Vet Med 13: 23-27.
18. Angesom H, Adem A, Fikru R (2013) Major prepartum and postpartum reproductive problems of dairy cattle in Central Ethiopia. J Vet Med Anim Health 5: 118-123.
19. Birhanu T (2012) Assessments of the risk factors and financial impacts of LSD in selected districts of Tigray and Afar Regional States, Northeastern Ethiopia. M.Sc. Thesis.
20. Moges N, Hailemariam T, Fentahun T, Chanie M, Melaku A (2012) Bovine Mastitis and Associated Risk Factors in Small Holder Lactating Dairy Farms in Hawassa, Southern Ethiopia. Global Vet 9: 441-446.
21. Wudu T (1999) Study on Bovine mastitis in and around Mekelle. DVM thesis, Faculty of Veterinary Medicine, Addis Ababa University, Ethiopia.
22. Mungube EO, Tenhagen BA, Regassa F, Kyule MN, Shiferaw Y, et al. (2005) Reduced milk production in udder quarters with subclinical mastitis and associated economic losses in crossbred dairy cows in Ethiopia. Trop Anim Health Prod 37: 503-512.
23. Sori H, Zerihun A, Abdicho S (2005) Dairy cattle mastitis in and around Sebeta, Ethiopia. Intern J Appl Res Vet Med 3: 332-338.

24. Birhanu S (1997) Bovine Mastitis in Dairy Farm in Dire Dawa Administrative Council and Western Harareghe Zone. Prevalence, isolation and *in vitro* antimicrobial susceptibility study. DVM thesis. Addis Ababa University, Faculty of Veterinary medicine, Ethiopia.

25. Workineh S, Bayleyegn M, Mekonnen H, Potgieter LN (2002) Prevalence and aetiology of mastitis in cows from two major Ethiopian dairies. Trop Anim Health Prod 34: 19-25.

26. Dego OK, Tareke F (2003) Bovine mastitis in selected areas of southern Ethiopia. Trop Anim Health Prod 35: 197-205.

27. Anteneh S, Guadu T, Fentahun T, Chanie M (2012) Incidence of Milk Fever on Dairy Cows and its Risk Factors in Gondar Town, Northwest Ethiopia. Int J Nat Sci 9: 659-662.

28. Horst RL (1986) Regulation of calcium and phosphorus homeostasis in the dairy cow. J Dairy Sci 69: 604-616.

29. Brandly CA, Cornelius CE (1969) Parturient Hypocalcaemia in Dairy Cows. Advances in Veterinary Science and Comparative Medicine. Academic press, USA, 15: 143-150.

30. Micheal K (2003) Major clinical reproductive problem of small holder dairy cows in and around Awassa. DVM Thesis, Addis Ababa University, Faculty of Veterinary Medicine, Debre Zeit, Ethiopia.

31. Adane H, Yisehak T, Niguse T (2014) Assessment of major reproductive disorders of dairy cattle in urban and per urban area of Hosanna, Southern Ethiopia. Animal Vet Sci 2: 135-141.

32. Hadush A, Abdella A, Regassa F (2013) Major prepartum and postpartum reproductive problems of dairy cattle in Central Ethiopia. J Vet Med Anim Health 5: 118-123.

33. Arthur G, Noakes D, Pearson H (1989) Veterinary Reproduction and Obstetrics. Theriogenology 6th edition. Baillier Tindall UK, Pp: 83-85.

34. Molalegne B, Shiv P (2011) Study on Major Reproductive Health Problems in Indigenous and Cross Breed Cows in and Around Bedelle, South West Ethiopia. J Anim Vet Adv 10: 723-727.

35. Mamo T (2004) Study on major postpartum reproductive problems of smallholder dairy cows in and around Debre Zeit. DVM Thesis, Addis Ababa University, Faculty of Veterinary Medicine, Debre Zeit, Ethiopia.

36. Gashaw A, Worku F, Mulugeta S (2011) Assessment of small holder dairy production system and their reproductive health problems in Jimma town Southwestern Ethiopia. Intern J Appl Res Vet Med 9: 80-86.

37. Tesfaye D, Shamble A (2013) Reproductive health problems of cows under different management systems in kombolcha, North east Ethiopia. Adv Biol Res 7: 104-108.

38. Noakes D (1986) Fertility and Obstetrics in cattle. Blackwell Science Publishers, Oxford, UK, Pp: 28-30.

39. Befekadu U (2007) A field investigation of delayed resumption of postpartum ovarian activity and prolonged postpartum anestrus in cross bred dairy cows in Debre Zeit dairy herds (Doctoral dissertation, MSc Thesis, Addis Ababa University, Faculty of Veterinary Medicine, Debre Zeit, Ethiopia).

40. Dinka H (2013) Major reproductive disorders of dairy cows in and around Asella town, Central Ethiopia. J Vet Med Anim Health 5: 113-117.

41. Kidusan K (2009) Study on major reproductive disorders of dairy cattle in and around Wukro. DVM Thesis, College of Veterinary Medicine, Mekelle University, Tigray, Northern Ethiopia.

42. Asrat M, Tadesse GH, Gounder RV, Nagappan R (2013) Prevalence and Treatment of Ketosis in Dairy Cows in and Around Addis Ababa, Ethiopia. Br J Dairy Sci 3: 26-30.

43. Blood D, Radostists O, Henderson J (1983) Veterinary Medicine. 6th edition. Bailiere Tindall, London and New York.

44. Mugerwa ME (1989) A review of reproductive performance of female Bos indicus (Zebu) cattle. ILCA monograph No. 6. ILCA, Addis Ababa.

45. Plan LM (2008) Livestock development master plan study-Phase 1 report: Data collection and analysis. Volume H-Animal Nutrition (November 2008).

46. Stevenson JS, Call EP (1988) Reproductive disorders in the periparturient dairy cow. J Dairy Sci 71: 2572-2583.

The Effect of Marketing System on Cattle Welfare in Mersa and Woldia Towns

Yidersal Erega and Solomon Tsegaye*

College of Agriculture, Woldia University, P.O. Box 400, Woldia, Ethiopia

Abstract

Cattle welfare is hindered by several factors such as lack of feed, water, shelter, rest and comfortable transportation facilities; the aim of this study was to assess the effect of marketing system on cattle welfare. The majority age of respondents was range from 31-45 (47.5%) and the analysis for educational status disclosed that 45% of the respondents were illiterates and majority of households owned cattle in the range between 1-3 (42.5%) cattle. Most of the market actors in the study area were farmers which covered 47.5% and 45% of total sellers and buyers respectively. The majority of households owned cattle in the range between 1-3 (42.5%) cattle per head. About 72.5% of the respondents confirmed that price of cattle is set by negotiation between buyers and sellers. Abusive handling by stakeholders was the most frequently observed behavior (48% and 45%) at Mersa and Woldia markets respectively. Highest expressed abusive behaviors by stakeholders were beating of body by stick 45% and 48% at Mersa and Woldia markets respectively. The aggressive behavior of the animals due to human intervention at Woldia and Mersa accounts about 37% and 42% respectively. Transportation system of cattle in the study area was mostly by foot 96% and 94% in Mersa and Woldia respectively. Hunger and thrust was leading welfare problem whereas naturalness is not the main problem. Generally the welfare of cattle at markets was very poor and animal transport conditions are inadequate which implies awareness creation is vital.

Keywords: Behavior; Cattle; Mersa; Market; Welfare; Woldia

Introduction

Ethiopia is known for diversified agricultural activities [1]. Agriculture is the main economic backbone for Ethiopian economy since more than 80% of people in Ethiopia depend on agriculture and contributes to almost 40% of total GDP (Gross Domestic Product) (around 20% of this comes from livestock and their products). Ethiopia is the leading country in livestock population in Africa and ranked tenth from world [2].

Animal welfare is described generally in terms of comfortable interaction of animals with their environment and measured in terms of physiological, psychological and behavioural systems [3]. Animals that are transported by foot to the market often walk for days without adequate rest, water or feed. The drivers of animals in Ethiopia force them to move faster. By the time the animals reach at markets they are exhausted and their physical condition has greatly deteriorated [4]. In developing countries like Ethiopia, the main welfare concerns of animals are mainly, long distance journey, forcing animals to cross big rivers that have no bridge and journey without sufficient food, water and resting time [5]. Further Animals are also exposed to high radiation in summer and heavy rain in the winter. Animals are transported from farms to market or other places usually by walking or by inappropriate vehicles [6].

In Ethiopia there are no animal welfare regulations or any constitution that protects animals from suffering [7] so, animal welfare has been compromised due to different reasons including, breeding procedures and consequent difficulties, ill treatment, neglect accidentally or due to lack of knowledge, in adequacy in design of housing including pens. Inadequate management system or poor husbandry on the farm, poor conditions and procedures in the following conditions during moving or loading, during transport, at market or at slaughter house also affect cattle welfare [5,8].

Stakeholders at markets are handling cattle abusively. This type of handling is correlated with higher frequencies of aggressive, stress related and resistance behaviours that animal express. In Ethiopia, the most common transport system of cattle to markets is by foot [3]. A high prevalence of dead and injured animals during transport is common depending on the type of transport and distance covered [8].

In Mersa and Woldia cattle markets, there are many cattle suppliers. There are also other market actors like traders, brokers, cattle trekkers and truckers. However, the market actors are not aware of animal welfare. In the same they have no any care for the welfare of animals rather they only focus on the marketing activity without considering economic importance of cattle welfare. Compromising cattle welfare at markets leads to the animals to high stress levels and to loss body condition up to injury and death, so these leads to higher economic lose for cattle producers and market actors as well as affects the economic growth of the country by reducing the contribution of livestock sector to the total GDP (Gross Domestic Product). Even though cattle needs feed, water, shelter, rest and comfortable transportation facilities market actors do not know how to manage and care their cattle during transportation and at markets. So far, no work has done on the effect of marketing system on cattle welfare in the study area. Therefore, this research was initiated to address this problem.

Therefore the objective of this study was

- To assess the effect of marketing system on cattle welfare in Mersa and Woldia towns.

***Corresponding author:** Solomon Tsegaye, College of Agriculture, Woldia University, P.O. Box 400, Woldia, Ethiopia
E-mail: solomontsegaye25@gmail.com

Materials and Methods

Description of the study area

This research was conducted in north Wollo Zone Mersa and Woldia town cattle markets in 2016/2017. Mersa is a town in north Wollo of the Amhara Region in Ethiopia. It has a latitude and longitude of 11°40′N 39°39.5′E, with an elevation of 1600 meters. The town is one of the larger areas in the Habru district. Mersa is located along Ethiopian Highway 2 [9]. Woldia is a hillside market town, capital of the north Wollo Zone, and woreda in northern Ethiopia. Located north of Dessie and southeast of Lalibela in the Amhara Region, this town has a latitude and longitude of 11°50′N 39°36′E and an elevation of 2112 meters above sea level [10].

Sample size and sampling technique

Simple random sampling was used to collect data using interviews, semi structured questionnaires and direct observation. Moreover, a total of 80 respondents (40 from Woldia and 40 from Mersa) who participate in cattle marketing were participate to know their opinion why they compromised cattle welfare in markets.

Data collection and source

Data was collected through interviews and questionnaires. Formal survey was conducted to study the effect of marketing system on cattle welfare in the study area by using questionnaire, interview and direct observations. Questionnaires were prepared to the respondents who were selected from cattle market actors. The interview was used to gather necessary information through asking questions and writing down the response of the respondents. On the other hand, direct observation was used by the researchers to obtain qualitative data. The researchers' personal observation and experience of the study helps to understand the effects of marketing system on cattle welfare in the study area. Two types of data sources, which are primary and secondary data was collected for this study. Primary data was obtained by direct observation, interview, and questionnaire on the cattle welfare in markets of the study area. Secondary data was collected from various books, similar research project papers, internet services and from documents of the towns' trade and transport office and also from trade and industry office of north Wollo zone. Both quantitative and qualitative data was gathered through direct observation, interview and questionnaire.

Data analysis

Data was analyzed by using Microsoft Excel computer program 2010 and descriptive statistics like tables, percentage, chart and figures were used to summarize information collected from a sample. Furthermore, compression between cattle welfare problems based on their dangerousness was ranked. A simple descriptive statistical technique was applied for the effect of marketing system on cattle welfare. The data was organized, summarized and analyzed using different statistical method. The level of practical knowledge and some other relationship was analyzed. The result was interpreted and presented to share findings with the scientific community.

Results and Discussion

Socioeconomic characteristics of respondents

The household characteristics of respondents (Table 1) revealed that the proportion of female respondents were less than males in both towns. The majority age of respondents was range from 31-45 (47.5%), these age category is related with poor cattle welfare by market actors because in our study we found that respondents with this age category teaser their cattle after the transaction ends and they drink alcohols but they give nothing for their cattle and thus the animals suffer different welfare problems up to night. The finding of Fufa et al. said that the largest proportion (82.8%) of the respondents was within the age group of 31-60 years [6]. The analysis for educational status disclosed that 45% of the respondents were illiterates. Reading and writing 30%, 12.5% had primary education and 12.5% of respondents had secondary education.

As indicated in Table 2 the majority of households owned cattle in the range between 1-3 (42.5%) cattle per head. These are destitute category households. These are closely followed by poor category households 40% and own 4-8 heads of cattle. About 7.5% of the respondents were categorized to medium with 10-30 heads of cattle. The rich and very rich households own cattle heads that range from 30-40 and >50 respectively with frequency observed 2.5% and 0% respectively mostly rich owners compromise welfare than poor ones because they (the former) are mostly enjoying more without any care for the animals than the later. Other study by Zekarias and Teshale, reported that the majority of households owned cattle in the range between 4-12 (45.29%) cattle per head [11]. These are poor category households. These are closely followed by medium category households 43% and own 13-43 heads of cattle. The rich and very rich households own cattle heads that range from 44-56 and 57-109 respectively. However, the proportion of these households is less than 3%.

Cattle marketing in the study area

The price setting activity of cattle in the study area was accomplished by various actors in the market. About 72.5% (Table 3) of the respondents confirmed that price of cattle is set by negotiation between buyers and sellers based on initial price given by sellers and final price from buyers. Lack of modern pricing like weighing affects animal welfare and we observed that above 70% of oxen forced to plough in frustrating place and time to test their ability as one pricing parameter. Some proportion of respondents recognized determination of price by brokers 15% and based on previous week market information 15%. This shows that market actors had different level of influence in the role they played for setting price. It is observed that every aspect of price setting mechanisms majorly was controlled by buyers and sellers.

Other study by Fufa et al. reported that the price setting activity of cattle in pastoralist area is known to be accomplished by various actors in the market [6]. According to the study about 62% of pastoralists confirmed that price of cattle is set by brokers based on initial price given by sellers and final price from buyers. The proportion of pastoralists recognized determination of price by buyers based on central market information, by brokers based on central area information and sellers by their own respectively is 22%, 10% and 6%.

As indicated in Table 3 the total cattle transactions, 47.5% have access to domestic market information where as 52.5% has no market information. So, most of them turn back their animals when the price is under their expectation and this highly compromise animal welfare. Along this, the result indicated that traders who have access to information about the domestic market paid (obtained) significantly lower prices than those who do not have any and the finding agrees with another study by Hailemariam et al. of the total cattle transactions, 66% were transacted by those who have no accesses to domestic market information [4]. The result indicated that traders who have access to information about the domestic market paid significantly lower prices in both shoat and cattle markets than those who do not have any.

From the samples 37.5% of the respondents said that the reason for

Variables		Towns				Total (N=80) percent
		Mersa (n=40)		Woldia (n=40)		
		Frequency	Percent	Frequency	Percent	
Sex of respondents	Male	30	75	32	80	77.5
	Female	10	25	8	20	22.5
Age of respondents(years)	15-30	6	15	6	15	15
	31-45	18	45	20	50	47.5
	46-60	12	30	10	25	27.5
	Above 60	4	10	4	10	10
Educational status of respondents	Illiterate	20	50	16	40	45
	Read &Write	12	30	12	30	30
	Elementary school	4	10	6	15	12.5
	High school	4	10	6	15	12.5

Table 1: Household characteristics.

		Towns				Total (N=80) percent
		Mersa (n=40)		Woldia (n=40)		
Average owned	Wealth category	Frequency	Percent	Frequency	Percent	
0	Very poor	4	10	2	5	7.5
1-3	Destitute	20	50	14	35	42.5
4-8	Poor	14	35	18	45	40
10-30	Medium	2	5	4	10	7.5
30-50	Rich	0	0	2	5	2.5
>50	Very rich	0	0	0	0	0

Table 2: Cattle ownership with respect to wealth classification.

selling their cattle is to cover house hold necessities followed by, income generation 32.5%, replace older stock 12.5%, cover health payment 7.5%, pay tax% 5 and cover school fee 5% (Table 3). In addition, cattle market used as input, capital, insurance and livelihood income base, social heritage capital, income source and livelihood base. Hailemariam et al. reported also, cattle marketing play a variety of roles for most rural people's livelihoods, particularly as insurance for disaster, income and livelihood base capital [4].

Most of the market actors in the study area were farmers Table 3 which covered 47.5% and 45% of total sellers and buyers respectively and they affect cattle welfare due to lack of awareness. Traders were the second contributors covered 27.5% of transaction activity, 12.5% of buyers were fatteners and they covered 17.5% of total sellers in the study area, 15% of buyers were butchers and hotel owners. Brokers also contributed as sellers about 7.5% (Table 3). The study by Zekarias and Teshale, also reported, market actors were producers, medium to large traders, middlemen/brokers, butchers, restaurant owners' farmers [11]. The study also fined that each actor has its own function.

As indicated above Table 4 the price of ox was range from 8000 Eth. Birr to 18000 Eth. Birr with average price 12,250 ETB per head. The average price of bull, cow, heifer and calf were 10500, 6500, 5250 and 3125 Eth. Birr per head respectively (Table 4). The finding disagreed from the study of DCA, which reported that the price of ox ranges from 2325 to 2850 Eth. Birr, cow 1425 to 1600 and heifers 975 to 1175 Eth. Birr [12].

The common cattle marketing channels in the study areas involve several marketing agents. During the weekly market day, producers supply cattle and sell them to traders or farmers and pastoralists. The producers often sell livestock directly to farmers or to traders. Sometimes brokers engage in the purchase of animals for resale. Regional buyers of oxen and cow collect animals from different agents and transport them to distant markets such as Mekele, Semera, Dessie and Addis Ababa by transporting cattle using vehicles. This also indicated by Harko, producers sell cattle to other producers, consumer traders, urban dwellers and new comers from surrounding highlands who buy cattle for festival consumption [13].

Cattle behaviour and human intervention

Behavioral studies were conducted by direct observation. The result was divided into five categories: natural behaviors, abusive handling by stakeholders, aggressive, stress-related- and resistance behaviors and 40 cattle were observed when showing different behaviors. Of the five categories: abusive handling by stakeholders was the most frequently observed with frequency of 48% and 45% at Mersa and Woldia markets respectively. Natural behaviors observed at frequency of 28% and 30%, at Mersa and Woldia markets respectively followed by aggressive 10% and 12%, stress-related 8% and 6% and resistance behaviors 6% and 7% were observed at Mersa and Woldia markets respectively.

From behavioral observations at Woldia and Mersa markets, the highest expressed abusive behaviors by stakeholders were beating of body by stick 45% and 48%, beating of head 37% and 32% tail pulling 10% and 12%, pushing animal forward 6% and 5%, forcing animals to fall 2% and 3% at Woldia and Mersa respectively were observed. Antonia, reported that the most frequent behaviours expressed by humans were "beating of the body" at a frequency of 46% and "beating of the head" with a frequency of 34%. These two behaviours were observed at significantly high levels and differ from the rest of the abusive handling behaviours in observed occurrence. The third most observed abusive behaviour was "tail pulling," but is yet only expressed 10% and therefore differs 24% from "beating of the head".

Aggressiveness with frequency of 37% and 42% at Woldia and Mersa respectively was the most observed animal aggressive behavior due to human intervention followed by moving forward (31% and 28%), fighting (30% and 26%) at Woldia and Mersa respectively. Mounting that was recorded at markets was 2% and 4% at Woldia and Mersa respectively was the lowest expressed aggressive behavior. Josefine, reported that the highest expressed aggressive behavior was moving

Variables		Towns				Total (N=80) percent
		Mersa (n=40)		Woldia (n=40)		
		Freq.	Percent	Freq.	Percent	
Types of buyers	Fatteners	4	10	6	15	12.5
	Farmers	22	55	14	35	45
	Traders	10	25	12	30	27.5
	Hotels and butchers	4	10	8	20	15
Types of sellers	Farmers	22	55	16	40	47.5
	Traders	10	25	12	30	27.5
	Brokers	2	5	4	10	7.5
	Fatteners	6	15	8	20	17.5
Market information	Have information	16	40	22	55	47.5
	Not have information	24	60	18	45	52.5
Sources of market information	Brokers	8	20	10	25	22.5
	Tax collectors	6	15	4	10	12.5
	Relatives	8	20	12	30	25
	Previous information	18	45	14	35	40
Reasons of cattle purchase	For fattening	8	20	10	25	22.5
	For breeding	6	15	8	20	17.5
	For farming	18	45	14	35	40
	Other	8	20	8	20	20
Reasons of cattle selling	To cover HH necessities	16	40	14	35	37.5
	To pay tax	2	5	2	5	5
	To cover school fee	4	10	2	5	7.5
	To cover health	2	5	2	5	5
	To replace older stock	4	10	6	15	12.5
	To earn income	12	30	14	35	32.5
Price determination	Brokers	4	10	8	20	15
	Buyer and seller	30	75	28	70	72.5
	Previous week price	6	15	4	10	12.5
Reasons for price variation	Holidays	14	35	16	40	37.5
	Drought time	12	30	12	30	30
	Farming season	8	20	8	20	20
	Number of buyers and sellers available	6	15	4	10	12.5

Table 3: General information on cattle marketing in the study area.

forward (41%), fighting (29%) and aggressiveness (27%) [8]. The least expressed behaviors by animals' were jumping (3%), stretching and balking which never was observed. Within the resistance behavior group, different behaviors were significantly expressed but most common were resistance to being pulled (30%, 28%), refusing to leave their original place (25%, 32%), reversing (20%, 20%), charging at stakeholders (20%, 18%), slips slightly of 4%, 2% were recorded at Woldia and Mersa respectively. Josefine, reported that of the resistance behaviors, occurrences of each behavior varied greatly between markets but most common were resistance to being pulled, charging at stakeholders and falling down on ground [8].

The stress-related behavior that was observed at the highest extent at both markets was moving forward 32%. The other stress related behaviors include head swings 25%, vocalization 20%, foaming 15%, and paralyzed respiration 8% in average from the two markets. According to the study of Antonia 2013, of the stress-related behaviors, panting (10%), moving forward (8%), vocalizing (6%) and head swinging (6%) were the most frequently observed behaviors in markets. The behaviors paralyzed respiration, stamping of feet was never seen and idling, foaming and stretching were expressed at less than 2%. In both Woldia and Mersa markets cattle expressed natural behaviors and watching around was the most significant observed behavior, with a frequency of 40%. The animals also expressed the behaviors ear erect at an incidence of 23%, vocalization at 16% and moving forward at 18%. However, the natural behavior ruminating was only observed at 3% in the both markets.

Other study by Josefine, reported that the natural behaviors that were highest expressed by animals were watching around, ear erecting, and eliminations. At market, rumination and ear erecting were more frequently observed and vocalization, turning and moving forward least observed.

Animal handling and transport

The transportation system of cattle in the study area was mostly by foot 96% and 94% in Mersa and Woldia respectively. The rest of transportation system was 4% and 6% in Mersa and Woldia respectively was by vehicles. Table 5 presents the recorded flow of animals from the vicinity of Woldia town. The cattle were brought from farms with average distance of 22.2 km, varying from 8 km to 40 km and they walked for 1 to 6 h.

During transport by foot to Woldia market, the animals were exposed to radiation; had no feed and water allowance. It was also observed that animals could be injured when forced to walk on asphalted road and the sharp gravel on the road which could injure animals' foot during long journey. Lameness and injury to bone, muscle, swelling of leg and sickness were widely seen during transportation by walking.

Types of cattle	Mersa			Woldia			Mean
	Minimum	Maximum	Average	Minimum	Maximum	Average	
Ox	8000	18000	13000	5000	18000	11500	**12250**
Bull	6000	15000	10500	5000	16000	10500	**10500**
Cow	4000	8000	6000	4000	10000	7000	**6500**
Heifer	3000	7000	5000	3000	8000	5500	**5250**
Calf	2000	4000	3000	2000	4500	3250	**3125**

Table 4: Price per head of cattle in Woldia and Mersa towns (ETB, Ethiopian Birr).

Animal category	No. of animals brought to market	Original place	Estimated distance, [Km]	Time taken for transport, [hr]
Farmer-1	2 oxen and 1 cow	Kalim	30	5
Farmer-2	1-ox	Sanka	25	4
Farmer-3	4-oxen	Girana	40	6
Farmer-4	3-oxen	Mersa	30	5
Farmer-5	2-cows	Dorogibir	12	2
Farmer-6	2-heifer	Gubarja	10	2
Farmer-7	2-oxen	Gedober	12	2
Farmer-8	6-bull	Woldiagebriel	8	1
Farmer-9	2-oxen	Kobo	40	6
Farmer-10	2-cows	Lemasolela	15	3

Table 5: Animals flow to Woldia market from different sources.

Five freedoms	Ranks based on severity	
	Mersa	Woldia
Hanger and thrust	1	1
Discomfort	2	2
Pain, injury and disease	4	3
Fear and distress	3	4
Naturalness	5	5

Table 6: Common cattle welfare problems at markets.

Possible reasons	Towns				Total (N=80) percent
	Mersa (n=40)		Woldia (n=40)		
	Freq.	Percent	Freq.	Percent	
Lack of awareness	20	50	14	35	42.5
Social and cultural problems	2	5	4	10	7.5
Carelessness	14	35	18	45	40
Economic problems	4	10	2	5	7.5
Others	0	0	2	5	2.5

Table 7: Reasons for poor welfare of cattle.

According to the report of Frimpong, the development of market infrastructure and market institution in the country is very important to reduce such economic loss in the animal supply chain [14]. During transport, as animals move from known to un- known environment, so better animal handling and logistics management are required to improve animal welfare.

Most cattle sources for Mersa and Woldia market are rural areas most of which have no asphalt road and about 75% of cattle owners said that lameness is the most common welfare problem due to long distance journey up to 40 Km on rocky roads for up to 6 h without provision of rest, food or water. About 70% of those rural cattle owners trek their animals by their own where as 20% of the owners trekked their cattle by rural trekkers who compromise welfare by beating the body 67%, beating head 18%, and tail pulling 10% and stoning 5%.

During transportation of cattle to markets and away from markets the most common welfare problems at both Woldia and Mersa are injury 30%; due to long distance journey inappropriate loading and unloading and transportation facilities, hunger and thrust 25%; discomfort 18%; due to sun attack and rough road, fear and distress 15%; due to mixing of different animals, confusion by the new environment and vehicles, inappropriate transportation vehicles, and disease due to the combined effect of those problems 12%. The finding is not supported by other studies numerically.

Cattle welfare problems at markets

Due to different reasons the five freedoms were compromised at both Woldia and Mersa markets. To study those problems we used direct observations, semi structured questionnaire and interviews.

There is no any feed or water in markets, sun attack, lack of rest, disturbance by human and other animals, beating by owners, fighting each other, stony market place, lack of veterinary care, beating by owners, ploughing, mixing of animals, new environment, bad treatment by owners, separation from their companions, not allowed for mounting, no grazing, no suckling all these factors affect cattle welfare in the study area.

Hunger and thrust was leading welfare problem followed by discomfort, pain injury and disease and fear and distress whereas naturalness is not the main problem as animals has mostly freedom to mix with other companions (Table 6). FAWC (Farm Animal Welfare Committee) also reported that the welfare situation for animals at markets was not in accordance with the Five Freedoms [15]. The markets in Ethiopia do not allow animals to have freedom from discomfort, or pain, injuries or diseases, or fear and distress.

Reasons for poor welfare of cattle in the study area

Lack of awareness with a frequency of 42.5% is the primary reason for poor welfare conditions of cattle in the study area closely followed by carelessness 40% (Table 7). Economic problems 7.5%, social and cultural problems 7.5%, and other factors 2.5% also contribute for poor welfare conditions of cattle. Lack of marketing facilities were economic problems because due to lack of standard measurements for cattle oxen were forced to plough at markets to test their ability as the main marketing parameter. The study of Broom and Fraser, 2007 also reported those problems with different rank from this study as economic problems 35%, lack of awareness 30%, carelessness 23%, social and cultural problems 7% and other factors 5%.

Conclusion and Recommendations

In the study area the concept, definition and importance of animal welfare is not well known by most cattle producers and market actors. Poor animal welfare is common in the study and lack of awareness was the primary reason closely followed by carelessness. Stakeholders at markets were handling animals abusively. Animals expressed different behaviours in markets due to human intervention: including natural behaviors, abusive handling by stakeholders, aggressive, stress-related- and resistance behaviors. The animal welfare at markets in the study area was very poor and animal transport conditions are inadequate with above 95% of transportation system was by foot. The welfare of cattle in the study area was compromised by long distance journey and abusive handling. Therefore, trainings and awareness creation on cattle production, handling, marketing and transportation should be provided for the society engaged in cattle production. Moreover, relevant information for cattle producers and market actors should be provided.

Acknowledgement

The authors would like to thank Woldia University specifically animal production and technology department for the support.

References

1. Stock F, Gifford-Gonzalez D (2013) Genetics and African Cattle Domestication. Afr Archaeol Rev 30: 51-72.
2. Mengistu A (2006) Country Pasture/Forage Resource Profiles. FAO, pp. 5-35.
3. Aleri JW, Nguhiu M, Mogoa EM, Mulei CM (2012) Welfare of Dairy Cattle in the Smallholder (Zero-grazing) Production Systems in Nairobi and its Environs. Livestock Research for Rural Development 24: 15-22.
4. Hailemariam T, Getachew L, Dawit A (2011) Market Structure and Function for Live Animal and Meat Exports in Some Selected Areas of Ethiopia. Research Report 79. Addis Ababa, Ethiopia 33p.
5. Broom DM, Fraser AF (2007) Domestic Animal Behaviour and Welfare, 4th Edn. Cambridge University press, Cambridge, UK. pp. 495-520.
6. Fufa S, Bulitta M, Girma G, Techane B (2012) Animal Handling during Supply for Marketing and Operations at an Abattoir in Developing Country: The Case of Gudar Market and Ambo Abattoir, Ethiopia. J Serv Sci Manage 5: 59-68.
7. Antonia G (2013) Animal Welfare in Ethiopia: Handling of Cattle During Transport and Operations at Kera Abattoir, Addis Ababa. Swedish University of Agricultural Sciences.
8. Josefine J (2013) Animal Welfare in Ethiopia: Transport to and Handling of Cattle at Markets in Addis Abeba And Ambo. Swedish University of Agricultural Sciences.
9. Yilmaz S, Venugopal, Varsha (2008) Local Government Discretion and Accountability in Ethiopia (PDF). Working Paper 08-38. International Studies Program, Andrew Young School of Policy Studies, Georgia State University.
10. Bahru Zewde (2001) A History of Modern Ethiopia. second edn. Oxford: James Currey. pp: 218.
11. Zekarias B, Teshale W (2015) Value Chain Analysis of the Cattle Trade in Moyale, Southern Ethiopia: An Economic Assessment in Oromiya Regional State. Country Report, London.
12. DCA (2008) Agricultural marketing in Ethiopia: The Case of Arrero, Goro and Dehana Districts. Dun Church Aid, Addis Ababa, Ethiopia.
13. Harko H (2015) Review of Beef Cattle Value Chain in Ethiopia. Ind Eng Lett 5: 10-22.
14. Frimpong S (2009) Effect of Pre-Slaughter Handling and Transport on Welfare and Meat Quality of Cattle: A Case Study of Kumasi Abattoir. Master's Thesis, Kwame Nkrumah University of Science and Technology, Kumasi.
15. Farm Animal Welfare Committee (FAWC). (2011).

Antioxidant Trace Elements and Oxidative Stress Levels Associated with Pasteurellosis in Camel-Calves (*Camelus dromedarius*)

Sherif Mohamed Shoieb[1], Hussam Mohamed Mohamed Ibrahim[2], Mohamed Sayed-Ahmed[2,3]* and Sabry Ahmed El-khodery[2]

[1]*Veterinary Teaching Hospital, Faculty of Veterinary Medicine, Mansoura University, Mansoura 35516, Egypt*
[2]*Department of Internal Medicine and Infectious Diseases, Faculty of Veterinary Medicine, Mansoura University, Mansoura 35516, Egypt*
[3]*Department of Clinical Pharmacy, College of Pharmacy, Jazan University, Jizan 45142, Saudi Arabia*

Abstract

The aim of the present study was to evaluate changes in the electrolyte and trace elements profiles, antioxidants and oxidative stress level associated with pneumonic pasteurllosis in camel-calves in Saudi Arabia. For this purpose, venous blood samples were obtained from 48 camel-calves with pneumonic pasteurellosis and 48 randomly selected clinically healthy camel-calves (control group). Serum trace elements including sodium, potassium, chloride, copper and zinc were assayed. Serum malondialdehyde and low-density lipoprotein levels as well as total antioxidant capacity; hydrogen peroxide concentration; and activity of reduced glutathione, catalase, and superoxide dismutase were measured. Moreover, copper/zinc ratio and oxidative stress index were calculated. In camel-calves with pnoumonic pasteurellosis, there was a significant ($P<0.05$) decrease in the level of serum sodium, potassium, chloride, copper and zinc; total antioxidant capacity; and the activity of reduced glutathione, superoxide dismutase and catalase when compared with control group. Meanwhile, there was a significant ($P<0.05$) increase in copper/zinc ratio; level of malondialdehyde and low density lipoprotein; concentration of hydrogen peroxide; and oxidative stress index in pneumonic camel-calves compared to control group. The results indicate that electrolyte profiles, trace element level and oxidants antioxidants balance are greatly disturbed in camel-calves with pasteurellosis.

Keywords: Respiratory diseases; Pasteurollosis; Antioxidants; Oxidants; Electrolytes; Trace elements; Camel-calves

Introduction

Nowadays, some interest and attention has been drawn toward camel because of its unique adaptive characteristics for survivability in harsh and difficult environment [1]. However, high mortality rate reported in camel-calves during the first three months of life is the major concern [2]. Respiratory airway diseases are encountered as an emerging health hazards to camel population worldwide due to significant mortalities and cost of treatment and vaccination [3]. The definite etiology of most respiratory tract diseases of camels has not yet been fully determined [4,5]. Moreover, several important predisposing factors as sudden climatic changes, poor management practices, exposure to various diseases, frequent travelling and poor nutrition may influence the occurrence of such diseases [2].

Pasteurellosis is a highly infectious, often fatal disease with very serious economic impact in feedlot animals [6,7]. It is the most common disease with wide prevalence and high mortality rate [8,9]. Septicaemic pasteurellosis affects mainly cattle, camels and to a lesser extent horse and sheep. *Pasteurella multocida* type B is the main cause, but type D and type E are occasionally isolated [6].

Several studies have reported that the imbalance between lipid peroxides and antioxidants in pneumonia may contribute to the damage of pulmonary endothelium [10]. Moreover, poor perfusion in pulmonary tissues may induce free radical processes and impairment of the antioxidant system with acceleration in the process of lipid peroxidation. The body is supported with a variety of antioxidants to overcome the toxic effects of these reactive oxygen species. Superoxide anions which are generated during metabolic processes are reduced to hydrogen peroxide in the presence of superoxide dismutase. Hydrogen peroxide was degraded in the presence of both catalase and glutathione peroxidase [11].

Oxidative stress is thought to play an important role in the pathogenesis of a number of lung diseases [12]. In respiratory tract infection, neutrophils are recruited to the pulmonary tissues to remove the invading micro-organisms by their phagocytic activity producing tissue damaging products such as reactive nitrogen species and nitric oxides modulating both acute and chronic inflammatory reactions [13]. When phagocytes are exposed to appropriate stimuli, they form large quantities of superoxide radical, an important precursor of other more reactive species that contribute to pulmonary damage [14].

Antioxidant trace elements produce consistent immune response and increase the resistance of calves against infection with *Pasteurella hemolytica* [15,16]. In calves with *Mycoplasma bronchopneumonia*, there was a significant alteration in major and trace elements in the bronchoalveolar lavage fluid [17]. In cattle, the oxidative stress level and antioxidant status have been described in bronchopneumonia caused by *Mycoplasma bovis* [18,19]. The camel, however, has been neglected for a long time and reports on pasteurellosis and their associated oxidant/antioxidant imbalance are scare. Therefore, the aim of the present study was to assess the alteration in electrolyte profile, trace element level and oxidative stress indices in camel-calves with pasteurellosis.

***Corresponding author:** Mohamed Zakaria Sayed-Ahmed, Department of Internal Medicine and Infectious Diseases, Faculty of Veterinary Medicine, Mansoura University, Mansoura 35516, Egypt, E-mail: drzakaria-infect@hotmail.com

Materials and Methods

Animals

A total of 96 camel-calves of both sexes at 3-11 months of age were studied. Of all, 48 camel-calves were exhibiting the clinical signs of pasteurellosis. In addition, other 48 apparently healthy camel-calves within the same age were randomly selected as a control group. The current study was carried out at three camel farms during 2013 in Shaqra, a town in central Saudi Arabia. The town is located near Ushaiger and about 190 kilometers north-west of the capital Riyadh. This study was approved by the Animal Welfare and Ethics Committee, Saudi Arabia, on December, 2012.

Clinical examination

Data concerned with the case history, clinical findings, and medical record for each camel-calf were recorded. A detailed clinical examination of camel-calves was carried out, and the clinical findings were recorded [6]. Camel-calves with pasteurellosis had clinical signs of anorexia, pyrexia (40-41°C), dullness, lethargy, mucopurulent nasal and occular discharges, cough, hyperpnea, tachycardia, dyspnea and recumbency. Mandibular and cervical lymph nodes become enlarged and painful. In the terminal stage, the animal lied down and stretched its neck straight along the ground in an effort to inhale with dilated nostrils and opened mouth and die within 24-48 hours from the initial occurrence of the illness (Table 1).

Blood samples

Via jugular vein puncture, two venous blood samples (10 mL each) were obtained from each camel-calf. The first blood sample was collected into anticoagulant containing tube (sodium ethylene diamine tetra-acetic acid, EMD Chemicals Inc., United States) for haematological examination. Meanwhile, the second blood sample was collected into a sterile tube without anticoagulant to obtain serum which was kept frozen at -80°C for further biochemical analysis.

Bacteriological isolation and identification

Isolation and identification of *Pasteurella multocida* was carried out from blood and tissue samples obtained from live and dead camel-calves based on morphology, cultural characteristic and staining by Leishman's staining as previously described [20]. All isolates were identified as gram-negative, bipolar-staining short bacilli. Furthermore, the colonies suggestive of *Pasteurella multocida* were subjected to biochemical tests [21] for identification using of API 20E system (BioMe´ rieux, Marcy-l'E´ toile, France).

Biochemical analysis

Sodium, potassium, chloride, copper and zinc levels were determined by established procedures of atomic absorption spectrometry (Visible Absorption Spectrometer PD-303 UV, APEL, Japan). In addition, total antioxidant capacity, hydrogen peroxide concentration, and activity of reduced glutathione, catalase, and superoxide dismutase as well as level of malondialdehyde and low density lipoprotein were measured spectrophotometerically following standard methods using commercially available test kits (Bio-diagnostic, Cairo, Egypt). As an indicator of the degree of oxidative stress, oxidative stress index (OSI) was calculated as the ratio of the total peroxide levels to the total antioxidant capacity. The OSI value was calculated as follows:

OSI=[(total peroxide mmol/L)/(total antioxidant capacity mmol/L) × 100].

Statistical analysis

Statistical analysis was carried out by using statistical software program (SPSS for Windows, version 16.0, SPSS Inc., Chicago, IL). Data were normally distributed; therefore, mean and standard deviation were statistically analyzed and presented. *Paired-sample T-test* was used to assess statistical differences between the groups. For all statistical examinations, results were considered significant at $P<0.05$.

Results and Discussion

Hemorrhagic septicemia, one of fetal diseases of ruminant animals, is caused by *Pasteurella multocida* serotype B; a gram-negative bacterium secretes endotoxins in the blood stream, which are responsible for all manifestations of the disease [7,22]. These endotoxins trigger arachidonic acid metabolites resulting in the production of prostaglandins and leukotrienes causing moderate to severe pyrexia which is a hallmark of this disease [23].

Clinically, there was a significant increase in both respiratory and heart rates in camel-calves with pneumonic pasteurellosis. Moreover, wheezing with a high pitched breath sound was also detected during thoracic auscultation indicating severe lung injury (Table 1). Furthermore, four camel-calves (8.3%) exhibited severe respiratory embaressment with deterioration of their health status and death occur within 24-48 hours from the initial occurrence of the illness. Such clinical findings were typical to the disease as described before in the previous reports [24-26]. Likewise, postmortem findings in camel-calves with pasteurellosis indicates septicemia. These findings were in agreement with those previously reported [7,27]. Depending on the recorded history, clinical findings, post mortem examination and results of bacteriological isolation and identification, these camel-calves were infected with *Pasteurella multocida*. The characters of the isolated colonies and their biochemical identification tests were in agreement with those previously reported [20]. However, in previous reports, several microorganisms including *Pasteurella hemolytica* were also recovered from lung of camels with pneumonic pasteurellosis [5], suggesting that other contributing factor may influence the severity of the disease.

Leukogram reflected a state of respiratory tract infection (Table 2), where leukocytosis could be an appropriate physiological response to an infectious or inflammatory process, which serves the sole job of killing bacterial infection. Similar findings were recorded in cattle [6], and horses with respiratory diseases [28]. Neutrophilia, lymphocytopenia and eosinophilia recorded in camel-calves with pasteurellosis indicates acute infection, and inflammation secondary to tissue injury, hypersensitivity reactions and stress. These findings were in agreement with those reported by Radostits et al. [6]. Meanwhile, the hematological findings in camel-calves with pasteurellosis revealed an increase of hemoglobin concentration, packed cell volume (PCV) %, mean corpuscular volume (MCV) % and mean corpuscular hemoglobin (MCH) % when compared to control group (Table 3). Such changes in hematological parameters could be attributed to dehydration and hypovolemia which accompany the endotoxemia occurring in camel-calves with hemorrhagic septicemia [27].

Biochemically, sodium, potassium and chloride levels were significantly ($P<0.05$) decreased in camel-calves with pasteurellosis when compared with control group (Table 4). This could be attributed to dehydration and endotoxemia associating respiratory diseases with a resultant alteration in electrolyte profile associating such conditions [6,29]. Furthermore, there was a significant ($P<0.05$) decrease in

Table 1: Clinical Findings in Camel-calves with Pneumonic Pasteurellosis.

Groups	Temperature (°C)	R.R. (Cycle/Min.)	H.R. (Beat/Min.)	Nasal discharge	Cough	Tracheal sound	Lung sound
Control *(n=48)*	37.4 ± 0.19 [a]	11.4 ± 0.34 [a]	51.9 ± 2.7 [a]	Absent (48/48)	Absent	Normal	Normal vesicular sound
Diseased *(n=48)*	39.3 ± 0.17 [b]	20.9 ± 0.6 [b]	78.0 ± 1.68 [b]	Mucoid (23/48) Muco-purulent (23/48) Absent (2/48)	Dry cough (8/48) Moist cough (33/48) Absent (7/48)	Tracheal rales (41/48)	Crackles (9/48) Wheezes (24/48) Exaggerated vesicular sound (9/48) Mixed (6/48)

Abbreviation: R.R: Respiratory Rate; H.R: Heart Rate
a, b: Means with different superscript letters in the same column are significantly different at P<0.05.

Table 2: Total and Differential Leukocytic Counts (mean values ± SD) in Clinically Healthy Camel-calves and in Those with Pneumonic Pasteurellosis.

Groups	TLC (count) × 10 [3]	Neutrophil %	Lymphocyte %	Monocyte %	Eosinophil %	Basophil %
Control *(n=48)*	13.77 ± 3.36 [a]	39.03 ± 4.63 [a]	49.79 ± 2.82 [a]	4.69 ± 1.66 [a]	5.63 ± 1.64 [a]	0.37 ± 0.21 [a]
Diseased *(n=48)*	17.26 ± 4.44 [b]	71.42 ± 10.44 [b]	22.75 ± 3.04 [b]	3.25 ± 2.12 [a]	1.73 ± 1.01 [b]	0.65 ± 0.93 [a]

Abbreviation: R.R: Respiratory Rate; H.R: Heart Rate
a, b: Means with different superscript letters in the same column are significantly different at P<0.05.

Table 3: Complete Blood Picture (mean values ± SD) in Clinically Healthy Camel-calves and in Those with Pneumonic Pasteurellosis.

Groups	RBCs (count) × 10[6]	Hb %	PCV %	MCV %	MCH %	MCHC %
Control *(n=48)*	13.70 ± 0.79	12.33 ± 0.77 [a]	23.45 ± 2.51[a]	19.32 ± 5.83 [a]	10.26 ± 2.44 [a]	38.96 ± 5.67
Diseased *(n=48)*	16.98 ± 1.75	18.90 ± 1.30 [b]	35.43 ± 3.51 [b]	31.96 ± 7.77 [b]	23.61 ± 9.63 [b]	38.08 ± 10.97

Abbreviations: RBCs: Red Blood Cells; Hb: Hemoglobin; PCV: Packed Cell Volume; MCV: Mean Corpuscular Volume; MCH: Mean Corpuscular Hemoglobin; MCHC: Mean Corpuscular Hemoglobin Concentration.
a, b: Variables with different superscript in the same column are significantly different at P<0.05.

Table 4: Electrolyte Profile and Trace elements status (mean values ± SD) in Clinically Healthy Camel-calves and in Those with Pneumonic Pasteurellosis.

Groups	Sodium (μM/L)	Potassium (μM/L)	Chloride (μM/L)	Copper (μM/L)	Zinc (μM/L)	Copper/zinc ratio
Control *(n=48)*	160.07 ± 13.2 [a]	4.58 ± 0.53 [a]	65.67 ± 6.23[a]	34.62 ± 1.65 [a]	42.81 ± 2.15 [a]	0.81 ± 0.10[a]
Diseased *(n=48)*	111.50 ± 10.40 [b]	2.30 ± 1.22 [b]	40.13 ± 2.92[b]	24.60 ± 1.85 [b]	22.81 ± 2.03[b]	1.08 ± 0.61[b]

a, b: Variables with different superscript in the same column are significantly different at P<0.05.

copper and zinc levels in camel-calves with pasteurellosis suggesting towards losses of these nutrients (Table 4). Indirect losses of these trace elements may be speculated during infectious diseases owing to accelerated metabolism or consumption, low intake due to inappetence or weakness, stress or pyrexia [30]. Moreover, copper/zinc ratio was significantly (P<0.05) increased in camel-calves with pasteurellosis compared with control group (Table 4). Serum zinc level was decreased more than copper. The significant changes of copper/zinc ratio with changes in the indices of oxidative stress suggest various degrees of airway inflammation. A similar finding of copper/zinc ratio has been recorded in horses with airway inflammation [28]. Furthermore, zinc and copper administration could modulate the humoral immune response to vaccines in cattle as recorded previously [31,32].

In pneumonic camel-calves, there was a significant (P<0.05) decrease in the total antioxidant capacity and activity of reduced glutathione, catalase, and superoxide dismutase when compared with control group (Table 5) indicating a worse state of oxidative stress. The antioxidant enzyme activities were decreased, and then the superoxide radical and hydrogen peroxide intermediate radicals accumulate. These oxygen free-radicals could undergo the Fenton's reaction, generating hydroxyl radicals, which may lead to lipid peroxidation in cells [33]. Therefore, the reason of increased lipid peroxidation in camel-calves with pasteurellosis may be related to decreased antioxidant enzymes activity. Furthermore, the decreased antioxidant enzymes activity, as found in the existing study, was attributed to its consumption in the protection of cells against oxidative injury by preventing the peroxidation process which is capable of inducing severe cellular damage [11]. In calves with bronchopneumonia, the reported decrease in the superoxide dismutase activity was correlated with high blood level of superoxide radicals as previously described [14]. Several studies have reported reduction of these antioxidant enzymes activities in horses with lower airway disease [28], and in human patients suffering pneumonia [34].

In the current investigation, there was a significant (P<0.05) increase in hydrogen peroxide concentration, levels of malondialdehyde and low density lipoprotein, and oxidative stress index in pneumonic camel-calves compared to their levels in healthy control group (Table 5). These findings were in agreement with those obtained in feedlot cattle with pneumonia caused by *Mycoplasma bovis* [19]. Hydrogen peroxide, which may be potentially dangerous for the lung, was produced normally by type II pneumocytes, endothelial cells and others [35-37]. In case of hypoxia, inflammation and insufficient antioxidant defense, hydrogen peroxide may initiate or intensify lung destruction. Furthermore, selenium deficiency with a resultant drastic decline in selenium dependent glutathione peroxidase activity produce a rise in cellular hydrogen peroxide concentration [28]. In a study conduced on buffaloes vaccinated against haemorrhagic septicaemia, polymorphonuclear cells generated significantly higher hydrogen

Table 5: Antioxidants Level and Other Oxidative Stress Markers (mean values ± SD) in Clinically Healthy Camel-calves and in Those with Pneumonic Pasteurellosis.

Groups	TAC (mmol/L)	GSH (mg/dL)	SOD (U/mL)	MDA (nmol/mL)	H_2O_2 (μM/L)	LDL (mmol/L)	CAT (U/L)	OSI
Control *(n=48)*	1.53 ± 0.48^a	8.19 ± 0.53 ^{a}	5.52 ± 0.72 ^{a}	11.26 ± 1.75^a	10.2 ± 4.5 ^{a}	0.55 ± 0.01^a	18.80 ± 0.63 ^{a}	0.74 ± 0.36 ^{a}
Diseased *(n=48)*	0.59 ± 0.21^b	3.12 ± 0.55 ^{b}	2.55 ± 0.23 ^{b}	24.46 ± 3.12^b	26.7 ± 5.2 ^{b}	2.28 ± 0.65 ^{b}	6.70 ± 1.56 ^{b}	4.18 ± 1.49 ^{b}

Abbreviations: TAC: Total Antioxidant Capacity; GSH: Reduced Glutathione; SOD: Superoxide Dismutase; MDA: Malondialdehyde; H_2O_2: Hydrogen Peroxide; LDL: Low Density Lipoprotein; CAT: Catalase; OSI: Oxidative Stress Index.

a, b: Variables with different superscript in the same column are significantly different at P<0.05.

peroxide and nitric oxide, suggesting that these polymorphonuclear cells possessed a potent oxidant defense system even in the presence of *Pasteurella multocida* lipopolysaccharide, an antiphagocytic bacterium [38]. The results of the present study indicate that the antioxidant defense system is compromised in camel-calves with pneumonic pasteurellosis, which is evidenced by decreased total antioxidant capacity and increased malondialdehyde level, which may indirectly indicate increased whole free radical activity with a resultant increased oxidative stress index. Such findings coincide with those reported previously in draft horses with inflammatory airway disease [28].

Conclusion

All the results point to camel-calves with pneumonic pasteurellosis as a significant factor in alteration of the electrolyte and trace elements profiles and indices of oxidative stress. This is clearly demonstrated by low level of trace elements and electrolytes and high oxidative stress index in camel-calves with pasteurellosis compared with healthy ones. Furthermore, to the best of our knowledge, this is the first report on camel-calves with pasteurellosis. Further studies are needed to asssess the effect of trace elements and antioxidants supplementation on the clinical outcomes and oxidant antioxidant balance in camel-calves with pasteurellosis.

Conflict of Interest

None of the authors of this paper has a financial or personal relationship with other people or organizations that could appropriately influence or bias the content of the paper.

References

1. Abdoun KA, Alsofi MA, Samara EM, Alhidary IA, Okab AB, et al. (2015) Evaluation of the effects of chromium supplementation on growth and nitrogen balance of camel calves under summer conditions. Trop Anim Health Prod 47: 619-621.
2. Kamber R, Farah Z, Rusch P, Hassig M (2001) Studies on the supply of immunoglobulin G to newborn camel-calves (*Camelus dromedarius*). J Dairy Res 68: 1-7.
3. Kebede F, Gelaye E (2010) Studies on major respiratory diseases of Camel (*Camelus dromedarius*) in Northeastern Ethiopia. Afr J Microbiol Res 4: 1560-1564.
4. Schwartz HJ (1992) Productive performance and productivity of dromedaries (*Camelus dromedarius*). Anim Res Dev 35: 86-98.
5. Wareth G, Murugaiyan J, Khater DF, Moustafa SA (2014) Subclinical pulmonary pathogenic infection in camels slaughtered in Cairo, Egypt. J Infect Dev Ctries 8: 909-913.
6. Radostits OM, Done SH (2007) Veterinary Medicine: A Textbook of the Diseases of Cattle, Sheep, Pigs, Goats, and Horses. Elsevier Saunders.
7. Hassan AKM, Mustafa AA (1985) Isolation of *Pasteurella multocida* type B from an outbreak of haemorrhagic septicaemia in camels in the Sudan. Rev Elev Med Vet Pays Trop 38: 31-33.
8. Mohamed RA, Abdelsalam EB (2008) A review on pneumonic pasteurellosis (respiratory mannheimiosis) with emphasis on pathogenesis, virulence mechanisms and predisposing factors. BJVM 11: 139-160.
9. Al-Rawashdeh OF, Al-Ani FK, Sharrif LA, Al-Qudah KM, Al-Hami Y, et al. (2000) A survey of camel (*Camelus dromedarius*) diseases in Jordan. J Zoo Wildl Med 31: 335-338.
10. Doelman CJA, Bast A (1990) Oxygen radicals in lung pathology. Free Radic Biol Med 9: 381-400.
11. Halliwell B (1994) Free radicals and antioxidants: a personal view. Nutr Rev 52: 253-265.
12. MacNee W (2001) Oxidative stress and lung inflammation in airways disease. Eur J Pharmacol 429: 195-207.
13. Lykkesfeldt J, Svendsen O (2007) Oxidants and antioxidants in disease: oxidative stress in farm animals. Vet J 173: 502-511.
14. Ledwozyw A, Borowicz B (1991) The influence of normobaric hyperoxia on antioxidant enzymes activities and peroxidation product levels in rat lungs. Arch Vet Pol 32: 135-141.
15. Gengelbach GP, Ward JD, Spears JW, Brown TT (1997) Effects of copper deficiency and copper deficiency coupled with high dietary iron or molybdenum on phagocytic cell function and response of calves to a respiratory disease challenge. J Anim Sci 75: 1112-1118.
16. Ward JD, Gengelbach GP, Spears JW (1997) The effects of copper deficiency with or without high dietary iron or molybdenum on immune function of cattle. J Anim Sci 75: 1400-1408.
17. Suzuki K, Higuchi H, Iwano H, Lakritz J, Sera K, et al. (2012) Analysis of trace and major elements in bronchoalveolar lavage fluid of *Mycoplasma bronchopneumonia* in calves. Biol Trace Elem Res 145: 166-171.
18. Hermeyer K, Jacobsen B, Spergser J, Rosengarten R, Hewicker-Trautwein M (2011) Detection of *Mycoplasma bovis* by *in-situ* hybridization and expression of inducible nitric oxide synthase, nitrotyrosine and manganese superoxide dismutase in the lungs of experimentally-infected calves. J Comp Pathol 145: 240-250.
19. Schott C, Cai H, Parker L, Bateman KG, Caswell JL (2014) Hydrogen peroxide production and free radical-mediated cell stress in *Mycoplasma bovis* pneumonia. J Comp Pathol 150: 127-137.
20. Mochabo MO, Kitala PM, Gathura PB, Ogara WO, Eregae EM, et al. (2006) The socio-economic impact of important camel diseases as perceived by a pastoralist community in Kenya. Onderstepoort J Vet Res 73: 269-274.
21. DeRosa DC, Mechor GD, Staats JJ, Chengappa MM, Shryock TR (2000) Comparison of *Pasteurella* spp. simultaneously isolated from nasal and transtracheal swabs from cattle with clinical signs of bovine respiratory disease. J Clin Microbiol 38: 327-332.
22. Horadagoda NU, Hodgson JC, Moon GM, Wijewardana TG, Eckersall PD (2001) Role of endotoxin in the pathogenesis of haemorrhagic septicaemia in the buffalo. Microb Pathog 30: 171-178.
23. Raza MA, Muhammad G, Athar M, Khan MZ (2000) Comparative efficacy of three protocols for the treatment of haemorrhagic septicaemia in buffaloes and cattle. Pak Vet J 20: 35-39.
24. Angle N, Hoyt DB, Coimbra R, Liu F, Herdon-Remelius C, et al. (1998) Hypertonic saline resuscitation diminishes lung injury by suppressing neutrophil activation after hemorrhagic shock. Shock 9: 164-170.
25. Rizoli SB, Kapus A, Fan J, Li YH, Marshall JC, et al. (1998) Immunomodulatory effects of hypertonic resuscitation on the development of lung inflammation following hemorrhagic shock. J Immunol 161: 6288-6296.
26. Rizoli SB, Rhind SG, Shek PN, Inaba K, Filips D, et al. (2006) The immunomodulatory effects of hypertonic saline resuscitation in patients sustaining traumatic hemorrhagic shock: a randomized, controlled, double-blinded trial. Ann Surg 243: 47-57.
27. Fraz MK (2011) Field epidemiology of an outbreak of hemorrhagic septicemia in

dromedary population of greater Cholistan Desert Pakistan. Pak Vet J 32: 31-34.

28. Youssef MA, El-Khodery SA, Ibrahim HMM (2012) Antioxidant trace elements in serum of draft horses with acute and chronic lower airway disease. Biol Trace Elem Res 150: 123-129.

29. Constable PD (1999) Hypertonic saline. Vet Clin North Am Food Anim Pract 15: 559-585.

30. Heidarpour M, Mohri M, Borji H, Moghdass E (2012) Oxidative stress and trace elements in camel (*Camelus dromedarius*) with liver cystic echinococcosis. Vet Parasitol 187: 459-463.

31. Salyer GB, Galyean ML, Defoor PJ, Nunnery GA, Parsons CH, et al. (2004) Effects of copper and zinc source on performance and humoral immune response of newly received, lightweight beef heifers. J Anim Sci 82: 2467-2473.

32. Nunnery GA, Vasconcelos JT, Parsons CH, Salyer GB, Defoor PJ, et al. (2007) Effects of source of supplemental zinc on performance and humoral immunity in beef heifers. J Anim Sci 85: 2304-2313.

33. Baskol G, Atmaca H, Tanrıverdi F, Baskol M, Kocer D, et al. (2007) Oxidative stress and enzymatic antioxidant status in patients with hypothyroidism before and after treatment. Exp Clin Endocrinol Diabetes 115: 522-526.

34. Cui H, Yin SA, Gao H, Li G (1997) The comparison of selenium status between the children suffered from pneumonia and the normal children from kindergarten. Wei Sheng yan jiu = J Hyg Res 26: 242-244.

35. Art T, Kirschvink N, Smith N, Lekeux P (1999) Indices of oxidative stress in blood and pulmonary epithelium lining fluid in horses suffering from recurrent airway obstruction. Equine Vet J 31: 397-401.

36. Deaton CM, Marlin DJ, Smith NC, Harris PA, Roberts CA, et al. (2004) Pulmonary epithelial lining fluid and plasma ascorbic acid concentrations in horses affected by recurrent airway obstruction. Am J Vet Res 65: 80-87.

37. Valko M, Leibfritz D, Moncol J, Cronin MT, Mazur M, et al. (2007) Free radicals and antioxidants in normal physiological functions and human disease. Int J Biochem Cell Biol 39: 44-84.

38. Roy SC, More T, Pati US, Srivastava SK (1996) Effect of *Pasteurella multocida* vaccination on buffalo polymorphonuclear hydrogen peroxide and nitric oxide production. Vet Immunol Immunopathol 51: 173-178.

The Major Cause of Lameness and Associated Risk Factors in Working Donkey in and around Hawassa Town, Ethiopia

Guluma Assefa[1], Birhanu Abera[2*], Ahmed Nur[1], Diriba Lemma[2], Lamessa Keno[1], Eyob Eticha[2], Gebeyehu Chali[3] and Mahammed Hussen[4]

[1]East Shoa Zone Livestock and Fishery Resource Office, Adama, Ethopia
[2]Asella Regional Veterinary Laboratory, Asella, Ethiopia
[3]Ilu Aba Bor Zone Livestock and Fishery Resource Office, Mattu, Ethioipia
[4]Buno Bedelle Zone Livestock and Fishery Resource Office, Bedelle, Ethiopia

Abstract

Across sectional study survey of the major work related lameness in donkey in and around Hawassa was under taken to determine the main causes of lameness in working donkeys and associated risk factor s. A total of 205 lame donkeys have been examined and their owners were interviewed to assess the possible cause of lameness and the type of management conditions. The result reveal that donkeys found in study area mainly cart pulling donkeys (96.5%) and about 99.5% of working donkeys are male. The result of questioner survey and visual study reveal that the main causes of lameness in donkey are ;28.3% is muscular and tendon problem,21.5% is joint problem,5.4% is bone problem, 20.0% is tendon problems,13.2% is hoof problem and 27.0% is other associated risk factor were shown to cause lameness in working donkey with the extreme significant ($p<0.0001$).the major types of lameness encountered during the study was supportive leg lameness (47.3%) and with the least of non weight bearing lameness were encountered with the significant of ($p<0.0001$).the result of this study suggested that in spite of varies use of donkey; they are confronted by series of health and welfare problem. Joint problem, tendon problem, hoof problem, bone problem and other relative risk factor; abusing, over loading, over working and unnecessary neglect and general maltreatment that are causing lameness are still prevalent health and welfare problem. The public veterinary clinic is almost lacking medical equipment and medicine; meant foot treating of lame donkey, therefore, further study on lameness and welfare constraints hindering the efficient use of donkey in region is of paramount importance.

Keywords: Donkey; Lameness; Risk factors; Hawassa; Ethiopia

Introduction

The equine population of the world was reported to be 122.4 million with 40 million donkeys, 15 million mules and 43.3 million horses. In the distribution pattern, 98% of all donkeys, 97% of all mules and 60% of all horses were noted to be found in developing countries [1]. The number of equines in Africa was in the range of 17.6 million comprising 11.6 million donkeys, 2.3 mullion mules and 3.7 million horses. Ethiopia possessed approximately half of Africa's equines population with 37%, 58% and 46% of all Africa, donkeys, horses and mules, respectively [2].

According to recent CSA (2014), there are about 2.03 million horses, 7.43 million donkeys, 0.4 million mules, and about 1.16 million camels in the sedentary areas of the country [3]. In Ethiopia the use of donkeys as pack animal or for pulling cart has enabled small scale farmers to participate in the market economy. Donkeys are used for fetching water, for household shifting, for carrying the sick to hospital, for carrying sick calves, for transportation, hoping and for pulling materials needed for construction [4]. Despite their remarkable contributions, donkeys in Ethiopia are the most neglected animals accorded low social status [5].

Although, equine play a significant role in the economy of the country, the government livestock development programs and those of aid agencies are aid toward increasing milk, meat, egg and wool production. Equines have been completely neglected and omitted from the agricultural system and their role in production is not yet well recognized and magnified. In country where there is less developed modern transportation and communication services. The natural choice rest on the use of human and pack animal mode of transport and it has been the case in the some part of the world. This is still remains true in Ethiopia context [6].

The donkey (equusasinus) is a domesticated race of African wild ass. The term ass is normally used for animal found in the wild where as the term donkey is used for domesticated animals. The donkey performs hard work under variable agro climate condition and withstands scarcity of feed. hardiness, little maintenance and low purchase price have made the donkey the cheapest and suitable means of transport over the centuries [7]. Generally the mountains and rugged trials of Ethiopia land scrape has treble time consuming and difficult which made equides remain the only means of transportation [8].

The donkey considered a better than other draught animals because of in heritance tolerant for dehydration, low sweat rate and good thermo ability. Donkeys are harder than mules and ponies under short term feed stress. Donkeys have been used to catty arms and ammunition to the different terrains that mechanized vehicles cannot reach easily [7]. Despite all this equids receive less attention in terms of feeding, health and management cares [9].

Equines assume an important place and act as multipurpose animals in the rural and urban society. however, management constraints like

***Corresponding author:** Birhanu Abera, Asella Regional Veterinary Laboratory, Asella, Ethiopia, E-mail: birhanuabera27@yahoo.com

feed shortage, traditional health care, absence of grooming and hoof care, housing problems and different cruelties on the animal together with occurrence of parasite, infectious disease and physical injuries render efficient use of donkeys impossible [10].

Hard working donkeys (pack and cart) were providing 1-3 kg concentrate rations, where as donkeys for light to moderate work were depend on grazing or inadequate fodder, donkeys were deprived of vaccination, deworming and veterinary aid, debility, wounds and abrasion, parasitic infestation, lameness, bite cases, respiratory and digestion disorders were the common ailments affecting 10-40% of the working donkeys [7].

A variety of disease condition hinders the utilization of donkey, among which lameness contributes a significant impact. Lameness is an indication of structural and functional disorders in one or more limbs that is manifested during progression or in standing position. Lameness cause animal acute pain in the foot, leg or joints, often resulting in lame. A sever case may mean that the animal is unable to bear the pain putting its hoof to the ground. Lameness can include hoof problem for example where they have picked up nail or other sharp objects through the sole after leading to infection, strained muscle or tendons; joint problems and traumatic injuries caused by accident. Lameness can be caused by trauma, congenital or acquire anomalies, infection. Metabolic disturbance, circulatory and nervous disorder or any combination of those.

Lameness is one of the most prevalent health problems in the donkeys. Lameness is not a disease, but a manifestation of either pain caused by any impediment in the musculoskeletal system or, if pain is not involved, of mechanical lameness, although a combination of the two frequently exists. Mechanical lameness is the best typified by fibrotic myopathy with its characteristic in gait abnormality, but can also be the result of restriction. Pain related lameness can be classified as weight bearing (supporting leg) or non-weight bearing (swinging leg) lameness. Although lameness most often is composed of both a supportive leg lameness may originate from anywhere in the limb (proximal or distal) while swinging leg lameness, although often believed to represent a proximal problem or distal [11]. Most important predisposing factors ultimately leading to hoof problems were found to be poor housing, standing in muddy areas for long period, disproportionate harnessing design unskilled furriers and neglect of the car accorded to the hoof [12].

The cause of lameness is multifactorial and its occurrence is associated with risk factors such as nutritional, climatic, housing, breed and age of animals and as squeal of other disease [13]. factors that predispose to lameness include physical immaturity e.g., bones that are anatomically normal but biochemically weak due to the animal at the onset of training or bone that is abnormally weak due to developmental orthopedic disease) and monotonous repetitive stresses on bones [11]. Lameness has got to be treated, otherwise the affected animal will not be able to get about grazing effectively, it may be bullied and it will be lose weight and because lameness is often associated with pain, it is usually on animal welfare problem. There are many possible causes of lameness but for many type, the earlier treatment is given the more likely it is result in permanent cure [14].

Although lameness has been reported as one of the health problem of working donkeys affecting their health and welfare, little attempt has been made to characterize the nature of lameness in working donkey in Ethiopia. Recognizing early assign of lameness is very helpful in reduction of loses due to lameness. Therefore the objective of this study is to identify the types and cause of lameness in working donkeys and to determine associated risk factors of lameness in study area.

Materials and Methods

Study area

The study was conducted in and around hawassa town, the capital city of sidama zone, which is located in the northern parts of southern nations, nationalities and people's region (SNNPR), Ethiopia and is located on the shore of rift valley lakes and found at 270 km south of Addis Ababa with a total land area 6793.6 km geographically the area lies between 427" and 8, 30'N latitude and 34, 21"E longitude [15]. During the study period, Hawassa received an annual average rain fall ranging from 0-3.4 mm and with a mean temperature of the area of 14°C-29.1°C with a mean relative humidity of 51.8%and with an average altitude of 1790 m above sea level (Meteorology, 2008) the average house hold size is 5-6 years. The total livestock population of Sidama zone is (including Hawassa is estimated to constitute 1,573,378 cattle, 183,462 goat, 221,505 sheep, 49,150 horse, 42,653 asses, 3,959 mule, 1,196,56 poultry and 73,479 bee hives [3].

Study population and sampling

The study animals were conducted on working donkeys that are found in and around hawassa town. The study was conducted from November 2007 to May 2008 in Hawassa town. In those months of study; donkeys that are brought to clinic and visits to certain area were examined for lameness. The study protocol or design were done by a questionnaire survey and physical examination techniques were used to study the types, cause and associated risk factors of lameness in working donkeys, purposive sampling technique was used. Donkeys presented to clinic were examined for lameness indicators. A total 205 lame sample size with expected prevalence of 16% using the formula [16].

$$n = \frac{1.96^2 \times Pexp\ (1 - Pexp)}{d^2}$$

Whereas; n=number of study population

Pexp=expected prevalence

d=desired Precision

Study methodology

Physical/visual examination: This is done on lame donkeys to generate categorical variables that help to quantify and describe the magnitude of musculoskeletal disorders. Visual examination, examination by manipulation and palpation was done in diagnosis of lameness. Clinical/ physical examination like;

Examination at rest: this examination was done at a distal, then up on close, viewing the animal from front, side and behind to asses symmetry of lameness, conformation, the condition and alteration in posture, weight shifting and pointing. At close observation each limb was observed and compared to its opposite.

Examination at exercise: This is to identify the lameness involved and the degree of lameness and in coordination in movement. Each selected donkey (lame donkey) was examined while it is walking and trotting, and to categorized the degree of lameness on examination and categorized as grade 1, grade 2, grade 3 and grade 4, following observation of the animal from a disease, close examination of the limbs by palpation and manipulation. While the animal is being trotted, to see whether the limb carried in straight line or adducted, abducted or circumducted during progration. Also look for any deviation in long axis of body during movement. When both limbs are lame they are carried stiffly and the group movements are not reliable for diagnosis of lameness. The head movement seen in lameness of one of the fore limbs may however be seen in case of lameness in opposite hind limb also at animal on one hind limb may be suspected to be lame on opposite forelimb this is called cross lameness. Correct diagnosis in cross lameness is made by observing the group movement also. When one fore limb and the opposite hind limb are lame the condition is called diagonal lameness.

Detail examination of lame limb: this examination is used to locate the exact seat of lameness. The various bones, joint, tendon and sheathe was palpated, flexed, abducted, adducted to know the exact seat of the area for the cause of lameness. Local inflammatory lesions were detected by this examination [17].

Questionnaire survey: This is a structured questionnaire is designed to collect data on information related to lameness like manage mental practices and associated risk factors. This interview was carried out donkey owners and cart drivers.

Data analysis: Data that are collected during study was computed and analyzed with Ms excel and using stat 7 software against all results that are collected from the study animal to determine significant differences among different causes.

Results

Questionnaire survey

The result of cross sectional study conducted from December 2007 to May 2008 to determine the causes of lameness in working donkeys and associated risk factor. A total of 205 working donkey owners were examined to investigate the cause of the lameness in working donkey that are found in and around hawassa town. as the involvement of limbs affected,50.24% is hind limb and 43.41% is fore limb and 6.34%is both limbs affected (Table 1). The pattern of foot inspection when donkey became lame is (96.6%), no inspection (2.0%) and immediately after work (1.4%) (Table 2). The duration of relative lameness >month is (52.7%), less than week (7.3%) and less than month (40.0%) (Table 3). The house types of working donkey, roofed is (59%) and open air (41%) (Table 4). The floor type of the donkey's house sand /soil type is (93.2%), concrete and stone layer is (3.4%) (Table 5). The driving speed of working donkey, the average speed is (74.1%), fast (17.5%) and slow (4.4%) (Table 6). The onset of lameness of working donkey (98.5%) is during work and after work (1.5%) (Table 7). The treatment of lame donkey by rest is (94.3%) and brand (5.7%) (Table 8).

Involved Limb	Frequency	Percentage
Fore limb	89	43.41
Hind limb	103	50.24
Both	13	6.34
Total(n=205)	**205**	**100**

Table 1: The lame donkeys in terms of limb affected.

Inspection pattern	Frequency	Percentage
No inspection	4	2.0
After work	3	1.4
When lame	198	96.6
Total	**205**	**100.0**

Table 2: The pattern of inspection of donkey's foot.

Duration of lameness	Frequency	Percentage
Less than a week	15	7.3
Less than a month	82	40.0
More than a month	108	52.7
Total	**205**	**100**

Table 3: Duration of lameness in working donkeys.

House Type	Frequency	Percentage
Open air	84	41
Roofed	121	59
Total	**205**	**100**

Table 4: The relative house type of working donkey.

Floor Type	Frequency	Percentage
Concrete	7	3.4
Sand/Soil	191	93.2
Stone	7	3.4
Total	**205**	**100**

Table 5: The relative floor types of donkey's house.

Driving Speed	Frequency	Percentage
Fast	36	17.5
Average	160	78.1
Slow	9	4.4
Total	**205**	**100.0**

Table 6: The relative speed of working donkey.

Onset of Lameness	Frequency	Percentage
During Work	202	98.5
After work	3	1.5
Total	**205**	**100**

Table 7: The relative on set of lameness on working donkey.

How alleviate Lameness	Frequency	Percentage
Branding	6	5.7
Rest	199	94.3
Total	**205**	**100.0**

Table 8: The donkey owner for the treatment of lame donkey.

The pattern of foot inspection when donkey became lame is when donkey became lame (96.6%), immediately after working (1.4%) and no inspection (2.0%) where recorded (Table 2).

Physical/visual examination

The type of lameness that was encountered during study period was 47.3% is supportive leg lameness. With the significant ($p<0.0001$) (Table 9). As the primary cause of lameness is working donkey 28.3% is muscle and ligament problem and other associated risk factor(mixed) is 27.0% with extreme significant of ($p<0.0001$) (Table 10). As use of working donkey in the study area is cart pulling (96.6%) and pack working donkey (3.4%) (Table 11).

Discussion

The overall prevalence of muscular skeletal disorder; including hoof over growth and inter digital skin hyperplasia that did not cause lameness, for all category of animals was 16.3% [13].

The result of this study revealed that lameness is of importance to

Types of lameness	Frequency	Percentage
Hanging	9	4.4
Lateral	5	2.4
Supporting	97	47.3
Pointed	82	40.0
Pointed	12	5.9
Total	**205**	**100**

X2=194.6, df=4, P<0.0001

Table 9: The relative types of lameness in working donkey.

Primary cause of lameness	Frequency	Percentage
Joint Problem	44	21.5
Bone Problem	11	5.4
Tendon Problem	41	20.0
Muscle and ligament	58	28.3
Hoof problem	27	13.2
Mixed	55	27.0

X2=38.3, df=5, P<0.0001

Table 10: The percentage of major cause of lameness in working donkey.

Use	Frequency	Percent
Cart	198	96.6
Pack	7	3.4
Total	**205**	**100.0**

Table 11: Number of lame donkeys that are examined during study period.

the healthy and wellbeing of working donkey. The higher percentage of affected leg is hind limb (50.24%), fore limb (43.42%) and in both (6.34%). The major cause of hind limb lameness is beating donkeys up on working and poor hygienic condition this result is the same with Bolbol and Sahel reported in upper Egypt [18].

The inventory of draught donkey kept by the owner is more of male donkeys (98%) because the draught power of male donkey is greater than female donkey and also the possible reason could be the economic return associated with their keeping.

During performing the draught work, those animals were subjected to different kinds of cruelties and stress by the owners due to varies reasons. They use beating for the highest speed and poor consideration of owner to the well being of donkey is evident. The reasons for this condition are the poor knowledge of animal health and the focus of owners only on the income.

The frequent occurrence oflameness is during work (98.5%) because of several cruelties and stresses by the owner during work due to varies causes the first and the major cause of lameness in working donkey is muscles and ligament problems (28.2%) may be due to short period of rest for donkeys, after rest starting with high speed and the presence of hoof over growth (33.2%), the highest duration of lameness due to other causes on the working donkey and over working, if duration of lameness is greater than a month (57.7%),this may be the main predisposing factor for tendon luxation together with hoof over growth and causing much of weight bearing on the un affected limb leading to atrophy of muscle of the opposite limbs and causes permanent lameness. The second most causes of lameness is joint problem. This may due to over working of the donkey and hoof over growth. The 3rd major cause is tendon problem (20.0%) the probable cause of this conditions is because of donkey exposed to over loading. The 4th major cause is hoof problem (13.2%). The percentage hoof problem in donkey by Addisalem (25.5%) is twice as recorded by this study (13.2%) but it is almost similar with (Moti,2005)(15%) were reported [10]. The possible reason for recording the low hoof problem is that the establishment of help aid in the town/zone and weekly treatment of donkey by donkey sanctuary in their site and the management aspect of the donkey is good(daily clearance of donkeys house (-%),59% of donkey is housed/roofed, high inspection of donkeys hoof immediately the donkey became lame(96.6%) and the highest working donkey on the soil(93.2%) rather than concrete (3.4%) and atone/asphalt(3.4%) (P<0.0001). The 5th rank is bone problems (5.4%) this is to indicate that fracture and related orthopedic problems. This low result is may be due to the donkeys' owners' care for breakage of donkey's legs by considering the economic impact for treatment of broken donkey.

As per type of lameness in working donkey on study is supportive leg lameness (47.0%), the possible cause of this is, the donkeys" owners work by lame donkey until it become unable to walk because of the owner purchase donkey with high cost and the donkey owners haven't any other possible income besides the knowledge of donkey owners on lameness identification earlier is low. The 2nd most common types of lameness is hinder leg lameness (40.0%) due to donkey suffering from lameness exhibit the clinical signs only during rest; which is show by pointing of leg while standing.

Lameness is one of the major factors for working equine leading to low power or energy generation and loss of animal and having high economic impact, this is true in all animals including dairy animals. Thus further studies must be conducted on lameness to overcome loss animal power and economy.

Conclusions and Recommendations

The result of the present study conducted on working donkeys for six months from November 2007 to May 2008 in and around Hawassa town showed that lameness of donkeys is one of the major conditions in study area affecting the well being of the animals. The major cause of lameness is working donkey in study area is muscle and ligament (28.3%) and joint problem (21.5%) and other associated mixed factors (27.0%) are encountered during the study period. The most common types of lameness were supportive leg lameness (47.3). This shows that lameness in the area becoming high prevalent, if no veterinary aid and attention of any help to alleviate these problems. Those lameness conditions have an impact on the power working of the animal. Therefore, based on the above conclusions the following recommendations are forwarded:

- Donkeys as drought animal will play a pivot role for many decades to come, therefore, it is necessary that a comprehensive research program for their ration and efficient use in future to be formulated.
- Short courses on drought donkey management, disease control, health cover, handling, training, welfare, housing, feeding and first aid should be launched in rural and urban area for drought animal power owners.
- There is dire need to conduct research on animal derived vehicles, implements and other equipment to make the more appropriate for animal from welfare point as well as the efficiency.
- There should be regular inspection of hoof, daily cleaning of house of donkey and trimming of the overgrown hoofs.
- The donkey sanctuary aid should be expanded throughout the country to achieve the wellbeing and health of working donkeys.

References

1. Wilson RL (1991) Equine in Ethiopia. In: Fieldings D, Pearson RA (eds.). Donkeys, mules and horses in tropical agricultural development. Preceding of colloquium help 3-6 september 1990, Edinbrough, Scotland, Center for tropical veterinary medicine, University of Edenborough, UK, pp: 33-47.
2. Blench R, Champman R, Slay Marker T (2003) A study of role of livestock inpoverty reduction strategy papers. pro-poor livestock initiative working paper, FAO, pp: 52.
3. CSA (2004) Ethiopia- Agricultural Sample Enumeration, Farm Practice 2001-2002 (1994 E.C) Authority, Federal Democratical of Ethiopia.
4. Pritchard JC, Lindberg AC, Main DCJ, Whay HR (2005) Assessment of the welfare of working horses, mules and donkeys using health and behavior parameters. Prev Vet Med. 12: 265-283.
5. Biffa D, Woldemeskel M (2006) Causes and Factors Associated With Occurrence of External Injuries in Working Equines in Ethiopia. International J Appl Res Vet Med. 4: 1-7.
6. Feseha GA,Yilma JM, Sevandense ED, Mohammed A (1991) Health problem of working donkey in Debre zeit and Menagesha region of Ethiopia in FAO.
7. Singh MK, Gupta AK, Yadav MP (2005) The donkey; its role and the scope for better management, Livestock International. 9: 18-20.
8. Hassen K (2000) A preliminary study on the socio economic importance, health problem and other management constraints of horses in mid and high land area of north Gonder, DVM thesis, FVM, AAU, Debre zeit, Ethiopia.
9. Gizaw (1987) Policy and strategy option to ward rapid development of Ethiopia livestock improvement conference, IAR, Ethiopia.
10. Addisalem H (2005) Assessment of health and welfare problems of donkeys and mules in SNNP region. DVM thesis, Faculty of veterinary Medicine, AAU, pp: 452-453.
11. Khan CM, Scott line (2005) The merck veterinary manual, 9th edn. Merck and Co., Inc., white house station, NJ, USA, pp: 618-619.
12. Moti Y (2005) Assessment of hoof associated problem in cart horses in five town of SPANA- Ethiopia operation sites. Centeral Ethiopia, DVM thesis. FVM. AAU. Debre zeit. Ethiopia, pp: 480.
13. Alemayehu L, Fikre Legabo, Azage Tegegn (1999) Lameness as a disease of intensification in dairy cattle under urban and peri urban production system in Addis Ababa milk shed. Bulletin of Animal Health and Production in Africa. 49: 254-261.
14. Marjories O (1993) Lameness is caused by many factors which differ between individual cows and farms. Reducing the number of lame cows on your farm therefore requires a long-term, planned approach that is supported by the whole farm team.
15. Ghirottic M (1995) Farming practices and pattern in coffe growing mid land Sidama-Ethiopia,Msc thesis, Haramaya University, pp: 1-11.
16. Thrusfield M (2007) Veterinary Epidemiology. 3rd edn, Blackwell Science Ltd, Oxford, pp: 244-245.
17. Kelly WR (1974)Veterinary clinical Diagnosis. 2nd edn., Pub Baillier Tindale, London, UK, pp: 335-346.
18. Bolbol AE, Saleh AS (1987) Survey on equine hoof affection in Upper Egypt (Abstract). Jounal of the egypt veterinary medicine association. 47: 545-553.

21

Evaluation of Different Calcium Sources on the Performance of Highly Prolific Lactating Sows

Barrilli LNE[1], Silva BAN[2]*, Maiorka A[1], Falleiros FT[3], Silva CC[3], Raidan FSS[2] and Araújo WAG[4]

[1]*Animal Science Department, Federal University of Paraná (UFPR), 80035-050, Curitiba, Paraná, Brazil*
[2]*Institute of Agricultural Sciences/ICA, Federal University of Minas Gerais (UFMG), 39404-547, Montes Claros, Minas Gerais, Brazil*
[3]*DSM Nutritional Products, Av. Engineer Billings 1729, 05321-010, São Paulo, Brazil*
[4]*Animal Science Unit, Federal Institute of Education, Science and Technology Northern Minas Gerais (IFNMG), 39480-000, Januária, Minas Gerais, Institute of Agricultural Sciences/ ICA, Federal University of Minas Gerais (UFMG), 39404-547, Montes Claros, Minas Gerais, Brazil*

Abstract

Improvements in sow productivity have raised questions regarding dietary mineral recommendations. Current calcium (Ca) levels and/or Ca sources might not support milk requirements of the larger litter in the modern sow. Therefore, four hundred and eighty mixed parity sows of a high prolificacy genetic line were used to evaluate the impact of the calcium source on the performance of highly prolific lactating sows. Sows were distributed in a completely randomized experimental design among six treatments containing different levels of inorganic Ca (INO) and organic calcium carbon-amino-phospho-chelate (CQT) inclusion. The sows were allocated to one of the six treatments represented by increased replacement ratios between sources of calcium: 100% INO; 100% CQT; 80% INO and 20% CQT; 60% INO and 40% CQT; 40% INO and 60% CQT; 20% INO and 80% CQT. Farrowing duration was not influenced (P>0.10) by the treatments, and averaged 185 minutes. Average daily voluntary feed intake did not differ (*P*>0.10) between treatments (5.54 kg d^{-1} on average). The lactation BW, backfat losses and chemical composition of body weight loss was not influenced (*P*>0.10) by the treatments. Litter size and average piglet weight at birth were not influenced (*P*>0.10) by the treatments (13.7 and 1.26 kg, on average). Litter weight gain, litter size and average piglet weight at weaning were also not influenced (*P*>0.10) by the treatments. The Treatments did not influence (*P*>0.10) estimated daily milk yield; which averaged 11.41 kg d^{-1}. The treatments tended to influence (P<0.10) urinary pH levels at day 7 of lactation, were 100% CQT sows had a lower pH value than other treatments (6.72 *vs.* 7.27). 100% CQT sows also showed a significantly lower pH level at d 14 and 21 when compared to the other treatments (6.44 *vs.* 7.09; *P*<0.05; and 6.48 *vs.* 7.14; *P*<0.01; respectively for d 14 and 21 of lactation). Free Ca and parathyroid hormone (PTH) serum levels were not affected (*P*>0.10) by treatments during lactation and averaged 1.38 mmol/L and 14.62 pg/ml, respectively. In conclusion, this experiment demonstrated that in diets for lactating sows an inorganic Ca source can be fully replaced by a more available Ca source (i.e., calcium carbon-amino-phospho-chelate), without negatively impacting the productive and reproductive performance of these animals or the performance of their litters.

Keywords: Sows; Calcium; Lactation; Milk production; Parathyroid hormone

Introduction

The productivity of sows has risen substantially during the past 10 years, mainly due to management and genetic advances and selection based on parameters such as litter size, weaning-estrus interval, and lactation efficiency. Although genetic advances have made sows more productive, they are more nutritionally demanding and less resistant to nutritional challenges. Mineral requirements have changed, as have other nutrient requirements. Average levels of digestible phosphorus (Pd) and calcium (Ca) recommended by the NRC in 2012 are higher than the levels practiced by the NRC in 1998.

Ca is enrolled with important metabolic functions and is closely related to Phosphorus (P) metabolism, regulation of Vitamin D absorption, parathyroid hormone (PTH) and Calcitonin [1]. Ca is also involved in extracellular functions such as blood clotting, maintenance and stability of cell membranes, structural integrity of bones and teeth, renal and respiratory function [2]. In addition to ATP metabolism, Ca affects muscle contraction, particularly during the parturition process, which is directly related to how long delivery takes and how many piglets are born alive, given that hypocalcemia reduces myometrium contractions. Furthermore, this mineral is also present in the sow´s milk, as one of the most important minerals secreted in milk [3].

The primary sources of Ca supplements for swine diets come from inorganic sources (e.g., rocks). Inorganic minerals have a structure that limits satisfactory absorption by the organism, therefore resulting in significant losses through feces [4]. Several studies have focused on finding new, more efficient mineral sources that are highly soluble, have a stable chemical structure, and are electrically neutral in the gastrointestinal tract, factors that would prevent reactions that could impair the absorption of other minerals [5]. For minerals to be absorbed, they must overcome an intestinal barrier, entailing factors such as physical and chemical conditions, pH and intestinal viscosity. In this context, researchers have focused on developing studies aiming towards the use of organic mineral sources. Organic minerals can be found in various forms, including compounds with amino acids, chelated amino acids, protein minerals and complex polysaccharide minerals [6]. Although some variance has been seen, it has been suggested that organic mineral forms offer higher bioavailability in animals [7].

***Corresponding author:** Bruno Silva, Institute of Agricultural Sciences/ ICA, Universidade Federal de Minas Gerais (UFMG), 39404-547, Montes Claros, Minas Gerais, Brazil, E-mail: BrunoSilva@ufmg.br

Some alternative organic ingredients have been explored to replace inorganic Ca sources (i.e., bone meal, meat and bone meal, ground shells and Ca from algae [5]. However, the main problem with using organic sources is the variation in composition, availability, and cost [8]. The use of chelated minerals comes as an alternative to inorganic sources of calcium. These are metallic ions chemically bound to an organic molecule, forming stable and highly bioavailable molecules and resulting in more efficient use by the animal [9].

Due to the evident importance of Ca for sows before farrowing and during lactation, the present study aimed to study the impact of a total and/or partial replacement of inorganic Ca with a more available source of Ca (i.e., calcium carbon-amino-phospho-chelate) on the productive performance of sows and their litters during the lactation period.

Materials and Methods

This study was conducted in compliance with and with approval from the Committee for Ethical Use of Animals at the Federal University of Paraná (UFPR) Agricultural Science Division, under the protocol number 016/2014.

Animals and experimental design

The study was performed in the facilities of a commercial sow unit, located in the South-eastern part of Brazil in the state of Minas Gerais, and was performed during summer, covering the period between January 2015 and March of 2015. According to the Köpen climate classification, the region is defined as Cwa (hot, temperate, rainy, and with a dry winter season and hot summer).

A total of 480 mixed parity sows of a high-prolificacy commercial genetic line (TOPIGS 20®) from four successive batches of 130 sows each were used in this study. Within each batch, sows were distributed in a completely randomized experimental design among six treatments containing different levels of inorganic Ca (INO) and organic calcium carbon-amino-phospho-chelate (CQT) inclusion according to parity order (1st, 2nd and 3rd-4th parity), body weight and backfat thickness at d 110 of gestation. The sows were allocated to one of the six treatments represented by increased replacement ratios between sources of calcium: 100% INO; 100% CQT; 80% INO and 20% CQT; 60% INO and 40% CQT; 40% INO and 60% CQT; 20% INO and 80% CQT. Each treatment consisted of 80 repetitions, and each sow was considered an experimental unit. Feed was formulated based on corn, soybean meal and soybean oil, and supplemented with industrial minerals, vitamins and amino acids to meet the requirements of this animal category according to recommendations in the feeding manual for the genetic breed (Table 1). For the ratios between essential amino acids and digestible lysine, the values indicated by Rostagno et al. were used as reference (Table 1) [10].

At 110 d of gestation, sows were weighed, backfat measured and transferred to the farrowing rooms and housed in farrowing crates (2.1 × 2.2 m) on fully slatted metal floor. During this period, the sows were fed the respective treatment diet as follows: day 110: 3.0 kg d^{-1}, 111: 2.80 kg d^{-1}, 112: 2.60 kg d^{-1}, 113: 2.40 kg d^{-1}, 114: 2.00 kg d^{-1}, and at d 115, if the sow had not yet farrowed, they were offered 1.50 kg d^{-1} until the farrowing day. The animals had *ad libitum* access to water throughout the entire experimental period.

Twenty-four hours after farrowing, all sows were again weighed, had their backfat measured (P2). Sows were then submitted to a step-up feeding regime to stimulate a gradual feed intake increase up to day 7 post-farrowing, starting with 2 kg on day 1 post-farrowing and reaching 8 kg d^{-1} on day 7. The allowance increased by 1 kg each day. This feeding management was applied to avoid over-consumption at the beginning of lactation and agalactia problems. After d 7 sows were fed 2 kg+0.5 kg piglet^{-1} d^{-1}.

After birth, piglets were handled for tooth clipping, umbilical cord treatment and ear tagged for labelling. On d 3, they received an intramuscular injection of 200 mg of iron dextran. As necessary, cross-fostering was conducted within the first 48 h after birth to standardize litter size at 13 piglets. On d 10, male piglets were castrated. Creep housing equipped with infrared lights provided supplemental heat for the piglets during the lactation period. The day prior to weaning (i.e., d 24), sows were allowed 5 kg of feed (i.e., at least 1.5 kg lower than their usual feed intake) to standardize consumption for all sows for determination of sow weight at weaning. At weaning, sows were again weighed and backfat measured and moved to a breeding facility and were presented to a mature boar twice daily to detect onset of standing estrus. Sows were inseminated when positive to the back-pressure test. During the weaning-to-estrus interval, all sows were submitted to the same feeding management, receiving 3.0 kg d^{-1} of their respective lactation diet.

Collected measurements and parameters

Variations in environmental conditions inside the farrowing barns were recorded daily using a thermo-hygrometer kept in an empty cage in the middle of the building, at the average midpoint of the animals' height. Temperature and humidity data were recorded daily at 0700; 1200; and 1700. Sows were weighed using a digital scale (Líder Balanças Ltda., Mod. LD 2000E, Araçatuba, SP, Brazil), and backfat thickness was measured at P2 (65 mm from the dorsal line) using ultrasound equipment (Renco Lean-Meater, Renco Corporation, Minneapolis, USA) at d 110, 24 h post-farrowing and at weaning in order to determine body weight and backfat thickness variation. The following litter parameters were collected at farrowing: total number of piglets born, born alive, stillborn, and mummies. Piglets were individually weighed using a digital scale (Líder Balanças Ltda., Mod. B150, Araçatuba, SP, Brazil) 24 h post-farrowing and at weaning to determine litter birth and weaning weights, and daily weight gain during lactation. All dead piglets during lactation were weighed in order to properly estimate growth rates and daily milk production.

Every morning, feed refusals were collected, and fresh feed was immediately distributed once per day between 0700 and 0800. Feed consumption was determined as the difference between feed allowance and the refusals collected on the next morning. Every day, one sample of feed and feed refusals were collected daily for DM content measurement, and successive samples were pooled and stored at 4°C for further analyses. The feed samples were analyzed for DM, ash, fat content (AOAC, 1990) and CP (N × 6.25 for feed) according to Dumas method (AOAC, 1990) and for crude fiber and for cell wall components (NDF, ADF, and ADL) according to van Soest and Wine (1967) at the Animal Nutrition Laboratory of Federal University of Paraná Animal Nutrition Laboratory (Curitiba, Brazil).

The impact of treatments on farrowing duration was evaluated by recording the time farrowing began, which was defined as the moment the first placenta break, and the time farrowing ended, which was defined as the moment the sow expelled the last placenta. To analyze the sows' urinary pH levels, urine samples were collected 24 hours after farrowing and at d 7,14 and 21 of lactation, in a predetermined subgroup of 20 sows per treatment. The subgroup consisted of sows chosen according to parity order to be the most representative samples of the treatments.

	Treatments[1]					
Ingredients	100% INO	100% CQT	80% INO 20% CQT	60% INO 40% CQT	40% INO 60% CQT	20% INO 80% CQT
Corn, kernel	52.38	52.27	52.36	52.34	52.32	52.30
Soybean meal 46%	25.00	25.00	25.00	25.00	25.00	25.00
Soybean hull	13.85	13.85	13.85	13.85	13.85	13.85
Soybean oil	4.94	4.94	4.94	4.94	4.94	4.94
Dicalcium phosphate	2.28	-	1.81	1.35	0.88	0.41
Calcitic limestone	0.30	-	0.25	0.19	0.14	0.08
Chelated Calcium[5]	-	2.70	0.54	1.08	1.62	2.16
Salt	0.48	0.48	0.48	0.48	0.48	0.48
Mineral mixture[2]	0.15	0.15	0.15	0.15	0.15	0.15
Vitamin mixture[3]	0.15	0.15	0.15	0.15	0.15	0.15
L-Lysine HCL 78%	0.24	0.24	0.24	0.24	0.24	0.24
L-Threonine	0.08	0.08	0.08	0.08	0.08	0.08
L-Tryptophan	0.02	0.02	0.02	0.02	0.02	0.02
L-Valine	0.06	0.05	0.06	0.06	0.06	0.06
DL-Methionine	0.02	0.02	0.02	0.02	0.02	0.02
TOTAL	100	100	100	100	100	100
	Analyzed composition as fed[4]					
Metabolizable Energy, Mcal/kg	3.40	3.40	3.40	3.40	3.40	3.40
Crude protein %	17.1	17.1	17.1	17.1	17.1	17.1
Digestible Lysine %	0.95	0.95	0.95	0.95	0.95	0.95
Digestible Met+Cys %	0.51	0.51	0.51	0.51	0.51	0.51
Digestible Threonine %	0.61	0.61	0.61	0.61	0.61	0.61
Digestible Tryptophan %	0.18	0.18	0.18	0.18	0.18	0.18
Digestible Valine %	0.74	0.74	0.74	0.74	0.74	0.74
Digestible Arginine %	1.00	1.00	1.00	1.00	1.00	1.00
Total Calcium %	0.86	0.86	0.86	0.86	0.86	0.86
Total Phosphorous %	0.73	0.63	0.71	0.69	0.66	0.64
Digestible Phosphorus %	0.39	0.39	0.39	0.39	0.39	0.39
Digestible Ca:P ratio %	2.2	2.2	2.2	2.2	2.2	2.2
Sodium %	0.22	0.22	0.22	0.22	0.22	0.22

[1]100% Inorganic Calcium source (INO); 100% organic calcium source (calcium carbon-amino-phospho-chelate = CQT); 80% INO and 20% CQT; 60% INO and 40% CQT; 40% INO and 60% CQT; 20% INO and 80% CQT. [2]Contents in 1 kg of feed: Iron, 100 mg; Copper, 10 mg; Cobalt, 1 mg; Manganese, 40 mg; Zinc, 100 mg; Iodine, 1.5 mg; and excipient q.s. [3]Contents in 1 kg of feed: Vit A - 8000 IU; Vit D3 - 1200 IU; Vit E - 20 IU; Vit K3 - 2 mg; Vit B1 - 1 mg; Vit B2 - 4 mg; nicotinic acid - 22 mg; pantothenic acid - 16 mg; Vit B6 - 0.50 mg; Vit B12 - 0.020 mg; folic acid - 0.4 mg; biotin - 0.120 mg; choline - 400 mg; and antioxidant – 30 mg. [4]Composition calculated per TOPIGS (2012). [5]Contents: 25% Ca and 12% P (digestible).

Table 1: Composition of the lactation experimental diets.

Sampling was standardized within 2 hours after meals, and a pH meter was used to measure sample pH immediately after collecting. On the d 14 and 21, blood samples were collected from the same subgroup of sows from which urine was collected. The sows were immobilized in their farrowing crates, and then 10 ml of blood were drawn from the jugular artery using a 40 mm × 12 mm needle. Blood samples were then sent to a laboratory, where they were centrifuged for 10 minutes at 3500 rpm for subsequent analysis of free Ca using the Selective Ion method, with ISELAB equipment – SL 0014 – DRAKE, and parathyroid hormone (PTH) using the Automated Chemiluminescent method, with Siemens IMMULITE 2000 equipment. The following parameters were assessed: time of farrowing duration, total feed intake of sows considering pre-farrowing and lactation, number of total born, live born, stillborn and mummified fetuses, birth weight of piglets, variations in the sows' physical conditions, variations in body composition, estimated milk production, piglet and litter weight gain, sow urinary pH levels, and circulating levels of free Ca and PTH (parathyroid hormone).

Calculations and statistical design

Daily maximum, minimum, mean, and variance of daily ambient temperatures and relative humidities were averaged and analysed for the entire experimental period. Body protein, fat, and energy contents at farrowing and at weaning were estimated according to the equations of Dourmad et al. [11]. Protein, lipid, and energy losses during lactation were estimated as the difference between calculated values determined at weaning and farrowing. Average daily milk production estimation was based on litter growth rate and size during lactation, according to the equations of Noblet and Etienne [12]. Data were submitted to normality tests and analysed using the generalized linear model procedure (GLM) and the mixed linear model (PROC MIX procedure) of SAS statistical package (SAS Inst., Inc, Cary, NC; version 9.2) and differences were considered significant at the P<0.05 level. The effects of parity order (O), batch (G) and treatments during lactation (TL) and litter size and weight as a covariate effect were included in the statistical model. Analyses were conducted using the following statistical model:

$$Y_{ijk}=\mu+A_i+B_j+C_k+D_l+E(X_{ijkl}-X)+F(Z_{ijkl}-Z)+e_{ijkl};$$

where μ=general average, A_i=fount type of Ca, B_j=parturition order, D_l=back fat, C_k=group effect, X_{ijkl}=observed value of the covariate "sow weight", X=average of the covariate "sow weight", E=regression coefficient between the covariate (X) and the response variable (Y), Z_{ijkl}=observed value of the covariate "litter weight", X=average of the covariate "litter weight", F=regression coefficient between the covariate (Z) and the response variable (Y), and e_{ijkl}=incidental residual effect of observation.

Results

The average maximum and minimum environmental temperatures and average maximum and minimum relative humidity recorded during the experimental period were 32.9 and 19.3°C and 86.6 and 58.8%, respectively. A total of 29 sows were removed from the experiment due to low litter size at weaning (<9 piglets) and/or health problems. According to the experimental design, the average parity order was 3.17 and did not differ (P>0.10) between treatments. No differences in lactation length were observed between treatments (24.5 d on average). Farrowing duration was not influenced (P>0.10) by the treatments, and averaged of 185 minutes.

Average daily voluntary feed intake did not differ (*P>0.10*) between treatments (5.54 kg d^{-1} on average; Table 2). The lactation BW and backfat losses were not influenced (*P*>0.10) by treatments (9.51 kg and 2.83 mm, on average), as shown in Table 3. The chemical composition of body weight loss was not influenced (*P*>0.10) by the treatments (7.64 kg; 2.36 kg; and 280 MJ; respectively for body protein, lipids and energy losses; Table 2).

Litter size and average piglet weight at birth were not influenced (*P*>0.10) by the treatments (13.7 and 1.26 kg, on average; Table 3). Litter weight gain during lactation was not influenced (*P*>0.10; Table 3) by the treatments and averaged 2.39 kg d^{-1}. Litter size and average piglet weight at weaning were also not influenced (*P*>0.10) by the treatments (12.2 and 6.29 kg on average, respectively; Table 3). The Treatments did not influence (*P*>0.10; Table 3) estimated daily milk yield; which averaged 11.41 kg d^{-1}.

The treatments tended to influence (P<0.10) urinary pH levels at day 7 of lactation, where treatment 2 sows presented a lower pH value than other treatments (6.72 *vs.* 7.27; Table 4). Treatment 2 sows also showed a significantly lower pH level at d 14 and 21 when compared to the other treatments (6.44 *vs.* 7.09; *P*<0.05; and 6.48 *vs.* 7.14; *P*<0.01; respectively for d 14 and 21 of lactation; Table 4). Free Ca and PTH serum levels were not affected (*P*>0.10; Table 4) by treatments during lactation and averaged 1.38 mmol/L and 14.62 pg/ml, respectively.

Discussion

The effects of high temperatures on the performance of lactating sows is well established [13]. In tropical climate conditions, the temperature observed in different seasons is always higher than the upper limit of the sows' thermoneutral zone (i.e., 22°C; Quiniou and Noblet, 1999). While conducting this study, the average maximum temperatures (26.1°C) exceeded 22°C. Therefore, lactating sows suffered from heat stress most of the time during our experiment.

There is quite extensive research on the benefits of chelated mineral sources in animal nutrition, in particular for non-ruminants [14-17]. These associated mineral sources have been reported to improve mineral absorption, and when replacing traditional inorganic mineral sources are capable of maintaining or improving performance [14,15]. However, the vast majority of studies focus their work on "trace" minerals like Cu, Zn, Fe, Mn and Se. Research focusing on the study of Ca sources chelated to organic molecules in animal feed is rare [15] and in particular those focusing on their effect on reproductive and productive aspects of pigs are nonexistent.

During the farrowing period, intramuscular Ca reserves are extremely important for uterine contraction and expulsion of the fetus, but over the course of the parturition the uterine musculature response tends to decrease due to muscle fatigue and decreased intramuscular Ca reserves, sometimes requiring the application of hormones like oxytocin or medication like Ca gluconate to prevent increased total

Variables	Treatments							
	100% INO	100% CQT	80% INO 20% CQT	60% INO 40% CQT	40% INO 60% CQT	20% INO 80% CQT	RSD[2]	Statistics[3]
Number of sows	76	74	73	76	75	77		
Parity order	3.1	3.1	3.1	3.1	3.2	3.2	1.2	
Lactation duration, d	24.7	24.6	24.4	24.5	24.5	24.3	1.2	
Av. daily feed intake (d 1 to weaning), kg d^{-1}	5.51	5.54	5.54	5.61	5.38	5.55	0.73	
Body weight, kg								
At farrowing,	226.6	234.1	224.1	222.0	224.9	227.2	29.1	OP***, G***
At weaning	219.2	225.2	218.8	219.7	223.7	220.3	3.2	OP*, G†
Weight loss	-7.41	-8.91	-5.34	-5.14	-5.16	-6.94	3.2	OP***, G***
Backfat thickness, mm								
At farrowing,	15.4	16.0	15.8	15.7	15.7	15.5	3.2	OP***
At weaning	12.6	13.1	12.9	12.9	12.6	12.8	2.8	OP*
Backfat loss	-2.8	-2.9	-2.9	-2.8	-3.1	-2.6	1.9	OP**, G*
Chemical composition of body weight loss[4]								
Protein, kg	-6.09	-10.35	-4.46	-2.02	-1.21	-2.72	2.38	OP***, G***
Lipids, kg	-2.19	-3.26	-1.63	-0.90	-0.97	-0.95	1.16	OP***, G**
Energy, MJ	-250.6	-326.7	-224.2	-178.1	-176.1	-183.5	59.5	OP***, G***
Weaning to insemination, d	3.8	4.0	3.8	3.8	3.6	3.9	0.5	
Parturition duration, min.	178.9	166.9	205.4	176.7	195.4	184.5	71.6	

[1]100% Inorganic Calcium source (INO); 100% organic calcium source (calcium carbon-amino-phospho-chelate=CQT); 80% INO and 20% CQT; 60% INO and 40% CQT; 40% INO and 60% CQT; 20% INO and 80% CQT. [2]RSD = Residual standard deviation. [3]Obtained from the analysis of variance (GLM including the effects of the parity order (OP), treatment during lactation (TL) and sow batch (G)). [4]Calculated based on the equations published by Dourmad et al. (1997). Protein (kg)=2.28 (2.22)+0.178 (0.017) × PV empty −0.333 (0.067) × P2 (*RSD=1.9*); lipids (kg) = −26.4 (4.5) + 0.221 (0.030) × PV empty + 1.331 (0.140) × P2 (*RSD = 6.1*); Energy (MJ) =−1.075 (159)+13.67 (1.12) × PV empty +45.98 (4.93) × P2 (*RSD=208*). PV empty (kg) = a × $PV^{1.013}$ (kg), where a = 0.912 at birth and a=0.905 at weaning. P2=P2 backfat thickness (mm) PV = live weight (kg). ***P<0.001; **P<0.01; *P<0.05; †P>0.05.

Table 2: Impact of Calcium source on the productive performance of sows during 24 days of lactation (least-square means)[1].

Variables	Treatments[1]							
	100% INO	100% CQT	80% INO 20% CQT	60% INO 40% CQT	40% INO 60% CQT	20% INO 80% CQT	RSD[2]	Statistics[3]
Number of litters	76	74	73	76	75	77		
Lactation duration, d	24.7	24.6	24.4	24.5	24.5	24.3	1.2	
Litter size								
At birth (liveborn)	13.69	13.71	13.47	13.93	13.81	13.54	1.35	
At weaning	12.04	12.41	12.06	12.18	12.00	12.05	1.22	OP***
Average piglet weight, kg								
At birth (liveborn)	1.27	1.33	1.27	1.21	1.24	1.24	0.20	OP**
At weaning	6.39	6.24	6.26	6.35	6.29	6.22	0.83	OP***
Litter weight, kg								
At birth	17.4	18.2	17.1	16.8	17.1	16.8	2.89	OP**
At weaning	76.6	77.1	75.1	77.1	75.1	74.5	10.8	
Litter weight gain, kg/d	2.40	2.38	2.38	2.46	2.36	2.38	0.43	
Milk production[4], kg/d	11.38	11.47	11.24	11.88	11.22	11.22	2.45	

[1]100% Inorganic Calcium source (INO); 100% organic calcium source (calcium carbon-amino-phospho-chelate = CQT); 80% INO and 20% CQT; 60% INO and 40% CQT; 40% INO and 60% CQT; 20% INO and 80% CQT. [2]RSD = Residual standard deviation [3]Obtained from the analysis of variance (GLM) including the effects of the parity order (OP), treatment during lactation (TL) and sow batch (G). [4]Daily milk production calculated based on the litter's weight gain, litter size, and milk MS (19%) using the Noblet and Etienne equation (1989). Milk yield (kg/d)=([0.718 × GPD − 4.9] × Number of piglets) / 0.19. ***P<0.001; **P<0.01.

Table 3: Impact of Calcium source for sows on the productive performance of their litters during 24 days of lactation (least-square means).

Variables	Treatments[1]							
	100% INO	100% CQT	80% INO 20% CQT	60% INO 40% CQT	40% INO 60% CQT	20% INO 80% CQT	RSD[2]	Statistics[3]
Number of sows	20	20	20	20	20	20		
pH								
On d 1	6.60	6.45	6.71	6.72	6.32	6.33	0.76	G*
On d 7	7.14	6.72	7.18	7.08	7.53	7.43	0.58	TL†
On d 14	7.25^{a}	6.44^{b}	7.26^{a}	7.18^{a}	6.91^{a}	6.85^{a}	0.71	TL*
On d 21	7.13^{a}	6.48^{b}	7.06^{a}	6.98^{a}	7.27^{a}	7.28^{a}	0.52	TL**
PTH[4], pg/ml								
On d 14	18.81	17.08	19.11	19.03	22.50	21.03	25.47	
On d 21	10.97	11.65	6.09	8.79	15.63	4.78	8.26	G*
Free Ca, mmol/L								
On d 14	1.40	1.36	1.38	1.35	1.36	1.36	0.07	G*
On d 21	1.41	1.39	1.36	1.42	1.38	1.37	0.09	

[1]100% Inorganic Calcium source (INO); 100% organic calcium source (calcium carbon-amino-phospho-chelate=CQT); 80% INO and 20% CQT; 60% INO and 40% CQT; 40% INO and 60% CQT; 20% INO and 80% CQT. [2]RSD=Residual standard deviation. [3]Obtained from the analysis of variance (GLM) including the effects of the parity order (OP), treatment during lactation (TL) and sow batch (G). [4]Parathyroid hormone. **P<0.01; *P<0.05; ∗P=0.0609.

Table 4: Impact of Calcium source for sows on the PTH and free Ca plasma levels and on pH of urine during 25 days of lactation (least-square means).

parturition time and consequently the incidence of higher stillborn rates. According to Frend et al. the increase in parturition duration from three to eight hours results in an increased stillborn piglet rate from 18.2 to 61.1%. On the other hand, Cunha et al. who evaluated total, ionic calcium and albumin serum levels in pregnant mixed-parity sows and their suckling piglets during lactation, found that the sows' average parturition duration was around 164 minutes, lower than the values found in our study (i.e., 185 min) [18]. This difference between studies can be attributed to the fact that the sows used by the previous authors farrowed on average 10.7 liveborn piglets while in our study the sows farrowed on average of 13.7 liveborn piglets, justifying the need for a longer delivery period. One benefit of using chelated Ca in the nutrition of sows is the role of Ca in activating oocytes during conception. Kishigami and Wakayama demonstrated that Ca chelation may induce meiosis activation after the second metaphase in the oocytes of mammals [19]. Studies on nutritional sources of chelated Ca are still rare and its responses in animal metabolism and performance are still unknown. More studies must therefore be conducted to better clarify its effects.

The lactation stage has often been investigated in swine nutrition, given that milk yield of sows is directly related to piglet weight gain. The lack of difference on average weight gain of litters and sow milk production between the different levels and sources of Ca is in agreement with the findings of Komegay and Kite and Kornegay et al. who evaluated the use of different Ca and P levels for sows and found no differences on litter size, birth weight nor weaning weight [20,21]. Similarly, Maxon and Mahan, studying first and second parity sows for two consecutive reproductive cycles using a Ca to P ratio of 1.3:1, also found no difference in litter parameters [22]. However, these same authors found that bone composition, litter size and weight are more closely related to sow body Ca than to dietary Ca.

In nature there are different forms of chelation between Ca and organic molecules [23] and their molecular nature and structure are still being studied, requiring new techniques in the field of biotechnology [24]. However, these chelation reactions do not always result in molecules with high nutritional bioavailability [25]. However, the association of Ca with organic molecules in the form of proteinate has shown this high bioavailability [15]. One of the points that should be noted in the methodology when studying chelated minerals is the recommended nutritional level. Many studies indicate that, due to increased bioavailability, lower levels of chelated minerals (compared to saline sources) would be sufficient to meet the animals' requirements [5,14,16,17]. Perhaps this explains the absence of difference in the performance of sows fed with organic and inorganic Ca sources in the present study. Therefore, one may hypothesize that due to the fact that in our study we did not work with different dietary Ca levels, the sows had their requirements met independent of Ca source. Similarly to this work, Acda and Chae, that studied the performance of sows fed chelated trace minerals (Fe, Cu, Zn and Mn), observed no improvement in reproductive and productive responses in the animals fed with high levels of chelated minerals [14]. These researchers also observed similar results among animals fed with high levels and reduced levels of chelated minerals, confirming our hypothesis. Similar results were also observed by Martin et al. these authors tested saline and chelated sources of trace minerals in diets for piglets in the nursery phase, and did not find any performance improvement in the animals fed with organic when compared to inorganic sources [26].

Differently from our findings, Mello et al. evaluating the supplementation of piglet nursery diets using a chelated trace source, found an optimal level by replacing the saline source for the organic source at approximately 25% substitution [13]. Working with Ca proteinate supplementation for turkey hens, Grimes et al. reported greater hatchability values in the incubated eggs [15]. The authors attributed these findings to greater Ca bioavailability when provided in the form of proteinate in diets. This greater bioavailability resulted in improved deposition in egg shells, thus giving embryos a lower late mortality rate during incubation. However, still there are contradictory researches on the effect of mineral source types, for instance, Creech et al. studied the nutritional response of chelated trace minerals on the performance of nursing gilts and found similar performance between gilts fed with low levels of inorganic and chelated sources and those supplemented with appropriate levels of inorganic sources [5]. Trace mineral deficiency can be difficult to detect, due to the fact that these may be supplemented via the presence of raw materials used as ingredients to prepare feed.

Ca is important not only during parturition and lactation, but also plays an important role in other functions, given that Ca is soluble in acid and precipitates in alkaline pH, as is the case of urinary pH in certain situations. In sows with urinary tract infections, we expect to find alkaline urine, due to the microbiota located in the urinary tract which synthesize the urease enzyme and transform urea into ammonia, resulting in alkalization [27]. However, urinary pH at 14 days of lactation was more acidic when sows were fed with 100% organic Ca sources. This may indicate that Ca carbon-amino-phospho-chelate can help prevent the proliferation of pathogenic bacteria in the urinary tract or even acidify if an infected environment already exists, thus potentially preventing reproductive problems. However urinary pH levels from 5.5 to 7.5 are considered normal for sows, and levels from 6.5 to 8 represent urinary tract infections, according to Sobestiansky [3]. Thus, the levels found in our study would be within the normal urinary pH range for sows. Furthermore, the previous author stated that sows with and without urinary tract infections can show average pH levels of 6.4 and 6.2, respectively.

Ca plays a key role in many physiological processes, and its concentration in the extracellular fluid is regulated very precisely. In plasma, Ca is distributed into three major fractions: a biologically active ionized fraction, which corresponds to 50% of total Ca; the fraction bounded to proteins, especially albumin, which represents approximately 40% of total Ca; and the fraction bounded to anionic substances in plasma and interstitial fluids, such as citrate and phosphate, which account for the remaining 9%. Its extracellular concentration results from the balance between intestinal absorption, renal excretion and bone release or uptake. These processes are regulated by Vitamin D, by parathyroid hormone (PTH) and by calcitonin, hormones that are directly related to Ca metabolism [2]. The Ca ion analyses at 14 and 21 days of lactation were performed to observe Ca level fluctuation during this period, with no difference found in relation to treatments and sampling dates. Cunha et al. analyzed the ionic Ca of lactating sows and found ionic Ca values of 0.82 mmol/L, levels lower than those found in our study (i.e., 1.36 and 1.38 mmol/L at 14 and 21 days of lactation, respectively) [18]. Another issue is the concentration of Ca^{2+} inside the kidney cells, Andreoli and Mcateer reported an increase in Ca^{2+} concentrations within epithelial cells of pig kidneys (LLC-PK_1) related to injury due to hydrogen peroxide exposure [28]. However, Golconda et al. related a decrease in damage to LLC-PK_1 DNA due to the use of chelating agents (BAPTA) in intracellular Ca [29]. This helps us infer that nutritional intake of Calcium in chelated form could help preserve the integrity of the renal mucosa.

Secretion of the PTH hormone is related to Ca metabolism. It is responsible for stimulating bone demineralization to increase circulating Ca levels, but despite not having seen a difference between treatments with respect to circulating PTH levels, we observed in our data higher PTH levels at 14 days of lactation when compared to 21 days [2]. One may hypothesize that this numerical difference between 14 and 21 days of lactation could be related to the impact of the high ambient temperature, and consequently to the limitation on voluntary feed intake and milk production yield. Together these factors might have influenced PTH levels, since lactation demands a large amount of Ca from the body reserves, a higher milk production would necessarily have required more Ca and, as a result, a higher hormonal PTH response.

In conclusion, this study showed that in diets for lactating sows an inorganic Ca source can be fully replaced by a more available Ca source, without negatively impacting on the productive and reproductive performance of these sows or the performance of their litters. However, further studies are needed to assess the benefits of using more available Ca sources and its interactions with the bioavailability and longevity of sows.

Acknowledgements

The authors gratefully acknowledge DSM and Tortuga for their technical and financial support; and gratefully acknowledge the farm owner for the opportunity of performing this study in their pig facilities.

References

1. Friend DW, Cunningham HM, Nicholson JW (1962) The duration of farrowing in relation to the reproductive performance of Yorkshire sows. Can J Comp Med Vet Sci 26: 127-130.
2. Guyton AC, Hall JE (2006) Textbook of Medical Physiology, 12th edition. Saunders Elsevier, PA, USA.
3. Sobestiansky J (1998) Causas e controle de descargas vulvares na suinocultura intensiva. In International Swine Seminar (Eds Gessulli), pp: 60-72. Porto Feliz Publishing, São Paulo, Brazil.
4. Herrick JB (1993) Minerals in animal health. In: The roles of amino acid chelates in animal nutrition (ed HD Ashmead), pp: 3-20. Noyes Publication, Park Ridge, NJ, USA.

5. Creech BL, Spears JW, Flowers WL, Hill GM, Lloyd KE, et al. (2004) Effect of dietary trace mineral concentration and source (inorganic vs. chelated) on performance, mineral status, and fecal mineral excretion in pigs from weaning through finishing. J Anim Sci 82: 2140-2147.

6. Spears JW (1996) Organic trace minerals in ruminant nutrition. Anim Feed Sci Technol 58: 151-163.

7. Schiavon S, Bailoni L, Ramanzin M, Vincenzi R, Simonetto A, et al. (2000) Effect of proteinate or sulphate mineral sources on trace mineral elements in blood and liver of piglets. J British Anim Sci 71: 131-139.

8. Fawcett RH, Wester M (1999) Variabilidade de alimento e dos ingredientes do alimento: impacto na performance de frangos e corte e lucro. In I Simpósio Internacional ACAV(Ed EMBRAPA– CNPSA), pp. 59-68. EMBRAPA– CNPSA, Concôrdia, Santa Catarina, Brazil.

9. Kratzer FH, Vohra P (1996) Chelates and chelation. In Chelates in nutrition (eds FH Kratzer and P Vohra), pp: 5-33. CRC Press, Boca Raton, FL, USA.

10. Rostagno HS (2011) Brazilian tables for poultry and swine: composition of feedstuffs and nutritional requirements. Ed: Horacio Santiago Rostagno, 3rd Edn, Press Universidade Federal de Viçosa (UFV), Viçosa, Brazil. P: 251.

11. Dourmad JY, Etienne M, Noblet J (1997) Reconstitution of body reserves in multiparous sows Turing pregnancy: Effect of energy intake Turing pregnancy and mobilization Turing the previous lactation. J Anim Sci 74: 2211-1997.

12. Noblet J, Etienne M (1989) Estimation of sow milk nutrient output. J Anim Sci 67: 3352-3359.

13. Mello G, Berto, DA, Tierzo LOV, Augusto RMN, Silva AMR, et al. (2012) Sources of organic trace minerals in diets for weaned piglets. Revista Brasileira de Zootecnia – Brazilian J Anim Sci 41: 1872-1877.

14. Acda ESP, Chae BJ (2002) Effects of Organic Trace Mineral Supplementation on Sows' Reproductive and Neonates' Growth Performance through 2 wk Postweaning. Asian-Australian J Anim Sci 15: 1312-1318.

15. Grimes JL, Noll S, Brannon J, Godwin JL, Smith JC, et al. (2004) Effect of a Chelated Calcium Proteinate Dietary Supplement on the Reproductive Performance of Large White Turkey Breeder Hens. J Appl Poultry Res 13: 639-649.

16. Vieira SL (2008) Chelated Minerals for Poultry. Brazilian J Poultry Sci 10: 73-79.

17. Thomaz MC, Watanabe PH, Pascoal LAF, Assis MM, Riuz US, et al. (2015) Inorganic and organic trace mineral supplementation in weanling pig diets. Academia Brasileira de Ciências 87: 1071-1081.

18. Cunha AA, Alberton GC, Filho A, Rocha RMVM (2005) Serum calcium levels in pregnant sows and in labor. Acta Sci Anim Sci 27: 333-339.

19. Kishigami S, Wakayama T (2007) Efficient strontium-induced activation of mouse oocytes in standard culture media by chelating calcium. J Reprod Dev 53: 1207-1215.

20. Komegay ET, Diggs BG, Hale OH, Handlin DL, Hitchcock JP, et al. (1985) Reproductive performance of sows fed elevated calcium and phosphorus levels during growth and development. J Anim Sci 61: 1460-1468.

21. Kornegay ET, Kite B (1983) Phosphorus in swine. VI. Utilization of nitrogen, calcium and phosphorus and reproductive performance of gravid gilts fed two dietary phosphorus levels for five parities. J Anim Sci 57: 1463-1470.

22. Maxson PF, Mahan DC (1986) Dietary calcium and phosphorus for lactating swine at high and average production levels. J Anim Sci 63: 1163-1172.

23. Van Gelder JM, Breuer E, Ornoy A, Schlossman A, Patlas N, et al. (1995) Anticalcification and antiresorption effects of bisacylphosphonates. Bone 16: 511-520.

24. Jin Y, Fu W, MA M (2011) Preparation and structure characterization of soluble bone collagen peptide chelating calcium. African J Biotechnol 10: 10204-10211.

25. Sellea PH, Cowieson AJ, Ravindranc V (2009) Consequences of calcium interactions with phytate and phytase for poultry and pigs. Livestock Science 124: 3126-3141.

26. Martin RE, Mahan DC, Hill GM, Link JE, Jolliff JS (2011) Effect of dietary organic microminerals on starter pig performance, tissue mineral concentrations, and liver and plasma enzyme activities. J Anim Sci 89: 1042-1055.

27. Coles EH (1989) Veterinary Clinical Pathology. Saunders/ Elsevier Inc., Philadelphia, PA, USA.

28. Andreoli SP, Mcateer JA (1990) Reactive oxygen molecule mediated injury in endothelial and renal tubular epithelial cells in vitro. Kidney Int 38: 785-794.

29. Golconda MS, Ueda N, Shah SV (1993) Evidence suggesting that iron and calcium are interrelated in oxidant-induced DNA damage. Kidney Int 44: 1228-1234.

Evalution of General Anesthesia Using Xylazine-Ketamine Combination with and without Diazipam for Ovariohysterectomy in Bitches

Ayalew Nesgash*, Belay Yaregal, Tesfamariam Kindu and Endalkachew Hailu

Faculty of Veterinary Medicine, College of Medical and Health Science, University of Gondar, PO Box 196, Gondar, Ethiopia

Abstract

Clinical anesthetic trial was conducted on twelve apparently healthy bitches presented to Gondar University Veterinary Clinic for ovariohysterectomy procedures. The aim of the study is to evaluate the effects of intravenous diazepam on physiological, hematological, and anesthetic parameters and also to assess anesthetic complications and develop anesthetic protocol for dogs. The bitches were randomly assigned into Group I and Group II. Anesthetic protocol was achieved by administration of atropine (0.04 mg/kg BW, S.C) immediately followed with xylazine-ketamine (1 mg/kg BW+10 mg/kg BW, I.M) for both groups but diazepam (0.5 mg/kg BW, I.V) was also given to Group I bitches when the bitches were attaining lateral recumbency. Physio-hematological and anesthetic parameters were recorded and analyzed. Quality of induction and recovery was statistically significant ($P<0.05$) difference between the groups. The mean of induction time was significantly ($P<0.05$) shorter in Group I. The mean time for loss of pedal reflex was found significantly ($P<0.05$) decreased in group I. Response to surgical incision and muscle relaxation was statistically significant ($P<0.05$) difference between groups. Duration of anesthesia, time of sternal recumbency, time of unassisted standing and duration of recovery were significantly ($P<0.05$) longer in Group I as compared Group II. Post anesthetic salivation was significantly ($P<0.05$) exhibited by Group I. No bitches were died during anesthesia or after recovery. In conclusion, atropine-Xylazine-ketamine-diazepam anesthesia does not affect physio-hematological parameter and is a very satisfactory anesthetic protocol for excellent induction, adequate muscle relaxation, longer duration of anesthesia and smooth recovery compared to atropine-Xylazine-ketamine anesthesia.

Keywords: Atropine; Bitch; Diazepam; General anesthesia; Ketamine; Ovariohysterectomy; Xylazine

Introduction

Anesthesia is a reversible process which is targeted to produce a convenient, safe, effective, yet inexpensive means of chemical restraint so that medical or surgical procedure may be conducted with minimum stress, pain, discomfort, and toxic side effects to the patients or to the anesthetist [1,2].

The selection of anesthetic drugs and techniques depends on species, breed, age, physical status, concurrent medications of the animal, personal knowledge and experience, availability and training of assistants, familiarity with available equipment, and length and type of operation or procedure performed. Pre-anesthetic medications are an essential part of safe anesthetic management and they minimize stress, cardiopulmonary depression, and the deleterious effect when used appropriately and associated with many intravenous (IV) and inhalation anesthetics [3].

Various sedatives and tranquilizing agents are used as pain killers and/or muscle relaxants while animals undergo minor or major surgeries. These drugs are needed in veterinary practice and are indispensable as they help in overcoming resistance of the animals during examination, maintaining depth of anesthesia, reducing the amount of anesthetic agents and increasing margins of safety. For these purposes, the commonest drugs used are Ketamine, Diazepam, Xylazine and Atropine sulphate [4].

Atropine is most commonly used in premedication in combination with acepromazine maleate to minimize or prevent vagal effects that may induce bradycardia and also this drug reduce potential muscles spasm gastrointestinal motility and secretion, salivation and animal respiratory secretion as well as decrease tear production during anesthesia [5]. Atropine has been used to prevent bradycardia caused by administration of α2- agonists in dogs [6].

Xylazine, an alpha-2 agonist used in animal experiments, stimulates alpha-2 adrenergic receptor in cerebral presynaptic nerve ends, inhibits release of cathecolamines and dopamine resulting in analgesic and sedative eff ects, and hinders nerve conduction in the central nervous system leading to relaxation of striated muscles. Xylazine is usually used in combination with ketamine during anesthetic applications [7].

Diazepam is a potent hypnotic-sedative that causes muscle relaxation. It is a long-acting drug as it is metabolized slowly, and it has relatively weaker cardiovascular effects as compared to other sedative drugs. In combined use with ketamine, diazepam alleviates unwanted cardiovascular effects of ketamine, and demonstrates anticonvulsive, amnestic and muscle relaxant effects [8].

Ketamine increases heart rate and mean arterial pressure, stimulates cardiovascular functions and when used alone. It can induce undesired effects such as muscular hypertonicity, myoclonus, and convulsions. To minimize these unwanted and restricting effects, ketamine is administered in combination with other drug groups such as benzodiazepines, and alpha-2 agonists [7,9]. Recently, depending on the species involved, the drug is commonly used in combination

***Corresponding author:** Ayalew Negash, Faculty of Veterinary Medicine, University of Gondar, Gondar, PO Box 196, Ethiopia
E-mail: ayalewnegash2014@gmail.com

with diazepam, alpha-2-adrenergic drugs [4]. Since, drugs manifested different effects when they were used separately or in combination, changes that occurred during use of combined-drug should be understood and recognized [7].

The UoG veterinary clinic receives large number of dogs for elective and emergency surgeries. There dogs which are highly aggressive and nervous, even the owner could not restrain them for premedication and general anesthetic administration. Almost all the general anesthetic protocols developed so far for small animal surgery utilizes intravenous administration of drugs. The available protocols are difficult to follow in such highly aggressive and nervous dogs. Hence considering the temperament the dogs, it is decided to induce balanced anesthesia with intramuscular injection of anesthetic agents. Therefore, this study is designed with the objective of developing a general anesthetic protocol suitable for aggressive and nervous dogs, studying the clinical, and hematological changes during general anesthesia and assessing the anesthetic complications during anesthesia and recovery if any.

Materials and Methods

The study was conducted from October 2015 to May 2016 in University of Gondar veterinary clinic, North Gondar, Ethiopia. Bitches that were brought to University of Gondar Veterinary Clinic for elective ovariohysterectomy were used for the study. Based on the physical examination and medical history, apparently healthy bitches alone were selected and the selected bitches (n=12) were randomly divided into two experimental groups using a Randomised Controlled Trials (RCT). All study bitches were assigned into two groups as Group I (with diazepam) and Group II (without diazepam group) each consisting of six based on the anesthetic drugs given; atropine, zylazine, ketamine and diazepam injected groups (G-I) and atropine, xylazine, and ketamine injected groups (G-II).

Assessing physiological parameters

The physiological parameters; (temperature in c_0), heart rate in beats min^{-1} and respiratory rate in breath min^{-1}) were studied before anesthesia, during anesthesia and after recovery. Temperature was taken by inserting a clinical digital thermometer (produce sound after manipulation for 2 minutes in the rectum) at least 1.5-2.0 cm length in to the rectum and keep it in the position. Heart rate and Respiratory rate were recorded by auscultation with a stethoscope place over the left side of chest and counting the abdominal movements respectively [10].

Assessment of hematological parameter

Blood samples (n=3) of 2 ml each was collected aseptically from cephalic vein of each experimental bitch before anesthesia, during anesthesia and after recover. Immediately after collection, the blood samples was transferred in a dry, clean and sterile test tube containing Ethylene Diaminetetra Acetic Acid (EDTA) as anticoagulant. It was used within 2 h after collection to determine Hemoglobin, PCV, TEC and DLC. Hemoglobin (Hb) in gm per dl, Total Erythrocyte Count (TEC) in thousands per cubic millimeters (10^3/cu mm), the Total Leukocyte Count (TLC) in thousands per cubic millimeters (10^3/cu mm) and Differential Leukocyte Count (DLC) in percentage (%) will be estimated as per standard methods using Automatic Blood Analyzer. The Packed Cell Volume (PCV) in percentage (%) will be estimated by microhaematocrit method. Butter fly catheter (21G and 0.75 inch length) or i.v canula (22G) was fixed in the cephalic vein on the dorsal aspects of the fore limb and taped it to the patient's skin using plaster.

Administration of anesthetic drugs

Drug administration: All bitches were randomly divided into two groups comprising of 6 animals in each group. **Group-I (G-I):** Anesthesia was achieved by administration of atropine (0.04 mg/kg body weight subcutaneously), immediately followed with xylazine-ketamine combination (in the same syringe) (1 mg/kg+10 mg/kg body weight intramuscularly) and after attaining lateral recumbency diazepam (at the rate of 0.5 mg/kg body weight intravenously) was given. **Group-II (G-II):** In this group, anesthesia was achieved by administration of atropine (0.04 mg/kg body weight subcutaneously), immediately followed with xylazine-ketamine combination (in the same syringe) (1 mg/kg+10 mg/kg body weight intramuscularly). The total dose of anesthetic drug required in mg, the total amount of anesthetic drug required in ml and the time of injection for each drug was recorded (Table 1).

The pedal reflex was assessed by deep pricking with a 1.0 inch length 24G hypodermic needle at the coronary band region [10] and the duration loss of pedal reflex was recorded. The total time taken for induction of anesthesia was recorded and calculated by considering time of loss of pedal reflex and time of injection of xylazine-ketamine anesthetics. Incremental dose was considered by adding additional dose of Ketamine @ dose rate of 5.0 mg/kg, i/v was administered if required, till the pedal reflex was completely abolished and the time of 1st and 2nd incremental dose if any was recorded.

Preoperative preparation of animals and ovariohysterectomy surgical procedure

Following anesthesia, all bitches were prepared aseptically for ovariohysterectomy by placing the bitch on surgical table, lying on her back and the surgical teams were prepared for the surgery with a meticulous hand scrubbing, followed by application of a sterile surgical gown and gloves thereby the surgery was started. The site (midline approach) was prepared by shaving or clipping hair aseptically in their respective direction with sterile surgical blade over the middle of the abdomen after scrubbing with surgical soap and the skin is scrubbed with antiseptics (Savlon) to disinfect the area for 5 min. A sterile drape was placed over the surgical site. A scalpel was used to incise the skin at the middle of the abdomen, and then the abdominal cavity was opened. The organs of the female reproductive tracts were identified and the major blood vessels supplying the ovaries and the uterus were ligated (tied off). Sutures (cat gut) that dissolve over time were used to tie off or ligate the blood vessels and also to close the uterus above the cervix. The abdominal incision was then closed with one or two layers of sutures. The outer layer of skin was closed with cotton suture and required to be removed in about 7 days based on clinical union.

Group	Induction of Anesthesia	Maintenance by incremental dose
G-I	a) Atropine 0.04 mg/kg, s.c immediately followed with; b) Xylazine 1 mg/kg, +Ketamine 10.0 mg/kg IM were given. After attaining lateral recumbency Diazipam 0.5 mg/kg, i/v was given	Ketamine 5.0 mg/kg, i/v
G-II	a) Atropine 0.04 mg/kg, s.c immediately followed with, b) Xylazine 1.0 mg/kg, +Ketamine 10.0 mg/kg i.m were given.	Ketamine 5.0 mg/kg, i/v

Table 1: Anesthetic protocol.

Assessment of anesthetic parameters

The anesthetic parameters include quality of induction, duration of anesthesia, complication of anesthesia, time for sternal recumbency, time for unassisted standing, quality and duration of recovery were recorded in all bitches. Type and time of induction of the animals were observed carefully from the moment of premedication thereby administration until the reflexes would be disappeared. Subjective evaluation of induction, muscle relaxation and recovery were monitored. The Induction time, time for sternal recumbency and time for unassisted standing were calculated as per the following guidelines using a stop watch [11].

Induction time and quality: The time interval in minute, between the time of ketamine administration and loss of pedal reflex was taken as induction time and recorded in all the animals. The quality of induction was graded based on scale of 1 (very poor) to 5 (excellent) represented as per the following signs noted in the table [12] (Table 2).

Quality of anesthesia: The quality of anesthesia was assessed based on adequacy of muscle relaxation and presence or absence of salivation, regurgitation and movement in response to surgical incision [13]. The adequacy of muscle relaxation was graded as adequate, if jaws could be opened at ease and abdominal muscles appeared relaxed and inadequate, if difficulty was encountered to open the jaws. The presence of salivation, regurgitation and movement in response to surgical incision, if any was recorded periodically [11].

Duration of anesthesia: The time interval in minute between the injection of anesthetics (time of injection of xylazine+ketamine) to the movement of the first spontaneous elevation of the dogs' head and limb which was recorded in all bitches [7].

Time for sternal recumbency: The time interval in minute, between the time of discontinuation of anesthesia and attainment of sternal recumbency was taken as time for sternal recumbency and was recorded in all the animals [7]. Time for unassisted standing: The time interval in minute between the time of discontinuation of maintenance administration and attainment of unassisted standing was taken as time for unassisted standing and was recorded in all the bitches [11].

Quality of recovery: The quality of anesthetic recovery was assessed and graded as smooth, if no excitement was noticed during recovery and rough if excitement was noticed during recovery.

Duration of recovery: The time interval in minute between the time of movement of the first spontaneous elevation of the dog's head and limb to unassisted standing was taken as time of recovery and was recorded in all bitches [7]. Assessment of post anesthetic complications: The anesthetic complications such as regurgitation, tympany, salivation, post-anesthetic mortality if any, were recorded in all the animals [14].

Data management and analysis

All the data collected during the study period was checked, coded and entered in to Microsoft Excel spreadsheet and analyzed using SPSS software version 20. Parametric variables were analyzed statistically using Student's independent-samples T-test was used to compare the effect of different treatments at each of the assessment time. Student's independent-samples T-test was used for comparison of mean values for HR, RR, temperature, Hemoglobin, PCV, TEC, TLC, DLC (neutrophil, lymphocyte, monocyte), induction time, duration of anesthesia, time of sternal recombency, time of unassisted standing and duration of recovery before, during and after anesthesia assessment between two treatment groups. Fisher's exact test (F) was used to compare the incidence of complication during and after anesthesia, quality of induction and quality of recovery. P-value <0.05 (at 5% level of significance) was considered as statically significant. All the data collected was statistically analyzed, compiled and reported.

Results

During the study period, animals remained hemodynamically stable and any problem requiring medical support was not seen. The mean (± SD) age of bitches was 2.17 ± 0.835 and the mean (± SD) BW of the bitches was 14.75 ± 0.965. Withholding of feed and water for 12 and 6 hours, respectively prior to induction anesthesia was found to be satisfactory. There was no statistically significant difference (p>0.05) between group I and group II bitches in mean of age and weight such that all the bitches (n=12) were found approximately equal weight and age.

Induction of anesthesia

The induction of anesthesia was induced by using atropine (0.04 mg/kg body weight subcutaneously), immediately followed with xylazine-ketamine combination (in the same syringe) (1 mg/kg+10 mg/kg body weight intramuscularly) and after attaining lateral recumbency diazepam (at the rate of 0.5 mg/kg body weight intravenously) for Group I and atropine (0.04 mg/kg body weight subcutaneously), immediately followed with xylazine-ketamine combination (in the same syringe) (1 mg/kg+10 mg/kg body weight intramuscularly) for Group II. The induction doses of the drugs atropine, xylazine and ketamine was not statistically significant (P>0.05) difference between G-I and G-II but diazepam was statistically significant (P<0.05) difference between the two groups.

Quality of induction: The quality of induction was assessed and graded as excellent, good, fair, poor and very poor. There was statistically significant difference (P<0.05) in quality of induction between group I and group II bitches. The quality of induction was excellent in 4 bitches from G-I but no from G-II, good in 2 bitches from G-I and G-II, fair and poor in 3 bitches and 1 bitch from G-II respectively. No bitch was found fair, poor or very poor induction from G-I.

Quality of anesthesia: The quality of anesthesia was assessed based on adequacy and inadequacy of jaw and abdominal muscle relaxation and presence or absence of salivation, regurgitation, urination, defecation and movement in response to pain stimuli. There was statistically significant difference (P<0.05) in muscle relaxation between group I and group II bitches. The abdominal muscle and jaw muscle relaxation was adequate in 5 bitches and two bitches from G-I

	Score	Description/sign
Induction	1	Very poor, unpredictable fall
	2	Poor, attaining recumbency unpredictably, but no injuries
	3	Fair, Bitches slowly attains sternal or lateral recumbency, marked paddling of limbs or shaking of head
	4	Good ,slowly attains recumbency, only slight paddling of limbs or shaking of the head
	5	Excellent, recumbency achieved slowly and smoothly, no paddling or head shaking

Table 2: Quality of induction.

and G-II respectively. However, the abdominal muscle and jaw muscle relaxation was also found inadequate in 1 bitch and 4 bitches from G-I and G-II bitches respectively. Salivation and vomiting were not statistically significant (P>0.05) difference between G-I and G-II in which salivation was encountered in 1 bitch from G-II and vomiting was encountered in 1 bitch from G-I during anesthesia. Regurgitation and urination during anesthesia were not also found statistically significant (P>0.005) between both groups but here was statistically significant (P<0.05) difference in response to surgical incision in response to pain stimuli between groups. Response to surgical incision was observed in 3 bitches from G-II but not observed in all bitches from G-I (n=6).

Anesthetic parameter

The anesthetic parameters: induction time, duration of anesthesia, time of return of pedal reflex, time of head right reflex, time for sternal recumbency, time for unassisted standing in munities recorded during the study were presented in Table 3.

Physiological parameters

The mean values of HR, RR and rectal temperature were differing before, during, after anesthesia. All parameter was assessed before during and after anesthesia and was not significantly decreased in group I bitches (P>0.05). The data for HR, RR and rectal temperature before, during and after anesthesia were summarized in Table 3 (Figure 1).

Hematological parameters

Hb, PCV, TEC, TLC and DLC were recorded and analyzed before anesthesia, during surgery and after recovery. Comparison of the mean (± SD) of Hb, PCV, TEC, TLC and DLC among the two groups revealed that there were significant differences (P<0.05) in PCV during anesthesia between group I and group II but no significance difference (p>0.05) were recorded in the other hematological parameters. The data were summarized in Figure 2.

Data on nature of recovery

The quality of recovery was assessed and graded as smooth and rough. The quality of recovery was found statistically significant (P<0.05) difference between group I and Group I. The quality of recovery was found almost smooth in G-I when comparison was considered with G-II in which all were appearing calm. However, during working time G-II bitches were experienced as transient excitement, struggle to stand, and moderate ataxia in which recovery was almost rough as compared with G-I.

Timing of anesthesia	Group	N	Mean ± Std. Dev	P-value
Induction of time	I II	6 6	6.00 ± 0.894 9.67 ± 1.211	0.000
Time of loss of pedal reflex	I II	6 6	3.00 ± 0.000 5.00 ± 0.894	0.003
Duration of anesthesia	I II	6 6	67.83 ± 2.994 59.17 ± 1.941	0.000
Time of sternal recombency	I II	6 6	12.17 ± 2.483 7.17 ± 1.47	0.002
Time of unassisted standing	I II	6 6	11.83 ± 2.483 6.33 ± 1.033	0.001
Time for duration of recovery	I II	6 6	17.67 ± 2.251 13.83 ± 1.169	0.004

Std. Dev.=Standard Deviations; Mean difference is significant (P<0.05); N=number of animals

Table 3: Mean (± SD) of Anesthetic parameter.

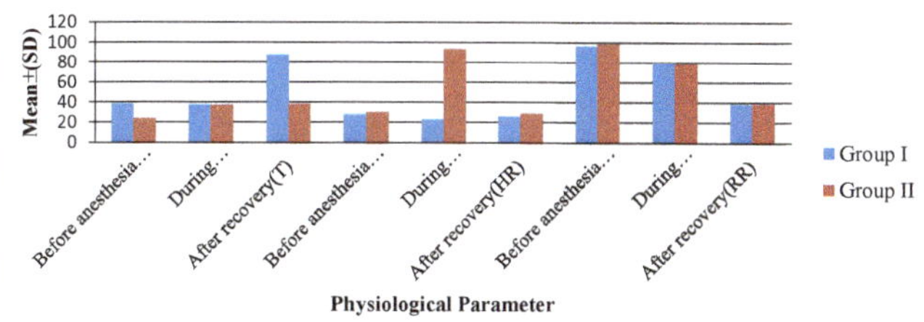

Figure 1: Mean ± (SD) rectal temperature (°C), heart rate (HR) (cycle/min) and respiration rate (RR) (beats/min) before anesthesia, during anesthesia and after recovery.

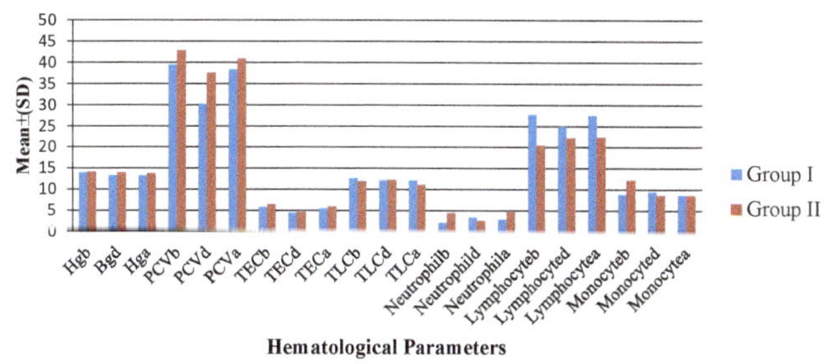

Figure 2: Mean ± (SD) Hg, PCV, TEC, TLC, DLC before (b) anesthesia, during (d) anesthesia and after (a) recovery of both groups.

Post anesthetic complication

Post anesthetic complications were assessed whether salivation, regurgitation, urination or mortality was encountered after recovery in both groups. Salivation was found statistically significant (P<0.05) in group I bitches as compared to Group II in which salivation was encountered in 5 bitches from G-I but 1 bitch from G-II. Regurgitation was not encountered at all in both groups. Urination was present in 1 bitches from G-I which was not significant (P>0.05). All bitches (n=12) were survived the surgery and recovered from anesthesia without any death.

Discussion

Various sedatives and tranquilizing agents are used as pain killers and/or chemical restraints while animals undergo minor or major surgeries. These drugs are needed in veterinary practice and are indispensable as they help in overcoming resistance of the animals during examination, maintaining depth of anesthesia, reducing the amount of anesthetic agents and increasing margins of safety [3]. The purpose of anesthesia is to provide reversible unconsciousness, amnesia, analgesia, and immobility with minimal risk to the patient [1].

Although the sedative and hemodynamic effect of diazepam has been reported previously, the sedative effect of simultaneous administration of diazepam and xylazine-ketamine in dogs has not been studied to current study knowledge. In present study, 12 indigenous bitches are taken with approximately equal age and body weight 2.17 ± 0.835 and 14.75 ± 0.965 respectively when comparison was considered. OHE was done using xylazine- ketamine with diazepam for Group I and xylazine- ketamine without diazepam for Group II provided that atropine was given for both groups as a premedication. This is in line of agreement with several studies using this mixture for general anesthesia in dog's anesthetic drug [15]. OHE was performed by xylazine- ketamine anesthesia with and without diazepam and this agreed with Delling [16] and William et al. [2].

In present study, xylazine-ketamine combination and diazepam is given as single IM and IV injections respectively in order to avoid distress caused by multiple injections. In the clinical setting, intramuscular injection is the preferred route of drug administration for sedation and premedication because minimal restraint is required. Besides, cardiovascular responses are attenuated when anticholinergics and α2-agonists are administered intramuscularly and when used in combination, the adverse actions of both drugs may be diminished due to the lower doses required [15].

The induction of anesthesia produced by G I was found fast, recumbency achieved slowly and smoothly as compared to G II. This result of the present study was in line with the findings of Azizpour and Hassani [12]. The fast induction of anesthesia result in G I was in contrary to the reports of the earlier studies in sheep [7] but because in the current study, there was no significant difference in age species and breed. This study was also investigated that loss of pedal reflex and duration of induction which was shown in Table 3 was significantly reduced. Because when diazepam and ketamine used together, they have a synergistic effect resulting in a smooth recovery and better muscle relaxation and their efficacy is enhanced whilst minimising their unwanted adverse effects which was in line of agreement with Sumitra et al. [17] conducted a research on male Wistar rats.

In this study, muscle relaxation was significantly ($p<0.05$) adequate in the G I than G II. Improvement of muscular relaxation in G I was associated with the muscle relaxant properties of diazepam. Diazepam has potent muscle relaxant and anticonvulsant properties and has been used in a wide range of wild and domestic animals and birds [18]. Jaw muscle relaxation was significantly ($P<0.05$) adequate in G I which was in accordance with earlier studies where resistance to open the mouth fully is lost in moderate anesthesia, hence jaw tone is considered to be a useful indicator of anesthesia [19,20]. In the present study, salivation, urination and vomition was not a significant difference between the two groups before anesthesia, during anesthesia and after anesthesia. This result demonstrated in accordance with the previous reports in which it has been demonstrated that anti-muscarinic drugs like atropine has decreasing effect on hyper secretion induced with ketamine [5,21]. In the present study, atropine was also incorporated in both groups as premedication which decreased hyper secretion which was induced during spontaneous breathing.

In the current study, duration of anesthesia for G I was found significantly longer as compare to G II which was in accordance with the previous studies where the highest duration of anesthesia was observed in the study of birds [8]. This might be due to wide-distribution of diazepam in the body, as because diazepam is highly soluble in lipid and can be redistributed into muscles and adipose tissues [22]. Furthermore, diazepam is a long-acting drug due to its slow-metabolism in the body as compared to the other sedatives [23]. The results obtained here were in line with the findings of Azizpour and Hassani [12] who performed general anesthesia in pigeons using a combination of ketamine HCL and diazepam. Lin et al. [24] investigated the effects of two different anesthetic regimens, namely ketamine-diazepam and ketamine- diazepam-xylazine combinations in sheep and found that the latter combination resulted in a longer duration of anesthesia.

In the present study, smooth recoveries were observed significantly in G I than G II which was in line with finding of Durrani et al. [8] and Mahmud et al. [4] that smooth recoveries were observed in diazepam-ketamine anesthesia. The longest recovery period was observed in the birds of diazepam-ketamine anesthesia, which was desirable since diazepam could augment ketamine's anesthetic effects decreasing its side effects; thus, it provided necessary depth and duration of anesthesia for the comfortable completion of surgeries [4,25]. Ketamine and diazepam induced a synergistic action producing a deep analgesia for long duration. Similar observations were also reported in pigeons using ketamine-diazepam [8,18]. This result is in line with the present study in which the duration of recovery of G I was significantly longer than G II.

Ketamine, in contrast to most of the anesthetic drugs, it has been shown to possess incremental effects on the heart rate, blood pressure and respiratory rate due to increase in sympathetic activation. It had also unwanted respiratory effects such as increase in respiratory secretions [21]. Diazepam decrease cardiovascular effects of ketamine [9]. Therefore the unwanted anesthetic effect of ketamine was compensated and balanced by xylazine and diazepam through lowering blood pressure and decreasing heart and respiratory rate.

In the current study, the mean ± (SD) of temperature, respiratory rate and heart rate of both groups before anesthesia, during anesthesia and after anesthesia were considered and compared between the groups. There were decrements of all the three parameters during anesthesia and came to the normal physiological range after recovery but the decrease in the physiological parameter was not found statistically significant ($P>0.05$) between the groups. These results were in accordance with previous studies as Coulson et al. [26] investigated cardiovascular effects of ketamine-diazepam in sheep and stressed lack of any meaningful effects on heart rates and respiratory rate. In this study, alterations in physiological parameter caused by both drug combinations remained within physiologic limits.

Demirkan et al. [27] and Atalan et al. [15] emphasized that rectal temperature decreased during the anesthesia. Anesthetic combination decreased significantly the mean rectal temperature during surgery and the decline was highly significant after surgery. However, in the present study of the mean ± (SD) of rectal temperature of both groups began to decrease during anesthesia but came to the physiological range after recovery and the difference between the groups was not significant ($P>0.05$). This finding is in agreement with previous reports [28].

The mean ± (SD) of the Haemoglobin, PCV, TEC, TLC and DLC were assessed before, during and after anesthesia and were slightly decreased for a short time in both groups during anesthesia but the alteration was not significant ($P>0.05$) between the groups. However, the values for PCV was significantly decreased ($P<0.05$) and the result was in accordance with previous studies [29,30]. Pooling of circulating blood cells in the spleen and other reservoirs secondary to decreased sympathetic activity could be the reason for a decrease in PCV. The decrease in PCV during the period of anaesthesia or sedation might be attributed to the shifting of fluid from extravascular compartment to intravascular compartment in order to maintain normal cardiac output in the animals [29].

The occurrence of post anesthetic complication in both groups were assessed and it was found not statistically significant ($P>0.05$) except salivation which was more experienced in G I than G II which is supported by previous reports [31]. Although diazepam is an initial cause of salivation, but the loss of spontaneous swallowing and the loss of spontaneous tongue reflex occurred during this study might be the cause of salivation observed after recovery as a result of diazepam injection.

Conclusion

The study was conducted on 12 female apparently healthy indigenous bitches which were randomly grouped in to Group I and Group II. Anesthesia was induced using atropine (0.04 mg/kg

BW, S.C) immediately followed with xylazine-ketamine (1.0 mg /kg/ BW+10.0 mg/kg BW, I.M) and after lateral recumbency, diazepam (0.5 mg /kg BW, i/v) was administered for G-I and atropine (0.04 mg/kg BW, S.C) immediately followed with xylazine-ketamine (1.0 mg /kg/ BW+10.0 mg/kg BW, I.M) for G-II. The anesthetic parameters; quality of induction, time loss for pedal reflex, induction time, duration of anesthesia, quality of anesthesia, time for sternal recumbency, time for unassisted standing, duration and quality of recovery were recorded and analyzed on both Group I and Group II and all the parameters were found statistically significant. The results of the present study concluded that atropinc-xylazinc ketamine diazepam combination is useful anesthetic protocol for excellent induction, adequate muscle relaxation, satisfactory duration of anesthesia and smooth recovery for OHE in bitches although it might result in prolonged recovery and some complication like salivation rarely as compared to atropine-xylazine-ketamine combination. Both drug combinations do not affect the physiological and hematological parameters of the animals during study time and both of them can be safe for OHE if used safely and appropriately. However, further studies are required to evaluate the effects on cardiopulmonary function of these drug combinations in detail.

Acknowledgements

We would like to express our heartfelt gratitude to our advisors' Prof. V. Ramaswamy and Prof. N. Rajendran for their unreserved crucial comments, valuable encouragement, and provision of necessary materials and sacrifice of their time to correct this manuscript. We would like to thank Dr. Ashenafi Assefa, head of the department of Veterinary Clinical Medicine for all the help and encouragement rendered by him throughout the study period. Our thanks go to Dr. Samson Leta for all his help in analyzing the research data and Getie Kindu, the surgery technicians for his help and cooperation rendered during the surgical procedures. We never forget to say thanks to University of Gondar Faculty of Veterinary Medicine microbiology and pathology laboratory staff workers for their help, patience permission and full information during my working period.

References

1. Thurmon JC, Tranquilli WJ, Benson GJ (1996) Lumb & Jones Veterinary Anesthesia. 3rd edn. Williams and Wilkins. Baltimore, Maryland, USA.
2. William WM, John AE, Richard MB, Roman TS (2007) Hand Book of Veterinary Anesthesia. 4th edn. Mosby Elsevier USA, Columbus, USA.
3. Habib S, Das BC, Islam MN, Hossain MK, Ahmed MF (2002) A Comparison of xylazine, diazepam, chlorpromazine and promethazine in relation to certain clinical and hematological parameters of indigenous sheep (Ovis aries). Pakistan J Biol Sci 5: 484-488.
4. Mahmud MA, Shaba P, Yisa HY, Gana J, Ndagimba R, et al. (2014) Comparative efficacy of Diazepam, Ketamine, and Diazepam-Ketamine combination for sedation or anesthesia in cockerel chickens. J Adv Vet Anim Res 1: 107-113.
5. Liga K, Edite B (2011) The effects of some premedication and general anesthesia drugs on intraocular pressure and pupil diameter in dog's eyes. LLU preclinical institute, LLU Raksti 26: 77-83.
6. Ko JC, Fox SM, Mandsager RE (2001) Effects of preemptive atropine administration on incidence of medetomidine-induced bradycardia in dogs. J Am Vet Med Assoc 218: 52-58.
7. Ozkan F, Cakir-Ozkan N, Eyibilen A, Yener T, Erkorkmaz U (2010) Comparison of ketamine-diazepam with ketamine-xylazine anesthetic combinations in sheep spontaneously breathing and undergoing maxillofacial surgery. Bosmian J Basic Med Sci 10: 297-302.
8. Durrani UF, Khan MA, Ahmad SS (2008) Comparative efficacy (sedative and anaesthetic) of detomidine, ketamine and detomidine-ketamine cocktail in pigeons (Columba livia). Pakistan Vet J 28: 115-118.
9. Dzikiti TB, Chanaiwa S, Mponda P, Sigauke C (2007) Comparison of quality of induction of anaesthesia between intramuscularly administered ketamine, intravenously administered ketamine and intravenously administered propofol in xylazine premedicated cats. J S Afr Vet Assoc 78: 201-204.
10. Amin A, Ali A, Al-Mutheffer E (2012) Clinical evaluation of TIVA by romifidine as a premedication, midazolam and ketamine in donkeys. In: Proceeding of the Eleventh Veterinary Scientific Conference, pp: 203-208.
11. Vishnugurubaran D (2013) Comparison of Diazepam and Midazolam as an adunct to xylazine- ketamine induction and isoflurane maintenance anaesthesia in goats. MVSc Thesis submitted to Tamil Nadu Veterinary and Animal Sciences University, Chennai, Tamil Nadu, India.
12. Azizpour A, Hassani Y (2012) Clinical evaluation of general anaesthesia in pigeons using a combination of ketamine and diazepam. J S Afr Vet Assoc 83: 12.
13. McKelvey D, Hollingshead KW (2003) Veterinary analgesia and anesthesia. 3rd edn. St. Louis, Missouri: United State of America.
14. Haliloglu M, Omur D, Yuksel TC, Alan C, Hanci V (2012) Post-Operative Effects: Anesthesia. J Anesth Clin Res 4: 291.
15. Atalan G, Uzun M, Demirkan I, Yildiz S, Cenesiz M (2002) Effect of medetomidine-butorphanol-ketamine anaesthesia and atipamezole on heart and respiratory rate and cloacal temperature of domestic pigeons. J Vet Med A Physiol Pathol Clin Med 49: 281-285.
16. Delling U (2005) The effects of xylazine, ketamine, diazepam anesthesia. Faculty of the Virginia Polytechnic Institute and State University, USA, p: 28.
17. Sumitra M, Manikandan P, Rao KVK, Nayeem M, Manohar BM, et al. (2004) Cardiorespiratory effects of diazepam-ketamine, xylazine-ketamine and thiopentone anesthesia in male Wistar rats-A comparative analysis. Life Sci 75: 1887-1896.
18. Lumeij JT, Deenik JW (2003) Medetomidine-ketamine and diazepam-ketamine anesthesia in racing pigeons (Columba livia domestica)-a comparative study. J Avian Med Surg 17: 191-196.
19. Tranquilli WJ, Thurmon JC, Grimm KA (2007) Injectable and alternative anaesthetic techniques. In: Veterinary Anaesthesia. 4th edn. Lumb WV, Jones EW (eds.). Blackwell Publishing, Ames, IA, USA, pp: 273-300.
20. Hopster K, Müller C, Hopster-Iversen C, Stahl J, Rohn K, et al. (2014) Effects of dexmedetomidine and xylazine on cardiovascular function during total intravenous anaesthesia with midazolam and ketamine and recovery quality and duration in horses. Vet Anaesth Analg 41: 25-35.
21. Ungern-Sternberg VBS, Regli A, Frei FJ, Ritz E, Jordi M, et al. (2007) A deeper level of ketamine anesthesia does not affect functional residual capacity and ventilation distribution in healthy preschool children. Pediatr Anesth 17: 1150-1155.
22. Bateson AN (2002) Basic pharmacologic mechanism involved in benzodiazepine tolerance and withdrawal. Current pharmaceutical design 8: 5-21.
23. Koshy TA, Mahabala TH, Srikantu J, Sanmathi S (2003) Thiopentone-midazolam mixture as an induction agent for general anesthesia on 'In-Patients'. Indian J Anaesth 47: 129-133.
24. Lin HC, Wallace SS, Tyler JW, Robbins RL, Thurmon JC, et al. (1994) Comparison of tiletamine-zolazepam-ketamine and tiletamine-zolazepam-ketamine-xylazine anesthesia in sheep. Aust Vet J 71: 239-242.
25. Muir WW, Hubbell JAE, Skarda RT, Bednarski RM (2000) Handbook of Veterinary Anesthesia. 3rd edn. Mobsy Inc., St. Louis.
26. Coulson NM, Januszkiewicz AJ, Dodd KT, Ripple GR (1989) The cardiorespiratory effects of diazepam-ketamine and xylazine-ketamine anesthetic combinations in sheep. Lab Anim Sci 39: 591-597.
27. Demirkan I, Atalan G, Gokce HI, Ozaydin I, Celebi F (2002) Comparative study of butorphanol-ketamin HCl and xylazine-ketamin HCl combinations for their clinical and cardiovascular/respiratory effects in healthy dogs. Turk J Vet Anim Sci 26: 1073-1079.
28. Davison KE, Lynne Hughes JM, Gormley E, Lesellier S, Costello E, et al. (2007) Evaluation of the anaesthetic effects of combinations of ketamine, medetomidine, romifidine and butorphanol in European badgers (Meles meles). Vet Anaesth Analg 34: 394-402.
29. Kilic N (2008) Cardiopulmonary, biochemical and haematological changes after detomidinemidazolam-ketamine anaesthesia in calves. Bull Vet Inst Pulawy 52: 453-456.
30. Pawde AM, Kinjavdekar P, Aithal HP, Pratap K, Bisht GS (2000) Detomidine-Diazepam-Ketamine Anaesthesia in Buffalo (Bubalus bubalis) Calves. J Vet Med A 47: 175-179.
31. Clarke KW, Taylor PM, Watkins SB (1986) Detomidine/ketamine anesthesia in the horse. Acta Vet Scand 82: 167-179.

Influence of the Live Weight of Incorporation of the Gilts on the Mortality and Productive Indicators of the Piglets

Caridad Suárez Machín[1*], Carmen Amarilys Guevara Rodríguez[1] and Juan Miguel Gómez Cama[2]

[1]*Cuban Research Institute of Sugar Cane (ICIDCA), Avenue White 804, Corner Central Road, San Miguel del Padrón, Havana, Cuba*
[2]*Universidad Nacional Autónoma de Honduras, UNAH, Havana, Cuba*

Abstract

A total of 80 gilts were selected and divided into two experimental groups of 40 animals each. Group I, grouped gilts with weights of 118 to 124 kg. And group II, those weighing more than 130 kg. The weight of incorporation of the gilts, as well as the litter size and the birth weight, at the weaning and average daily gain of the piglets, were controlled through simple ANOVA; in addition to relating the weight of incorporation of the gilts with the litter size, birth weight and weaning by linear regression, using the program Stagraphics plus 5.1. The results showed that there is a strong and positive relationship between the weight of incorporation of the gilts and the productive indicators of the piglets, which were always higher in the incorporated gilts weighing more than 130 kg. It was shown that more live piglets are born from incorporated gilts weighing more than 130 kg and that mortality is higher when the incorporation weights are lower than this. It was verified that in the incorporated gilts with less than 130 kg of live weight, 50575.00 Cuban pesos loosen benefits for fewer live born piglets.

Keywords: Gilts; Live weight; Productive indicators; Incorporation

Introduction

Feed for animal's crisis in the underdeveloped countries has increased and continues to grow in the production of proteins of high biological value necessary for man. The pork industry is an important solution, triggered by two variables that have strongly influenced the market. First: the challenge that has presented in recent years poultry, due to the appearance of bird flu; second, the sharp rise in the price of beef, which allows the pork industry to be the ideal to supply this demand in a short time and at affordable prices [1].

Taking into account the biological specificities of the swine species, particularly their high fertility, reproductive behavior constitutes an essential part of the species' productivity. It is therefore that any effort in order to increase the yield implies increasing fertility, prolificacy and productive expression of piglets [2].

Puberty is the stage in which animals become physiologically capable of reproducing and manifests itself before their anatomical development has been satisfactorily completed. This is why animals should not be incorporated into reproduction immediately after reaching puberty, as their subsequent development is compromised.

There are multiple factors involved in the appearance of oestrous in sows, marking the onset of puberty, as well as subsequent jealousy. Age, weight and growth rate; nutrition, genetics, environmental factors, housing conditions, prophylaxis, social environment and boar effect are the main aspects that directly influence the sexual behavior of the breeders [3].

The manual referred to above recognizes, in the category of gilts, females older than 7 months of age weighing not less than 95 kg., which maintain that condition until they are not service. These should have the following characteristics:

- Have had a good development in weight gain during growth, without over fatten. Must weigh not less than 110 kg. the first service.
- Do not have affections in the extremities.
- Not less than 10 breasts symmetrical (or blind or inverted).
- Healthy appearance.

For our country, it is a challenge to raise the productive yields of the gilts, as well as to reduce the mortality in these; currently it is established to server the gilts that have reached a weight greater than 110 kg. of live weight and more than 210 days of age. The objective of this research is to determine how influences the live weight of incorporation of gilts in the mortality and productive yields of its piglets.

Materials and Methods

The work was carried out in the pig unit La Guayaba, belonging to the Integral Military Farm "El Guatao", located in Guanabacoa municipality, province Havana. Eighty gilts, the race F1-Yorkland were intentionally selected, weighed and grouped according to their live weight in two groups of 40 animals each. In group I, the gilts with weights ranging from 118-124 kg were studied and in group II, those weighing more than 130 kg. The age of the animals ranged from 248 to 274 days, according to the controls of the farm.

Both experimental groups were subjected to the same conditions of exploitation and management. The feed offered was feed growth, with an average consumption of 2.7 kg/animal/day in a single ration, which does not coincide with the feeding norms established in the Manual de Crianza Porcina, which states that breeding should consume reproductive feed, supplied in 2 or 3 servings [4].

***Corresponding author:** Caridad Suárez Machín, Cuban Research Institute of Sugar Cane (ICIDCA), Avenue White 804, Corner Central Road, San Miguel del Padrón, Havana, Cuba, E-mail: caridad.suarez@icidca.azcuba.cu

The consumption of feed growth, by this category, is a critical aspect, because it is not able to contribute to the diet of these animals all the nutrients, nor in the adequate amounts, since the sows are too greasy and can have deliveries dystocia, problems with conception and reduce feed intake during the lactation period, affecting the development of their piglets.

The live weight of incorporation of the gilts was controlled, when they were service by direct mountaineering, performing two services to each female, with intervals of approximately 12 hours. The procedure after the service, was in accordance with what is regulated in the Manual de Crianza Porcina [4]. The piglets, born of the mothers that made up the experimental groups, were counted, thus determining the litter size, were then weighed at birth, whit in a weight of 50 kg of 1 kg ± appreciation and weaned (26-33 days), determining through these values the average daily gain (ADG) of the piglets through the formula, proposed by Romero et al. [5].

ADG=PF-PI/duration stage

Where:

ADG=Average daily gain; BW: Birth weight; WW: Weaning weight; Duration stage: Time from birth to weaning.

The analysis of the ADG, birth weight and weaning weight of the piglets, as well as the weight of incorporation of the gilts was performed through simple ANOVA, included in the statistical package Stagraphics plus 5.1 and linear regressions were made through the equation Y=a+b*x, where the weight of the gilts was the independent variable in the equation and the indicators of the piglets (litter size, birth weight and weaning weight) were dependent variables. The presentation of sick and dead piglets in each group was monitored through clinical examination, detecting any symptoms of disease and recording the incidences in the controls of the farm. With the help of the program COMPROP 1, the proportions of the number of sick and deaths piglets between groups were compared [6].

The economic valuation took into account the losses caused in the production of meat by the number of piglets live births in each group, taking into account the kilograms of meat that represents a greater number of live births. On the other hand were quantified the losses that represent the deaths produced by reason of the value of life of a piglet. Losses in meat gain were expressed in kg, while mortality losses were expressed in Cuban convertible pesos (CUC).

Results and Discussion

In the following Tables 1-5, is observed, the behavior of live weight of incorporation of the gilts in both experimental groups. The analysis shows that there are highly significant differences between live weights at the incorporation of gilts in the studied groups, with confidence levels of more than 99.9%, with differences of 18 kg between the means of both groups.

The following table shows the behavioral of the productive indicators of the piglets in each group studied. The results of the simple ANOVA to the productive indicators of the piglets, in general, showed superiority for the group of gilts that was incorporated in the reproduction with live weights superior to 130 kg., with confidence levels of more than 99.9%. These results coincide with that posed by Martin Rillo et al. when affirming that sows, when they increase their live weight, increase the size of the genital apparatus and have a greater capacity of ovulation and viability of the embryos, reason why they obtain greater litter [7].

Boyle et al. suggested that sows with a weight of 90-100 kg live weight tended to have a smaller number of piglets and with low birth weight, since the sows do not have the reserves necessary to develop piglets with optimal weights at and that piglets that are incorporated with low live weight are more likely to suffer physical disorders linked to reproductive life, which requires good physical and metabolic conditions to cope with the catabolic periods from which the reproductive must be replenished and reintroduce in the permissible time not to affect the zootechnical flow [8].

Faccenda pointed out that thin gilts do not manage to regain weight during lactation, thus compromising the success of subsequent pregnancies; being more susceptible to traumatic and decubitus injuries due to the shortage of fat, as well as frequent premature births and low birth weight piglets [9].

Wbrehme reports that the ideal weight of incorporation into reproduction is over 130 kg [10], to obtain piglets with better birth weights and, on the other hand, Quiniou et al. stated that piglets born with lower weight showed lower productive indicators than the rest of the piglets [11].

Regarding the ADG of the piglets, Aherne and Palomo highlighted the weight of mothers during breastfeeding as a defining element [12,13]. Casasola and Palomo stated that the weight with which the sows face gestation directly affects the quantity and quality of their dairy production and therefore the development of their piglets [14]. The following is the analysis of the influence of live weight of incorporation of the gilts on the litter size. For group I, 63.8% of variability of litter size and for group II was explained 50.6%, the correlation coefficient of 0.7 being expressed for both groups, indicating a moderately strong relation between the incorporation weight of the gilts and litter size.

These results coincide with what was proposed by Rodríguez et al. [15] who show that the gilts that receive the first service with lower weight obtain smaller litter, and with Romero [16], which affirms that the incorporation weight is an important factor to take into account since it influences the size of the litter. The following are the live weight of incorporation of gilts and the weight with which their piglets are born.

The results obtained show that birth weight is influenced by the incorporation weight of the gilts; on the one hand R^2 explains in group I 31.9% variability in birth weight and 12.2% group incorporated with greater weight. In group II, the correlation coefficient of 0.3 indicates a relatively weak relationship between the two variables under study and for group I, the correlation of 0.5 indicate a moderately strong relationship between these variables.

The results agree with the criteria of Merck, which states that birth weight is directly related to the live weight with which the gilts are incorporated [17]. This criterion coincides with Milkil, which emphasizes the need for the gilts to be incorporated with an adequate weight, since it is a determinant element in the weight of their cries at birth [18]. The following table shows the results of the regression analysis between the incorporation weight and the weights with which the piglets were weaned.

The R-square, explains 60.2% variability in group I and 19.3% in group II. The P value is less than 0.001, which shows that there are

Groups	Mean (kg)	SD	± SE	CV	Sig.
I	119.9	1.9	0.3	1.61%	***
II	137.9	3.3	0.5	2.39%	

***=P<0.001

Table 1: Analysis of live weight of incorporation.

Indicators	Mean		SD		± SE		Sig.	
	GroupI	Group II	Group I	Group II	Group I	Group II	Group I	Group II
LS	8.3	11.8	1.1	1.6	0.1	0.2	***	
BW	1.08	1.31	0.13	0.07	0.02	0.01		
WW	6.67	7.6	0.5	0.3	0.08	0.05		
ADG	169.2	190.6	15.2	9.3	2.4	1.4		

***=P<0.001; Legend: LS: Litter Size; BW: Birth weight; WW: Weaning weight; ADG: Average daily gain

Table 2: Behavior of the productive indicators of the piglets in each group.

Variables	Groups	R^2 %	r	± SE	Sig.
IW vs LS	I	63.8	0.7	0.6	*
	II	50.6	0.7	1.1	
Y=a+b*x (LS Group I=-48.03+0.047*IW); y=a+b*x (LS Group II=-36.6+0.35*IW)					

*=P<0.05; Legend: IW: Incorporation Weight of the gilts; LS: Litter size

Table 3: Relationship between incorporation live weight and litter size.

Variables	Groups	R^2 (%)	r	± SE	Sig.
IW vs BW	I	31.9	0.5	0.1	*
	II	12.2	0.3	0.07	
Y=a+b*x (BW Group I=-3.7+0.04*IW); Y=a+b*x (BW Group II 0.2+0.01*IW)					

*=P<0.05; Legend: IW: Incorporation Weight of the gilts; BW: Birth weight of piglets

Table 4: Relationship between birth weight of the piglets and incorporation weight the gilts.

Variables	Groups	R^2 (%)	r	± SE	Sig.
IW Vs. WW	I	60.2	0.7	0.3	***
	II	19.3	0.4	0.2	
Y=a+b*X (WW Group I=-19.2+0.2*IW); Y=a+b*X (WW Group II=-48.7+1.02*IW)					

***=P<0.001; Legend: IW: Incorporation weight of the gilts; WW: Weaning weight

Table 5: Relationship between live weight of incorporation and weaning weights.

highly significant differences with a confidence interval of more than 99.9%. Ponce de León states that the piglets born of sows with lower live weight consume milk with nutritional deficiencies qualitatively and quantitatively, since the sow needs to mobilize from its body reserves for milk production, decreasing its weight more and more live and therefore, producing less and less milk with less nutritional quality, so the piglets decrease their live weight [19].

These results are similar to those presented by Santiago who refers to the importance of live weight of the sows in the reproductive process [20]. In this regard, Casasola and Palomo argue that nutritional problems, during or before the gestation phase, can determine, in the sows, inferior weights to the ideals and then, in the affectation of the quantity and quality of their production milky and therefore in the development of their piglets [14]. The main causes of diseases and deaths were caused by colibacillosis, pneumopathies, crushes, umbilical hernias and perichartritis. The following figure shows the result of the comparison of proportions, among the groups studied, regarding the presentation of diseases and deaths.

Figure 1 shows the percentage that represents, in each of the groups, the sick and dead piglets of the total number of live born piglets (LBP). For group I was 332 and in group II of 472 LBP, with a difference between the groups of 140 piglets in favor of the group of gilts incorporated with more than 130 kg of live weight. The incidence of sick and dead piglets was always higher in group I, with high levels of significance, coinciding with what Alonso et al. when referring to the fact that when the age and incorporation weight are violated, the females do not reach a somatic development, which increases the probability of dystocical births and piglets more susceptible to diseases [21].

Qiles and Hebia for its part suggest that a low incorporation weight determines a poor productive yield, reflected in increased susceptibility and deterioration of the health status of their cries [22]. During the lactation period, low-weight snacks are forced to use body reserves (use of fat as a source of energy and muscle as a source of protein) in their dairy production, causing their bodily condition to be affected and therefore, the gradual deterioration of the health status of their piglets.

These criteria coincide with that proposed by Merck and Bernard, who refer to the mortality of pigs and other animals determined by the deterioration of the physical condition of their mothers, when crossing periods with high energetic requirements such as lactation [17,23].

Economic Valuation

When comparing the obtained productive results, in the studied groups, it is observed that, in general, the productive yields of the piglets born, of gilts with greater weight, were superior to those obtained in the group incorporated with lower average live weight, as well as the incidence of sick and deaths was more unfavorable in this group.

Based on the analysis, in the comparison of the live births in each groups, there is a difference of 140 more piglets obtained in the group of gilts incorporated with greater weight and considering that the live weight at slaughter, planned by the unit, is 85 kg, a total of 11 900 kg, which represents 50575.00 Cuban pesos (CUP) are no longer produced, only for this concept, in the group of gilts with lower weight

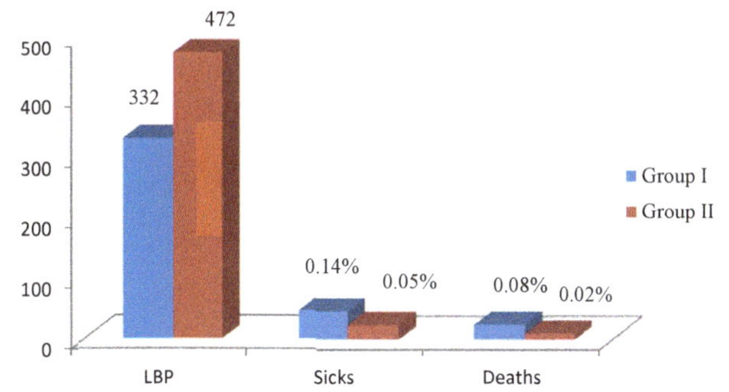

Figure 1: Proportion of sick and deaths piglets in the studied groups.

of incorporation. This is taking into account that the kg of standing meat has a value of 4.25 CUP.

In the group with less live weight, 25 deaths occurred, representing losses of 85.00 CUC, according to the current value of a piglet (3.40 CUC), while in the group with the highest live weight, only 10 deaths, with losses of 34.00 CUC, representing savings, only for this concept, of 50.60 CUC with respect to the group incorporated with lesser live weight.

Conclusions

- There is a relationship between the live weight of the piglets and the litter size, birth weight and weaning weight.
- Production indicators behaved higher in the group of gilts incorporated with more to 130 kg live weight.
- Were born, 140 piglets, less in the group of gilts incorporated with less than 130 kg, loosen benefits for 50 575CUP.

References

1. Machado G (2011) The pig is a member of the animal world, which falls within the category of mammals and whose meat is usually used.
2. Bourdon D, Février C, Pérez J, Lebas F, Leclerc B, et al. (1994) Raw materials. In: Feeding of monogastric animals: pig, rabbit and poultry. Paris: Blum JC. National Institute of Agronomic Research.
3. Manual of Reproduction and Artificial Swine Insemination (2008) Group of Biology Reproduction. Institute of Swine Research.
4. Manual of Technical Procedures for Pig Breeding (2008) Institute of Porcine Research. MINAGRI. CIMED Edition, Havana, Cuba.
5. Romero G, Andrial P, Tellechea G, Garzón B (2002) Multimedia educational veterinary (multivet). Section: Swine. Published: 2002 UNAH.
6. COMPROP 1 (2004) Statistical Package.
7. Martín Rillo S, De Alba C, Falato MV, Peralta W, Bustamante J (1999) Effect of the genital apparatus of the first-time mother on the productivity of the sow. VI International Symposium on Porcine Artificial Reproduction and Insemination. ANAPORC, Madrid, from 3 to 5 May.
8. Boyle LA, Leonard FC, Lynch PB, Brophy P (2009) Influence of housing system during gestation on the behavior and welfare of gilts in farrowing crates. Animal Science 71: 561-570.
9. Faccenda M (2005) Body condition of the sow. Delivery Room. The Pig Page.
10. Wbrehme H (2004) Maximizing weaning capacity: feeding of gilts during pregnancy. Part II. The Veterinary Portal of Chile. All Rights Reserved, Veternet. 2000-2009.
11. Quiniou N, Dagorn J, Gaudré D (2002) Variation of piglet's birth weight and consequences on subsequent performance. Livestock Production Science 78: 63-70.
12. Aherne F (1999) Feeding the lactation. Sow. Technique. Association of Animal's Productions 14: 29.
13. Palomo A (2013) Nutritional needs in gestation to maintain energy and protein reserves. Onlino: May 2013. Availablo at http://www.org/udoc/udoc/php.sec/industria/cerdo
14. Casasola F, Palomo Y (2003) Interaction between body condition at the level of dorsal fat and porcine reproductive efficiency. Anaporc Review of Porcinocultura, p: 234.
15. Rodríguez H (2005) Evaluation of the Reproductive and Developmental Risks of Caffeine. Birth Defects Res B Dev Reprod Toxicol 92: 152-187.
16. Romero M (2004) Study of the effect of weight, age and number on head to the incorporation on the reproductive behavior of piglets at the genetic center Porcino El Tigre. Diploma Thesis. Pinewood of the River.
17. Merck (2005) The Merck Manual of Veterinary Medicine. Madrid. 4th edn. Merck Veterinary Manual. Whitehouse Station, USA.
18. Milkil FP (2006) Determining Feeding to Maintain Body Condition of Sows Online (23-02-2006). Available from: http://www.3tres3.com/home/index.php (Consultation 2 May 2013).
19. Ponce de León R (1998) Consideration on some reproductive parameters. Cuban Journal of Agricultural Science 22: 9-15.
20. Santiago E (2006) Porcine production Body state, its importance in reproduction. Online April 2013.
21. Alonso R, Cama JM, Rodríguez J (2004) The pig. Editorial Félix Varela.
22. Quiles A, Hevia M (2004) Factors affecting neonatal mortality of piglets. Department of Animal Production. Veterinary School. University of Murcia: Campus of Espinardo. Murcia.
23. Bernard F (2006) The influence factors in the weight loss of animals. Available Online 2006.

The Zoonoses Data Collection in Italy: An Expert System for Data Quality Management and Improvement

Iannetti S[1]*, Cioci D[2], Falcone MG[3] and Colangeli P[2]

[1]*Veterinary Medicine, Istituto Zooprofilattico Sperimentale of Abruzzo and Molise G. Caporale, Campo Boario Teramo, Italy*
[2]*Computer Science, Istituto Zooprofilattico Sperimentale of Abruzzo and Molise G. Caporale, Campo Boario Teramo, Italy*
[3]*Veterinary Medicine, Ministry of Health, Office III DGSAF, Rome, Italy*

Abstract

The need to improve the quality of data for a better analysis and understanding of zoonoses' trend at country level has been increased year by year both by the EFSA and by reporting countries. In the framework of an EFSA's Grant project, aimed to complement the zoonoses historical database, an expert system based on logical rules of truth tables was put in place within the Italian information system for zoonoses data collection (SINZoo). During data entry, the truth tables check that, for each zoonoses, the combination of the area of interest, each possible sampling context, stage and sampling unit has been entered correctly, thus avoiding inconsistent data. Each combination available in the truth tables indicates the context, the stage, the sampling unit allowed for each zoonosis in a specific area and for a category of species. The goal of the project was achieved for most of the information to be retrieved: the 89% and the 83% of sampling contexts and stages respectively and the 100% of the other information were retrieved. To date, the truth tables developed for specific zoonoses have become integral part of SINZoo, allowing to avoid mistakes during data reporting. Data quality is the pillar for any analysis and to perform risk analysis: the logical rules of truth tables can be implemented in other information systems involved in data collection in the field of animal health and food safety, increasing both the consistence and the coherence of the data reported.

Keywords: Business rules; Data collection; Data quality; Data dictionary; Expert system; Information system; Zoonoses

Introduction

The European Union (EU) system for monitoring and collecting information on zoonoses is based on Directive (EC) n. 2003/99, which obliges the EU Member States to collect data on the occurrence of zoonoses, zoonotic agents, antimicrobial resistance, animal populations and food-borne outbreaks [1]. Moreover, under Regulation (EC) n. 178/2002, the European Food Safety Authority (EFSA) is assigned the tasks of examining these data and publishing annual European Union Summary Reports (EUSR) in cooperation with the European Centre for Disease Prevention and Control (ECDC), which provides and analyses the data on zoonotic infections in humans [2]. In order to collect data by the different Member States, which already have different systems to collect zoonoses data, EFSA developed a Zoonoses Data Model and a common dictionary (contained in pick lists) to be used by each reporting country, based on the Standard Sample Description, for all the items to be reported, with the aim of collecting data in a unique and uniform way and with the same semantic [3].

In Italy, the Italian Ministry of Health (MoH) is the national authority in charge of collecting data on zoonoses and zoonotic agents covered by Directive (EC) n. 2003/99 [4]. Since 2008, zoonoses data collection takes place at national level through the "national information system for zoonoses data collection", named SINZoo, developed in compliance with the Directive (EC) n. 2003/99 by the Istituto Zooprofilattico Sperimentale dell'Abruzzo e del Molise "G. Caporale" (IZSAM) on request of the MoH. Zoonoses data are registered into SINZoo by the regional veterinary services through different alternatives: on line forms, upload of XML files and Web Services [5]. A common dictionary was developed in SINZoo, integrated with the EFSA's one and with other categorizations specifically developed at national level. The database in SINZoo was established considering both the information debt toward the EFSA and the national needs and is made up of the following components:

- Zoonosis
- Tested species for animal prevalence data, species of origin of the food for food prevalence data, species of destination of feed for feed prevalence data
- Sampling Context
- Sampling Stage/Sample Type
- Sampling Unit

Each component includes a list of possible values which found the correspondence (mapping) of the values in the EFSA's catalogue [6].

SINZoo is strictly integrated with other national information systems already existent in animal health and food safety and is available on the website of the National Veterinary Information systems, thus avoiding double data entry and assuring data uniqueness and the coherence between dictionaries and definitions [7-9]. In fact, the national information debt towards the EFSA consists in aggregated data (i.e., not sample based) which come from the different national information systems:

- Data on animal population, available in the National veterinary database for livestock and holdings (BDN),
- Data on zoonoses and zoonotic agents in animal, food and feed,

***Corresponding author:** Iannetti S, Veterinarian, Doctor in Veterinary Medicine, Research Institute of Abruzzo and Molise G. Caporale, Campo Boario Teramo, Italy, E-mail: s.iannetti@izs.it

that represent the "prevalence data", entered in SINZoo by the authorised users,

- Data on Community co-financed eradication programs on sheep and goat brucellosis and bovine tuberculosis, collected by the Italian information system on Community co-financed eradication programmes (SIR),
- Data on the national *Salmonella* control program, collected by the Italian National information system for *Salmonella* control programme,
- Antimicrobial resistance data, which are provided by the national reference centre for antimicrobial resistance,
- Food-borne outbreak data, entered in SINZoo at outbreak level by the authorised users of the Local Health Units.

In order to improve data quality, a national Panel of 15 experts was appointed by the MoH for the evaluation of data collected prior to their submission to the EFSA. Despite this, during the first years, the lack of automatic controls increased data granularity and inconsistencies. Moreover, the need to improve data quality for a better analysis and understanding of the trend of zoonoses at country level increased year by year, both by the EFSA and by reporting countries: this was the reason why the EFSA launched in 2014 a Grant project within the article 36 of EFSA's Founding Regulation, to support the participating countries in updating and complementing their datasets in EFSA's historical databases. In the framework of this Grant project (Implementation and testing of electronic submission in XML, Excel and CSV formats of zoonoses, antimicrobial resistance and food-borne outbreak data and updating the historical dataset) the EFSA provided funds to the IZSAM for updating and revising the national historical dataset on zoonoses and zoonotic agents in animals from 2008 to 2011. In this context, an Expert system based on logical rules and truth tables was put in place in SINZoo for complementing the historical animal prevalence data and improving the overall data quality.

The aim of this paper is to describe the logical rules behind the Expert system and the results obtained.

Materials and Methods

The EFSA's historical database on animal prevalence data was firstly evaluated by year, then data with incorrect/missing values were identified and categorized. The inconsistencies consisted in missing or unspecified information to retrieve and wrong information to correct, in relation to the sampling context (which was split by EFSA during the reporting years in three fields: context, sampler, sampling strategy), sampling stage, sample type, sampling unit. The missing or unspecified information found were retrieved following a set of logical rules based on the legislation in place regarding the zoonoses covered by the project. After defined the logical rules, the removal of rows with clear errors in the EFSA's historical database was made possible by implementing in SINZoo truth tables customized for each zoonosis. In order to retrieve missing or incorrect data in the EFSA's historical database, it was considered worthwhile to analyse not all records, but only substantial combinations (SCs) of: matrix, sampling context, sampling strategy, sampler, sample type, sampling stage, sampling unit. Each SCs was substituted with a new combination where missing or incorrect field/s were replaced according to the logical rules. The SCs to be corrected were modified through a web interface, integrated with SINZoo, available only to users having a specific role (i.e., epidemiologists involved in the Grant project). The web interface allowed filtering the SCs through a search-form, to display them and to modify each combination manually. Once saved the correction, a pl/sql procedure verified if the new combination still contained errors/warning; in this case, the user was able to correct the SC for unlimited times. The data updating was performed in two different ways:

- Massive update: Allowed updating all rows belonging to a SC. Starting from a generic combination, the system allowed modifying (with the same criteria) all rows belonging to it.
- Single row update: Allowed updating a specific row which lies outside the rules foreseen for its SC and must be treated differently. Starting from the generic SC, the system allowed showing all single rows having that attributes' combination and permitted and modify a specific row in a way and all the others in a different way.

After data updating, some row amended could have been acquired the same SC belonging to other rows already existing into the EFSA's historical database. In this situation, data of the "new" and "old" combinations were automatically aggregated and total number of unit tested and total number of units positive was summed.

Examples of logical rules developed for missing, unspecified, wrong sampling context

In Italy, according to the Legislative Decree 4 April 2006 n. 191, the zoonoses to be monitored by the official competent authority are listed in the Annex I part A. Depending on the epidemiological situation of the region, other zoonoses shall be monitored and they are listed in Annex I part B. Therefore, for zoonoses and zoonotic agents listed in the Annex I part A, regarding animal area, when the sampler reported was "official sampling" and the context was "unspecified", the context was updated to "monitoring"; vice versa, when the context reported was "monitoring/ surveillance" and the sampler was unspecified, the sampler was updated to "official sampling".

National control and co-financed eradication programmes are in place for salmonellosis in *Gallus gallus*, tuberculosis due to M. bovis in cattle and water buffaloes, brucellosis in cattle, in water buffaloes and in sheep and goats. Thus, all the official sampling activities are carried out for the purpose of control and co-financed eradication programmes. When the context reported was "control and eradication programme" and the sampler was "official sampling", the missing sampling strategy was updated to "census", according to the legislation in place related to the national control and co-financed eradication programmes [10,11].

For official sampling activities in *Gallus gallus* and sampler "official sampling" the missing sampling context was updated to "control and eradication programme", and the sampling unit to "flock" if missing or reported with other values, since the controls are performed at flock level [12-15].

For trichinosis, according to Commission Regulation n. 2075/2005 and subsequent amendments laying down specific rules on official controls for *Trichinella* in meat, carcases of domestic swine shall be systematically sampled in slaughterhouses as part of the post-mortem examination [16]. Moreover, carcases of horses, wild boar and other farmed species susceptible to *Trichinella* infestation shall be systematically sampled in slaughterhouses, while carcases of wild animal shall be tested in game-handling establishments as part of the post-mortem examination. Therefore, the logic rule implemented for this zoonosis was: in farmed animals, when the sampler was "official sampling" the sampling strategy should be "census" and the sampling stage should be "at slaughterhouse", while in wildlife the sampling stage should be "at game handling establishments".

Data on *Toxoplasma, Yersinia, Staphylococcus, Campylobacter* and *Coxiella* in animals are mainly collected during clinical investigations, or surveys, since for the years covered by the project there was not a national monitoring system in place for these zoonoses in Italy. Therefore for such zoonoses the only possible sampling context in the EFSA's historical database could be "survey" or "clinical investigation". Clinical investigations are usually carried out for testing of symptomatic animals suspected to be affected by any zoonotic agent, therefore the sampling strategy was updated to "suspect sampling" when missing. The sampling context was also revised in case of mistakes: the main corrections regarded for instance official sampling activities reported wrongly with sampling context "monitoring" or "surveillance" for which the sampling context was amended and the sampling strategy was corrected to "objective sampling" or to "suspect sampling" in case of surveys or clinical investigations respectively.

Examples of logical rules developed for missing, unspecified, wrong sampling stage

The sampling stage was updated to "at farm" in case of farmed animals or of zoo animals, (since this stage in SINZoo was intended to be used for all type of premises keeping animals). As regards pets, in Italy most of them are investigated at private level; to date, EFSA does not include this stage in the pick lists, so it was left to "unspecified" in the EFSA's historical database. For wild animals, the only possible sampling stages could be "natural habitat", "conservation facilities" or "game handling establishments", depending on the zoonosis, the tested species and other rules described previously.

Examples of logical rules for generic species

EFSA implemented the matrix pick list within its catalogue, asking Member States to specify if a given species was farmed or wild, in order to obtain more and more detailed data. Therefore, a logical rule was implemented for wild boars and water buffaloes to decide whether the animals sampled were farmed or not. So, in case of water buffalo, this species was updated to "water buffalo-farmed" and the stage was updated to "at farm" when unspecified or missing, since this species in Italy is only farmed (Table 1). For *Echinococcus* and *Trichinella* in water buffaloes and in wild boars-farmed, the only possible sampling stage could be "at slaughterhouse", since according to the legislation, these species shall be systematically sampled at the slaughterhouse [16], while for wildlife-wild boars, the only possible sampling stage could be "natural habitat", where the animals can be hunted (Table 2). The correction of the reported species regarded "pigs-mixed herds-sows", which were corrected to "pigs - breeding animals - unspecified – sows" and "pigs-mixed herds-fattening pigs" were corrected to "pigs - fattening pigs – unspecified", since there are not mixed herds of farmed pigs in Italy.

Results

The logical rules described previously were used to create a truth table for each zoonosis to be reported to the EFSA. Each truth table was implemented taking into account the relationship between the zoonosis, the area of interest (animal, food, and feed) and each possible sampling context, stage and sampling unit. From Decoding menu of SINZoo, it is possible to download truth tables for each of the zoonoses to be reported to the EFSA according to the Dir. 2003/99/CE (Figure 2). The entire EFSA's historical database was processed by the truth tables in order to extract the rows containing combinations fields which were not admitted. Each time one or more row was updated, the system verified its correctness by checking the truth table for the zoonosis in question.

The database of SINZoo is logically structured within the entity-relationship (E/R) schemas (Figure 1). The truth table is linked, through foreign keys, to:

- zoonosis,

COD_EFSA	DESCR_EFSA	stage	stage update to:	species updated to:	species considered as:
A003581A	Wildlife - wild boars	unspecified or null	natural habitat		wild animals
A020861A	Wild boars - farmed	unspecified or null	at farm		Farmed/zoo animals
A010041A	Wild boars	at farm		wild boars - farmed	Farmed/zoo animals
A010041A	Wild boars	unspecified or null	natural habitat	Wildlife - wild boars	wild animals
A003581A	Wildlife - wild boars	at farm	natural habitat		wild animals
A020861A	Wild boars - farmed	natural habitat	at farm		Farmed/zoo animals
A006821A	Water buffalos	unspecified or null	at farm	Water buffalos - farmed	Farmed/zoo animals
A006821A	Water buffalos	at farm		Water buffalos - farmed	Farmed/zoo animals
A031641A	Water buffalos - farmed	unspecified or null	at farm		Farmed/zoo animals
A031641A	Water buffalos - farmed	natural habitat	at farm		Farmed

Table 1: Logical rules followed to update generic species.

COD_EFSA	DESCR_EFSA	stage	stage update to:	species updated to:	species considered as:
A003581A	Wildlife - wild boars	unspecified or null	natural habitat		wild animals
A003581A	Wildlife - wild boars	at farm	natural habitat		wild animals
A010041A	Wild boars	at farm	at slaughterhouse	wild boars - farmed	Farmed/zoo animals
A010041A	Wild boars	unspecified or null	natural habitat	Wildlife - wild boars	wild animals
A020861A	Wild boars - farmed	unspecified or null	at slaughterhouse		Farmed/zoo animals
A020861A	Wild boars - farmed	natural habitat	at slaughterhouse		Farmed/zoo animals
A006821A	Water buffalos	unspecified or null	at slaughterhouse	Water buffalos - farmed	Farmed/zoo animals
A006821A	Water buffalos	at farm	at slaughterhouse	Water buffalos - farmed	Farmed/zoo animals
A031641A	Water buffalos - farmed	unspecified or null	at slaughterhouse		Farmed/zoo animals
A031641A	Water buffalos - farmed	natural habitat	at slaughterhouse		Farmed/zoo animals

Table 2: Logical rules followed to update generic species in case of *Echinococcus* and *Trichinella*.

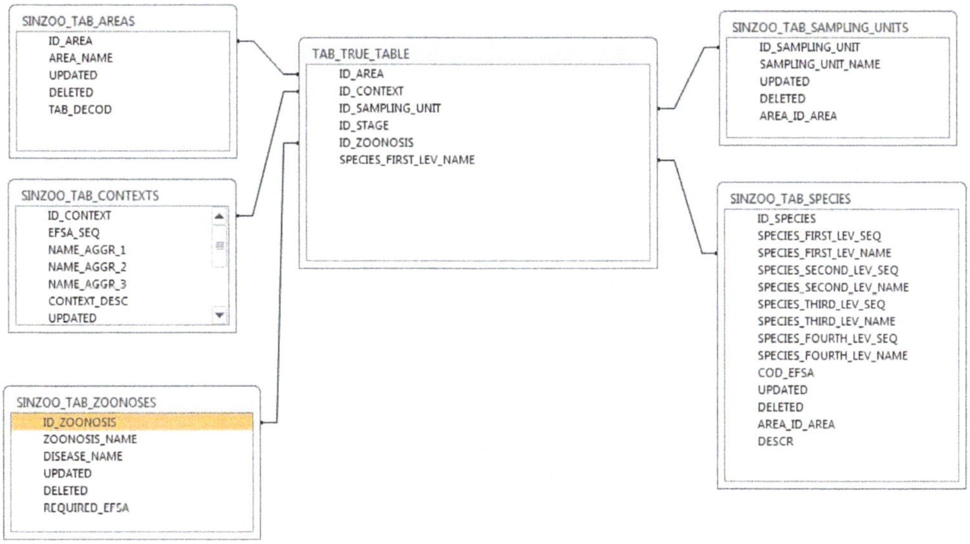

Figure 1: Entity-relationship (E/R) scheme.

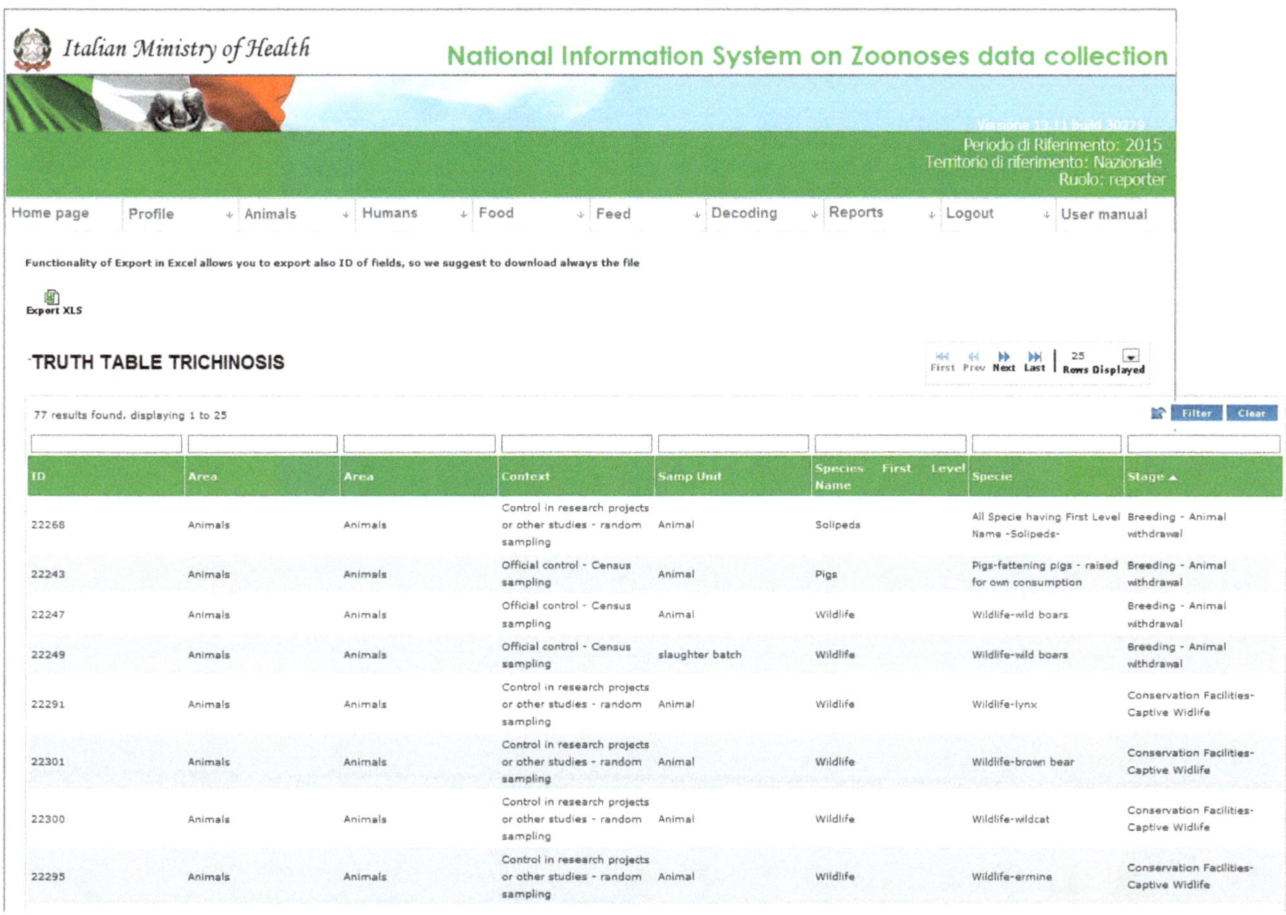

Figure 2: Truth table trichinosis.

- area,
- context,
- stage,
- sampling unit,
- Species (first level name): this field stands for the animal species if the reporting area is "Animal", the species of origin of the food if the area is "Food" and the species of destination of the feed if the area is "Feed".

Each combination available in the truth table indicates the context, the stage, the sampling unit allowed for the reported zoonosis in a specific area and for a category of species. Thanks to the logical rules and the truth tables, the missing/unspecified information was retrieved and the rows containing wrong combinations of zoonosis/ context/ stage/unit were corrected and updated. Overall, the goal of the Grant project was achieved for most of the information to be retrieved: the 89% and the 83% of sampling contexts and stages respectively and the 100% of the other information were retrieved (Table 3). The entire process was realised following logical rules both of the truth table and of the national legislation in place for the zoonoses covered by the project, thus ensuring the coherence of all the data retrieved. Also, the whole work was made easier by the implementation of the web interface shown in Figure 3: an alert "message" notified if the record selected had different or equal values for the fields composing the "context", i.e., sampler/ sampling context/ sampling strategy and what type of values. The user might change the selected values and by clicking on "Confirm select", saved the modification. Contextually, the system processed new combination and re-generates the comment field with success/error/ warning (Figure 3).

Examples of truth table developed for some specific zoonosis and zoonotic agent

***Toxoplasma, Yersinia, Staphylococcus, Campylobacter, Coxiella*:** National monitoring programme for *Toxoplasma, Yersinia, Staphylococcus, Campylobacter* and *Coxiella* in animals are not in place

Reporting Year	Sampling Context	Sampler	Sampling Strategy	Sampling Stage	Sample Type	Sampling Unit
2008	100%	100%	100%	80%	100%	-
2009	99%	100%	100%	86%	100%	-
2010	100%	100%	100%	80%	100%	100%
2011	87%	-	-	87%	100%	-
Total	**89%**	**100%**	**100%**	**83%**	**100%**	**100%**

Table 3: Percentage of retrieved information for each SCs.

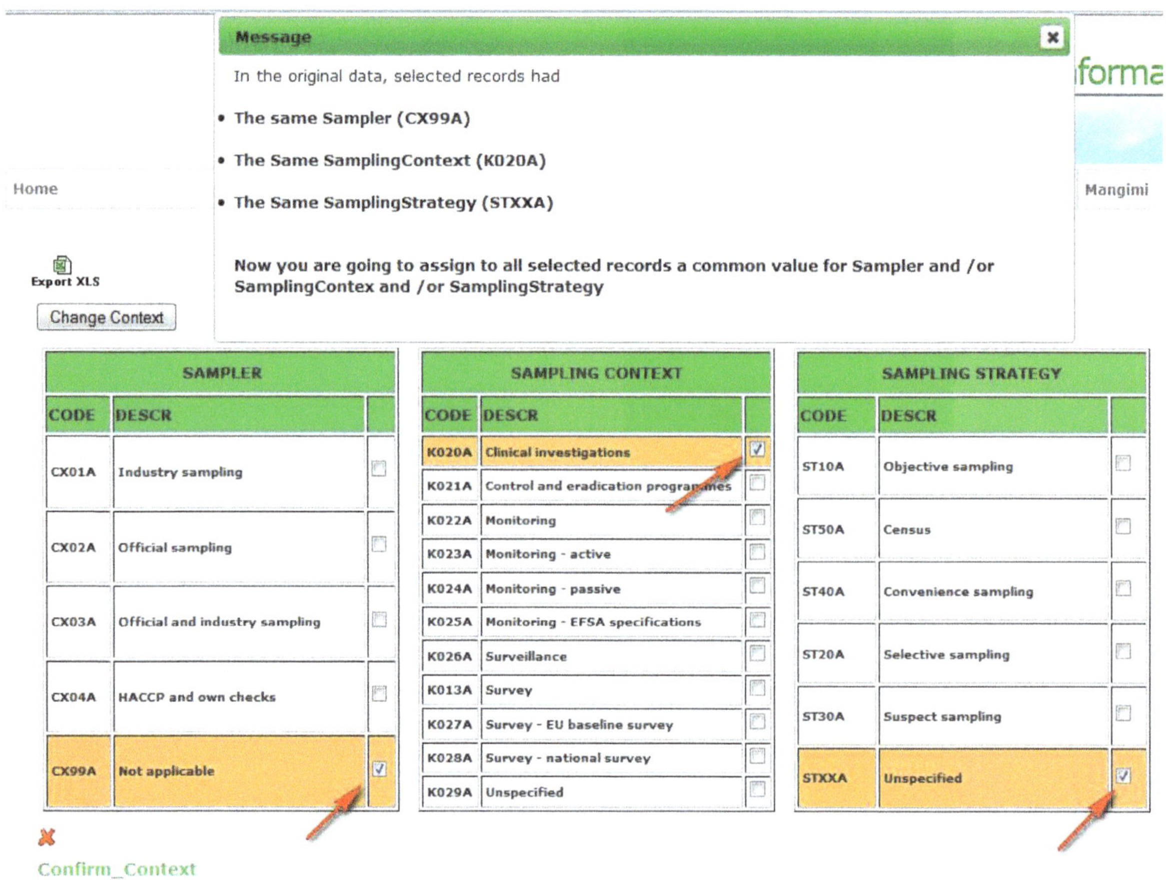

Figure 3: Web inferace.

for susceptible species, so most of the sampling activities are carried out during surveys or clinical investigations in animals suspected to be diseased, therefore for such zoonoses the truth tables admit only two sampling context (and only the susceptible species), "survey" or "clinical investigation". Moreover, in case of Campylobacter in poultry and birds, Campylobacteriosis does not cause clinical signs, therefore the truth table does not admit "clinical investigations" in these species. The sampling strategy admitted for clinical investigation is "suspect sampling", since the animals are controlled in case of suspectd disease. Also sample type admitted are coherent with the zoonosis: i.e., for Toxoplasma, typically blood (for intermediate hosts) is tested by serology, other samples could include abortion material (e.g., sheep) or faeces (e.g., cats); for Yersinia and Campylobacter, also faeces and environmental samples are admitted in the truth tables.

Echinococcus: Echinococcosis is one of the diseases listed in the Annex I part A, therefore it shall be monitored by the official competent authorities. In Italy, surveillance is performed during official meat inspection as part of Regulation (EC) No 854/2004 of the European Parliament and of the Council of 29th April 2004 laying down specific rules for the organisation of official controls on products of animal origin intended for human consumption [17]. Some regional programmes are in place on the national territory and official sampling activities take place at slaughterhouse as part of the post-mortem examination for all farmed animals. Therefore for echinococcosis the truth table admits the context "monitoring", sampler "official sampling", sampling strategy "census" and sampling stage "at slaughterhouse", according to Regulation (EC) No. 854/2004. The sample type admitted is "animal sample-organ/tissue". The sample unit is always "animal" since the unit tested in the framework of the monitoring programme is always the animal.

Brucella: The truth table for brucellosis does not admit official sampling activities carried out on cattle, sheep and goats and farmed water buffaloes, since these data are provided by the Italian information system on Community co-financed eradication programmes (SIR). Clinical investigations are admitted for other susceptible species, with sampling strategy "suspect sampling": for instance, pets may be subjected to clinical investigations carried out in case of suspect of disease, especially for dogs living on a farm. The sampling context "survey" is admitted for animal species susceptible to Brucella, with sampler "objective sampling". For sample type, typically blood is tested by serology; other animal samples could include abortion material. Sampling stage "natural habitat" is admitted for wild animals and "at farm" for farmed or zoo animals.

Trichinella: According to Regulation (EC) n. 2075/2005, the competent authority should implement a monitoring programme covering domestic swine, horses and other susceptible animal species coming from holdings or categories of holdings recognised as free from *Trichinella* or from regions where the risk of *Trichinella* in domestic swine is recognised as negligible, in order to verify that the animals are effectively free from *Trichinella*. To that end, meat samples shall be collected and examined for presence of Trichinella parasites. The truth table developed for trichinosis in animals admits only "animal" as sampling unit, "monitoring" as sampling context, "official sampling" as sampler and "census sampling" as sampling strategy. Since trichinosis is asymptomatic in most of the animal species, the context "clinical investigations" is not admitted.

Discussion

Data reported by the Member States and other reporting countries annually are stored in the EFSA's Zoonoses databases and used for the production of the annual European Union Summary Report (EUSR), other scientific or technical reports [18,19], and for supporting risk analysis carried out by EFSA's scientific panels [20,21]. Since changes in the historical datasets of Member States occurred over the years and the standardisation of the data reporting improved during the past years, needs to update and complement the national historical datasets in the EFSA's Zoonoses databases were required. This was to guarantee the correctness of the data and the subsequent accuracy of the analyses based on the national data. The work done during the Grant project permitted to trace, wherever possible, the missing right information and to improve, overall, the quality of data reported to the EFSA from 2008 to 2011. The need to retrieve historical data led to improve the rules of the national data collection foreseen by the truth tables and to define new logics and algorithms that may be used and improved for each reporting.

In conclusion, the work done during the project permitted to trace, wherever possible, the missing right information and to improve, overall, the quality of data reported to the EFSA from 2008 to 2011. The Italian team developed an expert, flexible system, using business rules (i.e., truth tables) able to support the annual collection both at aggregate level and sample based level. From the Grant project until the last reporting season (2015 zoonoses data collection) the implementation of the truth tables in SINZoo allowed checking the correctness of the data reported, thus avoiding rough mistakes during the system's feeding. To date, the truth tables contain all the valid combination of context, stage, sampling unit allowed for a given zoonosis in a given area (animal, food, and feed) and for a category of species. During zoonoses data entry, the truth table checks that, for each zoonosis, the combination of the area of interest, each possible sampling context, stage and sampling unit has been entered correctly, thus avoiding inconsistent data. Moreover, the truth tables are under revision annually by the national Panel of expert: the revision takes into account any possible change in the national or EU legislation and also the addition of new combinations for which the experts decide the cogency.

In the absence of any structured information system, data collection would be prone to delays, errors and omissions. In fact, the same information could be requested several times and in different formats, causing confusion for the lack of a unique data collection.

This Grant project highlighted the importance of data quality during the collection and feeding of any information system. Data quality is the pillar for any epidemiological analysis and to perform risk analysis: logical rules of truth tables can be implemented in other information systems involved in data collection in the field of animal health and food safety, increasing both the consistence and the coherence of the data reported.

Ensure the quality of the data collected is the basis for any subsequent processing. For this reason, the efforts go towards the integration of the various information systems, avoiding duplication of the same data in different systems. The data is entered only in one spot, usually by those who created it and is made available to those who need it (interoperability). Moreover, the existing national information systems shifted their ability over time from operational applications (collecting data in course of normal business operation) to decision support systems having primarily the purpose to collect appropriate data of high quality and presenting the results of data analysis to stakeholders and decision makers.

Acknowledgements

The authors would like to thank the European Food Safety Authority for funding the Grant project "Implementation and testing of electronic submission in XML, Excel and CSV formats of zoonoses, antimicrobial resistance and food-borne outbreak data and updating the historical dataset" under which this research was carried out.

References

1. European Parliament, Council of the European Union (2003) Directive 2003/99/EC of the European Parliament and of the Council of 17 November 2003 on the monitoring of zoonoses and zoonotic agents, amending Council Decision 90/424/EEC and repealing Council Directive 92/117/EEC, pp: 31-40.
2. European Parliament, Council of the European Union (2002) Regulation (EC) No 178/2002 of the European Parliament and of the Council of 28 January 2002 laying down the general principles and requirements of food law, establishing the European Food Safety Authority and laying down procedures in matters of food safety, pp: 1-24.
3. EFSA (European Food Safety Authority) (2010) Standard sample description for food and feed. EFSA Journal 8: 1457.
4. Legislative Decree No. 191 of 4th April (2006) Implementation of Directive 2003/99/EC on the monitoring of zoonoses and zoonotic agents. Italian Official Gazette no. 119 of 24 May 2006.
5. Colangeli P, Iannetti S, Ruocco L, Forlizzi L, Cioci D, et al. (2012) The Italian Information System on Zoonoses Data Collection. Zoonoses Public Health 60: 182-188.
6. European Food Safety Authority (EFSA) (2014) Manual for reporting on zoonoses and zoonotic agents, within the framework of Directive 2003/99/EC and on some other pathogenic microbiological agents for information deriving from the year 2015. 573: 107.
7. Colangeli P, Iannetti S, Cerella A, Ippoliti C, Di Lorenzo A, et al. (2011) The National information system for the notification of animal diseases in Italy. Vet Ital 47: 303-312.
8. Iannetti S, Malizia E, Sorgente A, Ricci A, Cibin V, et al. (2015) The Integrated Management System for Salmonella Control Plan in Italy. J Health Med Informat 6: 199.
9. Napoli C, Iannetti S, Rizzo C, Bella A, DiSabatino D, et al. (2014) Vector borne infections in Italy: results of the integrated surveillance system for West Nile Disease in 2013. BioMed Res International. 2015: Article ID 643439.
10. Commission Decision No. 2007/851/EC of 10 December 2007 amending Decisions 2006/687/EC, 2006/875/EC and 2006/876/EC as regards the reallocation of the Community's financial contribution to certain Member States for their programmes for the eradication and monitoring of animal diseases and for checks aimed at the prevention of zoonoses for 2007 (notified under document number C (2007) 5985).
11. Commission implementing Decision No. 2011/807/UE of 30 November 2012 approving annual and multiannual programmes and the financial contribution from the Union for the eradication, control and monitoring of certain animal diseases and zoonoses presented by the Member States for 2013 and following years.
12. Commission Regulation (EC) No. 1003/2005 implementing Regulation (EC) No. 2160/2003 of the European Parliament and of the Council as regards a Union target for the reduction of the prevalence of certain Salmonella serotypes in breeding flocks of Gallus gallus and amending Regulation (EC) No. 2160/2003.
13. Commission Regulation (EU) No. 1190/2012 of 12 December 2012 concerning a Union target for the reduction of Salmonella Enteritidis and Salmonella Typhimurium in flocks of turkeys, as provided for in Regulation (EC) No 2160/2003 of the European Parliament and of the Council Text with EEA relevance.
14. Commission Regulation (EC) No. 646/2007 of 12 June 2007 implementing Regulation (EC) No 2160/2003 of the European Parliament and of the Council as regards a Community target for the reduction of the prevalence of Salmonella Enteritidis and Salmonella Typhimurium in broilers and repealing Regulation (EC) No 1091/2005.
15. Commission Decision No. 2007/848/EC of 11 December 2007 approving certain national programmes for the control of Salmonella in flocks of laying hens of Gallus gallus.
16. Commission Regulation (EC) No. 2075/2005 of 5 December 2005 laying down specific rules on official controls for Trichinella in meat.
17. Regulation (EC) of the European Parliament and of the Council No. 854/2004 (EC, 2004) of 29th April 2004 laying down specific rules for the organisation of official controls on products of animal origin intended for human consumption.
18. EFSA (European Food Safety Authority) and ECDC (European Centre for Disease Prevention and Control) (2016) The European Union summary report on trends and sources of zoonoses, zoonotic agents and food-borne outbreaks in 2015. EFSA Journal. 14: 04634.
19. European Food Safety Authority (EFSA), Boelaert F, Hugas M, Ortiz Pelaez A, Rizzi V, Stella P et al. (2016) The European Union summary report on data of the surveillance of ruminants for the presence of transmissible spongiform encep halopathies (TSEs) in 2015. EFSA Journal. 14: 4643.
20. Opinion of the Scientific Panel on Biological Hazards on "Risk assessment of a revised inspection of slaughter animals in areas with low prevalence of Trichinella". The EFSA Journal 200: 1-411.
21. Scientific Opinion of the Panel on Biological Hazards on a request from EFSA on Surveillance and monitoring of Toxoplasma in humans, foods and animals (2007) The EFSA Journal 583: 1-64.

Effects of Dietary Protein Content on Milk Composition of Mixed Parity Lactating Sows in a Tropical Humid Climate

Silva BAN[1,2*], Gourdine JL[2], Corrent E[3], Primot Y[3], Mourot J[4], Noblet J[4] and Renaudeau D[2,4]

[1]*Institute of Agricultural Sciences/ICA, Federal University of Minas Gerais (UFMG), 39404-547, Montes Claros, Minas Gerais, Brazil*
[2]*INRA UR 143 Zootechnical Research Unit, F-97170 Petit Bourg, Guadeloupe, France*
[3]*Ajinomoto Eurolysine S.A.S. 153, Rue de Courcelles, F-75817 Paris Cedex 17, France*
[4]*INRA, UMR Breeding Systems, Animal and Human Nutrition INRA UMR 1079, 35590 St Gilles, France*

Abstract

Eighteen multiparous Large White sows were used to determine the effects of dietary protein content and lactation stage on milk composition during a 28-d lactation under humid tropical climatic conditions. This study was conducted at the INRA facilities in Guadeloupe, French West Indies (latitude 16°N, longitude 61°W). The average minimum and maximum ambient temperatures and average daily relative humidity during the trial were 22.7 and 29.4°C, and 93.7%, respectively. The dietary experimental treatments were a normal protein (NP, 17.3%) diet and a low protein (LP, 14.1%) diet supplemented with essential amino acids. The ADFI tended to be higher for the sows fed the LP diets when compared with the NP treatment (i.e., +9%, $P<0.10$). Litter BW gain and mean BW of piglets at weaning were not affected by dietary protein level ($P>0.10$). The treatments did not influence ($P>0.10$) sow body weight loss during lactation. The sows fed LP diets tended to show lower backfat thickness losses when compared to the sows fed NP diets (2.4 vs. 6.3 mm, respectively; $P<0.10$). Milk production and composition were not affected by dietary treatments ($P>0.10$). Milk dry matter and ash contents linearly increased according to lactation stage (17.6 to 19.9%, and 0.72 *vs.* 97%, respectively from d 7 to d 27; $P<0.01$). Lactose content increased from d 7 to d 14 (3.95 *vs.* 4.91; $P<0.01$) and thereafter remained constant. Fat content did not change during lactation and averaged 7.5%. The amino acid concentrations in milk protein were affected by the lactation stage: methionine, threonine, tryptophan, valine, and alanine concentrations decreased ($P<0.05$) but glycine and glutamic acid contents increased ($P<0.05$) from d 7 to d 27. Fatty acids milk profile was not influenced ($P>0.10$) by lactation stage. Maternal BW loss during lactation was negatively correlated with the average daily feed intake (r=-0.76; $P<0.05$) and positively correlated with backfat thickness loss (r=0.55; $P<0.05$). A positive correlation between milk production and body reserves mobilisation (r=0.82; $P<0.05$) was also observed. Polyunsaturated fatty acid content in milk fat was positively correlated with ADFI and negatively correlated to maternal BW loss (r=0.62 and r=-0.60; $P<0.05$). In conclusion, reducing dietary protein content can be an alternative to attenuate the negative effects of heat stress by increasing ADFI. Milk composition changes significantly according to lactation stage and the ability of sows to produce milk will depend on their capacity to mobilize body reserve for providing milk precursors.

Keywords: Sow; Lactation; Milk; Amino acids; Fatty acids

Implications

Heat stress is a constant problem in many tropical and subtropical areas. Under heat stress, sows reduce their appetite in order to reduce their metabolic heat production due to the thermic effect of feed. This reduced feed intake has negative consequences on body reserves mobilization and milk yield and composition. The way the sow's milk composition and production is affected by heat stress implicates in the need of new nutritional strategies to attend the current lactating sow's daily needs and a better understanding of the consequences of this stress towards metabolism.

Introduction

The growth rate of nursing piglets is mainly determined by milk nutrient output by the dam. As a consequence, the quantity and the composition of milk produced by sows are key factors to reach a successful piglet production. Milk production appears to be highly variable and depends on many factors. It can be affected by sow characteristics (genotype, litter size, parity number, and lactation stage) and by environmental factors (feeding management, photoperiod, climatic parameters) [1]. Under tropical conditions, we estimated that milk yield was reduced by at least 30 to 50% in comparison with data obtained in temperate countries [2]. This result is mainly connected to the combined negative effect of high ambient temperature and relative humidity resulting in a concomitant reduction of voluntary feed consumption and milk production combined with the reduced ability of the sow to mobilize maternal body reserves. In fact, under tropical conditions, because of opened or semi-opened buildings, animals are more directly exposed to nycthemeral variation of the outside climatic conditions [3,4]. While there is substantial information on milk composition from sows raised under temperate climate [5], data on milk composition obtained in tropical countries are scarce and limited to the general composition (total solids, protein, fat and ash contents) [3,6]. The objective of our study was to evaluate the amino acid and fatty acid profile of sow's milk composition according to the lactation stage and dietary protein content under tropical humid conditions. In

***Corresponding author:** Bruno Silva, Institute of Agricultural Sciences/ ICA, Universidade Federal de Minas Gerais (UFMG), 39404-547, Montes Claros, Minas Gerais, Brazil, E-mail: BrunoSilva@ufmg.br

the present paper, the relationship between sow's performance and milk composition are also analysed.

Materials and Methods

Care and use of animals were performed according to the certificate of authorization to experiment on living animals issued by the French Ministry of Agriculture to the head of the experimental facilities.

Animals and experimental procedure

The study was conducted during the year of 2007 at the INRA facilities in Guadeloupe, French West Indies (latitude 16°N, longitude 61°W) characterized as having a tropical humid climate. A total of eighteen Large White mixed parity sows from 3 successive replicates of 6 sows each were used in this study. Within each replicate, sows were distributed in a completely randomized experimental design between two dietary treatments according to parity order, BW and backfat thickness after farrowing.

The dietary experimental treatments were: a normal protein diet (NP) and a low protein diet (LP) supplemented with essential AA. The experimental diets (Table 1) were formulated using corn, wheat middlings, and soybean meal, which met or exceeded AA requirements of lactating sows (NRC, 1998). The NP and LP diets contained the same levels of standardized digestible lysine (i.e., 0.80 g/MJ of NE). The ratio between digestible essential amino acids and digestible lysine in the experimental diets were maintained by synthetic AA complementation (DL-methionine, L-threonine, L-tryptophan, L-isoleucine, L-valine) to ensure that they were not below that of the ideal protein recommended for this animal category [3]. Diets were offered as pellets. Diets were prepared for the three successive replicates and stored in a temperature-controlled room (24°C, 50 to 60% RH).

During the gestation period, sows were housed in open-fronted gestating pens in groups of 5 sows each and restrictively fed a conventional diet containing 13 MJ DE/kg, 140 g CP/kg, based on maize, wheat middling and soybean meal. Feed allowance during the first 30 d after mating was calculated to standardize body condition at farrowing, according to the model proposed by Dourmad et al. [7]. The feeding level was fixed at 2.5 kg/d from the 30th to the 114th of gestation. Ten days before parturition, sows were moved to open-fronted farrowing pens (2.1 × 2.2 m) on a slatted metal floor. Variations in ambient temperature, relative humidity, and photoperiod closely followed outdoor conditions. On d 1 postpartum, sows received 1 kg of the standard gestation diet and the allowance increased by 1 kg each day until d 4 of lactation to avoid over-consumption at the beginning of lactation and agalactia problems. The proportion of gestation diet decreased progressively over the 4-d postpartum (100, 75, 50 and 25% on d 1, 2, 3 and 4, respectively), and sows were fed only the lactation diet on d 5. From d 6 to 26 postpartum, sows were allowed to consume feed ad libitum. The day prior to weaning (i.e., d 27), sows were allowed 3 kg of feed (i.e., at least 1.5 kg lower than their usual feed intake) to standardize consumption for all sows for determination of sow BW at weaning.

After birth, piglets were handled for tooth cutting, umbilical cord treatment and ear tagged for labelling. On d 3, they received an intramuscular injection of 200 mg of iron dextran. When necessary, cross-fostering was conducted within the first 48 h after birth to standardize litter size at 11 piglets. On d 14, male piglets were castrated. After 21 d of lactation, piglets were offered creep feed containing 15.3 MJ of DE/kg, 20% CP, and 1.47% total lysine. Infrared lights provided supplemental heat for the piglets during the first 21 d of the lactation period.

Measurements and chemical analysis

Sows were weighed after farrowing and at weaning. Backfat thickness measurements were taken ultrasonically (Agroscan, E.C.M., Angoulême, France) at 65 mm from the midline at the point beside the shoulder and at the last rib on each flank 2 d before farrowing and at weaning. The total number of piglets born, born alive, stillborn, and piglet deaths during lactation were recorded for each litter. Piglets were individually weighed at birth, at d 14 and 21 of lactation and at weaning. Every morning, feed refusals were collected, and fresh feed was immediately distributed once per day between 0700 and 0900. Feed consumption was determined as the difference between feed allowance and the refusals collected on the next morning. Every day, one sample of feed and feed refusals were collected daily for DM content measurement, and successive samples were pooled and stored at 4°C for further analyses.

At d 7, 14, 21 and 27 piglets were separated from the sows after suckling, and 50 min later (i.e., equivalent to average suckling interval) [8], the sow was injected with 10 IU of oxytocin (Intervet, Angers, France) in an ear vein and all functional mammary glands were hand milked. Samples (approximately 150 to 200 mL) were immediately stored at -20°C for further analyses. At the end of the experiment, all samples were freeze dried and analyzed for moisture, ash, and N contents according to AOAC methods [9]. Lactose content was measured using an enzymatic method (ENZYPLUS EZS784, BioControl Systems, Inc.). The amino acids contents were determined by ion-exchange liquid chromatography (Biochrom 20, Pharmacia, Saclay, France) after a 24 h-hydrolysis in HCl (6 mol/L). For sulfur AA, the hydrolysis was performed by a performic oxidation. Tryptophan was hydrolyzed only for feed and milk in barium hydroxide solution (1.5 mol/L) for 20 h, separated by HPLC, and detected fluorimetrically (Waters 600E, St Quentin en Yvelines, France). The total lipid content was determined following a chloroform/methanol (2:1) extraction method according to Folch et al. [10]. Fatty acid methyl esters were prepared with 20% boron trifluoride/methanol solution according to Morrison and Smith, the fatty methyl esters were separated on a gas chromatograph equipped with a SP-2330 capillary column (30 m × 0.25 mm internal diameter) with a non-bonded poly (80% biscyanopropyl/20% cyanopropylphenyl siloxane) stationary phase (a 0.20- μm film thickness) [11]. Furnace temperature was 180°C, and injector and detector temperatures were 240°C.

Feed (two samples per diet and per replicate) samples were analyzed for DM, ash, fat content (AOAC) and CP (N × 6.25 for feed and N × 6.38 for milk) according to Dumas method (AOAC) and analyzed for crude fiber and for cell wall components (NDF, ADF, and ADL) according to Van Soest and Wine [9]. Feed AA contents were analyzed by Ajinomoto Eurolysine (Amiens, France) using ion-exchange chromatography, except for tryptophan, which was analyzed using HPLC and fluorimetric detection (Waters 600E, St. Quentin en Yvelines, France).

Calculation and statistical analysis

Daily maximum, minimum, mean, and variance of daily ambient temperatures and relative humidities were averaged for each replicate. Milk production was estimated from litter growth rate and litter size between d 1 and d 21, and milk DM using the equation from Noblet and Etienne [12]. The effects of diet composition, replicate, parity number, and their interactions on performance of sows and litters were tested the GLM procedure of SAS. The effect of lactation stage on daily feed intake was tested with a mixed linear model (Mixed procedure of SAS) for repeated measurements with diet composition, batch and parity

Ingredients, %	Normal protein	Low protein
Corn	59.5	67.4
Soybean meal	24.4	10.6
Wheat middlings	8.4	14.3
Soybean oil	3.4	2.4
L-lysine HCL	0.020	0.415
DL-methionine		0.109
L-threonine		0.175
L-tryptophan		0.064
L-isoleucine		0.127
L-valine		0.140
Monocalcium phosphate	1.0	1.0
Calcium carbonate	2.1	2.1
Salt	0.1	0.1
Minerals and vitamins[2]	1.1	1.1
Analyzed composition		
Crude protein	17.3	14.1
Starch	39.0	45.2
Ether extract	4.3	5.6
NDF	10.0	10.8
Calculated composition		
SID amino acids, %[2]		
Lysine	0.80	0.80
Methionine + cystine	0.49	0.48
Threonine	0.54	0.54
Tryptophan	0.18	0.17
Isoleucine	0.63	0.54
Leucine	1.36	1.07
Valine	0.71	0.65
Fatty acids (FA), % total[3]		
Saturated FA		
C16	11.1	11.4
C18	2.9	2.6
Total	14.6	14.6
Monounsaturated FA		
C16:1	0.2	0.3
C18:1	23.4	23.6
Total	24.5	24.8
Polyunsaturated FA		
C18:2	54.6	55.1
C18:3	5.0	4.2
Total	60.9	60.6
Calculated nutritional values[3]		
Net energy, MJ/kg	10.2	10.1
Digestible lysine, g/MJ of NE	0.80	0.80

[1]Adjusted for 88% DM; [2]Standardized ileal digestible (SID) AA contents were calculated from the analyzed AA content and estimated standardized digestibility coefficients of the raw materials from INRA Tables (Sauvant et al.); [3]Fatty acids composition and NE values was estimated from the chemical composition of the diet and the equation of Noblet et al.

Table 1: Composition of lactation diets, as fed basis and analyzed chemical composition of the lactation diets[1].

number as main effects. The least square means procedure (PDIFF option) was used to compare means when a significant F-value was obtained. Milk composition data were submitted to a linear mixed model including the effect of diet, batch, and lactation stage as main effects. In this later model, the sow was considered as a random effect and the repeated measurement option of the mixed procedure of SAS was used with an autoregressive covariance structure to take into account the correlations between repeated measurements on the same animal. Means comparison was performed according to the Pdiff option of SAS procedure using Tukey test for contrasts. Residual values were computed from the preceding models (without the random sow effect) and residual Pearson correlations between lactating performance and mean milk composition parameters were calculated using the CORR Procedure of SAS/STAT.

	Diet		RSD[1]	Statistics[2]
	Normal protein	Low protein		
No. of sows	9	9		
Parity no.	2.5	3.0	-	
Body Weight (BW), kg				
At farrowing	224	226	31	
Loss during lactation	29	21	9	
Backfat thickness, mm				
At farrowing	19.1	17.2	4.5	
Loss during lactation	6.3	2.4	3.6	D[t]
ADFI, g/d	4162	4555	653	D[t]
Litter BW gain, g/d	2142	1967	349	B[t]
Milk production, g/d[3]	7800	7170	1450	B*

[1]Residual Standard Variation; [2]From an analysis of variance including the effect of diet (D), batch (B) and parity as main effects. Statistical significance: [t] $P<0.10$; * $P<0.05$; [3]Milk production during lactation was calculated from litter BW gain, litter size between d 1 and 27 using the equation from Noblet and Etienne.

Table 2: Effects of dietary protein content on performance of lactating sows over a 28-d lactation (least square means).

Results and Discussion

Average minimum and maximum ambient temperatures and average daily relative humidity measured during the experimental period were 22.7 and 29.4°C, and 93.7%, respectively. After farrowing, sows were restrictively fed for 5 d according to the same feeding plan and the increase of ADFI was similar for both treatments until d 4. After d 4, ADFI tended to be higher for LP diet as compared to the NP diet during the lactation (i.e., 4.55 vs. 4.16 kg/d, respectively; $P=0.08$; Table 2).

Similarly to our findings, Renaudeau and Noblet evaluating the effect of protein reduction (14.2 vs. 17.6%) also reported a numerical increase of ADFI in heat stressed (29°C) sows (fed LP diet (+0.639 kg/d) [13]. Lynch also observed an increased feed consumption (+0.700 kg/d) in multiparous lactating sows fed a low CP diet (14 vs. 20%) under heat stress conditions (i.e., 28°C) [14]. In contrast, Quiniou and Noblet did not report any effect of diet on performance of lactating sows kept at 29°C when dietary protein content was reduced from 17 to 14% [15]. According the later authors, the results could be due to the lack of interaction between temperature and diet to the low number of observations and (or) the deficiency in sulphur AA and Trp the low CP diet. The reduction of dietary protein content with a supplementation of industrial AA leads to an increase in the ratio between Trp and branched chain AA (LNAA: Leu, Ile, Val, Phe, Tyr) (i.e., 4.52 vs. 5.37% in NP and LP diet, respectively). According to Trottier and Easter, the reduction in the Trp:LNAA ratio through dietary addition of LNAA decreased feed intake of primiparous lactating sows [16]. Thus, it could be suggested that the increased ADFI in LP treatment may also be related to a reduced Trp:LNAA ratio. Tryptophan and LNAA share the same neutral carrier system to cross the blood-brain barrier, and they compete for uptake by the brain [17]. Serotonin and its precursor, Tryp, are known to be involved in the control of feed intake; an increased ratio of Tryp:LNAA is reported to increase appetite linearly in growing finishing pigs [18].

Litter BW gain, milk production and composition were not influenced by dietary CP content. Milk production from farrowing to d

27 and litter growth rate for the overall lactation period averaged 7,485 and 2,055 g/d, respectively. Similarly, Johnston et al. and Renaudeau et al. in lactating sows kept at 29°C, showed no change in litter BW gain when dietary CP level was decreased (from 16.7 to 13.3%; and from 17.6 to 14.2%, respectively) [13,19]. Lactation BW loss was not influenced statistically by treatments (*P*>0.10), but numerically, the LP sows lost 8 kg less than the NP sows in agreement with previous results [13]. The LP sows also tended to show a numerically lower backfat loss than NP sows (2.4 vs. 6.3 mm; *P*<0.10; Table 2). According to several authors theses findings can be attributed to the higher feed intake observed for the LP sows, which probably contributed for the sow to maintain its body condition [8,13,15].

The macro composition of milk is shown in Table 3. According to our findings, dietary protein content did not affect general milk composition and amino acids (AA) milk composition (Table 4). Similar results were reported by Dourmad et al. in primiparous lactating sows when dietary crude protein (CP) level was reduced from 17.1 to 15.5% without change in lysine concentration (0.77%) [7]. For a more severe restriction of dietary CP (15 to 5% and 23.8 to 6.3%, respectively), Elliott et al. and King et al. showed reduced fat and protein milk contents in low CP treatment [20,21]. In these latter studies, the milk AA composition expressed as a proportion of nitrogen content was slightly affected by protein supply. In particular, they reported a lower proportion of glutamic acid only in milk from sows receiving a diet with less than 10% dietary CP.

In the present study, milk DM and ash contents linearly increased with the advancement of lactation from 17.6 to 19.9% and from 0.72 to 0.97%, respectively between d 7 and d 27 (*P*<0.01). Lactose content

No. obs.	Lactation day, d				RSD	Statistics
	7	14	21	27		
	18	18	18	18		
Chemical composition, %						
Dry matter	17.6[a]	19.3[b]	18.7[b]	19.9[b]	1.2	S**, B**
Ash	0.72[a]	0.80[b]	0.88[c]	0.97[d]	0.06	S**
Nitrogen	0.82[ab]	0.80[a]	0.83[ab]	0.87[b]	0.07	S*, B**
Lipids	7.12	8.00	7.07	7.65	1.06	
Lactose	3.95[a]	4.91[b]	4.88[b]	4.90[b]	0.36	S**

[1]Residual Standard Variation; [a, b, c]Within a line, means with different superscripts are significantly affected by treatment; [2]From an analysis of variance with a general linear model including the effect of diet (D) and batch (B), lactation stage (S) and their interactions as fixed effects. Repeated measurements of milk chemical composition were analysed using an unstructured covariance structure with sows within batch as a subject. Statistical significance: **P*<0.05, ***P*<0.01.

Table 3: Effect of lactation stage on sows milk chemical composition (Least Square Means).

	Lactation day, d				RSD	Statistical analysis
	7	14	21	27		
No. observations	18	18	18	18		
Essential amino acids, g/16 g N						
Lysine	7.21	7.27	7.27	7.20	0.36	
Methionine	1.80	1.81	1.83	1.82	0.07	
Cystine	1.43[a]	1.39[b]	1.36[b]	1.29[c]	0.05	S***
Threonine	4.13[a]	4.04[ab]	4.01[ab]	3.98[b]	0.15	S*
Tryptophan	1.34[a]	1.29[b]	1.28[b]	1.28[b]	0.06	S*
Valine	5.24[a]	5.14[b]	5.12[b]	5.08[b]	0.12	S*
Leucine	8.43	8.38	8.36	8.32	0.17	B*
Isoleucine	4.00	3.98	3.97	3.92	0.19	
Histidine	2.58	2.59	2.58	2.57	0.10	
Tyrosine	4.18	4.14	4.13	4.11	0.23	
Phenylalanine	4.02	4.01	4.02	3.96	0.11	
Total	44.4	44.0	43.9	43.5	1.4	
Non essential amino acids, g/16 g N						
Arginine	4.64	4.59	4.58	4.65	0.11	B*
Glycine	3.08[a]	3.07[a]	3.11[ab]	3.20[b]	0.14	S*
Alanine	3.63[a]	3.56[ab]	3.54[ab]	3.50[b]	0.08	S**
Serine	5.14	5.11	5.14	5.12	0.15	
Aspartic acid	8.05	7.95	7.97	7.96	0.19	
Glutamic acid	19.2[a]	19.6[ab]	19.8[b]	19.7[b]	0.50	S*
Proline	10.1	10.3	10.5	10.7	0.53	
Total	53.8	54.2	54.6	54.8	1.3	

[1]Residual Standard Variation; [a, b, c]Within a line, means with different superscripts are significantly affected by treatment; [2]From an analysis of variance with a general linear model including the effect of diet (D) and batch (B), lactation stage (S) and their interactions as fixed effects. Repeated measurements of milk chemical composition were analysed using an unstructured covariance structure with sows within batch as a subject. Statistical significance: * *P*<0.05, ** *P*<0.01.

Table 4: Effect of lactation stage on sows milk protein amino acid composition (Least Square Means).

increased from d 7 and d 14 (3.95 to 4.91%, $P<0.01$) and thereafter remained constant. Whatever the stage of lactation, the percentage of fat in milk was constant and averaged 7.46%. Nitrogen milk concentration was significantly affected by stage of lactation being minimum on d 14 and maximum on d 27. Our results for the overall milk composition are essentially the same as those reported by Salmon-Legagneur, Elliott et al., Klobasa et al. and Csapó et al. [20,22-24].

In our study, the AA composition of milk protein generally agreed with those presented by King et al. and Dourmad et al. (Table 4) [7,21]. Milk proteins were particularly rich in glutamic acid, proline, leucine, and aspartic acid (19.6, 10.4, 8.4, and 8.0 g/16 g N, respectively). In contrast, tryptophan, cystine, and methionine were present in a least amount in milk (1.3, 1.4 and 1.8 g/16 g N, respectively). The AA concentration in milk was affected by the stage of lactation: whereas sulfur AA, threonine, tryptophan, valine, and alanine concentrations decreased ($P<0.05$) but glycine and glutamic acid contents increased ($P<0.05$) from d 7 to d 27. Similar results were reported by Csapó et al. and Elliott et al. [21,24]. As the AA are derived from milk proteins, changes in AA patterns during lactation reflect a change in the relative distribution of milk proteins with different AA pattern. According to Klobasa et al. the relative proportion of caseins to whey proteins such as immunoglobulins and α-lactalbumin increases during lactation in the sow´s milk [23]. In fact, whey proteins in general have a lower concentration of glutamic acid, proline and methionine, and are richer in cysteine, threonine, and valine compared to caseins proteins [5]. From these results, it can be suggested that changes in AA pattern during lactation could be explained by the presence to some extent of immune proteins in mature milk produced after the colostrum stage. On average lysine milk content concentration was not affected by stage of lactation ($P>0.05$) and averaged 7.24 g/ 16 g N; this value is rather similar to the levels reported by Elliott et al., King et al., and Dourmad et al. (7.30, 6.95, and 7.39 g lysine / 16 g N, respectively) [7,20,21].

The fatty acids composition of milk fat is presented in Table 5. In agreement with data previously published in the literature, more than 80% of the fatty acids in sow's milk fat were palmitic (16:0), oleic (18:1) and linoleic acids (18:2) (Miller et al., Csapó et al. and Gerfault et al.) [24-26]. According to Darragh and Moughan, most of the fatty acids founds in milk reflect closely those in the blood triacylglycerol which in turn are influenced by the type of dietary fat ingested by the sow and/ or the amount of mobilized maternal fat tissue [5]. In the present study, fatty acids composition in milk fat was not influenced ($P>0.05$) by the stage of lactation. Similarly, Bee did not report any change in fatty acids concentration in milk sampled on d 9, 16 or d 23 [27]. In contrast, Miller et al. and Csapó et al. showed that the proportion of linoleic acids (C18:2) was reduced whereas that of palmitoleic acid (C16:1) increased during lactation [24,25]. The discrepancy between the studies can be explained by differences in animal characteristics (genotype, milk production, ability to mobilize body reserves), in animal management (amount and FA composition of the diet; Rosero et al. [28]) or in the method of milk collection [5].

Residual correlations between sow performance and milk composition are presented in Table 6. Logically, the maternal BW loss during lactation was negatively correlated with ADFI (r=-0.76) and positively correlated with backfat thickness loss (r=0.55). In addition, there was a positive correlation between milk production and body reserves mobilisation (r=0.82). This result would suggest that in our experimental conditions in which appetite was limited by the hot environment, the ability of sows to produce milk depends of their capacity to mobilize body reserve for providing milk precursors. The polyunsaturated FA (PUFA) content in milk fat was positively correlated with ADFI and negatively correlated to maternal BW loss (r=0.62 and r=-0.60). The PUFA deposited in milk fat originated

	Lactation day, d				RSD	Statistical analysis
	7	14	21	27		
No. observations	18	18	18	18		
Saturated fatty acids, mg/L						
C12:0	14	17	17	15	4	
C14:0	178	195	201	179	36	
C16:0	1711	1814	1869	1783	295	
C18:0	287	262	258	246	50	
C20:0	13	16	16	15	7	
Total	2207	2307	2364	2240	362	
Total, %	37.1	38.0	38.9	38.0	2.6	
Monounsaturated fatty acids, mg/L						
C14:1	11	13	13	12	3	
C16:1	474	483	515	456	99	
C18:1	1799	1721	1751	1624	426	
C20:1	19	20	21	20	7	
Total	2313	2245	2308	2121	464	
Total, %	38.3	36.8	37.1	35.6	4.4	
Polyunsaturated fatty acids, mg/L						
C18:2	1274	1335	1306	1359	212	
C18:3	92	102	95	103	22	
C20:2	26	24	27	26	12	
C20:4	37	33	32	32	9	
Total	1410	1528	1497	1567	245	
Total, %	24.8	25.4	24.4	26.7	3.2	

[1]Residual Standard Variation; [2]From an analysis of variance with a general linear model including the effect of diet (D) and batch (B), lactation stage (S) and their interactions as fixed effects. Repeated measurements of milk chemical composition were analysed using an unstructured covariance structure with sows within batch as a subject. Statistical significance: * $P<0.05$, ** $P<0.01$.

Table 5: Effect of lactation stage on sows milk fatty acid composition (Least Square Means).

	ADFI	dlys intake	BW loss	BT loss	Milk
ADFI, g/d	1.00	–	–	–	–
dlys intake, g/d	**0.92**	1.00	–	–	–
BW loss, g/d	**-0.76**	**-0.55**	1.00	–	–
BT loss, g/d	-0.39	-0.29	**0.62**	1.00	–
Milk, g/d	**-0.49**	-0.34	**0.82**	0.40	1.00
Dry matter, %	0.14	0.10	0.05	0.37	0.09
Ash, % DM	0.02	0.05	-0.33	**-0.51**	-0.42
Crude protein, % DM	-0.17	0.01	0.08	-0.43	0.19
Fat, % DM	0.16	0.12	0.13	0.39	0.21
Lactose, % DM	0.07	0.16	-0.37	-0.08	-0.26
SFA, mg/L	0.38	0.42	-0.02	0.22	-0.15
MUFA, mg/L	-0.41	-0.21	**0.78**	0.41	**0.73**
PUFA, mg/L	**0.62**	**0.47**	**-0.60**	-0.33	**-0.69**
Lysine, g/16 g N	-0.39	**-0.53**	-0.04	-0.31	-0.20
Sulfur AA, g/16 g N	-0.14	-0.25	-0.33	-0.39	**-0.61**
Threonine, g/16 g N	-0.16	-0.33	-0.31	-0.40	**-0.49**
Tryptophan, g/16 g N	-0.32	**-0.49**	-0.17	**-0.54**	-0.27
Leucine, g/16 g N	**0.58**	0.41	**-0.74**	-0.09	**-0.79**
Isoleucine, g/16 g N	-0.30	-0.41	-0.06	-0.24	-0.23
Valine, g/16 g N	0.05	-0.09	**-0.46**	-0.30	**-0.67**
Arginine, g/16 g N	0.01	-0.22	0.07	-0.07	0.39
Histidine, g/16 g N	**-0.65**	-0.31	-0.12	-0.21	-0.26

[1]Sow performance: ADFI (average daily feed intake), Dlys (digestible lysine) intake, BW (body weight) loss, BT (backfat thickness) loss and milk (milk production). SFA, MUFA, and PUFA for saturated fatty acids (FA), monounsaturated FA, and polyunsaturated FA, respectively. Correlation coefficient in bold was significantly different from 0 ($P<0.05$).

Table 6: Residual correlation coefficients between lactation performance and chemical composition of milk of sows over a 28-d lactation[1].

mainly from dietary FA because animals cannot synthesize them, while saturated FA (SFA) and monounsaturated FA (MUFA) are derived from diet, mobilisation of fat tissue, or *de novo* synthesis. As a result, when sows are in a negative energy balance, a large amount of body reserves are mobilized and then exogenous PUFA are diluted with endogenous *de novo* synthesised fatty acids (SFA and MUFA). Finally, except for arginine, negative correlations were reported between milk production and AA concentration; the correlation coefficients were significantly different from zero only for sulphur AA, threonine, branched chain AA (leucine and valine). According to these results, changes in milk production would affect the AA composition of milk proteins. In conclusion, reducing dietary protein content can be an alternative to attenuate the negative effects of heat stress by increasing ADFI. Milk composition changes significantly according to lactation stage and the ability of sows to produce milk will depend on their capacity to mobilize body reserve for providing milk precursors.

Acknowledgements

The authors gratefully acknowledge Ajinomoto Eurolysine (Paris, France) for their financial support and for measurement of amino acid contents in feeds and in milk; the authors also gratefully acknowledge C. Anäis, M. Bructer, K. Benoni, T. Etienne for their technical assistance.

References

1. Etienne M, Dourmad JY, Noblet J (1998) The influence of some sow and piglet characteristics and of environmental conditions on milk production. The Lactating Sow, pp: 285-299.
2. Gourdine JL, Renaudeau D, Noblet J, Bidanel JP (2004) Effects of season and parity on performance of lactating sows in a tropical climate. Anim Sci 79: 273-282.
3. Renaudeau D, Anaïs C, Noblet J (2003) Effects of dietary fiber on performance of multiparous lactating sows in a tropical climate. J Anim Sci 81: 717-725.
4. Silva BAN, Noblet J, Oliveira RFM, Donzele JL, Primot Y, et al. (2009) Effects of dietary protein level and amino acids supplementation on the feeding behavior of multiparous lactating sows in a tropical humid climate. J Anim Sci 87: 2104-2112.
5. Darragh AJ, Moughan PJ (1988) Composition of sow' colostrum and milk. In: Verstegen MW, Moughan PJ, Schrama JW (eds.), The Lactating Sow. Wageningen Pers, Wageningen, pp: 1-19.
6. Gourdine JL, Bidanel JP, Noblet J, Renaudeau D (2005) Effects of breed and season on performance of lactating sows in a tropical humid climate. J Anim Sci 84: 360-369.
7. Dourmad JY, Noblet J, Etienne M (1998) Effect of protein and lysine supply on performance, nitrogen balance, and body composition changes of sows during lactation. J Anim Sci 76: 542-550.
8. Renaudeau D, Noblet J (2001) Effects of exposure to high ambient temperature and dietary protein level on sow milk production and performance of piglets. J Anim Sci 79: 1540-1548.
9. AOAC (1990) Official Methods of Analysis. 15th edn. The Association of Official Analytical Chemists, Washington, DC. P1106.
10. Folch J, Lee M, Sloane Stanley GH (1967) A simple method for the isolation and purification of total lipids from animal tissues. J Biol Chem 226: 497-509.
11. Morrison WR, Smith LM (1964) Preparation of fatty acid methyl esters and dimethylacetals from lipids with boron fluoride methanol. J Lipid Res 5: 600-608.
12. Noblet J, Etienne M (1989) Estimation of sow milk nutrient output. J Anim Sci 67: 3352-3359.
13. Renaudeau D, Quiniou N, Noblet J (2001) Effects of exposure to high ambient temperature and dietary protein level on performance of multiparous lactating sows. J Anim Sci 79:1240-1249.
14. Lynch PB (1989) Voluntary food intake of sows and gilts. In: Smith AT, Lawrence TLJ (eds.), Pig Housing and the Environment. British Society of Animal Production, Edinburgh, UK, pp: 71-77.
15. Quiniou N, Noblet J (1999) Influence of high ambient temperatures on performance of multiparous lactating sows. J Anim Sci 77: 2124-2134.
16. Trottier NL, Easter RA (1995) Dietary and plasma branched-chain amino acids in relation to tryptophan: Effect on voluntary feed intake and lactation metabolism in the primiparous sow. J Anim Sci 73: 1086-1092.
17. Tackman JM, Tews JK, Harper AE (1990) Dietary disproportions of amino acids in the rats: effects on food intake, plasma and brain amino acids and brain serotonin. J Nutr 120: 521-533.

18. Henry Y, Séve B (1993) Feed intake and dietary amino acid balance in growing pigs with special reference to lysine, tryptophan and threonine. Pig News Info 14: 35-43.

19. Johnston LJ, Ellis M, Libal GW, Mayrose VB, Weldon WC, et al. (1999) Effect of room temperature and dietary amino acid concentration on performance of lactating sows. J Anim Sci 77: 1638-1644.

20. Elliott RF, Vander Noot GW, Gilbreath RL, Fisher H (1971) Effect of Dietary Protein Level on Composition Changes in Sow Colostrum and Milk. J Anim Sci 32: 1128-1137.

21. King RH, Toner MS, Dove H, Atwood CS, Brown WG (1993) The response of first-litter sows to dietary protein level during lactation. J Anim Sci 71: 2457-2463.

22. Salmon-Legagneur E (1965) Some aspects of nutritional relationships between pregnancy and lactation in the sow. Ann Zootech 14: 1-137.

23. Klobasa F, Werhahn E, Butler JE (1987) Composition of sow milk during lactation. J Anim Sci 64: 1458-1466.

24. Csapó J, Martin TG, Csapó-kiss ZS, Hjzas Z (1996) Protein, fats, vitamin and mineral concentrations in porcine colostrum and milk from parturition to 60 days. Int Dairy J 6: 881-902.

25. Miller GM, Conrad JH, Harrington RB (1971) Effect of Dietary Unsaturated Fatty Acids and Stage of Lactation on Milk Composition and Adipose Tissue in Swine. J Anim Sci 32: 79-83.

26. Gerfault V, Mourot J, Etienne M, Mounier A (1999) Influence of the source of lipids added to the sow pregnancy diet on reproductive performance and on body composition of piglets at birth. Journées de la Recherche Porcine en France 31: 191-197.

27. Bee G (2000) Dietary conjugated linoleic acids alter adipose tissue and milk lipids of pregnant and lactating Sows. J Nutr 130: 2292-2298.

28. Rosero DS, Odle J, Mendoza SM, Boyd RD, Fellner V, et al. (2015) Impact of dietary lipids on sow milk composition and balance of essential fatty acids during lactation in prolific sows. J Anim Sci 93: 2935-2947.

Higher Intake of Milk-Replacer Pre-Weaning Enhances Post-Weaning Insulin-Like Growth Factor 1 Levels in Japanese Black Cattle

Hideyuki Takahashi[1]*, Atsuko Matsubara[1], Akira Saito[2], Ouanh Phomvisith[1], Akari Shiga[1], Ha T Mai[1], Toshihisa Sugino[3], Christopher D McMahon[4], Tetsuji Etoh[1], Yuji Shiotsuka[1], Ryoichi Fujino[1], Mitsuhiro Furuse[1] and Takafumi Gotoh[1]*

[1]*Kuju Agricultural Research Center, Kyushu University, 878-0201 Kuju-cho, Oita, Japan*
[2]*Zenrakuren, Shiba 4-17-5, Minato-ku, 108-0014 Tokyo, Japan*
[3]*Graduate School of Biosphere Science, Hiroshima University, Higashi-Hiroshima, Higashi-Hiroshima-shi, 739-8528 Hiroshima, Japan*
[4]*AgResearch Ltd, Private Bag 3123, Hamilton, New Zealand*

Abstract

Alterations in early pre-natal nutrition of Japanese Black calves influence the glucose and lipid metabolism after weaning. However, the effects of early nutritional status on the endocrine system in later life stages in Japanese Black cattle are unknown. This study examined how post-weaning plasma levels of growth hormone (GH), insulin-like growth factor 1 (IGF-1), and blood insulin, which are hormones affecting growth and meat quality, and metabolites were affected by feeding 1800 g versus 500 g of milk replacer to Japanese Black cattle (5 per group) during nursing. Up to weaning (90 days post-birth), all calves received calf starter and hay *ad libitum*, and post-weaning, they received a concentrate feed and hay *ad libitum*. Plasma concentrations of GH and IGF-1 were greater at weaning in the high-milk-replacer group ($P<0.1$ and $P<0.01$, respectively), and elevated IGF-1 concentrations persisted until the study end (210 d) ($P<0.05$), suggesting that the levels were sustained independent of the influences of both GH and nutrient intake. Blood insulin and metabolites (plasma glucose, beta-hydroxybutyric acid, and non-esterified fatty acids) were not significantly different between the two groups. The results of this study suggest that feeding calves a high volume of milk replacer during nursing will increase IGF-1 secretion well beyond weaning.

Keywords: Japanese Black cattle; Growth hormone; Insulin-like growth factor 1; Milk replacer; Ruminant growth rate

Abbreviations: GH: Growth hormone; IGF-1: Insulin-like growth factor 1; CP: Crude protein; CF: Crude fat; TDN: Total digestible nutrients; TR-FIA: Time-resolved fluoroimmunoassay.

Introduction

Nutrient composition and availability during the early growth phase affects tissue composition and metabolism at adulthood in mammals [1]. A high plane of nutrition during the initial growth phase affects meat quantity and quality in 10-mo-old crossbred steers (Japanese Black male × Holstein female) [2]. In addition, feeding high quantities of milk to Japanese Black cattle until 150 d of age increases post-weaning growth, glucose concentrations and lipid metabolism [3]. However, there is a lack of information about the effect of a high plane of nutrition pre-weaning on the endocrine system in post-weaning of Japanese Black cattle.

In ruminants, changes to the nutritional status and nutrient intake of feed alter hormone secretion [4,5]. Specifically, increased concentrations of growth hormone (GH) trigger the secretion of insulin-like growth factor 1 (IGF-1) in rats [6,7] and in beef cattle [8]. Increased concentrations of both hormones in blood are linked to muscle growth and, thus, the amount of lean meat in cattle [9,10]. Based on the afore mentioned findings, we hypothesized that a high plane of nutrition offered pre-weaning might affect post-weaning secretion of GH and IGF-1 in Japanese Black cattle. Previously, we reported positive correlations between the pre-weaning period of nutrition, plasma insulin and blood metabolite levels (plasma glucose, beta-hydroxybutyric acid [β-HBA], non-esterified fatty acids [NEFAs]) and post-weaning growth rate in these calves [2,3]. Therefore, in this study, we sought to assess how a high-nutrient feed affects the relationship between hormones, blood metabolites and growth rate.

Materials and Methods

Experimental animals

All experimental procedures, including animal care and handling, were performed in accordance with guidelines from the Committee for Animal Welfare of Kyushu University.

Ten Japanese Black male calves were randomly assigned to two groups. The calves of both groups were fed milk replacer containing 26% crude protein (CP), 25.5% crude fat (CF) and 116% total digestible nutrients (TDNs). The quantity of milk replacer was determined according to a previous study [3]. Five control calves (initial body weight; 32.7 ± 1.19) were provided with 500 g/d of milk replacer from 14 to 90 d of age. Five calves in the experimental group (initial body weight; 33.6 ± 1.90) received 800 g/d until 14 d of age. Between 4 and 27 d, the amount of milk replacer was progressively increased to 1800 g/d and maintained at this level until 72 d. From 73 to 85 d, milk replacer was gradually reduced to 800 g/d, where it remained until weaning at

***Corresponding authors:** Hideyuki Takahashi, Kuju Agricultural Research Center, Kyushu University, 878-0201 Kuju-cho, Oita, Japan
E-mail: takahashi@farm.kyushu-u.ac.jp

Takafumi Gotoh, Kuju Agricultural Research Center, Kyushu University, 878-0201 Kuju-cho, Oita, Japan, E-mail: gotoh@farm.kyushu-u.ac.jp

90 d. Both experimental and control calves were fed calf starter (TDN, 72%; CP, 18%; ether extract, 2%) from 30 to 90 d. Between 90 to 210 d, calves were fed concentrate (CP, 16%; CF, 2.5%; TDN, 68%). The calves and cattle were fed concentrate at quantities necessary for individual weight gain of 1 kg/d, as recommended by the Japanese Feeding Standard for Beef Cattle [11] and hay (CP, 13.4%; CF, 3.6%; TDN, 59.3%) *ad libitum*. Body weight was measured at 90 and 210 d of age.

Blood samples

The secretion of GH in cattle is pulsatile [12]; therefore, a single blood sample may not reflect the average concentration of GH in blood. To reduce variability, we took advantage of the fact that GH release is synchronized around feeding, with a burst immediately prior, followed by no secretion during or for at least 1 h after feeding [13]. Therefore, we collected blood samples to coincide with the pre-feeding secretory episode.

Blood samples were collected from the jugular vein into heparinized tubes with aprotinin (500 kallikrein inhibitory units/mL of blood; Sigma-Aldrich Inc., Tokyo, Japan) before calves were provided their morning feed at 90, 150, and 210 d of age. Blood samples were centrifuged at 2330 × g at room temperature for 30 min and stored at -40°C until analysis. Concentrations of GH and IGF-1 were measured using a time-resolved fluoroimmunoassay (TR-FIA) as previously described [4,14]. Intra- and inter-assay coefficients of variability (CVs) for GH were 2.6% and 3.6%, respectively; for IGF-1, they were 6.9% and 5.5%, respectively. The lowest detectable doses of GH and IGF-1 in this assay were 0.158 ng/mL and 0.053 ng/mL, respectively. Insulin, glucose, β-HBA and NEFA concentrations were measured, respectively, with a bovine insulin enzyme-linked immunosorbent assay kit (Mercodia, Uppsala, Sweden), glucose oxidase enzymatic method (glucose B-test; Wako Pure Chemical, Osaka, Japan), β-HBA enzyme-linked immunosorbent assay kit (Cusabio Biotech, Wuhan, China), and acyl-CoA synthetase-acyl-CoA oxidase enzymatic method (FFAC; Wako Pure Chemical Industries Ltd., Osaka, Japan), following manufacturer protocols.

Statistical analyses

Body weight gain, milk replacer, CP and CF intake, and plasma GH and IGF-1 concentrations are presented as mean ± SEM. StatView 5 (SAS Institute Inc., Cary, NC, USA) was used for statistical analyses of GH and IGF-1 concentrations. Post-hoc comparisons between the control and experimental groups were performed with two-tailed, unpaired Student's t-tests. Data for GH, IGF-1, and insulin and blood metabolite profiles were analyzed using the MIXED procedure in SAS (SAS Institute Inc.) in which the treatment was a fixed effect while cattle and feeding period were random effects. For statistical analyses of plasma hormones and metabolite concentrations, the interaction of sampling time by treatment was added to the model.

Results and Discussion

At 90 d, mean concentrations of GH tended to be higher in the experimental group than in the controls ($P<0.1$), but these differences disappeared by 150 and 200 d of age (Figure 1a). Overall, concentrations of GH varied with dietary treatment (P=0.03) and age ($P<0.01$), although the interaction of age and treatment was not significant ($P=0.15$) (Figure 1a). These results are in accordance with previous reports wherein changing the amount of milk replacer have little influence concentrations of GH in nursing Holstein bull calves [15], but that basal and growth hormone-releasing hormone (GHRH)-induced GH concentrations decline with age in dairy cattle

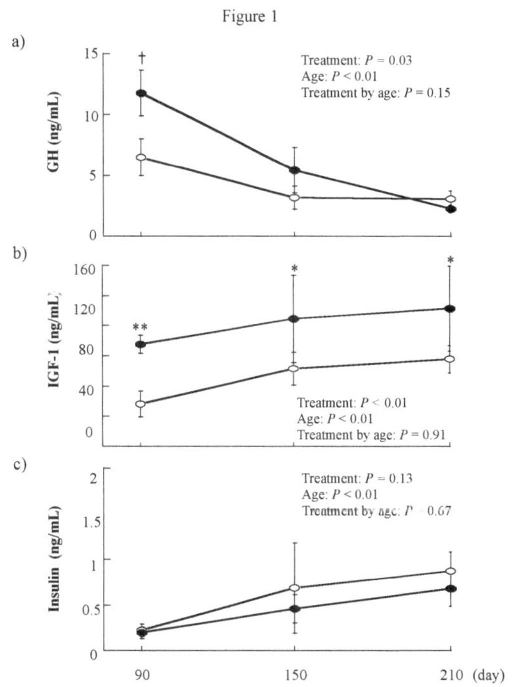

Figure 1: Plasma concentrations of (a) growth hormone (GH), (b) insulin-like growth factor 1 (IGF-1), and (c) insulin in control (○) and experimental (•) groups at 90, 150, and 210 d of age. Values are means ± SEM (n=5/group). **$P<0.01$; *$P<0.05$; †$P<0.1$.

[16]. Therefore, age may influence the secretion of GH more than the amount of milk consumed in nursing and just-weaned calves.

Plasma concentrations of IGF-1 were significantly greater in the experimental group than in the controls at all measured time points ($P<0.05$; Figure 1b). Moreover, although total intake of CP did not differ between the two groups at 90 d, experimental animals had a higher intake of CP from the milk replacer than the control animals ($P<0.01$; Table 1). Our findings are in agreement with work showing that both GH and dietary CP regulate secretion of IGF-1 in beef cattle [8]. The increased concentrations of IGF-1 in the experimental calves could thus be attributed to increased protein content ingested from the high-milk-replacer diet, which is easily digested and absorbed (compared with other protein sources such as soy), resulting in superior calf performance (in male Holsteins; [17]). However, we also found that experimental calves maintained higher concentrations of IGF-1 after weaning ($P<0.01$). Additionally, concentrations of IGF-1 increased in both groups with age ($P<0.01$), but there was no age by treatment interaction ($P=0.91$) (Figure 1b). Given the lack of differences in GH concentrations and CP intake after weaning between the two groups (Table 1 and Figure 1a), these data suggest that GH and CP intake may actively regulate IGF-1 secretion during nursing while also priming an independent mechanism to maintain post-weaning secretion. Our previous studies similarly revealed that a high volume of milk replacer fed to nursing calves influenced both meat quality and the expression of genes related to post-weaning nutrient metabolism [3,18,19].

Moreover, research in humans has shown that individuals that were fed milk replacer during infancy ingested more protein and exhibited higher IGF-1 concentrations at 6 mo compared with breastfed individuals [19]. A subsequent study confirmed the influence of early-life protein consumption: infants fed high-protein milk replacer had higher concentrations of IGF-1 in blood compared with

	Control	Experimental
Body weight (at 90 d, kg)	90.8 ± 4.80	118.7 ± 8.33*
Body weight (at 210 d, kg)	226.6 ± 9.51	249.2 ± 13.90
Average daily gain (kg/d)	0.92 ± 0.04	1.03 ± 0.06
Pre-weaning (0-90 d, kg)		
Milk replacer intake		
DM	38.26 ± 0.57	93.94 ± 6.97**
CP	9.95 ± 0.15	24.42 ± 1.81**
CF	9.76 ± 0.15	23.95 ± 1.78**
Calf starter intake		
DM	59.56 ± 3.15	18.21 ± 1.29**
CP	10.72 ± 0.57	3.28 ± 0.23**
CF	1.19 ± 0.10	0.36 ± 0.03**
Hay intake		
DM	31.97 ± 1.69	14.84 ± 1.05**
CP	4.28 ± 0.23	1.98 ± 0.14**
CF	1.15 ± 0.06	0.53 ± 0.04**
Total intake		
CP	24.95 ± 0.77	29.69 ± 2.18
CF	12.10 ± 0.17	24.85 ± 1.84**
Post-weaning (90-210 d, kg)		
DM	344.2 ± 14.40	346.5 ± 19.30
CP	62.58 ± 2.63	63.01 ± 3.51
CF	9.78 ± 0.41	9.85 ± 0.55
Hay intake		
DM	228.7 ± 9.6	263.2 ± 14.7
CP	36.6 ± 1.53	42.1 ± 2.35
CF	9.83 ± 0.41	11.3 ± 0.63
Total intake		
CP	99.15 ± 4.16	105.09 ± 5.86
CF	19.60 ± 0.82	21.15 ± 1.18

Table 1: Average weight gain and daily intake of Japanese Black calves fed milk replacer, calf starter, concentrate, and hay as well as nutritional components (CP and CF). DM: Dry matter; CP: Crude protein; CF: Crude fat; Data for feed intake are expressed as the mean ± SEM (n=5). ***P*<0.01, **P*<0.05.

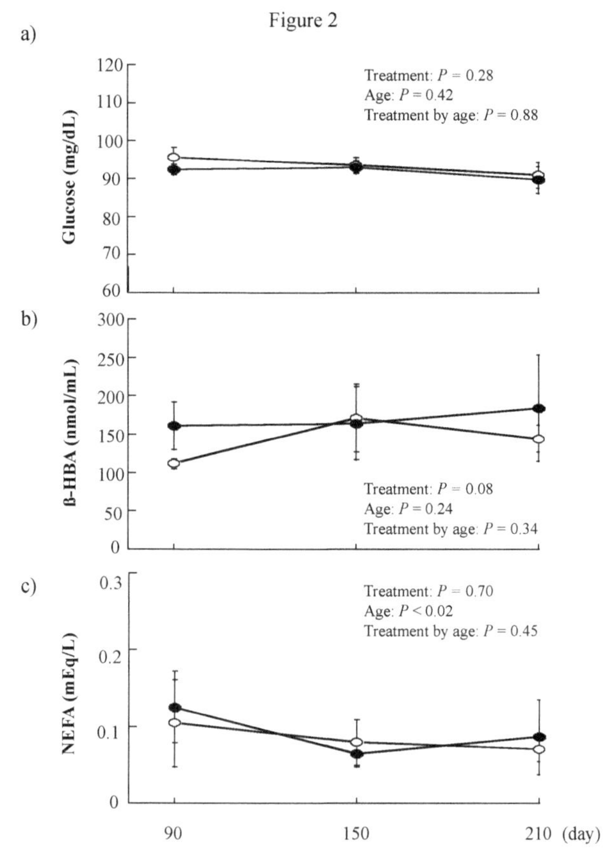

Figure 2: Plasma concentrations of (a) glucose, (b) beta-hydroxybutyric acid (β-HBA), and (c) non-esterified fatty acids (NEFAs) in control (○) and experimental (●) groups at 90, 150, and 210 d of age. Values are means ± SEM (n=5/group).

those fed low-protein milk replacer, and elevated concentrations of IGF-1 persisted through to adolescence [20]. Together, current and previous observations are consistent with nutritional programming, a phenomenon wherein nursing-diet quality or quantity (e.g., more high-protein milk replacer) has a persistent post-weaning effect [21]. Future studies should, therefore, focus on elucidating the mechanisms underlying the nutritional programming of IGF-1 secretion in Japanese Black cattle, specifically verifying the potential link with a high-milk-replacer diet during nursing.

In the current study, concentrations of insulin did not differ between the two groups (P=0.13), although it did vary with age (P<0.01), and the age by treatment interaction was not significant (P=0.67) (Figure 1c). Thus, the observed changes were the result of age alone. Our results are in accordance with previous work showing a positive correlation between age and insulin concentrations in the blood of Japanese Black cattle [22].

Calves in the experimental group weighed more than control calves at 90 d, although these differences disappeared by 210 d (Table 1). Moreover, a higher amount of milk appeared to have negligible effects on blood metabolite concentrations (Figure 2). In contrast, our previous study showed that feeding high volumes of milk replacer to nursing Japanese Black cattle increased growth performance and blood metabolite (glucose, β-HBA, NEFA) concentrations compared with the control (data not shown). Post-weaning up-regulation of glucose/lipid-metabolism-related gene expression subsequently decreased blood metabolites in the experimental group [3]. These differences may be due to variations in feeding periods; calves received a high-milk-replacer diet for 48 d over the 90-d feeding period in this study, whereas they received milk replacer for 90 d over a 150-d feeding period in Matsubara et al. [3]. These results combined suggest that a 48-d maximum nursing period is not sufficient and that the duration should be extended beyond 90 d to improve the growth performance, as well as glucose and lipid metabolism, of Japanese Black calves.

Although we had previously demonstrated that a high-milk-replacer treatment increased concentrations of β-HBA and NEFA (data not shown), we did not observe a significant difference in lipid concentrations between groups in this study despite high CF intake during nursing (Figures 2b and 2c). Equivocal results from fat-supplemented diets have been reported elsewhere. For example, such diets increased concentrations of β-HBA and NEFA in some dairy cattle (Holstein cows [23]), but not in others [24]. Given these inconsistent effects of CF intake on concentrations of β-HBA and NEFA, further research is required to explore how milk fat influences lipid metabolism in calves.

In conclusion, a high milk-replacer diet more strongly affected plasma IGF-1 concentrations than GH concentrations in Japanese Black cattle. Furthermore, the plane of nutrition during nursing may program post-weaning regulation and secretion of IGF-1 resulting in prolonged or permanent changes to secretion patterns. Further studies are warranted to determine the mechanisms by which IGF-1 secretion is maintained in ruminants fed high volumes of milk replacer and whether such changes affect body composition at maturity. Data from this study provides direction for the effective regulation of early feeding regimes to improve meat quantity and quality in the cattle industry.

Acknowledgements

We thank Dr. AF Parlow and the National Hormone and Pituitary Program at the National Institute of Diabetes and Digestive and Kidney Diseases (NIDDK) for bovine GH protein and antibodies. This study was supported by Zenrakuren, Japan and Ito-Kinen-Zaidan, Japan.

References

1. Sinclair KD, Lea RG, Rees WD, Young LE (2007) The developmental origins of health and disease: current theories and epigenetic mechanisms. Soc Reprod Fertil Suppl 64: 425-443.
2. Ebara F, Inada S, Morikawa M, Asaoka SH, Isozaki Y, et al. (2013) Effect of nutrient intake on intramuscular glucose metabolism during the early growth stage in cross-bred steers (Japanese Black male × Holstein female). J Anim Physiol Anim Nutr 97: 684-693.
3. Matsubara A, Takahashi H, Saito A, Nomura A, Sithyphone K, et al. (2016) Effects of a high milk intake during the pre-weaning period on nutrient metabolism and growth rate in Japanese Black cattle. Anim Sci J 87: 1130-1136.
4. Takahashi H, Kurose Y, Suzuki Y, Kojima M, Yamaguchi T, et al. (2009) Ghrelin differentially modulates the GH secretory response to GHRH between the fed and fasted states in sheep. Domest Anim Endocrinol 37: 55-60.
5. Laarman AH, Ruiz-Sanchez AL, Sugino T, Guan LL, Oba M (2012) Effects of feeding a calf starter on molecular adaptations in the ruminal epithelium and liver of Holstein dairy calves. J Dairy Sci 95: 2585-2594.
6. Roberts CT Jr, Brown AL, Graham DE, Seelig S, Berry S, et al. (1986) Growth hormone regulates the abundance of insulin-like growth factor I RNA in adult rat liver. J Biol Chem 261: 10025-10028.
7. Isgaard J, Nilsson A, Vikman K, Isaksson OGP (1989) Growth hormone regulates the level of insulin-like growth factor-I mRNA in rat skeletal muscle. J Endocrinol 120: 107-112.
8. Elsasser TH, Rumsey TS, Hammond AC (1989) Influence of diet on basal and growth hormone-stimulated plasma concentrations of IGF-I in beef cattle. J Anim Sci 67: 128-141.
9. Florini JR, Ewton DZ, Coolican SA (1996) Growth hormone and the insulin-like growth factor system in myogenesis. Endocr Rev 17: 481-517.
10. Gotoh T, Takahashi H, Nishimura T, Kuchida K, Mannen H (2014) Meat produced by Japanese Black cattle and Wagyu. Anim Front 4: 46-54.
11. Agriculture, Forestry and Fisheries Research Council Secretariat, Ministry of Agriculture, Forestry and Fisheries (MAFF) (2000) Available from URL: http://www.maff.go.jp/e/
12. Gluckman PD, Breier BH, Davis SR (1987) Physiology of the somatotropic axis with particular reference to the ruminant. J Dairy Sci 70: 442-466.
13. McMahon CD, Radcliff RP, Lookingland KJ, Tucker HA (2001) Neuroregulation of growth hormone secretion in domestic animals. Domestic Animal Endocrinology 20: 65-87.
14. Sugino T, Hasegawa Y, Kikkawa Y, Yamaura J, Yamagishi M, et al. (2002) A transient ghrelin surge occurs just before feeding in a scheduled meal-fed sheep. Biochem Biophys Res Comm 295: 255-260.
15. Quigley JD, Wolfe TA, Elsasser TH (2006) Effects of additional milk replacer feeding on calf health, growth, and selected blood metabolites in calves. J Dairy Sci 89: 207-216.
16. Hodate K, Johke T, Kawabata A, Fuse H, Ohashi S (1988) Age-associated changes in bovine growth hormone release via human growth-releasing factor. Japanese J Zootech Sci 59: 285-291.
17. Silva AG, Huber JT, DeGregorio RM (1986) Influence of substituting two types of soybean protein for milk protein on gain and utilization of milk replacers in calves. J Dairy Sci 69: 172-180.
18. Gotoh T (2010) Metabolic imprinting effects in grass-fed Wagyu (Japanese Black) beef production. FASEB 24: 90-94.
19. Scheffler JM, McCann MA, Greiner SP, Jiang H, Hanigan MD, et al. (2014) Early metabolic imprinting events increase marbling scores in fed cattle. J Anim Sci 92: 320-324.
20. Socha P, Janas R, Dobrzańska A, Koletzko B, Broekaert I, et al. (2005) Insulin like growth factor regulation of body mass in breastfed and milk formula fed infants. Data from the EU Childhood Obesity Programme. Adv Exp Med Biol 569: 159-163.
21. Larnkjaer A, Ingstrup HK, Schack-Nielsen L, Hoppe C, Mølgaard C, et al. (2009) Early programming of the IGF-1 axis: negative association between IGF-1 in infancy and late adolescence in a 17 year longitudinal follow-up study of healthy subjects. Growth Horm IGF Res 19: 82-86.
22. Martin PM, Holly JM, Smith GD, Ness AR, Emmett P, et al. (2005) Could associations between breastfeeding and insulin-like growth factors underlie associations of breastfeeding with adult chronic disease? The Avon Longitudinal Study of Parents and Children. Clin Endocrinol 62: 728-737.
23. Matsuzaki M, Takizawa S, Ogawa M (1997) Plasma insulin, metabolite concentrations, and carcass characteristics of Japanese Black, Japanese Brown, and Holstein steers. J Anim Sci 75: 3287-3293.
24. Skaar TC, Grummer RR, Dentine MR, Stauffacher RH (1989) Seasonal effects of prepartum and postpartum fat and niacin feeding on lactation performance and lipid metabolism. J Dairy Sci 72: 2028-2038.

Study of Ruminant Fasciolosis in Selected Districts in Upper Awash River Basin, South Western Shoa, Ethiopia

Melaku Taye[1], Teshome Jagema[2], Asefa Tadese[3], Endalu Mulatu[4], Kumela Lelisa[5] and Delesa Damena[6]*

[1]*South West Shoa Livestock Development and Fishery Office, Woliso, Oromia, Ethiopia*
[2]*Oromia Livestock Development and Fishery Office, Finfinne, Oromia, Ethiopia*
[3]*Ambo University, College of Agriculture, Ambo, Oromia, Ethiopia*
[4]*Bedelle College of Agriculture and Forestry, Mettu University, Bedelle, Oromia, Ethiopia*
[5]*National Institute for Control and Eradication of Tsetse Fly and Trypanomosis, Addis Ababa, Ethiopia*
[6]*National Animal Health Diagnostic and Investigation Center, Sebeta, Oromia, Ethiopia*

Abstract

A cross-sectional study was conducted in February 2013 to determine the prevalence of fasciolosis in cattle and sheep in areas adjacent to the upper Awash River basin, South Western Shoa, Ethiopia. A total of 399 (308 bovine and 91 ovine) faecal samples were collected from Illu and Sebeta Hawas districts and microscopically examined using sedimentation techniques. Eggs of *Fasciola* species were identified based on their characteristic morphology and colour. Besides, a gross pathological examination was conducted on a total of 237 livers of slaughtered animals at Sebeta municipal abattoir to identify *Fasciola* species and assess the extent of infection. Coprological examinations revealed that, significantly higher prevalence (48.4%) in sheep than in cattle (36.7%). Similarly, a prevalence rate recorded in Illu district (45.6%) was significantly higher than that of Sebeta Hawas district (34.7%). Out of a total of 237 livers examined, 38.4% (91) were infected by one or more *Fasciola* species. The majority (54.9%) of the infection was caused by *F. hepatica* followed by *F. gigantica* (28.6%) and mixed species (16.5%). This study showed that, fasciolosis is exerting a significant impact on livestock production and productivity in the study areas. Therefore, proper control scheme should be designed and implemented in areas adjacent to the upper Awash River basin to minimize the burden of fasciolosis.

Keywords: Prevalence; Fasciolosis; Bovine; Ovine; South West Shoa; Ethiopia

Introduction

Ethiopia is endowed with high livestock population with 54 million heads of cattle and 25.5 million sheep; the large proportions of which are kept in traditional extensive production system [1]. Despite the large population of animals, productivity in Ethiopia is low and below the average compared to most countries in Sub-Saharan Africa. This is mainly due to poor nutrition, reproduction insufficiency, management constraints and animal diseases [2].

Fasciolosis is one of the most important parasitic diseases that hamper livestock production in Ethiopia [3]. *F. hepatica* (the high land) and *F. gigantica* (low land) types of liver flukes cause severe economic losses in different parts of the country. Effects of fasciolosis are usually expressed in terms of liver condemnation at slaughter houses, infertility, reduction in traction power and low weight at birth and mortality [4-7]. It occurs in water logged and marshy grazing areas, particularly along the Abay (Blue Nile) river basin. It is also highly prevalent in the high land and low land areas of Oromia regional state [2]. The intermediate hosts for both *F. hepatica* and *F. gigantica* are snails of the family Lymnaesidae. *L. truncatula* is the most important and common intermediate host for *F. hepatica* in different parts of Ethiopia [4].

Understanding the local epidemiology of fasciolosis could help to device and implement effective control programs [8]. Sebeta Hawas and Illu districts also known as Bacho, constitute a significant part of the upper Awash River basin. In these districts, Awash River is known to cause annual over flooding of wide areas during long Ethiopian rainy season leaving large water bodies and swampy areas for an extended period into the dry season. Although this creates a favourable environment for breeding of snail hosts, information is lacking on the extent and magnitude of Fasciolosis in the areas. Therefore, this study was initiated with the aim of determining the prevalence of bovine and ovine fasciolosis and assessing associated risk factors in Sebeta Hawas and Illu districts of central Ethiopia.

Materials and Methods

Study location

The study was carried out in Sebeta Hawas and Ellu districts of South Western Shoa, located adjacent to uplands of the Awash River basin, 50 kms west of Addis Ababa. The area has an altitude of 1800-3385 meters above sea level (masl) and is characterized by long rainy season (June - September), short rainy season (March- may) and a dry season (October- January). The average annual rain fall, annual temperature and relative humidity are 866-1200 mm, 11.3-28°C and 49.3% respectively. Awash River floods the areas during the long Ethiopian rainy season and leave large water bodies and swampy places for an extended period into the dry season. Mixed agriculture is the mainstay of the livelihood of the society where crop and livestock production play integral roles. Small scale irrigation is wide spread for production of cash crops in the areas.

Study animals

The study population constituted of indigenous zebu cattle and sheep. The animals are kept under traditional extensive husbandry system with communal grazing lands and watering points. Animal

***Corresponding author:** Delesa Damena, National Animal Health Diagnostic and Investigation Center, Sebeta, PO Box 04, Oromia, Ethiopia
E-mail: delesa_damenaa@yahoo.com

population of the district consisted of 33,610 cattle, 1,945 goats, 6,202 sheep, and 6,753 equines.

Sampling and sample size determination

A cross-sectional study was conducted in February 2013 to estimate the prevalence of fasciolosis and assess associated risk factors. The study sites were selected based on their accessibility to transport and availability of suitable habitat for snail host and the parasite. Owners were informed one day a head of sample collection to gather their animals at one place and simple random sampling technique was employed to select the study from the population. The sample size required was calculated at 50% prevalence with level of precision at 5% and 95% confidence interval using a formula described by Thrusfield [9]. As the actual prevalence was unknown, 50% was used to produce the largest sample size possible. Therefore, a total of 384 animals were needed to sample. However, a total of 399 (308 cattle and 91 sheep) were sampled to increase the precision of the study. Age, sex and body condition score of the studied animals were recorded during sampling. The age was estimated by means of dentition. Cattle were grouped as calf (up to 1 year), young (1-3 years) and adult above 3 years while sheep were grouped as lamb (up to 6 months), young (6-12 months) and adult above 1 year [10]. The body condition status of selected animals was assessed and ranked as good, medium and poor [11]. Besides, growth pathological examination was conducted on 237 bovine livers at Sebeta municipal abattoir.

Coprological study

For coprological examination, faecal samples were collected directly from rectum early in the morning, preserved in 10% formalin and transported to the National Animal Health Diagnostic and Investigation Centre (NAHDIC) for laboratory diagnosis. Faecal examination for *Fasciola* eggs was carried out using sedimentation method as described by Hansen and Perry [12]. 2 grams of faeces was added to 42 ml of water in a graduated cylinder. The contents were then mixed thoroughly using a glass rod, and were poured through a tea strainer to remove large debris. The solution was then further passed through a sieve (mesh aperture 210 mm) into a conical flask and water was run through the sieve to ensure no eggs remained attached to the sieve. The filtrate was then allowed to sediment for 3 min after which the supernatant was siphoned off taking care not to disturb the precipitated matters. The latter was stained with two drops of methylene blue and the entire sediment placed on slide covered with a cover slip and viewed under a compound microscope (Labomed). Eggs of *Fasciola* species were identified by their characteristic morphology and colour.

Abattoir survey

In abattoir survey, livers of slaughtered animals were registered and examined according to the description given by Dwinger et al. [13]. The affected liver was designated as lightly affected: if none or only enlarged bile duct was seen or if the quarter of the liver was affected before cutting on the visceral surface, cutting reveals enlarged bile ducts and/or flukes. **Moderately affected:** If half of the organ was affected and more than one enlarged bile ducts were visible before cutting. **Severely affected:** If the entire organ was involved or if the liver was cirrhotic. Additionally, the gall bladder was removed from the rest of the liver and the contents were checked for the presence of adult *Fasciola* species. The bile duct was carefully opened with scissors and searched for adult flukes. The rest of the liver was cut into an approximate size of 1 cm thick slices and pressed between fingers to expose flukes lodged in small liver ducts. Identification of recovered fluke species was done as described by Urquhart et al. [14].

Data analysis

Raw data were entered into a Microsoft Excel spreadsheet and descriptive statistics were used to summarize the data. STATA® version 11.0 statistical software programs were used to analyze the data. The prevalence was calculated for all data as the number of infected positives divided by the total number examined and multiplied by 100. The association between the prevalence of Fasciolosis and risk factors were assessed by chi-square test (χ^2). The test result was considered significant when the calculated p-value was less than 0.05 at 95% confidence interval.

Results

An overall prevalence of 36.7% (113/399) was recorded in this study. The prevalence of fasciolosis was significantly higher in ovine species (48.4%) than in bovine species (36.7%) as shown in Table 1. Similarly, a prevalence recorded in Illu district (45.6%) was significantly higher than that of Sebeta Hawas district (34.7%) (Table 2).

In abattoir survey, out of a total of 237 livers examined, 38.4% (91) were infected by one or more *Fasciola* species. The majority (54.9%) of the infection was caused by F. hepatica followed by *F. gigantica* (28.6%) and mixed species (16.5%) as shown in Table 3. The majority (48.5%) of the infected livers were moderately affected (Table 4). Variables such as age and sex were not significantly associated with the prevalence of fasciolosis.

Discussions

The current study revealed that fasciolosis is among economically important diseases in the study area. Coprological examination revealed a prevalence rate of 36.7% in cattle and 48.4% in sheep. This finding is higher than the results of most of the earlier studies in Ethiopia [15,16]. However, studies in different parts of Ethiopia showed a huge variation of prevalence rate ranging from 20.3% to 90.7% [8,17-19]. This disparity could have been attributed to the differences in climatic and ecological conditions, study methodology and sampling strategy. In addition to the variations in climatic and ecological conditions, the seasons in which the studies were conducted could contribute to the variations that exist among different findings in different areas [20]. In dry seasons, snails are forced to undergo aestivation deep in the mud in search of moisture. Only those snails in permanent water source have the opportunity to shed cercariae and hence low prevalence rate in dry season [20,21].

The higher prevalence recorded in dry season in this study suggests the presence of a suitable habitat for breeding of the snails and development of the parasites throughout the year. In addition to the presence of large swampy areas, the presence of small scale irrigation in some places could have been contributed in making favourable environment for snails; consequently leading to the wide spread distribution of the disease. Irrigation has a huge potential to facilitate transmission of water borne human and animal diseases. Aquatic or amphibian intermediate host transmit diseases such as malaria, fasciolosis and shistosomiasis [22].

The prevalence in Illu district (45.6%) was significantly higher than that of Sebeta Hawas district (34.7). This could be due to the presence

Species	n	Positives	Prevalence (%)	P-value
Bovine	308	113	36.7	0.03
Ovine	91	44	48.4	

Table 1: Prevalence of fasciolosis in Sebeta Hawas and Ellu districts of south west shoa, Ethiopia.

Species	Variable	Category	Number examined	Number of Positive	Prevalence (%)	Chi-sq result	*P- value*
bovine	Age	Calf Young Adult	24 66 218	7 26 80	29.2 39.4 36.7	0.793	0.673
	Sex	Female Male	132 176	50 63	37.9 35.8	0.141	0.707
	Site	Sebeta Ellu	166 142	52 61	31.3 43.0	4.458	0.035
ovine	Age	Lamb Young Adult	21 25 45	9 13 22	42.9 52 48.9	0.392	0.822
	Sex	Female Male	52 39	25 19	48.1 48.7	0.004	0.925
	Site	Sebeta Ellu	62 29	27 17	43.5 58.6	1.797	0.180

Table 2: Associations of different risk factors with ruminant fasciolosis assessed by Chi-square.

Species of parasite	Number of liver (%)	P value
F. gigantica	26(28.8%)	0.045
F. hepatica	50(54.9%)	
Mixed infection	15(16.5%)	

Table 3: Relative distribution of *Fasciola* species among examined livers.

Lesions	n	%	Average fluke burden
Light	27	29.7%	39.1
Moderate	44	48.5%	80.0
Severe	20	21.8%	53.5
Total	91	100%	57.5

Table 4: Degree of liver lesion and average fluke burden.

of relatively larger swampy areas in Illu district resulting from over flooding of Awash River during the rainy season. These areas remain wet for long periods during the dry season. Swampy areas are favourable for breeding of snails [4,14,20]. Seasonal movement of animals could also play an important role in the epidemiology of fasciolosis in this district. During the rainy season, animals move to the neighbouring hill side (high lands) for grazing and move back during the dry season to the marshy lands in search of pasture.

In this study, the prevalence of fasciolosis in sheep (48.3%) was significantly higher than that of cattle (36.7%). Variations between different species (bovine and ovine) could have been arisen from the differences in host susceptibility to the infection. Sheep's don't normally develop a protective immune response to reinfection while cattle have the ability of developing protection against reinfection with *Fasciola* species [20]. The prevalence rate in between different sex and age groups showed no significant variations. Similar finding was reported from Ethiopia [23,24]. This indicates that both sexes and different age groups are equally susceptible to fasciolosis.

In the current abattoir survey, out of a total of 237 livers examined, 38.4% (91) were infected by one or more *Fasciola* species. The majority (54.9%) of the infection was caused by *F. hepatica* followed by *F. gigantica* (28.6%) and mixed species (16.5%). Consistent to our findings, abattoir surveys in different parts of Ethiopia reported the predominance of *F. hepatica* over *F. gigantica* [17,18,25,26]. This might be associated with the existence of favourable ecological conditions for lymnea truncatula, the intermediate host for *F. hepatica* [14]. Flood-prone areas and low lying marshy and drainage ditches are ideal for breeding of lymnea truncatula [20].

In this study, the fluke count in moderately affected livers was higher than the count in severely affected livers. This could be due to severe fibrosis in the latter that potentially impede the movements of immature flukes; making the liver less attractive to newly the invading flukes [20]. A high fluke burden (57.5 per affected liver) was recorded in this study. This finding was in close agreement with earlier studies in Ethiopia [15,27]. Presence of more than 50 flukes per liver indicates high pathogenicity [17]. The more flukes an animal has, the more blood it losses and the more anaemic it becomes [14].

In conclusion, fasciolosis is a wide spread ruminant health problems and cause significant economic losses both in terms of production loss and liver condemnation in the study areas. This study provides important information on epidemiology of ruminant fasciolosis and highlights the urgency of proper intervention strategy to minimize the burden of the disease.

References

1. Central Statistical Agency (2013) Agricultural Sample Survey (2012/13) Volume II. Report on Livestock and Livestock Characteristics. Statistical Bulletin, 570. Addis Ababa, Ethiopia.
2. DACA (2006) Standard Veterinary Treatment Guideline for Veterinary practice. 1st edn. Drug Administration and Control Authority, Addis Ababa, Ethiopia.
3. OIE (2011) World Animal Health Information Database (WAHID) Interface.
4. Graber MM (1975) Helminths and Helminthiasis of different domestic and wild animals of Ethiopia. Bulletin of Animal Health and production in Africa 23: 57-86.
5. Adem A (1994) Prevalence of bovine and ovine fasciolosis: A preliminary survey around Ziway Region (Shewa). DVM Thesis, Faculty of Veterinary Medicine Addis Ababa University Debre Zeit, Ethiopia.
6. Ngategize PK, Bekele T, Tilahun G (1993) Financial losses caused by ovine fasciolosis in the Ethiopian highlands. Trop Anim Health Prod 25: 155-161.
7. Njau BC, Scholtens RG (1991) The role of traditional harvested hay in the transmission of ovine fasciolosis in Ethiopian highlands. Vet Res Com 15: 369-372.
8. Yilma JM, Malone JB (1998) A geographic information system forecast model for strategic control of fasciolosis in Ethiopia. Vet Parasitol 78: 103-127.
9. Thrusfield M (2005) Veterinary Epidemiology. 3rd edn. Blackwell Science, Oxford, UK, Pp: 233.
10. Pasquini C, Spurgeon T, Pasquini S (2003) Anatomy of Domestic Animals: Systemic and Regional Approach. 10th edition. Sudz Publishing, USA, Pp: 255.
11. Nicholson MJ, Butterworth MH (1986) A guide to condition scoring of Zebu cattle. International Livestock Center for Africa (ILCA), Addis Ababa, Ethiopia.
12. Hanson J, Perry B (1994) The Epidemiology, Diagnosis and Control of Helminth Parasites of Ruminants. A Hand Book. International Laboratory for Research on Animal Diseases. Food and Agricultural Organization of the United Nations, Rome, Italy, Pp: 72-89.
13. Graber MM (1975) Helminths and helminthiasis of domestic and wild animals of Ethiopia. Bull Anim Health Prod 23: 57-86.

14. Armour JL, Duncan JL, Dunn AM, Jennings FW, Urquhart GM (1997) Veterinary Parasitology. 2nd edn. Blackwell Publishers, London, UK, Pp: 103-113.

15. Sintayehu M (2007) Bovine fasciolosis in and around sebeta on field and abattoir survey in Ethiopia.

16. Hymanot A (1990) Prevalence survey of Bovine Fasciolosis in Easte Hararghe administrative region. DVM thesis, Faculty of Veterinary Medicine, Addis Ababa, Debre Zeit, Ethiopia. Pp: 21.

17. Aragaw K, Negus Y, Denbarga Y, Sheferaw D (2012) Fasciolosis in slaughtered cattle in Addis Ababa Abattoir, Ethiopia. Global Vet 8: 115-118.

18. Berhe G, Berhane K, Tadesse G (2009) Prevalence and economic significance of fasciolosis in cattle in Mekelle Area of Ethiopia. Trop Anim Health Prod 41: 1503-1505.

19. Woldemariam S, Wossene A (2007) Effects of a strategic anthelmintic treatment intervention bovine Fasciolosis: A study conducted in facilities endemic area in north western Ethiopia. Ethiop Vet J 11: 59-68.

20. Soulsby FJL (1982) Helminths, Arthropoda and Protozoa of domestic animals. 7th edn. Lea and Febiger, Pp: 44-51.

21. Constable PD, Hinchcliff KW, Gruenberg W, Done SH (1994) A text book of the disease of cattle, sheep, goats, pigs and horse: Veterinary Medicine. 8th edn. Elsevier Health Sciences, London, UK. Pp: 1015-1026.

22. Traore A (1989) Incidence and control of faciolosis around Niono, Central Mali. ILCA Bulletin No. 33, Pp: 18-20.

23. Yehenew M (1985) Prevalence of Fasciolosis at Gondor clinic in and around Lake Tana. DVM thesis, Faculty of Veterinary Medicine, Addis Ababa University, Debre Zeit, Ethiopia. Pp: 25.

24. Dagne M (1994) Survey on prevalence and economic significance of bovine Fasciolosis in Debre Berhan Region. DVM Thesis, Addis Ababa University, Debre Zeit, Ethiopia.

25. Tolosa T, Tigre W (2007) The Prevalence and Economic Significance of Bovine Fasciolosis at Jimma Abattoir, Ethiopia. The Internet J Vet Med, p: 3.

26. Ibrahim NP, Wasihun W, Tolosa T (2010) Prevalence of Bovine Fasciolosis and Economic Importance due to Liver Condemnation at Kombolcha Industrial Abattoir, Ethiopia. The Internet J Vet Med 8: 1-7.

27. Mesfin AY (1999) Study on the prevalence of bovine fasciolosis and morph Metric analysis of liver fluke populations in North Gondar area, Ethiopia. DVM Thesis, Faculty of Veterinary Medicine, Addis Ababa University, Debre Zeit, Ethiopia.

Effect of Feeding Enriched Mutton on Blood Lipid-Mineral Parameters and Cardio Vessel Changes in Male Sprague-Dawley Rats

Meng GY[1,2], Rajion MA[1], Jafari S[1,3], Ebrahimi M[1*] and Torshizi MAK[3]

[1]*Department of Veterinary Preclinical Sciences, Universiti Putra Malaysia, 43400 Serdang, Selangor, Malaysia*
[2]*Institute of Tropical Agriculture, Universiti Putra Malaysia, 43400 Serdang, Selangor, Malaysia*
[3]*Department of Poultry Science, Faculty of Agriculture, Tarbiat Modares University, PO Box 14115-336, Iran*

Abstract

Sixty male *Sprague-Dawley* rats aged six to seven months were allotted randomly into five groups of 12 animals each to evaluate the effects of mutton with altered fatty acid profiles on blood plasma lipid parameters and aortic intima changes. The five experimental diets were, the oil palm frond (OPF) meat pellet (from sheep fed 80% OPF+20% (% w/w) commercial concentrate), HAF meat pellet (from sheep fed 50% OPF+50% (% w/w) commercial concentrate), COC meat pellet (from sheep fed 100% commercial concentrate), COM meat pellet (prepared using commercially available mutton as its ingredient) and CON (standard rat chow pellet fed as the control group). The feeding trial lasted for 6 weeks. Blood and arterial tissue samples were obtained at two, four and six weeks after the onset of the trial. Results showed that COC increased the rat serum HDL-Cholesterol significantly ($P<0.05$) compared to CON group at different weeks of sampling. Conversely, CON had the highest triglyceride value among the treatments at 6th week of feeding. The results on arterial lesions were inconclusive. It is concluded that meat-based diets could raise serum HDL- Cholesterols in rats compared to a plant-based standard rat chow diet.

Keywords: Blood; Lipid profile; Mineral; Mutton; Rat

Introduction

Cholesterol is required for cell growth and replacement, steroid hormone genesis, bile acid synthesis and it is also involved in the pathway of vitamin D production [1]. However, increased blood cholesterol level is considered to be a risk factor for heart-related diseases [2]. Increased blood cholesterol level can also disturb triglyceride metabolism causing fatty liver diseases [3]. The low density lipoprotein (LDL) - cholesterol particles are the major cholesterol carriers in humans which carry cholesterols from the digestive system to the cells and thus are the key players of cholesterol transfer and metabolism [4]. The high density lipoprotein (HDL)-cholesterol is thought to be involved in reverse cholesterol transport from the tissues to the liver [5]. High LDL-Cholesterol levels are associated with higher risks of developing coronary heart diseases [1]. Contrastingly, higher levels of HDL-Cholesterol are protective against these diseases [5].

Serum magnesium and calcium levels have shown to affect lipid metabolism, particularly the LDL portion [6]. In fact, magnesium deficiency was known to cause hypercholesterolemia, hypertriglyceridaemia and dyslipoproteinaemia characterized by an increase of LDL-Cholesterol as well as decrease of HDL-Cholesterol in rats [7]. Calcium was known to modulate lipid metabolism in experimental animals by promoting fecal excretion of saturated fatty acid [8].

Rats have long been preferred species for biomedical research animal models due to their physiological, anatomical, and genetic similarity to humans. Advantages of rats include their short life cycle, small size, ease of maintenance, and abundant genetic resources [9]. Rat models have also being used extensively for vascular studies to investigate atherosclerosis [10].

The objectives of the current study were to describe the effects of the consumption of modified mutton by rats, particularly the changes in their serum lipid-mineral profiles. The gross arterial intimal changes were also surveyed. It was hypothesized that modified mutton in the rat diet would raise the rats' serum HDL-Cholesterol, while lowering the serum LDL-Cholesterol.

Materials and Methods

Animals and diets

Sixty individually-housed male *Sprague-Dawley* rats aged between six to seven months were used for this seven-week feeding. Animals were allotted randomly into five groups of 12 animals each based on the treatment diet offered. The five experimental diets were, the oil palm frond (OPF) meat pellet (from sheep fed 80% OPF+20% (% w/w) commercial concentrate), HAF meat pellet (from sheep fed 50% OPF+50% (% w/w) commercial concentrate), COC meat pellet (from sheep fed 100% commercial concentrate), COM meat pellet (prepared using commercially available mutton as its ingredient) and CON (standard rat chow pellet fed as the control group). The mutton-based pellets for the rat diets were prepared from lamb carcass based on the technique developed in the Medical Physiology Laboratory, Department of Biomedical Sciences, University of Putra in Malaysia. Four rats from each treatment group were selected randomly at fortnightly intervals for blood sampling, and then sacrificed for their aortic tissues. All the procedures and techniques related to the use, care of animals for

***Corresponding author:** Dr. Mahdi Ebrahimi, Faculty of Veterinary Medicine, Department of Veterinary Preclinical Sciences, Universiti Putra Malaysia, 43400 UPM, Serdang Selangor Darul Ehsan, Malaysia
E-mail: mehdiebrahimii@gmail.com

research, and the experimental design were undertaken following the guidelines of the research policy of the University Putra Malaysia on animal ethics.

Chemical analyses of experimental diets

The standard method of AOAC was followed to determine the proximate chemical composition of food samples [11]. Samples of experimental diets were dried in a forced-air oven at 105°C for 24 h. Nitrogen was determined by Kjeltec Auto Analyzer and then converted to crude protein (CP=N × 6.25). Ether extract (EE) was determined by extracting the sample with petroleum ether (40-60°C) using a Soxtec Auto Analyzer. Crude fiber was obtained from the loss in weight on ignition of dried residue remaining after digestion of fat free samples with 1.25% each of sulfuric acid and sodium hydroxide solutions. Each analysis was performed in triplicate. Samples were then ashed in a muffle furnace at 550°C for 4 h to determine the ash content.

The fatty acid content in experimental diet samples were extracted as described by Jafari et al. [12]. In brief, chloroform/methanol 2:1 (v/v) containing butylated hydroxy toluene was used for the extraction of fat. An internal standard, heneicosanoic acid (Sigma Chemical, St. Louis, MO, USA), was added to each sample before transmethylation to determine the individual fatty acid concentration within the sample. Transmethylation of the extracted fatty acid to their fatty acid methyl esters (FAME) was carried out using potassium hydroxide in methanol and 14% methanolic boron trifluoride. The FAME was separated by gas chromatography (Agilent 5890A), using a Supelco SP 2560 capillary column of 30 cm × 0.25 mm ID × 0.2 µm film thickness (Supelco, Bellefonte, PA, USA). The fatty acid concentrations were expressed as g/100 g of identified fatty acid.

Sampling procedure and serum lipid-mineral determination

Blood sampling was carried out on three animals from each group sacrificed serially at two, four or six weeks after the adjustment period. Blood samples were collected via the abdominal aorta of the rats and allowed to clot overnight to obtain serum samples. The serum was then analyzed for total cholesterol, HDL-Cholesterol, LDL-Cholesterol, triacylglycerols, serum magnesium and serum calcium using analytical kits (Pointe Scientific Inc, Michigan, USA), determined colorimetrically on a Cobas Mira chemistry analyzer (Roche International, Basel, Switzerland).

Staining of the rat aorta

Following the blood sampling and immediately after euthanasia by an overdose of sodium pentobarbitone, the entire length of the aorta (base of the aortic arch to the aorta-illiac bifurcations) was taken. The aorta was excised and pinned on wooden dissection boards to expose their intimal surfaces. It was then fixed with formaldehyde for 24 h. Sudan staining was then performed and the stained aorta was viewed under a stereomicroscope. This was to determine the percentage of sudanophilic positive area over total aortic intimal surface observed using a custom-made plastic 1 mm × 1 mm measuring grid. The procedures and sample site selection described were as detailed in the methods and recommendations by Yang et al. [13]. However, due to the absence of intimal sudanophilia in the vast majority of the experimental animals (more than 95%), the intimal surface was only designated as positive or negative for sudanophilia.

Statistical analysis

All results (serum total cholesterol levels, triacylglycerol, HDL-Cholesterol, LDL-Cholesterol, magnesium, calcium levels and aorta) were analyzed using a two-way ANOVA to compare the effects of treatment diets and treatment weeks. The significant difference ($P<0.05$) among means was further tested by Duncan's multiple range test using SPSS for Windows version 16.0 (SPSS Inc. 2007, Chicago, USA) [14].

Results

Nutrient composition of the rat diets

The nutrient composition of the rat pellets is given in Table 1. Dry matter content was significantly lower ($P<0.05$) in the standard rat chow compared with the other meat-based pellets. Crude protein was similar in the four meat-based pellets (OPF, HAF, COC and COM), but was 50% lower in CON.

Similarly, the ash content was also significantly high ($P<0.05$) only in CON. Crude fiber content for the HAF, COC and COM was low, but significantly higher ($P<0.05$) in the OPF. The CON group which was formulated mostly from plant materials had higher ($P<0.05$) crude fiber content. The EE was lowest in CON, moderately high ($P<0.05$) in both the OPF meat and HAF meat diets and highest ($P<0.05$) in the COC and COM. In terms of energy content, CON had the lowest ($P<0.05$) gross energy content.

The fatty acid profiles of the rat experimental diets are also shown in Table 1. The COC contained a significantly higher ($P<0.05$) amount of palmitic and oleic acids compared to both CON and OPF. The stearic acid content was lowest ($P<0.05$) in the COC followed by HAF, COM and OPF, respectively. The linoleic acid content of all treatment diets was also significantly different ($P<0.05$).

The CON had the highest linoleic acid ($P<0.05$) while COM had the lowest ($P<0.05$) amount of linoleic acid among the treatment groups. Total unsaturated and saturated fatty acid contents were significantly highest and lowest in CON group compared to other treatment groups ($P<0.05$). The total monoene content of the COM was similar to that of the COC and HAF but significantly ($P<0.05$) higher by more than 10% when compared to both OPF and CON groups.

Blood lipid parameters in rats

In the week 2nd and 6th, the COM rats had the highest serum total cholesterol (Table 2) compared to all the other groups ($P<0.05$). In these weeks (2nd and 6th), CON had also the lowest total cholesterol.

The serum HDL-Cholesterol levels were elevated ($P<0.05$) in all treatment groups except those fed the CON group after six weeks of treatments (Table 2). In fact, the serum HDL-Cholesterol values were significantly increased ($P<0.05$) in the COC meat treated group as early as the Week 2nd of the experiment. Rats fed on HAF, COC and OPF had significantly ($P<0.05$) higher LDL-Cholesterol values compared with other treatment groups at 6th week of feeding. The effect of the treatment diets on serum triacylglycerol was also at 4th week of feeding as shown in Table 2. Feeding CON to the rats resulted in an increased serum triacylglycerol levels after four week ($P<0.05$).

Blood serum magnesium and calcium levels in rats

Serum magnesium levels (Table 3) were only significantly ($P<0.05$) different across treatment groups after 6th week of feeding. At this point both the OPF and HAF groups had significantly ($P<0.05$) lower magnesium levels compared with the other treatment groups.

At the end of the feeding, all treatment groups had similar ($P>0.05$) amounts of calcium in their serum. However, at the 4th week of feeding, HAF had the lowest concentration of calcium among the treatments.

Treatments	CON	COM	COC	HAF	OPF
Constituents					
Dry Matter (g/kg)	909.5 ± 34.8^{b}	935.5 ±10.3^{ab}	956.4 ± 37.4^{a}	956.8 ± 28.7^{a}	948.4 ± 45.9^{a}
Crude Protein (g/kg)	226.9 ± 21.8^{b}	417.5 ± 37.9^{a}	460.9 ± 51.6^{a}	445.4 ± 53.2^{a}	450.0 ± 37.0^{a}
Crude Fibre (g/kg)	4.5 ± 3.2^{c}	4.8 ± 0.3^{b}	5.7 ± 1.7^{b}	5.1 ± 0.6^{b}	7.5 ± 1.1^{a}
Ether Extract (g/kg)	23.5 ± 4.1^{c}	152.8 ±11.1^{a}	138.5 ± 9.6^{a}	100.2 ± 7.2^{b}	92.4 ± 4.6^{b}
Ash (g/kg)	62.7 ± 2.9^{a}	39.9 ± 1.4^{b}	41.1 ± 2.6^{b}	42.5 ± 5.7^{b}	42.6 ± 2.5^{b}
Gross Energy (MJ/kg)	15.54 ± 0.53^{c}	22.55 ±1.15^{a}	20.89 ± 1.59^{b}	21.15 ± 1.27^{ab}	20.51 ± 0.79^{b}
Fatty acid (g/100g FA)					
Palmitic Acid (16:0)	18.2 ± 3.4^{c}	21.9 ± 1.2^{b}	26.7 ± 3.1^{a}	24.2 ± 2.0^{a}	22.0 ± 2.1^{ab}
Palmitoleic Acid (16:1n-7)	0.5 ± 0.2^{c}	1.8 ± 0.4^{a}	1.8 ± 0.3^{a}	1.8 ± 0.4^{a}	1.1 ± 0.3^{b}
Stearic Acid (18:0)	5.1±3.0^{c}	25.0 ± 3.8^{a}	18.7 ± 1.9^{b}	20.9 ± 2.2^{b}	27.5 ± 4.1^{a}
Oleic Acid (18:1n-9)	30.0 ± 2.9^{b}	42.7 ± 4.0^{a}	42.4 ± 3.2^{a}	41.1 ± 6.7^{a}	30.3 ± 5.6^{b}
Linoleic Acid (18:2 n-6)	43.4 ± 7.7^{e}	6.7 ± 2.1^{d}	8.9±0.7^{c}	10.3 ± 0.9^{b}	16.3 ± 4.4^{a}
Linolenic Acid (18:3 n-3)	2.4 ± 0.3^{a}	0.7 ±0.4^{c}	0.5 ± 0.3^{c}	0.6 ± 0.2^{c}	1.1 ± 0.4^{b}
Arachidic Acid (20:0)	0.4 ± 0.1^{ab}	0.6 ± 0.2^{a}	0.2 ± 0.1^{b}	0.2 ± 0.1^{b}	0.3 ± 0.2^{b}
Arachidonic Acid (20:4 n-6)	ND	0.6 ± 0.2^{b}	0.6 ± 0.1^{b}	0.9 ± 0.4^{a}	1.4 ± 0.3^{a}
Total Saturated Fatty Acids	23.7 ± 3.0^{c}	47.6 ± 5.2^{ab}	45.6 ± 3.7^{b}	45.2 ± 2.1^{b}	49.9 ± 4.1^{a}
Total Unsaturated Fatty Acids	76.3 ± 8.8^{a}	52.4 ± 4.3^{b}	54.4±2.9^{b}	54.8 ± 3.1^{b}	50.1 ± 2.7^{b}
Total Monoenes	30.5 ± 5.6^{b}	44.5 ± 3.5^{a}	44.3 ± 6.6^{a}	43.0 ± 5.8^{a}	31.4 ± 4.7^{b}
Total PUFA n-3	2.4 ± 0.3^{a}	0.7 ±0.4^{b}	0.5 ± 0.3^{b}	0.6 ± 0.2^{b}	1.1 ± 0.4^{ab}
Total PUFA n-6	43.4 ± 7.7^{a}	7.3 ± 1.9^{c}	9.5 ± 1.6^{c}	11.2 ± 1.3^{b}	17.7 ± 2.8^{b}

CON (standard rat chow pellet fed as the control group), COM meat pellet (prepared using commercially available mutton as its ingredient), COC meat pellet (from sheep fed 100% commercial concentrate), HAF meat pellet (from sheep fed 50% OPF+50% (% w/w) commercial concentrate), OPF meat pellet (from sheep fed 80% OPF+20% (% w/w) commercial concentrate). Total saturated fatty acids=sum of C16:0+C18:0. Total unsaturated fatty acids=sum of C16:1+C18:1+C18:2n-6+C18:3n-3+C20:1. Total monoens=sum of C16:1+C18:1+C20:1. Total PUFA n-3=sum of C18:3n-3+C20:5n-3+C22:5n-3+C22:6n-3. Total PUFA n-6=sum of C18:2n-6+C20:4n-6. C18 PUFA: sum of (C18:3n-3+C18:2n-6+C18:1n-9). ND: not detected. Different letters ($^{a,\ b\ and\ c}$) in each row denote significant difference at P<0.05.

Table 1: Chemical composition of the experimental diets (Mean ± SD).

Treatment Weeks	CON	COM	COC	HAF	OPF
Total Cholesterol					
0	1.26 ± 0.24	1.26 ± 0.24	1.26 ± 0.24	1.26 ± 0.24	1.26 ± 0.24
2	1.14 ± 0.15^{b}	1.62 ± 0.06^{a}	1.41 ± 0.24^{ab}	1.44 ± 0.31^{ab}	1.39 ± 0.11^{ab}
4	1.35 ± 0.24	1.70 ± 0.33	1.71 ± 0.41	1.59 ± 0.18	1.61 ± 0.20
6	1.46 ± 0.15^{b}	1.75 ± 0.11^{a}	1.69 ± 0.21^{ab}	1.71 ± 0.22^{ab}	1.67 ± 0.09^{ab}
HDL- Cholesterol					
0	0.59 ± 0.16	0.59 ± 0.16	0.59 ± 0.16	0.59 ± 0.16	0.59 ± 0.16
2	0.58 ± 0.14^{c}	0.94 ± 0.09^{ab}	1.08 ± 0.12^{a}	0.73 ± 0.42^{ab}	0.74 ± 0.09^{ab}
4	0.69 ± 0.23^{b}	0.76 ± 0.09^{ab}	1.00 ± 0.14^{a}	1.02 ± 0.05^{a}	0.88 ± 0.09^{ab}
6	0.83 ± 0.18^{b}	0.79 ± 0.10^{b}	1.09 ± 0.31^{a}	1.05 ± 0.20^{a}	1.00 ± 0.09^{a}
LDL-Cholesterol					
0	0.25 ± 0.05	0.25 ± 0.05	0.25 ± 0.05	0.25 ± 0.05	0.25 ± 0.05
2	0.27 ± 0.08	0.29 ± 0.10	0.22 ± 0.07	0.24 ± 0.07	0.31 ± 0.06
4	0.26 ± 0.04	0.28 ± 0.04	0.26 ± 0.10	0.27 ± 0.10	0.39 ± 0.08
6	0.22 ± 0.08^{b}	0.31 ± 0.03^{ab}	0.36 ± 0.05^{a}	0.41 ± 0.09^{a}	0.32 ± 0.05^{a}
Triacylglyceride					
0	0.42 ± 0.10	0.42 ± 0.10	0.42 ± 0.10	0.42 ± 0.10	0.42 ± 0.10
2	0.35 ± 0.07	0.35 ± 0.06	0.46 ± 0.15	0.44 ± 0.06	0.35 ± 0.10
4	0.45 ± 0.04^{a}	0.26 ± 0.05^{b}	0.34 ± 0.03^{b}	0.30 ± 0.05^{b}	0.33 ± 0.09^{b}
6	0.46 ± 0.16	0.53 ± 0.15	0.43 ± 0.09	0.53 ± 0.17	0.35 ± 0.12

Table 2: Effect of supplemented diets on blood serum lipid parameters in rats (Mean ± SD mmol/L). CON (standard rat chow pellet fed as the control group), COM meat pellet (prepared using commercially available mutton as its ingredient), COC meat pellet (from sheep fed 100% commercial concentrate), HAF meat pellet (from sheep fed 50% OPF+50% (% w/w) commercial concentrate), OPF meat pellet (from sheep fed 80% OPF+20% (% w/w) commercial concentrate). Different letters ($^{a,\ b\ and\ c}$) in each row denote significant difference at P<0.05.

Effect of supplemented diets on aortic intima

The aortic intima changes are as shown in Table 4. The results appeared inconclusive. All groups apart from the animals fed the COC and COM had at least one animal showing sudanophilic reaction on its aortic intima.

Discussion

Nutrient composition of the rat diet

Based on Atwater's calculation methods, the total fats contribute about 17% of the total energy [15]. In the current study, the mean of total fat in mutton-based pellets were 22.77% of total energy. Total fats from the CON diet contributed about 5.6% of the total dietary gross energy. The high dietary lipid content in the mutton-based pellets had an adverse effect on the rat serum lipids as a whole when compared against the CON diet. The fat content of each diet was not standardized as the main focus was to investigate the overall effect of consuming these meats on the blood lipids. Apart from the level of dietary fat inclusion, the levels of the individual classes of fatty acids would also contribute to the modulation of blood lipids [16].

Blood lipid parameters of rats

Fatty acids in dietary lipids have been implicated in the response of serum lipids to feeding different oils and fats [17]. The current study attempted to examine the probable benefits of the modified mutton on the rat serum lipids. This study is also unique in which the rats are fed whole mutton samples rather than purified diets and supplementary oils with limited dietary fatty acid mix.

Although the latter approach was beneficial in compartmentalising and segregating the effects of individual fatty acids on the serum lipids, it offered little to illustrate the overall effects of the particular meat/diet fatty acid mix and its interaction with the hosts' serum lipids, as meat is consumed whole together with its unique mix of lipid properties.

Furthermore, Karupaiah and Sundram postulated different triacylglycerols absorbability between those of plant oils and beef tallow in rat intestines [18]. The serum total cholesterol values from the control rats in this study were similar to that of the control (non-castrated) rats used by Ima-Nirwana et al. which was kept and fed under similar Malaysian conditions [19]. However, at the end of the six-week trial, rats fed mutton-based pellets generally had higher serum total cholesterol levels. The rats fed commercial meat pellets in particular had higher levels of serum total cholesterols compared to the controls. There was no difference in the serum cholesterol levels within the four groups of rats given mutton-based pellets. A report by Ali also supported the fact that rats fed four different plant oils at the same dietary inclusion levels for seven weeks had similar total serum cholesterol values [20]. The difference in the total serum cholesterol levels between the CON rats fed a plant-based diet and the four groups of rats fed mutton-based diets in this study was perhaps due to the dietary fat inclusion levels, and to a less extent differences in the fat absorption tendencies between plant-based and animal-based triacylglycerols as reported by Massera et al. [21]. Compared with the values of the CON animals, the serum triacylglycerol remained within normal limits throughout the trial for the mutton-fed rats. The constant serum triacylglycerol levels may help

Treatment Weeks	CON	COM	COC	HAF	OPF
Magnesium					
0	0.37 ± 0.03	0.37 ± 0.03	0.37 ± 0.03	0.37 ± 0.03	0.37 ± 0.03
2	0.34 ± 0.05	0.41 ± 0.08	0.38 ± 0.07	0.39 ± 0.09	0.42 ± 0.09
4	0.37 ± 0.08	0.33 ± 0.06	0.37 ± 0.02	0.32 ± 0.04	0.39 ± 0.07
6	0.36 ± 0.04[a]	0.38 ± 0.07[a]	0.37 ± 0.06[a]	0.29 ± 0.02[b]	0.27 ± 0.03[b]
Calcium					
0	2.39 ± 0.80	2.39 ± 0.83	2.39 ± 0.78	2.39 ± 0.68	2.39 ± 0.70
2	2.17 ± 0.30	2.37 ± 0.28	2.06 ± 0.38	2.25 ± 0.38	2.41 ± 0.28
4	2.42 ± 0.40[a]	2.18 ± 0.38[b]	2.26 ± 0.38[ab]	2.11 ± 0.36[b]	2.39 ± 0.4[a]
6	2.11 ± 0.16	1.96 ± 0.18	1.94 ± 0.28	2.02 ± 0.10	1.77 ± 0.12

CON (standard rat chow pellet fed as the control group), COM meat pellet (prepared using commercially available mutton as its ingredient), COC meat pellet (from sheep fed 100% commercial concentrate), HAF meat pellet (from sheep fed 50% OPF+50% (% w/w) commercial concentrate), OPF meat pellet (from sheep fed 80% OPF+20% (% w/w) commercial concentrate). Different letters [a, b] in each row denote significant difference at P<0.05.

Table 3: Effect of supplemented diets on blood serum magnesium and calcium in rats (Mean ± SD mmol/L).

Treatment Weeks	Sudanophilic changes	CON	COM	COC	HAF	OPF
0	Positive			1(30%)		
	Negative			14		
2	Positive	1 (21%)	0	0	0	0
	Negative	3	4	4	4	4
4	Positive	0	0	0	0	1 (17%)
	Negative	4	4	4	4	3
6	Positive	0	0	0	1 (42%)	0
	Negative	4	4	4	3	4

CON (standard rat chow pellet fed as the control group), COM meat pellet (prepared using commercially available mutton as its ingredient), COC meat pellet (from sheep fed 100% commercial concentrate), HAF meat pellet (from sheep fed 50% OPF+50% (% w/w) commercial concentrate), OPF meat pellet (from sheep fed 80% OPF+20% (% w/w) commercial concentrate). Numbers in parenthesis indicate the % of the aortic intimal area that was sudanophilic.

Table 4: Sudanophilic changes on the rat aortic intima.

to rule out the effects of triacylglycerols on lipoprotein metabolism, as the rat is equally efficient in processing dietary fats in its intestines compared to humans at 135 mol/h, thereby increasing serum fatty acid levels [20].

Increased serum fatty acid levels would acutely increase triacylglycerol synthesis [21]. This in turn would derange the metabolism of LDL and HDL cholesterols [1]. The serum HDL-Cholesterol values in all the mutton-fed groups were significantly elevated at week 6th compared to the initial baseline values. It is known that all fatty acids (both saturated and unsaturated) elevate HDL-Cholesterol when they replace carbohydrates as the energy source in diets. However, the effects diminished with increasing saturation of the fatty acids [1]. The results showed that rats fed COC had elevated serum HDL-Cholesterol, which was the highest of all treatment groups and significantly different compared to the rats fed commercially available mutton. The COC meat pellets reputably had the highest absolute concentration of total unsaturated fatty acid among all treatments. This is an important finding because a slight increase in serum HDL-Cholesterol levels was assumed to be synonymous with a lower risk for cardiovascular disease in humans [7].

Blood serum magnesium and calcium levels in rats

Serum magnesium and calcium levels were minimally affected during the course of treatment. This at least assured that there was minor interference in the rats' lipid metabolism from these metals.

Magnesium deficiency in rats is known to affect the apolipoprotein composition of LDL and HDL [22]. In humans, these would have decided the development of cardiovascular diseases since low levels of dietary magnesium enhanced, whereas high levels of dietary magnesium retarded the development of atherogenic lesions. Apart from interfering with the lipoprotein metabolism, serum magnesium would also affect the rate of calcium uptake into soft tissues, an important event during atherosclerosis [22].

Serum calcium is only important in the late stages of atherosclerosis and therefore minimal changes were expected in healthy rats throughout the course of the trial. However, calcium ions in the gut have been known to promote fecal excretion of long chain fatty acid by forming insoluble and non-absorbable salts [8].

Effect of supplemented diets on aortic intima

Only about 5% of the rats used in this study developed detectable gross lesions on the aortic intima. Although the lesion distribution seemed to be random, animals fed COC and COM did not exhibit any lesions at all. Incidentally, these groups were among those that received highest absolute concentration of unsaturated fatty acid. At this stage it was concluded that these were incidental findings as this was only a six-week trial. In fact, in rabbits, Hur et al. reported a poor correlation between the extent of atherogenic lesions and the levels of serum cholesterols alone [23]. In nature, most animal species have relatively low serum cholesterol concentrations and develop only occasional arterial lesions with advancing age [24]. In this study, only sudanophilic lesions were detected, which were among the most studied lesions. Nevertheless, presence of microscopic changes, which were not studied, must not be ruled out. Jang et al. gave an excellent and detailed account of the various types of arterial lesions [25]. The arterial lesion formation was thought to involve a series of cellular level changes modulated by oxidized-LDL particles and a host of cellular components before it finally becomes an atheroma.

Conclusion

In the current study, it was shown that the modified mutton (from the COC sheep) exhibited a probable cardio-protective effect based on its action in elevating the serum HDL-Cholesterol levels. It was also shown that meat-based diets would raise serum HDL- Cholesterols in rats compared to when a plant-based standard rat chow (CON) was fed. It was a surprise this happened without changing the blood triacylglycerols levels. No significant distribution/occurrence of gross aortic lesions was also detected.

Acknowledgements

The authors are thankful to the Faculty of Veterinary Medicine, Faculty of Agriculture, Universiti Putra Malaysia and Faculty of Agriculture, Tarbiat Modares University.

References

1. Jeong H, Yang BK, Jeong YT, Kim GN, Jeong YS, et al. (2007) Hypolipidemic effects of biopolymers extracted from culture broth, mycelia, and fruiting bodies of auricularia auricula-judae in dietary-induced hyperlipidemic rats. Mycobiology 35: 16-20.
2. Pande S, Platel K, Srinivasan K (2102) Antihypercholesterolaemic influence of dietary tender cluster beans (Cyamopsis tetragonoloba) in cholesterol fed rats. Indian J Med Res 135: 401-406.
3. Wang YM (2010) The mechanism of dietary cholesterol effects on lipids metabolism in rats. Lipids Health Dis 9: 4.
4. Hevonoja T, Pentikainen MO, Hyvonen MT, Kovanen PT, Ala-Korpela M (2000) Structure of low density lipoprotein (LDL) particles: Basis for understanding molecular changes in modified LDL. Biochim Biophys Acta 1488: 189-210.
5. Mikhailidis DP, Wierzbick AS (2000) HDL-cholesterol and the treatment of coronary heart disease : contrasting effects of atorvastatin and simvastatin. Curr Med Res Opin 16: 139-146.
6. Kiss SA, Galbács Z, Galbács G (2006) The role of magnesium in the supposed mechanism of anaesthesia. J Elementol 11: 521-532.
7. Manju L, Renuka N (2006) Magnesium deficiency augments myocardial response to reactive oxygen species. Ca J Physiol Pharmacol 84: 617-624.
8. Teegarden D, White KM, Lyle RM, Zemel MB, Van LMD, et al. (2008) Calcium and dairy product modulation of lipid utilization and energy expenditure. Obesity 6: 1566-1572.
9. Bryda CE (2013) The Mighty Mouse: The Impact of Rodents on Advances in Biomedical Research. Mo Med 110: 207-211.
10. Ellenbroek B, Youn J (2016) Rodent models in neuroscience research: is it a rat race?. Dis Model Mech 9: 1079-1087.
11. AOAC (1990) Official method of analysis. 15th edn. Arlington, VA: Association of Analytical Chemists.
12. Jafari S, Goh YM, Rajion MA, Jahromi MF, Ebrahimi M (2016) Manipulation of rumen microbial fermentation by polyphenol rich solvent fractions from papaya leaf to reduce green-house gas methane and biohydrogenation of C18 PUFA. J Agri Food Chem 64: 4522-4530.
13. Yang S, Li X, Chao B, Wu L, Cheng Z, et al. (2014) Abdominal aortic intimal flap motion characterization in acute aortic dissection: assessed with retrospective ecg-gated thoraco abdominal aorta dual-source ct angiography. PLoS ONE 9: e87664.
14. SPSS (2007) SPSS for Windows. Version 16.0, SPSS Inc., Chicago, USA.
15. Novotny JA, Gebauer SK, Baer DJ (2012) Discrepancy between the Atwater factor predicted and empirically measured energy values of almonds in human diets. Am J Clin Nutr 96: 296-301.
16. Haber EP, Procópio J, Carvalho CR, Carpinelli AR, Newsholme P, et al. (2006) New insights into fatty acid modulation of pancreatic beta-cell function. Int Rev Cytol 248: 1-41.
17. Kerr BJ, Kellner TA, Shurson GC (2015) Characteristics of lipids and their feeding value in swine diets. J Anim Sci Biotechnol 6: 30.

18. Karupaiah T, Sundram K (2007) Effects of stereospecific positioning of fatty acids in triacylglycerol structures in native and randomized fats: a review of their nutritional implications. Nutr Metab 4: 16.

19. Ima-Nirwana S, Jamaluddin M, Khalid B, Merican Z, Baharom S (1995) Serum lipids of castrated rats given hormonal replacement and fed diets with added soybean oil or palm oil. Asia Pacific J Clinical Nutri 4: 244-248.

20. Ali RFM (2016) Hypocholesterolemic effects of diets containing different levels of kishk as a dried fermented milkewhole wheat mixture in experimental rats. J Ethn Foods 3: 117-123.

21. Massera D, Graf L, Barba S, Ostfeld R (2016) Angina rapidly improved with a plant-based diet and returned after resuming a Western diet. J Geriatr Cardiol 13: 364-366.

22. Olatunji LA, Soladoye AO (2007) Increased magnesium intake prevents hyperlipidemia and insulin resistance and reduces lipid peroxidation in fructose-fed rats. Pathophysiology 14: 11-15.

23. Hur SJ, Min B, Nam KC, Lee EJ, Ahn DU (2013) Effect of Dietary Cholesterol and Cholesterol Oxides on Blood Cholesterol, Lipids, and the Development of Atherosclerosis in Rabbits. Int J Mol Sci 14: 12593-12606.

24. Svindland A, Berg K, Eliassen K, Lawn RM, Djurovic S, et al. (2000) Histopathology of arterial lesions in LPA transgenic mice on cholesterol-enriched chow. Atherosclerosis 153: 349-354.

25. Jang IK, Tearney GJ, MacNeill B, Takano M, Moselewski F, et al. (2005) In vivo characterization of coronary atherosclerotic plaque by use of optical coherence tomography. Circulation 111: 1551-1555.

Prevalence of Ovine Fasiolosis in Jimma and Selected Rural Kebeles Near Jimma, Southwest Ethiopia

Awol Ibrahim[1], Dagmar Nölkes[2], Elias Gezahegn[3]* and Mekuriya Taye[4]

[1]*Dawe Kechen District Pastoral Area Development Office, Ethiopia*
[2]*College of Veterinary Medicine, Haramaya University, Dire Dawa, Ethiopia*
[3]*Bale Zone Pastoral Area Development Office, Ethiopia*
[4]*Mede Welabu District Pastoral Area Development Office, Ethiopia*

Abstract

A cross-sectional study was conducted to determine the prevalence of ovine Fasciolosis in Jimma and nine selected rural kebeles near Jimma from November 2011 to April 2012 by coprological examination. A total of 384 samples were collected from different kebeles near Jimma. Out of the total sampled 164 (42.71%) were positive for Fasciolosis. According to coprological examination, variation in prevalence among the localities was not statistically significant (p>0.05). The result also revealed no statistically significant difference between sexes and ages (p>0.05). Infection rate in poor body condition animals (74.80%) was significantly higher (p<0.05) than good body condition animals (12.20%) and this indicates that the importance of Fasciolosis in causing weight loss and weakness, a characteristic of sign of chronic Fasciolosis. Results obtained in this area were discussed in comparisons with the finding of other research works. Appropriate strategies for the control of ovine Fasciolosis are recommended by considering the limiting local factors of the study area.

Keywords: Coprological examination; Fasciolosis; Jimma; Ovine; Prevalence

Introduction

Ethiopia has the largest livestock population in Africa including more than 38,749,320 cattle, 18,075,580 sheep, 14,858,650 goats, 456,910 camels, 5,765,710 Equines and 30,868,540 chickens with ownership currently contributing to live hoods of an estimated 80% of rural population (CSA, 2009). In Ethiopia sheep are among the dominant livestock species providing up to 63% of cash income and 23% of food subsistence value obtained from livestock production. Despite the animal and the contribution of this sub sector to the nation's economy is relatively low.

Endoparasitic infection and management problems are known to be the main factors that affect productivity. Among endoparasitic infection Fasciolosis is one of the difficult problems in helminthology [1]. Fasciolosis is caused by Fasciolidae trematodes of the genus *Fasciola; Fasciola hepatica* and *Fasciola gigantica* which migrate in the hepatic parenchyma and establish themselves and develop in the bile ducts. It causes significant morbidity and mortality [2,3]. The clinical features of fasciolosis can have acute, sub-acute and chronic forms [4].

In Ethiopia *F. gigantica* is found at altitude below 1800 masl. While *F. hepatica* is found at altitude between 1200-2560 masl [5]. Mixed infection by both species of *Fasciola* may occur where the ecology is conducive for replication of both intermediate hosts [1].

The snails of genus *Lymnaea* are mainly involved as an intermediate host in the life cycle of *Fasciola* [6]. *Lymnaea truncatula* is the most common intermediate host for *F. hepatica* in different parts of the world [7]. The most important intermediate host for *F. gigantica* is *L. natalensis* and *L. auriallaria* [8].

The economic impact of Fasciolosis may vary greatly from year to year depending on the climate, management, level of infection, host immunity status and the age of animals [9]. Ovine Fasciolosis losses were estimated at 48.4 million Ethiopian birr per year of which 46.5%, 48.8% and 4.7% were due to mortality, productivity (weight loss and reproductive wastage) and liver condemnation respectively [10]. In Ethiopia, Fasciolosis is mainly an animal disease, causing a great economic burden in the highland areas of the country [11].

Several control methods against ruminant Fasciolosis such as avoiding the predisposing risk factors like marshy areas, grazing the animals in the irrigation points and drained water bodies. Other methods include a reduction in the number of intermediate snail host by chemical or biological means and strategic application of antihelmintics [12].

Therefore the objective of this study is to know the prevalence of ovine Fasciolosis in Jimma and selected rural kebeles near Jimma so as to generate base line data for future research and recommend control strategies applicable to the study area.

Materials and Methods

Study area

The study was conducted from November 2011 to April 2012 in Jimma and selected rural kebeles near Jimma to study the prevalence of ovine fasciolosis. Geographically the area is found in Jimma zone, Oromia regional state, southwestern Ethiopia. It is located about 346 km southwest of Addis Ababa, the Capital city of Ethiopia at 7°36'-8°56' N latitude and 35°52'-37°37' E longitude. Jimma area poses highland and lowland areas. In Jimma and its surrounding elevation ranges from

***Corresponding author:** Elias Gezahegn, Bale Zone Pastoral Area Development Office, Ethiopia, E-mail: eluccaa@gmail.com

880-3360 meter above sea level. The study area receives a mean annual rainfall of about 1530 mm which from long and short rainy season. The average minimum and maximum annual temperature ranges between 14.4 and 26.7°C, respectively [13]. Mixed agriculture is the main occupation of the population of the area. The major livestock reared in the area are sheep, goat, cattle and equine. According to statistical data, Jimma zone has livestock population of 2,016,823 cattle, 288,411 goats, 942,908 sheep, 74,574 horses, 49,489 donkeys, 28,371 mules and 1,139,735 poultry [14].

Study animals

The study was conducted on local breeds of sheep which were selected by simple random sampling technique in the study area. A total of 384 sheep were randomly examined following coproscopic procedures. All these animals were privately owned by smallholder farmers. The management system was traditional extensive system with minimum or no supplementary feed and veterinary care.

Sample size determination

To determine the sample size, a prevalence rate of 50% was taken into consideration since there was no published research work on ovine fasciolosis done in the area. The desired sample size for the study was calculated by using the formula given by Thrusfield [15] with 95% Confidence interval and 5% absolute precision.

$$N = \frac{(1.96)^2 \times P_{exp}\left(1 - P_{exp}\right)}{D^2}$$

Where, N=Sample size; P_{exp}=Expected prevalence; D^2=Absolute precision;

Then,

$$N = \frac{(1.96)^2 \times 0.5(1-0.5)}{(0.05)^2} = 384$$

Accordingly the estimated sample size was 384 animals.

Study design

A cross sectional study was conducted from November 2011-April 2012. Animals were selected by simple random sampling.

Coproscopic examination

Fecal samples from a total of 384 sheep were collected directly from the rectum of each animals using disposable plastic gloves with strict sanitation and placed in clean screw capped universal bottles. Each sample was clearly labeled with animal identification, place of collection, body condition score, deworming history, sex and age. Based on their dental eruption formula the age of the animal was determined and they were classified as young (less than two years) and adult (greater than two years) [16]. Then the sample was transported to Jimma University, College of Agriculture and Veterinary Medicine, parasitology laboratory, for detailed coproscopic examination. To detect fasciola eggs, sedimentation technique was as described by Hanson and Perry [17]. To detect fasciola eggs, sedimentation technique was employed as described earlier [18,19].

Data analysis

The result obtained were recorded and this data were entered in to Microsoft excel spread sheet. The data fed in to excel sheet were analyzed by JMP 5 statistical software. Descriptive statiststics like percentage, Pearsons Chi^2 (χ^2) test and p-value were used.

Site	Number of examined animals	Prevalence n (%)
Bosakito	60	27 (45.00)
Babala Kara	33	12 (36.36)
Jiren	48	24 (50.00)
Garuke Furdisa	39	16 (41.03)
Gudata Bula	40	15 (37.50)
Sumudo	44	20 (45.45)
Kochi	41	17 (41.46)
Umuganole	50	22 (44.00)
Setosamaro	29	11 (37.93)
Total/Overall prevalence	384	164 (42.71)

Pearson chi^2 (8)=2.6695; p=0.953

Table 1: Prevalence of ovine fasciolosis at selected kebeles near Jimma.

Results

Fecal examination conducted from November 2011 to April 2012 shows that from a total of 384 fecal samples examined, 164 (42.71%) was found to be positive for fasciola eggs (mean 0.4271, standard error 0.0253, 95% CI 37.74-47.68%). The prevalence variation between study kebeles (Table 1) shows the highest at 50% in Jiren and the lowest at 36.36% in Babala Kara. The differences were not statistically significant. Infections between sexes of animals were compared. The statistical indicated that 39.68% of males and 45.64% of females were positive for the infection (Tables 2-4). This difference was not statistically significant (p=0.238).

The prevalence among different age groups were adult (44.67%) and young (39.29%) and also showed no significant difference (p=0.304). On subjective evaluation of body condition to see the effect on prevalence of fasciolosis animals in poor (74.80%), medium (40.30%) and good (12.20%) body condition showed statistically significant difference (p=0.0001).

Discussion

Fasciolosis caused by *F. hepatica* and *F. Gigantica* is one of the most prevalent helimenths infectious of ruminants in the different part of the world it causes significant morbidity and mortality [2]. Ovine Fasciolosis exist in almost all regions of Ethiopia [19]. However, the prevalence rate, epidemiology and *Fasciola* species involved vary with locality. This is mainly attributed to the variation in the climatic and ecological conditions such as altitude, rainfall, humidity, temperature and management system of livestock.

The result of the present study conducted from November 2011 to April 2012 in Jimma and in nine selected rural kebeles near Jimma indicated that ovine fasciolosis is a wide spread with over all prevalence rate of 42.71%. High prevalence rate of ovine fasciolosis has been reported by other workers such as 56.3% in upper Awash river region [20], 49% in Dawa Cheffa district of Amhara regional state [21], 56.8% in Ziway [22], 70.2% in Lalo Midir district [23], 84.6% at Addis Ababa [24], 84% in Western Shoa [25], and 68% in and around Kombolcha [26]. When compared with the present result there is great difference. This great difference may be due to awareness of the people about the disease, expansion of veterinary clinics at different parts of the country, establishment of private veterinary drug shop at different parts of the country and some ecological change which cause the destruction of suitable environment which is used for the multiplication of intermediate host. The present study was higher as compared with the previous study where 14.5% were reported by Daniel [27] at Dire Dawa municipal Abattoir, 15.97% reported by Wassie at Nekemte and 31.8% reported by [28] at Assela. This difference may be due to ecological,

Sex	Number of examined animals	Prevalence n (%)
Male	189	75 (36.68)
Female	195	89 (45.64)
Total / overall prevalence	384	164 (42.71)

Pearson Chi^2 (1)=1.3926; p=0.238

Table 2: Prevalence of ovine fasciolosis on sex basis.

Age	Number of examined animals	Prevalence n (%)
Adult	244	109 (44.67)
Young	140	55 (39.29)
Total /overall prevalence	384	164 (42.71)

Pearson Chi^2 (1)=1.0548; p=0.304

Table 3: Prevalence of ovine fasciolosis on age basis.

Body condition	Number of examined animals	Prevalence n (%)
Poor	127	95 (74.80)
Medium	134	54 (40.30)
Good	123	15 (12.20)
Total/Overall prevalence	384	164 (42.71)

Pearson Chi^2(2)=100.57; p=0.0001

Table 4: Prevalence of ovine fasciolosis on body condition basis.

climatic differences and altitude among the localities.

Infection rate of ovine fasciolosis in the present study in Jimma (50%) was relatively higher than the other eight studied sites. This may be attributed to the existence of more favorable environment for both the snail intermediate host and the parasite which has small irrigation points and marshy area for long periods during the dry season. There is also small stagnant water in this area near the pasture where samples were collected from animals (personal observation).

Prevalence rate of 45.64% and 39.68% was recorded in female and male animals respectively. There was no statistically significant difference (p=0.238) between the two sexes. This signifies that sex has no impact on the infection rate and both female and male animals are equally susceptible and exposed to the disease. Similar results that support the present finding were reported by Dinka [29] and Molalegn et al. [21]. This might be due to grazing of both sexes in contaminated grazing pastures and both male and females stay out door due to the reason of no feed supplied at home.

However, some workers found higher prevalence rate in the male than female and their justification were related to management system with longer exposure of males outdoors when females are kept indoors at the end of pregnancy and at the beginning of lactation [29]. The prevalence between different age groups of animals were found to be statistically not significant (p=0.304). This might be due to grazing of young animals with the adults early after some days of parturition. However the results of Dinka [28] were contradictory to the present study. The highest prevalence was seen in the adults and relatively lowers in the young animals. Their justification was associated with the fact that young animals are not usually allowed to go far with adults for grazing. So the chance of exposure to infective metacercaria was very low as compared with adult animals.

The infection rate of ovine Fasciolosis was statistically analyzed on the basis of body condition to study the impact of disease on infected animals. The results of the study indicated that infection rates in poor body condition animals were significantly higher ($p<0.0001$) than that of good body condition animals, similar to the study done by Molalign et al. [21]. This signifies the importance of fasciolosis in causing weight loss and is the characteristic sign of the disease. Chronic fasciolosis is the commonest form of the disease in ruminants and one of the characteristics sign is weight loss (poor body condition) [30-32].

Conclusion and Recommendations

The present prevalence rate is 42.71% (overall prevalence) and conclude that fasciolosis is a widespread parasitic disease affecting the health and productivity of sheep. This is supported by the markedly higher prevalence among animals in poor body condition. The present study showed that the control program in the region may be ineffective. Therefore, proper attention should be paid to this parasitic problem and control strategies should advice at least to reduce the infection rate to economically tolerable level.

Based on the above conclusions the following recommendations are forwarded:

- Awareness creation to livestock owners to avoid risk factors, drain water bodies and proper deworming.
- Since the area is endowed with a lot of watery points feeding management should be implemented at their shades together with forage production.
- Strategic control of Intermediate host should be implemented in various methods according to feasibility.

Acknowledgements

The authors would like to thank the Jimma University, School of Veterinary Medicine and Haramaya University, College of Veterinary Medicine staffs for their cooperation and support.

Conflict of Interest

The authors declare that they have no conflict of interest.

References

1. Taylor MA, Coop RL, Wall RL (2007) Veterinary Parasitology. Blackwell Publishing, Oxford, England, UK, pp: 85-90.
2. Okewole EA, Ogunipe GA, Adejinmi JO, Olaniyasi AO (2000) Clinical evaluation of three chemoprophylactic regimes against ovine helminthiasis in Fasciola. endemic farm in Ibadan, Nigeria. Israel J Vet Med 56: 15-28.
3. WHO (World health organization) (1995) Control of food borne trematode infections. Technical Report series 849.
4. Radostits OM, Gray CC, Hichcliff KW, Constable PD (2007) Disease Associated with trematodes and cestodes. In: Veterinary Medicine, Textbook of the diseases of cattle, horses, sheep, pigs and goats, 10th edn, Elsevier, Amsterdam, Netherlands, pp: 1576-1580.
5. Yilma JM, Malone JB (1998) A Geographic information system forcast model for strategic control of fasciolosis in Ethiopia. Elev Vet Parasitology 78: 103-123.
6. Kahn CH (2005) The Merck Veterinary Manual. 9th edn, Fluke infection in Ruminants, Merck and Co, White House Station NJ, USA, pp: 273-276.
7. Nijau BC, Scholtens RG (1991) The role of traditional harvested hay in the Transmission of ovine fasciolosis in the Ethiopian highland. Veterinary Research Communication 15: 369-372.
8. Urquhart GM, Armour J, Duncan JL, Dunn AM, Jennings FW (1996) Veterinary parasitology. Oxford, Longman Scientific and Technical Press, UK, pp: 100-109.
9. Bowman DD (2003) Parasitology for veterinarians. 8th edn. Elsevier, pp: 115-122.
10. Negatisize PK, Bekele T, Tilahun G (1993) Financial losses caused by ovine fasciolosis in the Ethiopian highland. Trop An Health Prod 31: 155-161.
11. Mekete G, Mohammed AA (2003) Parasitology for medical laboratory technology students. Jimma University, Faculty of Public Health, pp: 42-44.
12. Mitchell GB (2003) Treatment and control of liver fluke in sheep and cattle. Technical Notes. West main roads, Edinburgh, UK.

13. Tolossa T, Tigre W (2007) The prevalence and economic significance of Bovine Fasciolosis at Jimma Abattoir. Int J Vet Med 3: 1-8.

14. JZAO (Jimma Zone Agricultural Office) (2010) Jimma.

15. Thrustfield M (2005) Veterinary epidemiology. 3rd edn. Blackwell Science, pp: 230-233.

16. Cringoli G, Rinaldi L, Veneziono V, Capelli G, Malone J (2002) A cross-sectional Coprological Survey from an area of southern Italian Apennines. Veterinary Parasitology 108: 137-143.

17. Hanson J, Perry B (1994) The epidemiology, diagnosis, and control of helminth parasites of ruminants. A handbook of animal production and health division, FAO, Rome.

18. Gupta SK, Singla LD (2012) Diagnostic trends in parasitic diseases of animals. In: Veterinary Diagnostics: Current Trends. Satish Serial Publishing House, Delhi, India, pp: 81-112.

19. Ahmed EK, Marcvitchtr K, Jumwasorn S, Koonawoot, Rittriron S, et al. (2007) Prevalence of Fasciola species infection in middle Awash river Basin, Ethiopia. Southeast Asian J Trop Med. Public Health 38: 51-57.

20. Michael A, Beyene P, Yilma J (2005) Infection prevalence of ovine fasciolosis in small scale Irrigation schemes along the upper Awash river basin. J Ethio Vet Asso 9:19-27.

21. Molalegne B, Nuradis I, Nahili A (2010) Study on the prevalence of Ovine fasciolosis in and around Dawa-Cheffa, Kemissie. African Journal of Agricultural Research 5: 2981-2985.

22. Adem A (1994) Prevalence of bovine and ovine fasciolosis: A preliminary survey around Zuway region, Shoa, Ethiopia. DVM Thesis, Faculty of Veterinary Medicine, Addis Ababa University, Debre Zeit, Ethiopia.

23. Chanie M, Begashaw S (2012) Assesment of the economic impact and prevalence of ovine fascilosis in Menz Lalo Midir District, North east Ethiopia. Vet World 5: 261-264.

24. Mezgabu M (1995) A survey on ovine fasciolosis and lung infestation in Addis Ababa and the surrounding highland area. DVM Thesis, Faculty of Veterinary Medicine, Addis Ababa University, Debrezeit, Ethiopia.

25. Yadata B (1994) Epidemiology of bovine and ovine Fasciolosis and distribution of its snail intermediate host in western Shewa. DVM Thesis, Faculty of Veterinary Medicine, Addis Ababa University, Debrezeit, Ethiopia.

26. Birhan T (2008) Prevalence of small ruminants' fasciolosis in and around Kombolcha. DVM Thesis, Haramaya University, Haramaya, Ethiopia.

27. Daniel F (1995) Economic importance of organs condemnation due to fasciolosis and hydatidosis in cattle and sheep slaughtered at Dire Dawa Abattoir. DVM Thesis, Faculty of Veterinary Medicine, Addis Ababa University, Debrezeit, Ethiopia.

28. Dinka A (1996) Preliminary study on prevalence of small ruminant fasciolosis in and around Assela. DVM Thesis, Faculty of Veterinary Medicine, Addis Ababa University, Debrezeit, Ethiopia.

29. Balock FC, Arthur RJ (1995) A survey of fasciolosis in beef cattle killed at Abattoir in Southern Queensland. Aust Vet J 62: 320-326.

30. Graber M (1995) Helimenths and Helimenthiasis of domestic and Wild Animals of Ethiopia. Bulletin of Animal Health and Production in Africa 23: 57-86.

31. Urquhart G, Armour J, Duncan A, Jennings F (1994) Veterinary parasitology. Longman Scientific and Technical Press, UK, pp: 159-165.

32. Central Statistical Authority (CSA) (2009) The federal democratic republic of Ethiopia, Central Statistical Authority, Agricultural sample survey 2008/2009 [2001 E.C]: Report on livestock Characteristics (privet peasant holdings), Addis Ababa, Ethiopia, p: 120.

Effect of Semen Diluents, Dilution Rates, and Storage Periods on Spermatozoa Motility of Different Varieties of Guinea Fowl

Keerthy AJ[1], Omprakash AV[2], Churchil RR[3] and Hudson GH[4]*

[1]*Directorate of Animal Husbandry, Kerala, India*
[2]*Poultry Research Station, Madhavaram Milk Colony, Chennai, Tamil Nadu, India*
[3]*Institutional Livestock Farm Complex, Veterinary College and Research Institute, Orathanadu, Thanjavur, Tamil Nadu, India*
[4]*Department of Poultry Science, Madras Veterinary College, Chennai, Tamil Nadu, India*

Abstract

Twelve number of healthy male guinea fowls from each variety of pearl, white, white breasted and lavender were selected based on the phenotypic characters and trained for semen collection by abdominal massage technique. Pooled semen from each variety, were diluted with the Lakes Semen Extender, Modified Beltsville Poultry Semen Extender, and Beltsville Poultry Semen Extender each in the ratio of 1:3, 1:4 and 1:5. The spermatozoa motility was assessed at 0, 1, 2, 4 and 6 hours of storage. Maximum per cent motility of 83.33, 86.67 and 79.19 were observed in the semen of pearl, white breasted and lavender varieties of guinea fowl diluted Beltsville Poultry Semen Extender in the ration 1:4 at 6 h of storage. Maximum spermatozoa motility with white guinea fowl variety at maximum storage period was observed with the semen diluted (1:3) with Beltsville Poultry Semen Extender (81.67%). The current study will be of immense useful for the selection of semen diluents for better fertility through artificial insemination in guinea fowls.

Keywords: Spermatozoa motility; Guinea fowl; Fertility

Introduction

Guinea fowls are hardy, semi wild poultry that are yet to be genetically improved for commercial meat and egg production. The fertility in guinea fowls is low which forms the major constraint for its genetic improvement and commercial exploitation. In addition, sexing problems [1], seasonality of breeding [2-4], monogamous behavior [5] may also contribute to lower fertility rates. Artificial insemination is the novel tool for improving the fertility in domestic animals and poultry. The technology can be successful only with superior semen quality. Spermatozoa motility is the important parameter that determines the movement of spermatozoa in the female oviduct. It was reported that the number of progressively motile sperm per ejaculate was the most consistent and reliable trait correlated with fertility [6]. Positive correlations between spermatozoa motility and fertility have been reported by several authors in different species of poultry [7,8]. Poultry spermatozoa are fragile, and the semen quality of raw semen deteriorates within one hour of collection [9]. Although published reports regarding the seminology of guinea fowls are less, the advantages of using the semen diluents in other poultry species were reviewed. The semen diluents are reported to be used to extend semen, maintain the livability and fertilizing capacity *in vitro*, and maximize the number of hens that can be inseminated [10]. Therefore the efficiency of different semen diluents in maintaining the spermatozoa motility of different varieties of Guinea Fowl namely the pearl, white, white breasted and lavender, under short term storage was studied.

Three semen diluents namely the Lakes Semen Extender (LSE), Modified Beltsville Poultry Semen Extender (MBPSE) and Beltsville Poultry Semen Extender (BPSE) were used for the current study. The spermatozoa motility of raw semen of pearl, lavender and white varieties was reported as 87.00 ± 4.40, 90.11 ± 3.70 and 84.34 ± 5.11 respectively [11]. The superiority of BPSE over many othersemen diluents were also reported in different poultry species [12-14]. The decrease in spermatozoa motility with increase in the dilution ratio and storage periods were reported with BPSE and IMV diluents in the ratio 1:2 and 1:3 stored for up to six hours [13]. No works regarding MBPSE with guinea fowl semen could be traced. The current study was carried out during October- December months where the average daily high temperature in the study area (13.1623°N, 80.2433°E) was was between 22oC and 31oC. The birds used for the study were housed in individual cages and maintained under standard feeding and manage mental conditions.

Materials and Methods

Initially 12 healthy, mature male guinea fowls aged eight months were selected based on their phenotypic characters from each variety of guinea fowl namely the pearl, white, white breasted and lavender. They were housed in individual cages providing a floor space of 1 sq. ft. per bird. Breeder ration containing 17% crude protein, 2700 kcal of Metabolisable Energy, 3% calcium, 1% lysine and 0.50% methionine was provided at *ad libitum* with free access to drinking water. The feathers around the vent region of the birds were clipped off and were trained for semen collection for a period of about one month.

Semen was collected during early hours of the day between twice a week following abdominal massage technique [14]. Pooled semen sample collected was then diluted with three different diluents namely the LSE [15], MBPSE [16] and BPSE [17]. The pH and osmolarity were measured and adjusted to standard levels using DALAL pH meter and OSMOMAT 030 cryoscopic osmometer respectively.

Exactly 100 μL of raw semen was diluted with 200 μL, 300 μL and 400 μL of each diluent in sterile eppendorf tubes to get the final dilution of 1:3, 1:4 and 1:5 respectively. The tubes were then stored at 5°C and the spermatozoa motility were analyzed at zero, one, two, four

***Corresponding author:** Hudson GH, Department of Poultry Science, Madras Veterinary College, Chennai, Tamil Nadu, India
E-mail: hudson.bvsc@gmail.com

and six hours of storage. A drop of diluted semen with the aid of a micropipette was placed on a microscope slide, which was then covered with a glass cover slip and examined under 400 x magnifications in a light microscope. The motility determination was carried out by taking into consideration subjective measurements based on the judgment of individuals making the determination. The motility was expressed as the percentage of cells that are motile under their own power [18].

The statistical analysis of the data was carried out by one way ANOVA using Statistical Package for the Social Sciences 20.0 software [19].

Results

Effect of different semen extenders, dilution ratio and storage periods on motility of pearl, white, white breated and lavender guinea fowl spermatozoa at 5°C (Mean ± SE) were presented from Tables 1- 4 respectively.

Pearl variety

The duration of storage had a significant ($P \leq 0.05$) effect in semen diluted with LSE and MBPSE in 1:3 dilution rates with significant ($P \leq 0.05$) reduction after 4 h post-dilution. However there was no significant ($P \geq 0.05$) difference between storage periods in semen diluted with BPSE at 1:3 dilution rates. At 1:4 dilution rates, significant change in motility was observed in semen diluted with LSE ($P \leq 0.01$) and BPSE ($P \leq 0.05$) but not with MBPSE. The reduction of motility became significant ($P \leq 0.05$) at 2 and 4 h post-dilution in LSE and MBPSE respectively. In case of 1:5 dilution rates, significant ($P \leq 0.01$) reduction in motility was noticed only in semen diluted with LSE.

Irrespective of the dilution rates, there observed significant difference ($P \leq 0.05$) between the extenders at 6 h of storage with BPSE maintaining significantly ($P \leq 0.05$) higher motility compared to other two semen extenders. The different dilution rates with a particular semen extender at any particular storage period did not have any significant effect on motility.

White variety

The duration of storage had a significant effect in both semen

Treatment combinations (n=6)	LSE	MBPSE	BPSE	F value
1:3,0 hour	$90.00^{b} \pm 4.66$	$88.33^{c} \pm 2.79$	91.67 ± 2.79	**0.265** ^{NS}
1:3,1 hour	$82.50^{ab} \pm 6.92$	$85.00^{bc} \pm 2.24$	88.33 ± 3.80	**0.719** ^{NS}
1:3,2 hours	$79.17^{ab} \pm 6.11$	$82.50^{abc} \pm 2.50$	86.67 ± 2.79	**0.843** ^{NS}
1:3,4 hours	$70.83^{a} \pm 6.11$	$80.00^{ab} \pm 2.24$	83.33 ± 2.11	**2.773** ^{NS}
1:3,6 hours	$64.17^{Aa} \pm 6.38$	$74.17^{ABa} \pm 2.39$	$81.67^{B} \pm 2.79$	**4.471** *
F value	**3.669** *	**3.464** *	**1.880** ^{NS}	
1:4,0 hour	$90.00^{c} \pm 3.87$	88.33 ± 4.01	$93.33^{b} \pm 2.11$	**0.390** ^{NS}
1:4,1 hour	$85.83^{bc} \pm 3.96$	85.00 ± 4.28	$90.00^{ab} \pm 1.83$	**0.520** ^{NS}
1:4,2 hours	$81.67^{ab} \pm 3.33$	80.83 ± 4.73	$89.17^{ab} \pm 2.01$	**1.763** ^{NS}
1:4,4 hours	$76.66^{ab} \pm 3.33$	77.50 ± 4.79	$86.67^{a} \pm 1.05$	**2.989** ^{NS}
1:4,6 hours	$69.17^{Aa} \pm 2.39$	$75.00^{AB} \pm 5.16$	$83.33^{Ba} \pm 2.11$	**4.695** *
F value	**5.137** **	**1.796** ^{NS}	**3.596** *	
1:5,0 hour	$87.50^{d} \pm 3.35$	84.17 ± 3.01	91.67 ± 2.79	**1.992** ^{NS}
1:5,1 hour	$85.00^{cd} \pm 2.58$	79.17 ± 4.17	90.00 ± 3.16	**2.884** ^{NS}
1:5,2 hours	$80.83^{bc} \pm 2.01$	75.83 ± 4.55	87.50 ± 4.03	**2.859** ^{NS}
1:5,4 hours	$75.83^{ab} \pm 1.54$	72.50 ± 5.13	83.33 ± 3.80	**2.397** ^{NS}
1:5,6 hours	$67.50^{Aa} \pm 1.12$	$70.00^{A} \pm 5.00$	$81.67^{B} \pm 4.60$	**3.867** *
F value	**10.198** **	**1.791** ^{NS}	**1.157** ^{NS}	

Ratio	0 hour	1 hour	2 hours	4 hours	6 hours
LSE ,1:3	90.00 ± 4.66	82.50 ± 6.92	79.17 ± 6.11	70.83 ± 6.11	64.17 ± 6.38
LSE ,1:4	90.00 ± 3.87	85.83 ± 3.96	81.67 ± 3.33	76.67 ± 3.33	69.17 ± 2.39
LSE ,1:5	87.50 ± 3.35	85.00 ± 2.58	80.83 ± 2.01	75.83 ± 1.54	67.50 ± 1.12
‘F’ value	**0.396** ^{NS}	**0.077** ^{NS}	**0.061** ^{NS}	**0.538** ^{NS}	**0.348** ^{NS}
MBPSE,1:3	88.33 ± 2.79	85.00 ± 2.24	82.50 ± 2.50	80.00 ± 2.24	74.17 ± 2.39
MBPSE,1:4	88.33 ± 4.01	85.00 ± 4.28	80.83 ± 4.73	77.50 ± 4.79	75.00 ± 5.16
MBPSE,1:5	84.17 ± 3.01	79.17 ± 4.17	75.833 ± 4.55	72.50 ± 5.12	70.00 ± 5.00
‘F’ value	**0.677** ^{NS}	**0.911** ^{NS}	**0.745** ^{NS}	**0.802** ^{NS}	**0.387** ^{NS}
BPSE,1:3	91.67 ± 2.79	88.33 ± 3.81	86.67 ± 2.79	83.33 ± 2.11	81.67 ± 2.79
BPSE,1:4	93.33 ± 2.11	90.00 ± 1.83	89.17 ± 2.01	86.67 ± 1.05	83.33 ± 2.11
BPSE,1:5	91.67 ± 2.79	90.00 ± 3.16	87.50 ± 4.03	83.33 ± 3.80	81.67 ± 4.60
‘F’ value	**0.039** ^{NS}	**0.114** ^{NS}	**0.254** ^{NS}	**0.347** ^{NS}	**0.047** ^{NS}

Means bearing different superscripts in uppercase letter in a row and lowercase letter in a column differ significantly. **Highly significant ($P \leq 0.01$), * Significant ($P \leq 0.05$), ^{NS}- Not significant ($P > 0.05$).

Table 1: Effect of different semen extenders- dilution ratio and storage periods on motility of pearl guinea fowl spermatozoa at 5°C (Mean ± SE).

Treatment combinations (n=6)	LSE	MBPSE	BPSE	F value
1:3,0 hour	80.00^{Ac} ± 1.29	88.33^{Bb} ± 2.79	91.67^{B} ± 2.79	**9.312^{**}**
1:3,1 hour	78.33^{Ac} ± 1.67	86.67^{Bb} ± 2.11	88.33^{B} ± 3.81	**9.646^{**}**
1:3,2 hours	74.17^{Abc} ± 2.39	81.67^{Bab} ± 2.47	86.67^{B} ± 2.79	**9.382^{**}**
1:3,4 hours	70.00^{Ab} ± 2.58	77.50^{ABab} ± 4.96	83.33^{B} ± 2.11	**5.144^{*}**
1:3,6 hours	63.33^{Aa} ± 2.11	70.83^{ABa} ± 7.12	81.67^{B} ± 2.79	**4.430^{*}**
F value	**10.868^{**}**	**3.012^{*}**	**1.880^{NS}**	
1:4,0 hour	83.33^{Ac} ± 2.79	90.83^{Bb} ± 2.39	90.83^{Bc} ± 0.83	**4.386^{*}**
1:4,1 hour	79.17^{Abc} ± 3.01	90.00^{Bb} ± 2.58	88.33^{Bbc} ± 1.05	**6.456^{**}**
1:4,2 hours	77.50^{Abc} ± 3.60	85.00^{Bab} ± 2.24	86.67^{Bb} ± 1.05	**4.047^{*}**
1:4,4 hours	72.50^{Aab} ± 2.50	84.17^{Bab} ± 2.71	81.67^{Ba} ± 1.05	**7.634^{**}**
1:4,6 hours	68.33^{Aa} ± 2.79	79.17^{Ba} ± 1.54	78.33^{Ba} ± 1.67	**8.530^{**}**
F value	**4.370^{**}**	**4.348^{**}**	**18.369^{**}**	
1:5,0 hour	82.50^{c} ± 1.71	87.50 ± 4.23	92.50^{b} ± 2.81	**3.179^{NS}**
1:5,1 hour	80.00^{bc} ± 1.83	83.33 ± 3.58	88.33^{ab} ± 2.79	**2.556^{NS}**
1:5,2 hours	75.83^{b} ± 1.54	81.67 ± 4.22	85.83^{a} ± 2.01	**3.286^{NS}**
1:5,4 hours	69.17^{Aa} ± 2.39	78.33^{AB} ± 4.01	83.33^{Ba} ± 2.79	**5.035^{*}**
1:5,6 hours	63.33^{a} ± 2.47	70.00 ± 6.71	79.17^{a} ± 3.01	**3.372^{NS}**
F value	**14.293^{**}**	**2.205^{NS}**	**3.861^{*}**	

Ratio	0 hour	1 hour	2 hours	4 hours	6 hours
LSE,1:3	80.00 ± 1.29	78.33 ± 1.67	74.17 ± 2.39	70.00 ± 2.59	63.33 ± 2.11
LSE,1:4	83.33 ± 2.79	79.17 ± 3.01	77.50 ± 3.59	72.50 ± 2.50	68.33 ± 2.79
LSE,1:5	82.50 ± 1.71	80.00 ± 1.83	75.83 ± 1.54	69.17 ± 2.39	63.33 ± 2.47
'F' value	**0.857^{NS}**	**0.162^{NS}**	**0.487^{NS}**	**0.490^{NS}**	**1.394^{NS}**
MBPSE,1:3	88.33 ± 2.79	86.67 ± 2.11	81.67 ± 2.47	77.50 ± 4.96	70.83 ± 7.12
MBPSE,1:4	90.83 ± 2.39	90.00 ± 2.58	85.00 ± 2.24	84.17 ± 2.71	79.17 ± 1.54
MBPSE,1:5	87.50 ± 4.23	83.33 ± 3.58	81.67 ± 4.22	78.33 ± 4.01	70.00 ± 6.71
'F' value	**0.241^{NS}**	**1.602^{NS}**	**0.360^{NS}**	**0.808^{NS}**	**0.757^{NS}**
BPSE,1:3	92.50 ± 1.71	89.17 ± 1.54	87.50 ± 1.71	85.00 ± 1.83	81.67 ± 2.79
BPSE,1:4	90.83 ± 0.83	88.33 ± 1.05	86.67 ± 1.05	81.67 ± 1.05	78.33 ± 1.67
BPSE,1:5	92.50 ± 2.81	88.33 ± 2.79	85.83 ± 2.01	83.33 ± 2.79	79.17 ± 3.01
'F' value	**0.742^{NS}**	**0.069^{NS}**	**0.255^{NS}**	**0.751^{NS}**	**0.534^{NS}**

Means bearing different superscripts in uppercase letter in a row and lowercase letter in a column differ significantly, **Highly significant (P≤0.01), *Significant (P≤0.05), ^{NS}-Not significant (P>0.05).

Table 2: Effect of different semen extenders - dilution ratio and storage periods on motility of white guinea fowl spermatozoa at 5°C (Mean ± SE).

diluted with LSE (P ≤ 0.01) and MBPSE (P ≤ 0.05) at 1:3 dilution rates. However there was no significant (P>0.05) difference in semen diluted with BPSE at 1:3 dilution rate. Significant (P ≤ 0.01) reduction in motility observed in semen diluted with LSE, MBPSE and BPSE at 1:4 dilution rate from 0 to 6 hours of storage. The reduction in motility became evident (P ≤ 0.05) at 4 h post-dilution in LSE and BPSE and 6 h post-dilution in MBPSE. At 1:5 dilution rate there was no significant reduction in motility in semen diluted with MBPSE, however there was significant reduction in motility in semen diluted with LSE (P≤0.01) and BPSE (P ≤ 0.05). Further semen diluted with BPSE at 1:3 and BPSE and MBPSE at 1:4 dilution rate maintained higher motility at 6 h storage period.

The superiority of BPSE over other diluents was much evident with 1:3 and 1:4 dilutions, irrespective of the storage periods. Whereas, with 1:5 dilution, significant difference in spermatozoa motility, was observed only at 4 hours of storage. The dilution rate alone did not show any significant difference between storage periods for each semen extender.

White breasted

The duration of storage had a significant (P≤0.05) effect on the spermatozoa motility of the white breasted Guinea Fowl semen diluted with LSE at 1:3 dilution rate and MBPSE at 1:3 and 1:5 dilution rates with reduction in motility from 0 h to 6 h of storage. With respect to BPSE, highly significant (P≤0.01) reduction in motility was observed from from 0 h to 6 h of storage in all the dilution rates under study. Further, irrespective of dilution rates, the semen diluted with BPSE had maintained superior spermatozoa motility at 6 h of storage compared to LSE and MBPSE diluents.**Lavender**

The duration of storage had high significant (P ≤ 0.01) effect in all other combinations except for LSE in 1:3 dilution rates. Further BPSE has maintained higher motility at 6 h storage period at all dilution rates compare to other semen extenders. There was significant difference observed in motility for semen diluted with LSE, MBPSE and BPSE except for 1:4 at 4 h of storage period. The dilution rate alone showed significant (P ≤ 0.05) difference in semen diluted with MBPSE at 0 and 6 h and BPSE at 1 and 2 h. The dilution rate alone showed highly significant (P ≤ 0.01) difference for MBPSE at 1 h and BPSE at 0 h of storage period. LSE was not influenced by dilution rate for different storage periods. After dilution, the motility was progressively reduced in all semen extenders and the reduction was significant (P ≤ 0.05) at 2 and 6 h post-dilution in 1:4 and 1:5 ratios with LSE, at 2, 4 and 6 h in all dilutions (1:3, 1:4 and 1:5). The addition MBPSE at 1:3 ratios has resulted in time-related reduction in spermatozoa motility at time intervals of post-dilution, 1 and 4 h at 1:4 ratio and 2 and 4 h at 1:5 dilution rates.

Discussion

Based on the dilution studies it was interpreted that among the diluents, the BPSE has shown its superiority over other diluents

Treatment combinations (n=6)	LSE	MBPSE	BPSE	F value
1:3,0 hour	90.00^{Ac} ± 4.08	87.50^{Ab} ± 2.81	97.50^{Bb} ± 1.12	**5.935***
1:3,1 hour	85.00^{Abc} ± 5.16	85.00^{Ab} ± 3.87	95.83^{Bb} ± 1.54	**4.393***
1:3,2 hours	76.67^{Aab} ± 6.01	84.17^{ABab} ± 2.39	91.67^{Bb} ± 1.05	**4.768***
1:3,4 hours	71.67^{Aab} ± 5.87	79.17^{ABab} ± 2.39	87.50^{Ba} ± 2.50	**4.703***
1:3,6 hours	67.50^{Aa} ± 5.74	75.00^{Aa} ± 2.58	85.00^{Ba} ± 1.83	**6.424****
F value	**3.830***	**3.052***	**8.667****	
1:4,0 hour	87.50 ± 5.59	90.83 ± 4.55	98.33^{c} ± 1.05	**3.293^{NS}**
1:4,1 hour	84.17 ± 7.24	85.83 ± 4.55	95.83^{b} ± 0.83	**2.489^{NS}**
1:4,2 hours	79.17 ± 6.25	82.50 ± 4.79	92.50^{ab} ± 1.12	**2.941^{NS}**
1:4,4 hours	75.00 ± 5.92	79.17 ± 5.23	88.33^{a} ± 1.05	**2.568^{NS}**
1:4,6 hours	70.00^{A} ± 5.92	75.83^{AB} ± 5.39	86.67^{Ba} ± 2.11	**3.837***
F value	**1.735^{NS}**	**2.287^{NS}**	**13.847****	
1:5,0 hour	85.83^{A} ± 5.23	87.50^{Ac} ± 3.82	96.67^{Bc} ± 1.67	**4.825***
1:5,1 hour	83.33^{A} ± 5.73	83.33^{Abc} ± 4.01	94.17^{Bbc} ± 1.54	**3.706***
1:5,2 hours	77.50 ± 5.59	77.50^{abc} ± 5.29	90.00^{ab} ± 0.00	**3.442^{NS}**
1:5,4 hours	70.83^{A} ± 5.39	71.67^{Aab} ± 4.60	85.83^{Ba} ± 2.01	**4.962***
1:5,6 hours	67.50^{A} ± 5.74	68.33^{Aa} ± 4.94	83.33^{Ba} ± 2.79	**4.399***
F value	**2.620^{NS}**	**3.039***	**8.671****	

Ratio	0 hour	1 hour	2 hours	4 hours	6 hours
LSE ,1:3	90.00 ± 4.08	85.00 ± 5.16	76.67 ± 6.01	71.67 ± 5.87	67.50 ± 5.74
LSE ,1:4	87.50 ± 5.59	84.17 ± 7.24	79.17 ± 6.25	75.00 ± 5.92	70.00 ± 5.92
LSE ,1:5	85.83 ± 5.23	83.33 ± 5.73	77.50 ± 5.59	70.83 ± 5.39	67.50 ± 5.74
'F' value	**0.249^{NS}**	**0.043^{NS}**	**0.073^{NS}**	**0.195^{NS}**	**0.078^{NS}**
MBPSE,1:3	87.50 ± 2.81	85.00 ± 3.87	84.17 ± 2.39	79.17 ± 2.39	75.00 ± 2.58
MBPSE,1:4	90.83 ± 4.55	85.83 ± 4.55	82.50 ± 4.79	79.17 ± 5.23	75.83 ± 5.39
MBPSE,1:5	87.50 ± 3.82	83.33 ± 4.02	77.50 ± 5.29	71.67 ± 4.60	68.33 ± 4.94
'F' value	**0.863^{NS}**	**0.151^{NS}**	**0.634^{NS}**	**1.164^{NS}**	**0.940^{NS}**
BPSE,1:3	97.50 ± 1.12	95.83 ± 1.54	91.67 ± 1.05	87.50 ± 2.50	85.00 ± 1.83
BPSE,1:4	98.33 ± 1.05	95.83 ± 0.83	92.50 ± 1.12	88.33 ± 1.05	86.67 ± 2.11
BPSE,1:5	96.67 ± 1.67	94.17 ± 1.54	90.00 ± 0.00	85.83 ± 2.01	83.33 ± 2.79
'F' value	**0.273^{NS}**	**0.325^{NS}**	**2.059^{NS}**	**0.388^{NS}**	**0.524^{NS}**

Means bearing different superscripts in uppercase letter in a row and lowercase letter in a column differ significantly, ** Highly significant (P≤0.01), * Significant (P≤0.05), ^{NS}- Not significant (P>0.05).

Table 3: Effect of different semen extenders-dilution ratio and storage periods on motility of white breasted guinea fowl spermatozoa at 5°C (Mean ± SE).

in maintaining the motility of guinea fowl different varieties of spermatozoa under short term storage. The results obtained were in agreement with the previous studies in turkey semen [8,12]. In addition, higher fertility percentage were reported in turkey semen diluted with BPSE extender stored for 24 hours [14] which may also be attributed to superior motility compared to IMV and MTGA diluents. However, the superiority of CARI diluent over BPSE, LSE and normal saline for a 24 hour storage period were also interpreted with higher fertility rates in guinea fowls [20]. The varying values obtained between the extenders may be due to different pH, composition of the diluents, metabolites released upon storage etc.

Irrespective of the diluents and dilution rates, the **spermatozoa motility** showed a declining trend, as storage time progresses from 0-6 hours. Similar results were also reported in Helmeted guinea fowl semen preserved in powdered coconut water [21] and turkey semen diluted (1:2) with poultry semen extender [22]. Complementary results were also obtained in guinea fowl semen in CARI (24 h), BPSE (6 h) and IMV (6 h) diluents in guinea fowl semen [13,23]. The reduction in motility may be attributed to the release of sperm metabolites which alter the nutrient composition of the medium. Further, storage alters the osmolarity [24] of the medium, which leads to various sperm abnormality, which further reduces the progressive motility. It was reported that storage of fowl semen in ringer's solution causes increased production of chloride ions which increases the spermatozoa abnormality [25]. The similar ionic changes that affect spermatozoa motility in guinea fowl semen needs to be further investigated with specific diluents under consideration. Identification of these attributes in future, may lead to efficient long term liquid storage of guinea fowl semen.

The dilution rate did not showed any significant difference between storage periods irrespective of the extenders and the guinea fowl varieties. However, the superior per spermatozoa motility at lower dilution (1:2 and 1:3) were reported with BPSE and IMV diluents [13]. The non-significant effects of dilution rates may be due to higher dilution rates used in the current study.

Conclusion

The dilution studies revealed that, the semen diluted with BPSE (1:4) and MBPSE (1:4) or BPSE (1:3) in pearl and white variety of guinea fowls respectively, and BPSE (1:4) in white breasted and lavender varieties, stored for 6 h is recommended, as the above combinations maintained superior motility, which may further yield better fertility through artificial insemination in Guinea Fowls.

Acknowledgements

The authors are highly thankful to Dean, Madras Veterinary College, Chennai and Hon'ble Vice Chancellor, Tamil Nadu Veterinary and Animal Sciences University for providing all the necessary support and facilities for conducting this study.

Treatment combinations (n=6)	LSE	MBPSE	BPSE	F value
1:3,0 hour	$82.50^{A} \pm 2.81$	$85.83^{ABd} \pm 2.01$	$90.83^{Be} \pm 0.83$	**4.751^{*}**
1:3,1 hour	$78.33^{A} \pm 2.79$	$83.33^{Ad} \pm 1.05$	$88.33^{Bd} \pm 1.05$	**9.026^{**}**
1:3,2 hours	$76.67^{A} \pm 3.58$	$78.33^{Ac} \pm 1.67$	$85.00^{Bc} \pm 0.00$	**4.453^{*}**
1:3,4 hours	$74.17^{A} \pm 3.96$	$73.33^{Ab} \pm 1.67$	$81.67^{Bb} \pm 1.05$	**3.752^{*}**
1:3,6 hours	$70.00^{A} \pm 4.08$	$61.67^{Aa} \pm 1.67$	$76.67^{Ba} \pm 1.05$	**8.782^{**}**
F value	**2.041^{NS}**	**31.176^{**}**	**34.855^{**}**	
1:4,0 hour	$86.67^{Ac} \pm 1.67$	$88.33^{Ad} \pm 1.05$	$93.33^{Bc} \pm 1.05$	**8.585^{**}**
1:4,1 hour	$81.67^{Abc} \pm 1.67$	$85.00^{Bcd} \pm 0.00$	$90.00^{Cb} \pm 0.00$	**24.222^{**}**
1:4,2 hours	$79.17^{Ab} \pm 2.39$	$80.00^{Abc} \pm 1.29$	$87.50^{Bb} \pm 1.12$	**8.227^{**}**
1:4,4 hours	$75.00^{ab} \pm 2.58$	$76.67^{b} \pm 3.33$	$82.50^{a} \pm 1.71$	**2.511^{NS}**
1:4,6 hours	$70.00^{Aa} \pm 2.58$	$70.00^{Aa} \pm 3.16$	$79.17^{Ba} \pm 2.01$	**4.447^{*}**
F value	**8.832^{**}**	**13.361^{**}**	**18.861^{**}**	
1:5,0 hour	$85.83^{Bc} \pm 0.83$	$82.50^{Ad} \pm 1.12$	$88.33^{Bc} \pm 1.05$	**8.291^{**}**
1:5,1 hour	$80.83^{Ab} \pm 0.83$	$80.83^{Acd} \pm 0.83$	$86.67^{Bbc} \pm 1.05$	**12.940^{**}**
1:5,2 hours	$79.17^{Ab} \pm 0.83$	$78.33^{Ac} \pm 1.05$	$84.17^{Bb} \pm 0.83$	**13.058^{**}**
1:5,4 hours	$73.33^{Aa} \pm 1.67$	$72.50^{Ab} \pm 1.12$	$80.83^{Ba} \pm 0.83$	**13.769^{**}**
1:5,6 hours	$70.83^{Aa} \pm 2.39$	$66.67^{Aa} \pm 1.05$	$78.33^{Ba} \pm 1.05$	**13.283^{**}**
F value	**18.195^{**}**	**36.826^{**}**	**17.199^{**}**	

Ratio	0 hour	1 hour	2 hours	4 hours	6 hours
LSE,1:3	82.50 ± 2.81	78.33 ± 2.79	76.67 ± 3.58	74.17 ± 3.96	70.00 ± 4.08
LSE,1:4	86.67 ± 1.67	81.67 ± 1.67	79.17 ± 2.39	75.00 ± 2.58	70.00 ± 2.58
LSE,1:5	85.83 ± 0.83	80.83 ± 0.83	79.17 ± 0.83	73.33 ± 1.67	70.83 ± 2.39
'F' value	**1.244^{NS}**	**0.794^{NS}**	**0.288^{NS}**	**0.104^{NS}**	**0.022^{NS}**
MBPSE,1:3	$85.83^{ab} \pm 2.01$	$83.33^{b} \pm 1.05$	78.33 ± 1.67	73.33 ± 1.67	$61.67^{a} \pm 1.67$
MBPSE,1:4	$88.33^{b} \pm 1.05$	$85.00^{b} \pm 0.00$	80.00 ± 1.29	76.67 ± 3.33	$70.00^{b} \pm 3.16$
MBPSE,1:5	$82.50^{a} \pm 1.12$	$80.83^{a} \pm 0.83$	78.33 ± 1.05	72.50 ± 1.12	$66.67^{ab} \pm 1.05$
'F' value	**4.106^{*}**	**7.308^{**}**	**0.535^{NS}**	**1.196^{NS}**	**3.910^{*}**
BPSE,1:3	$90.83^{ab} \pm 0.83$	$88.33^{ab} \pm 1.05$	$85.00^{a} \pm 0.00$	81.67 ± 1.05	76.67 ± 1.05
BPSE,1:4	$93.33^{b} \pm 1.05$	$90.00^{b} \pm 0.00$	$87.50^{b} \pm 1.12$	82.50 ± 1.71	79.17 ± 2.01
BPSE,1:5	$88.33^{a} \pm 1.05$	$86.67^{a} \pm 1.05$	$84.17^{a} \pm 0.83$	80.83 ± 0.83	78.33 ± 1.05
'F' value	**6.502^{**}**	**3.750^{*}**	**4.839^{*}**	**0.472^{NS}**	**0.819^{NS}**

Means bearing different superscripts in uppercase letter in a row and lowercase letter in a column differ significantly, **Highly significant ($P \leq 0.01$), *Significant ($P \leq 0.05$), ^{NS}- Not significant ($P > 0.05$).

Table 4: Effect of different semen extenders-dilution ratio and storage periods on motility of lavender guinea fowl spermatozoa at 5°C (Mean ± SE).

References

1. Abdul-Rahman II, Awumbila B, Jeffcoate IA, Robinson JE, Obese FY (2015) Sexing in guinea fowls (*Numida meleagris*). Poult Sci 94: 311-318.
2. Ayorinde KL (1989) Effect of semen dosage and insemination frequency on the fertility of local pearly Guinea Fowl in Nigeria. Trop Agric 66: 135-136.
3. Konlan SP, Avornyo FK, Karbo N, Sulleyman A (2011) Increasing guinea fowl eggs availability and hatchability in the dry season. J World's Poult Res 1: 1-3.
4. Premavalli K (2013) Influence of strain, age and system of management on the productive and reproductive performance of Guinea Fowl. PhD Thesis submitted to the Tamil Nadu Veterinary and Animal Sciences University, Chennai.
5. Aire TA, Ayeni JSO, Olowo-Okorun MO (1983) Some aspects of the reproductive biology of the guinea fowl (*Numida meleagris galeata Pallas*). The Helmet Guinea Fowl (*Numida meleagris galeata Pallas*) in Nigeria, Kainji Lake Research Institute, New Bussa, Nigeria, pp: 189-193.
6. Kammerer DM, Moreng RE, Muller HD, Hobbs HW (1972) Turkey semen evaluation for fertility prediction. Poult Sci 51: 77-82.
7. Wishart GJ, Palmer FH (1986) Correlation of the fertilizing ability of semen from individual male fowls with sperm motility and ATP content. Br Poult Sci **27**: 97-102.
8. Venkatesh G (2005) Effect of pre- Insemination vaginal douching and different semen extenders on fertility and hatchability in turkeys. MVSc Thesis submitted to the Tamil Nadu Veterinary and Animal Sciences University, Chennai.
9. Carter RD, McCartney MG, Chamberlin VD, Wyne JW (1957) The effect of storage time and temperature on fertilizing capacity of Turkey semen. Poult Sci 36: 618-621.
10. Lake PE (1956) A retarding factor in the problem of fowl semen storage. In: Proc. of 3rd International Congress on Animal Reproduction. 3: 104-106.
11. Mohan J, Sharma SK, Kolluri G, Singh RP, Tyagi JS, et al. (2016) Semen quality characteristics and seasonality in different varieties of male Guinea fowl. Adv Anim Vet Sci 4: 320-326.
12. Iaffaldano N, Rosato MP, Manchisi A, Centoducati G, Meluzzi A (2010) Comparison of different extenders on the quality characteristics of turkey semen during storage. Ital J Anim Sci 4: 513-515.
13. Hudson GH (2015) Fertility Parameters through artificial insemination in Guinea Fowl. M.V.Sc Thesis submitted to the Tamil Nadu Veterinary and Animal Sciences University, Chennai.
14. Burrows WH, Quinn JP (1937) The collection of spermatozoa from the domestic fowl and turkey. Poult Sci 16: 19-24.
15. Lake PE, Ravie O (1982) Effect on fertility of storing turkey semen for 24 hours at 10°C in fluids of different pH. Br Poult Sci 23: 41-47.
16. Kumararaj R, Omprakash AV (1996) Effect of different diluents, cryoprotectants and equilibration period on freezing of poultry semen. In: Proceedings of XX World Poultry Congress. Delhi, India, pp: 555-568.
17. Sexton TJ, Giesen AF (1982) Beltsville Poultry Semen Extender. 6. Holding turkey semen for 6 hrs at 15°C. Poult Sci 61: 1202-1208.
18. Parker JE, McKenzie FF, Kempster HL (1942) Fertility in the male domestic fowl. Research Bulletin 347: 1-50.
19. Snedecor GW, Cochran WG (1994) Statistical methods. IX edition. Oxford and IBH publishing & Co., Kolkata, India.
20. Mohan J, Sharma SK, Kolluri G, Tyagi JS (2015) Selection of Diluent for Short Term Preservation of Guinea Fowl Semen. Asian J Anim Vet Adv 10: 360-364.

21. Lavor CTB, Câmara SR, Bandeira BM, Salgueiro CDM, Castro EV, et al. (2012) Powdered coconut water as preservation medium of guinea fowl (*Numida meleagris*) sperm. In: Ciência Animal 22: 79-81.

22. Słowińska M, Liszewska E, Dietrich GJ, Ciereszko A (2012) Characterization of proacrosin/acrosin system after liquid storage and cryopreservation of turkey semen (*Meleagris gallopavo*). Theriogenology 78: 1065-1077.

23. Mohan J, Khanday JM, Singh RP, Tyagi JS (2013) Effect of Storage on the Physico-Biochemical Characteristics and Fertility of Guinea Fowl Semen. Adv Anim Vet Sci 1: 65-68.

24. Clark RN, Bakest MR, Ottinger MA (1984) Morphological changes in Chicken and Turkey spermatozoa incubated under various conditions. Poult Sci 63: 801-805.

25. Saeki Y (1960) Crooked-Necked Spermatozoa in Relation to Low Fertility in the Artificial Insemination of Fowl. Poult Sci 39: 1354-1360.

A Preliminary Comparison of Semen Quality between Competing and Non-Competing Equine Stallions

Megan Wilson and Anke Twigg-Flesner*

Performance in Equestrian Sport Research Group, Hartpury University Centre, Hartpury College, Gloucestershire, GL19 3BE, UK

Abstract

Rationale: Artificial insemination allows sport horse stallions within breeding programmes to breed and compete concurrently. The level of exercise of stallions complete during the breeding season is a controversial subject. Daily exercise at low intensities is important for the mental and reproductive well-being of the stallion, however higher intensities of exercise, as seen in competing stallions, may have detrimental effects on seminal quality. The purpose of this study was to gain a greater understanding into the effects of competition and discipline on equid stallion semen through analysis of seminal parameters. The identification of optimal competition management for breeding stallions may lead to increased stallion fertility and economic gain.

Methods: This retrospective study evaluated the seminal data of 1130 stallion collections from two UK based stud farms between 2009 and 2015. Seminal volume, concentration and progressive motility were analysed for differences between competing and non-competing stallions, then for differences between stallion disciplines.

Results: Competing stallion semen concentration and progressive motility was significantly lower than non-competing stallions ($p<0.05$). Semen volume was significantly higher in competing stallions ($p<0.05$) than non-competing stallions. Non-competing stallion semen count was significantly higher than that of competing stallions ($p<0.05$).

Conclusion: The difference in semen quality between competing and non-competing stallions, as well as the difference between disciplines suggests endocrinological and physiological changes occur in relation to training intensity and competition. Further research into semen quality considering exercise and competition will allow for contextualisation as to why these differences occurred.

Keywords: Stallion; Semen; Equine breeding; Semen quality

Introduction

Within equine breeding programmes, some stallions are non-competing or retired from competition, but the majority of sport horse stallions are expected to breed and compete concurrently, which increases their value within reproduction through sporting achievements [1-3]. Stallion competition performance within any discipline is considered one of the main criterion for breeding potential, with many stallions put through intensive performance testing before being accepted into stud books [4]. Clients often prefer stallions that are consistently performing at high levels within the competition sphere, with the intention of increasing genetic progress and ultimately obtaining high achieving offspring [5]. The increasing concentration on performance could however lead to reduced reproductive viability in stallions as impacts on the reproductive physiology and psychology be overlooked [6,7].

Daily exercise is thought to be important for the mental and reproductive well-being of stallions [8-10], with the amount of exercise necessary differing, dependent on individual factors such as genetics, nutrition and season [11]. Any stallion within a breeding programme should be in good health, with muscle tone maintained by exposing them to turnout or low intensity exercise on a regular basis. Competing stallions exercise more frequently and at higher intensities within training in order to achieve a higher level of performance [12]. It is therefore in the interest of stallion owners to recognise whether consistent high-level competition and repeated exercising of the stallion has a detrimental effect on semen quality and therefore breeding efficiency, potentially leading to a decrease in profit.

Within the human population, males who exercise regularly and live a healthy balanced lifestyle have better quality semen than those not exercising on a regular basis [13]. Exercise and other stressors can influence human endocrinology and fertility [14], with links to improved libido and a positive effect on hormone levels [15]. Physical activity increases the male anabolic hormone environment and therefore an increase in semen production occurs [16]. Semen parameters significantly decline with long-term strenuous exercise when compared with those exercising at moderate intensities [17]. Once exercise is reduced, impairments seen within the reproductive system gradually recover. Similar research suggests that intensity and volume of exercise is negatively correlated to seminal quality, concluding that careful attention should be paid to these variables when designing training programmes to ensure reproductive function is not compromised [18,19].

Limited research of the effects of intense exercise on stallion fertility is available; an early study evaluated the effect of controlled exercise on daily semen output in 2-year-old stallions [20]. Whilst no difference between exercised and non-exercised stallions was found, the young age and sexual inexperience of the stallions does not allow conclusions to be

***Corresponding author:** Anke Twigg-Flesner, Performance in Equestrian Sport Research Group, Hartpury University Centre, Hartpury College, Gloucestershire, GL19 3BE, UK, E-mail: Anke.Twigg-Flesner@hartpury.ac.uk

drawn for mature and established stallions. Moderate intensity exercise, walking for 30 minutes 4 days per week, has since been shown to have no impact on seminal parameters or the endocrinology of the stallion [21]. Elite-level stallion training would deem this research intensity to be very light rather than moderate, reducing the applicability of this research to the wider competing stallion population. Research on Icelandic stallion fertility rates indicated that high intensity training resulted in higher fertility rates than those in moderate intensity exercise or no exercise, with moderate intensities providing the lowest fertility rates [22]. However, this study was based on fertility rates and individual semen parameters and seminal quality were not taken into account. Controversially, where stallions were undergoing intensive exercise, two days per week, significant stress responses were induced, including increases in heart rate, plasma cortisol, lactate and testosterone concentrations [23]. Hence, excessive physical stress has a negative effect on stallion semen viability and productivity for up to one month after intensive periods of exercise.

The lack of research into the effects of competition on spermatozoa and the amount of conflicting studies into the effects of exercise on stallion semen quality suggests further research is needed within this sector of the equine reproductive industry. The identification of optimal competition management of stallions may help to educate owners, riders and grooms with the potential to lead to increased stallion fertility and economic gain.

The aim of this study was to gain a greater understanding of the effect that exercise and competition has on stallion semen quality.

Methods

This retrospective study used data from past semen collections of stallions that were being used within artificial insemination breeding programmes at two UK based stud farms between 2009 and 2015. Of the 102 stallions selected for participation in the study, 61 were competing and 41 were non-competing. The stallions were aged between 3 and 21 years old, of various breeds. Prior to data collection, all owners/ representatives of the stallions completed the appropriate consent and data protection forms. The stud farms provided data from each stallion, such as: age, breed and level of competition (higher or lower), if applicable. Alongside this, semen quality assessment information was provided which included: volume of the semen sample (ml), progressive motility (%) of the spermatozoa, concentration of spermatozoa ($\times 10^6$/ml) within the sample, the total sperm count ($\times 10^9$) and the date in which the semen sample had been collected. Stallions were categorised based on whether they were competing or non-competing and further by ages.

Throughout the study period, the stud farms gave access to data from 1130 semen collections, 798 of which were from competing stallions and 332 from non-competing stallions. All of the samples were collected and assessed by DEFRA approved equine artificial insemination technicians at professional stud farms, ensuring at the time of collection animal welfare was not compromised and limiting ethical considerations.

Statistical analysis

Data were analysed using IBM SPSS (version 24.0). The data within this study were found to be not normally distributed following the Kolmogorov Smirnov test, hence non-parametric statistical tests were to be performed. A series of Mann-Whitney U Tests compared semen volume, concentration, progressive motility and total sperm count between competing and non-competing stallions to determine if a difference existed between the two groups. A Kruskal-Wallis test of difference was used to determine if a difference existed in semen parameters between the stallion's level of competition. A Kruskal-Wallis test was used to identify if any differences occurred between stallion ages and breeds and semen quality. Data are presented as mean ± S.E.M. A significance value of $P<0.05$ was used throughout.

Results and Discussion

Stallion semen quality, in relation to exercise and competition, is not a topic within the equine industry where much research is available. The few studies analysing this association have shown inconsistent results [18-21]. Therefore, the purpose of this study was to investigate stallion semen quality in relation to competition participation and level.

Volume

The mean average for each seminal parameter was calculated for competing (n=798) and non-competing stallions (n=332). The average values of non-competing stallions ranged from 6.00 ml to 120.00 ml (Figure 1a) and competing stallions ranged from 3.00 ml to 182 ml (Figure 1a). The semen volume was significantly different (P=0.000) between competing and non-competing stallions.

Values in stallions competing at lower levels of competition (n=228) ranged from 6.00 ml to 182.00 ml and stallions at higher levels (n=570)

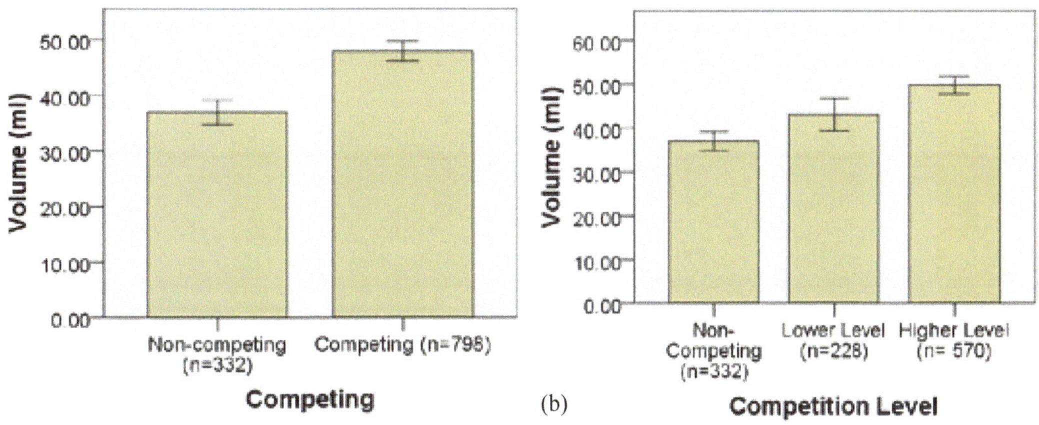

Figure 1: Mean semen volume of (a) competing and non-competing stallions; (b) stallion competition level. Significant = $P<0.05$.

ranged from 3.00 ml to 180.00 ml, with non-competing stallions (n=332) ranging from 6.00 ml to 120.00 ml (Figure 1b). Semen volume increased significantly between non-competing and competing stallions, and significantly increased with competition level (p=0.000).

Research carried out with human participants supports the present findings, stating that physical activity has a significant positive effect on seminological attributes including seminal volume, suggesting the outcome is due to the favourable homeostatic balanced of LH and testosterone [16,24]. Contrastingly, earlier research found no association between physical activity and semen volume, but as the sample consisted of males that were considered infertile, comparability is reduced [25].

In stallions, improvements in seminal volume are associated with increased teasing [26]. This may be a reason behind the increases in competing stallions due to the collection process differences between the two stud farms, with only one farm using a teaser mare. More concerningly, the mean seminal volumes of both competing and non-competing stallions were below that of the AI referencing ranges (60-120 ml). Fertility is not directly affected by seminal volume [27]; suggesting that it is more desirable to have lower seminal volumes with higher concentrations of spermatozoa [28]. Therefore, even though lower seminal volumes were observed, the participating stallions may still be sufficiently fertile dependent on the measurements obtained through analysis of additional semen parameters, such as total sperm count and progressively motility, which are considered to be main parameters in semen quality assessment.

Progressive motility

Values ranged from 1.00% and 95.00% in non-competing stallions (n=332) (Figure 2a) and in competing stallions (n=798) values ranged from 0.00% and 85% (Figure 2a). The progressive motility of competing and non-competing stallions was found to be significantly different (p=0.011).

Progressive motility ranged from from 1% to 95% in non-competing stallions (n=332), 10% to 80% in stallions at lower levels of competition (n=228) and 0% to 85% in higher levels of competition (n=570) (Figure 2b). Statistical analysis revealed a significantly lower progressive motility in competing stallions compared to non-competing stallions (p=0.000).

The outcomes from this research conform to observations from previous research, which reported a significant decrease in progressive motility of spermatozoa with moderate and high intensity exercise over a prolonged duration, concluding that progressive motility and exercise are negatively correlated [29]. Earlier research also supports these results, stating that training volume has a significant negative correlation to spermatozoa progressive motility, further suggesting that this could be due to low testosterone levels [18]. However, research that is more recent contradicts this, finding testosterone levels increase significantly following exercise and these are positively correlated with progressive motility [30]. Exercise plasma testosterone concentrations were increased, but progressive motility was negatively affected by the intensity of the exercise performed [23].

In humans, lower progressive motility of spermatozoa has been reported within competition periods of endurance athletes, proposing that this could be due to increased intra-scrotal temperatures [31]. Thermal stress has more recently been associated with decreased semen parameters, including progressive motility [32,33]. In equine research, thermal stress is a debated topic area with no conclusive results [34], suggesting further research into the effect of testicular thermal stress with regards to semen quality and exercise could be completed.

Concentration

Values in non-competing stallions (n=332) ranged from 77 × 10^6 to 852 × 10^6 (Figure 3a) Competing stallions' (n=798) values ranged from 11 × 10^6 and 811 × 10^6 (Figure 3a). A significant reduction in sperm concentration (P=0.000) was found between non-competing and competing stallions. Sperm concentration significantly decreased as competition level increased (p=0.000) (Figure 3b).

The results of this research support findings within human studies, showing decreases in semen concentration of men under high intensity exercise programmes [35]. Semen concentration was impaired with long term, moderate and high intensity exercise, with a decline from a 57.1 million/ml baseline to 21.7 million/ml at the lowest point [29]. Hence, it was concluded the intensity of exercise and semen parameters are negatively correlated. Research in ovine reproduction supports this, reporting that prolonged daily exercise negatively affects semen concentration is negatively [36].

Suggesting these effects could be due to declined testosterone levels and increases in cortisol, as, more recently, a significant decrease in spermatozoa concentration within males over long durations of high intensity exercise has been reported [37]. This would support previous research findings that psychological stress causes imbalances of the endocrine system which has negative implications on semen quality [38,39]. It was also hypothesised that decreases in seminal concentration could be caused by increases of seminal reactive oxygen species (ROS) following exercise [37,40]. Although ROS damage of spermatozoa

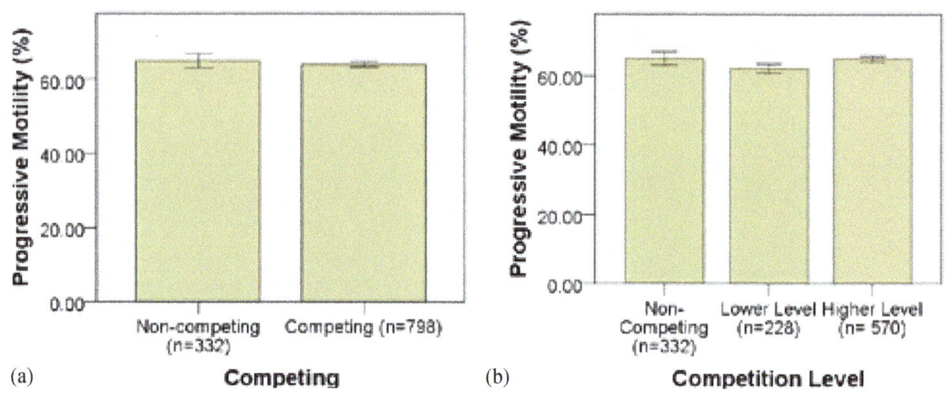

(a) (b)

Figure 2: Mean progressive motility of (a) competing and non-competing stallions; (b) stallion competition level. Significant – $P<0.05$.

with regards to seminal processing has been researched [41-43]; limited research investigating the effects of exercise and ROS damage in equine semen is available. In humans, sufficiently elevated levels of ROS to disrupt reproductive functions are seen following exercise [40]. However, equine research has not established adverse ROS levels, as only limited increases have been reported, which are unlikely to have significant effects on seminal quality [44]. The potential effects of oxidative stress on stallion semen require further contextualisation in order to understand the impact of elevated ROS levels.

Concerningly, all groups contained stallions, which were well under the minimum referencing ranges for artificial insemination (100-350 $\times 10^6$/ml). Therefore, would be classed as infertile, posing the ethical questions as to whether these stallions should be part of a breeding programme.

Total sperm count

The total sperm count values for competing stallions ranged from 0.38×10^9 and 39.00×10^9. The minimum value for non-competing stallions was 1.06×10^9 and the maximum value was 60.24×10^9. A significant difference (p=0.000) between competing (n=798) and non-competing (n=332) stallions' total sperm count was found (Figures 4a and 4b). A significant reduction in total sperm count occurs between non-competing and competing stallions, but moderate competition values were significantly lower than higher level competition total sperm counts (p=0.000).

The total number of spermatozoa in a stallion's ejaculate typically ranges from 3×10^9 to 20×10^9. Within the current research, values under these ranges were observed in both competing and non-competing stallions. It is important to consider that these stallions are used in artificial insemination programmes, where the minimum doses are 600×10^6, 300×10^6 and 250×10^6 total progressively motile spermatozoa in chilled, fresh and frozen semen respectively [27]. Therefore, provided minimum progressive motility standards were met, the stallions would be classed as fertile within a commercial artificial insemination programme.

The results of the current study are similar to previous research within human reproduction which established that intense training and competition correlates to decreases in total number of spermatozoa within an ejaculate. Recreationally active athletes are found to have the highest total sperm count [45], in contrast with the results in the present study. Other conflicting research states that higher levels of physical exertion increase spermatozoa numbers [46]. The inconsistencies in current human research that explores the effects of exercise on total sperm count, highlights the need for further research of the impact of exercise intensity on stallion semen quality.

Semen quality

Semen quality depends on biological, environmental and management practices within the stallion. In order to calculate semen quality and the reproductive capability of a stallion many seminal parameters can be taken into account [47-49]. This study only reports

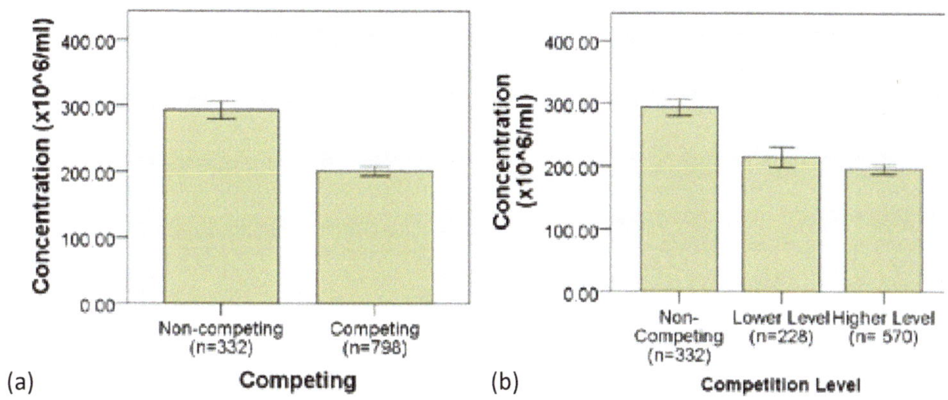

Figure 3: Mean semen concentration of (a) competing and non-competing stallions; (b) stallion competition level. Significant – *P*<0.05.

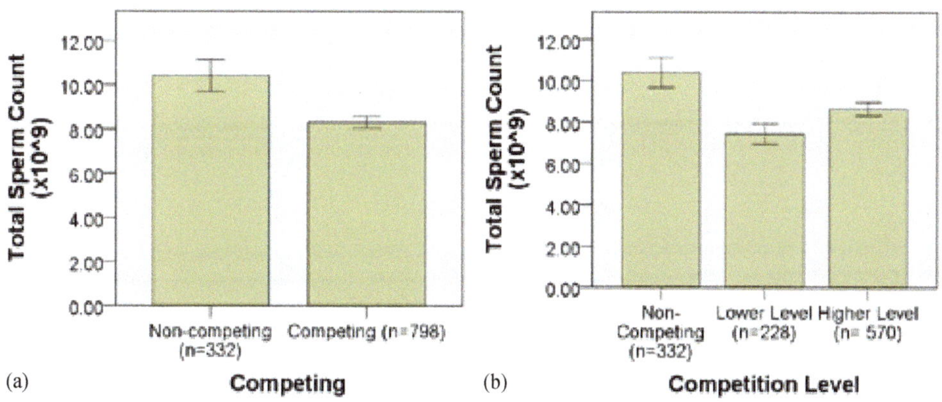

Figure 4: Mean total sperm count of (a) competing and non-competing stallions; (b) stallion competition level. Significant – *P*<0.05.

on volume, concentration, progressive motility and total sperm count as a measure of semen quality. Therefore, competing stallions have lower semen quality than non-competing stallions due to lower mean values of spermatozoa concentration, progressive motility and total sperm count. It should however be taken into account that stallion semen parameters do not necessarily correlate to stallion fertility, with conventional assessment of semen not capturing 100% of the fertilising potential of spermatozoa [50]. It is suggested that the assessment of many seminal attributes and the combination of results will improve the reliability of fertility prediction [51,52]. Within industry spermatozoa morphology is used to observe defects in the physiology of the spermatozoa [1,53] and, along with bacterial status, is seen as a key parameter when predicting the fertilising potential of semen [1,54,55]. The most important measurements for estimating stallion fertility is total sperm count alongside progressively motility.

Due to the retrospective design of this study, access to these factors was not available and many of the above semen parameters that could have assisted with the validation of seminal quality were not recorded. Further research should therefore consider the analysis of a wider range of seminal attributes to overcome this limitation.

The retrospective design of the current study meant a lack of standardisation compared to that of controlled experiments. The control of these variables would be unrealistic due to the individual needs of the stallions. The current study may lack standardisation due to these variables, but it allows for a true representation of the industry.

Breed type and age

Confounding variables such as management protocols, diet, collection technique and environmental factors could have had potential effects on the results obtained [54,55]. Stallion semen parameters are shown to vary significantly dependent on breed and age [56], both of which were confirmed within the present research.

There were significant differences (p=0.000) across all parameters between age categories, although no linear trends were identified, and changes for each parameter followed a different pattern for the different age groups (Table 1). The most notable finding is the reduction in mean concentration in stallions who would be considered to be in their prime in an athletic and reproductive sense (6-10 years). In contrast to previous research, PM was highest in stallions of 16 years and older. Breed type has a significant impact on all semen quality parameters (p=0.000), although no linear patterns were established (Table 2).

The retrospective design of the current study meant a lack of standardisation compared to that of controlled experiments. Variables which had the potential to effect semen quality such as environmental and management factors were unable to be regulated. The control of these variables would be unrealistic due to the individual needs of the stallions; control was further limited by the retrospective study design. The current study may lack standardisation due to these elements, but it allows for a true representation of the industry. The current results showing significant differences in semen quality between the ages and breeds of the stallion amplifies the importance of taking these factors into consideration when conducting future investigations into this topic area.

Conclusion

The research indicates that competition stallions had lower quality of semen than non-competing stallions, this may be due to an accumulation of both physiological and endocrinological factors. It is not possible from this research to state the reason behind the results obtained as much of the research into stallion semen quality is conflicting.

In both competing and non-competing stallions some individuals had semen parameters lower than the referencing ranges for AI, this should be a cause for concern within the equestrian breeding industry

			Volume (ml)	Progressive motility (%)	Concentration (× 10^6/ml)	Total sperm count (× 10^9)
Age	1-5 (n=225)	Mean	34.84	64.62	248.89	7.65
		S.E.M	1.25	0.94	8.97	0.30
	6-10 (n=598)	Mean	47.80	63.46	225.76	9.40
		S.E.M	1.04	0.49	4.85	0.22
	11-15 (n=201)	Mean	52.58	64.50	204.65	9.28
		S.E.M	1.90	0.73	7.19	0.27
	16-20 (n=26)	Mean	40.73	67.50	261.19	10.63
		S.E.M	4.30	2.71	16.37	1.40
	21+ (n=80)	Mean	30.73	68.45	238.46	7.55
		S.E.M	1.55	1.57	10.83	0.57

Table 1: Mean values of semen parameters for each stallion age category.

			Volume (ml)	Progressive motility (%)	Concentration (× 10^6/ml)	Total sperm count (× 10^9)
Breed	WB (n=491)	Mean	51.24	65.21	190.74	8.88
		S.E.M	1.07	0.51	4.10	0.20
	Arab (n=411)	Mean	39.45	62.96	246.56	8.49
		S.E.M	1.07	0.58	6.15	0.20
	Native (n=192)	Mean	42.18	65.70	283.76	10.34
		S.E.M	2.19	1.17	9.75	0.55
	TB (n=19)	Mean	28.21	60.26	204.42	6.21
		S.E.M	2.22	1.30	24.29	1.12
	Polo Pony (n=17)	Mean	29.59	60.88	273.82	7.95
		S.E.M	4.77	1.23	21.22	1.39

Table 2: Mean values of semen parameters for each stallion breed.

and more care is needed to ensure only high quality semen is being used within AI programmes to increase fertility rates.

Overall, it has been shown that careful attention needs to be paid to stallion management in order to properly balance exercise and competition with reproduction. Thus, maximal reproductivity is achieved leading to increased economic gain and maintaining high animal welfare standards.

References

1. Brito LFC (2007) Evaluation of stallion sperm morphology. Clin Tech Equine Pract 6: 249-264.
2. Strickland C (2011) Dual-career stallions: balancing showing and breeding. Horse Sport. February, pp: 38-40.
3. Sairanen, J, Katila T, Virtala AM, Ojala M (2011) Effects of racing on equine fertility. Anim Reprod Sci 124: 73-84.
4. Lange J, Matheja S, Klug E, Aurich C, Aurich JE (1997) Influence of training and competition on the endocrine regulation of testicular function and on semen parameters in stallions. Reprod Domest Anim 32: 297-302.
5. Manafi M (2011) Artificial insemination in farm animals. Rijeka, Croatia: InTech.
6. Colleoni S, Lagutina I, Lazzari G, Rodriguez-Martinez H, Galli C, et al. (2011) New methods for selecting stallion spermatozoa for assisted reproduction. J Equine Vet Sci 31: 536-541.
7. Varner DD, Gibb Z, Aitken RJ (2014) Stallion fertility: A focus on the spermatozoon. Equine Vet J 47: 16-24.
8. Davies Morel MC (2008) Equine reproductive physiology, breeding and stud management. Wallingford: CAB International, UK.
9. Samper JC, Donley S, McKinnon AO, Pycock JF (2003) Equine breeding management and artificial insemination. Can Vet J 44: 332.
10. Fraser AF (2010) The behaviour and welfare of the horse. 2nd edn. CAB International Oxfordshire, UK.
11. Pickett BW (2000) Exercise for the stallion. J Equine Vet Sci 20: 567.
12. Kuipers H, Keizer HA (1988) Overtraining in elite athletes. Sports Medicine 6: 79-92.
13. Homan GF, Davies M, Norman R (2007) The impact of lifestyle factors on reproductive performance in the general population and those undergoing infertility treatment: A review. Hum Reprod Update 13: 209-223.
14. Lange J, Matheja S, Klug E, Aurich C, Aurich JE (1997) Influence of training and competition on the endocrine regulation of testicular function and on semen parameters in stallions. Reprod Domest Anim 32: 297-302.
15. Wogatzky J, Wirleitner B, Stecher A, Vanderzwalmen P, Neyer A, et al. (2012) The combination matters - distinct impact of lifestyle factors on sperm quality: A study on semen analysis of 1683 patients according to MSOME criteria. Reprod Biol Endocrinol 10: 115.
16. Vaamonde D, Da Silva-Grigoletto ME, García-Manso JM, Barrera N, Vaamonde-Lemos R (2012) Physically active men show better semen parameters and hormone values than sedentary men. Eur J Appl Physiol 112: 3267-3273.
17. Safarinejad MR, Azma K, Kolahi AA (2008) The effects of intensive, long-term treadmill running on reproductive hormones, hypothalamus-pituitary-testis axis, and semen quality: A randomized controlled study. J Endocrinol 200: 259-271.
18. De Souza M, Arce J, Pescatello L, Scherzer H, Luciano A (1994) Gonadal hormones and semen quality in male runners. Int J Sports Med 15: 383-391.
19. Vaamonde D, Da Silva-Grigoletto ME, García-Manso JM, Vaamonde-Lemos R, Swanson RJ, et al. (2009) Response of semen parameters to three training modalities. Fertil Steril 92: 1941-1946.
20. Dinger JE, Noiles EE, Hoagland TA (1986) Effect of controlled exercise on semen characteristics in two-year-old stallions. Theriogenology 25: 525-535.
21. Gordon RK, Mawyer JD, Cavinder CA, Sigler DH, Blanchard TL, et al. (2014) Effects of moderate exercise on semen parameters and serum LH and cortisol concentrations in stallions. J Equine Vet Sci 34: 65.
22. Davies Morel MC, Gunnarsson V (2000) A survey of the fertility of Icelandic stallions. Anim Reprod Sci 64: 49-64.
23. Janett F, Burkhardt C, Burger D, Imboden I, Hässig M, et al. (2006) Influence of repeated treadmill exercise on quality and freezability of stallion semen. Theriogenology 65: 1737-1749.
24. Rosety-Rodriguez M, Rosety JM, Fornieles G, Rosety MA, Diaz AJ, et al. (2014) Home-based treadmill training improved seminal quality in adults with type 2 diabetes. Actas Urol Esp 38: 589-593.
25. Wise LA, Cramer DW, Hornstein MD, Ashby RK, Missmer SA (2011) Physical activity and semen quality among men attending an infertility clinic. Fertil Steril 95: 1025-1030.
26. Sieme H, Katila T, Klug E (2004) Effect of semen collection practices on sperm characteristics before and after storage and on fertility of stallions. Theriogenology 61: 769-784.
27. McKinnon AO (2010) Assisted Reproduction Techniques (ART) in the horse – a review from artificial insemination to cloning. BEVA.
28. Jasko DJ, Martin JM, Squires EL (1992) Effect of insemination volume and concentration of spermatozoa on embryo recovery in mares. Theriogenology 37: 1233-1239.
29. Hajizadeh Maleki B, Tartibian B (2015) Long-term low-to-intensive cycling training: impact on semen parameters and seminal cytokines. Clin J Sport Med 25: 535-540.
30. Cavinder CA, Zoller JL, Briers G, Sigler DH (2010) Sexual behaviour and blood hormone profiles around the time of ejaculation and subsequent sperm characteristics in stallions. Prof Anim Scientist 26: 540-546.
31. Lucia A, Chicharro JL, Perez M, Serratosa L, Bandres F, et al. (1996) Reproductive function in male endurance athletes: sperm analysis and hormonal profile. J Appl Physiol 81: 2627-2636.
32. Lue Y, Wang C, Liu YX, Hikim APS, Zhang XS, et al. (2006) Transient testicular warming enhances the suppressive effect of testosterone on spermatogenesis in adult Cynomolgus monkeys (Macaca fascicularis). J Clin Endocrinol Metab 91: 539-545.
33. Kim B, Park K, Rhee K (2012) Heat stress response of male germ cells. Cell Mol Life Sci 70: 2623-2636.
34. Mawyer JD, Cavinder CA, Vogelsang MM, Sigler DH, Love CC, et al. (2012) Thermoregulation of the testicle in response to exercise and subsequent effects on semen characteristics of stallions. J Anim Sci 90: 2532-2539.
35. Vaamonde D, Da Silva M, Poblador M, Lancho J (2006) Reproductive profile of physically active men after exhaustive endurance exercise. Int J Sports Med 27: 680-689.
36. Thwaites CJ (1995) The comparative effects of undernutrition, exercise and frequency of ejaculation on the size and tone of the testes and on semen quality in the ram. Anim Reprod Sci 37: 299-309.
37. Möstl E, Palme R (2002) Hormones as indicators of stress. Domest Anim Endocrinol 23: 67-74.
38. Walker WH (2009) Molecular mechanisms of testosterone action in spermatogenesis. Steroids 74: 602-607.
39. Gondim FJ, Zoppi CC, Reis Silveira L dos, Pereira-da-Silva L, Vaz de Macedo D (2009) Possible relationship between performance and oxidative stress in endurance horses. J Equine Vet Sci 29: 206-212.
40. Ball B (2000) The effect of oxidative stress on equine sperm function, semen storage and stallion fertility. J Equine Vet Sci 20: 95-96.
41. Ball BA (2008) Oxidative stress, osmotic stress and apoptosis: Impacts on sperm function and preservation in the horse. Anim Reprod Sci 107: 257-267.
42. Aitken RJ, Lambourne S, Gibb Z (2014) The John Hughes memorial lecture: Aspects of sperm physiology - oxidative stress and the functionality of stallion spermatozoa. J Equine Vet Sci 34: 17-27.
43. Andriichuk A, Tkachenko H, Tkachova I (2016) Oxidative stress biomarkers and erythrocytes hemolysis in well-trained equine athletes before and after exercise. J Equine Vet Sci 36: 32-43.
44. Hajizadeh Maleki B, Tartibian B, Eghbali M, Asri-Rezaei S (2012) Comparison of seminal oxidants and antioxidants n subjects with different levels of physical fitness. Andrology 1: 607-614.
45. Gaskins AJ, Mendiola J, Afeiche M, Jorgensen N, Swan SH, et al. (2015) Physical activity and television watching in relation to semen quality in young men. Br J Sports Med 4: 265-270.

46. Graham JK (2001) Assessment of sperm quality: A flow cytometric approach. Anim Reprod Sci 68: 239-247.

47. Kastelic J, Thundathil J (2008) Breeding soundness evaluation and semen analysis for predicting bull fertility. Reprod Domest Anim 43: 368-373.

48. Věžník Z, Švecová P, Zajícová A, Přinosilová P (2004) Repetitorium: Spermatology and Andrology and Sperm Analysis Methodology (in Czech). Brno, Czech Republic, p: 197.

49. Magistrini M, Vidament M, Clement F, Palmer E (1996) Fertility prediction in stallions. Anim Reprod Sci 42: 181-188.

50. Colenbrander B, Gadella B, Stout T (2003) The predictive value of semen analysis in the evaluation of stallion fertility. Reprod Domest Anim 38: 305-311.

51. Rodriguez-Martinez H (2003) Laboratory semen assessment and prediction of fertility: Still utopia? Reprod Domest Anim 38: 312-318.

52. Love CC (2011) Relationship between sperm motility, morphology and the fertility of stallions. Theriogenology 76: 547-557.

53. Samper JC, Pycock JF, Estrada A (2004) Evaluation of the stallion for artificial insemination with cooled shipped semen. Equine Vet Educ 16: 144-149.

54. Contri A, De Amicis I, Molinari A, Faustini M, Gramenzi A, et al. (2011) Effect of dietary antioxidant supplementation on fresh semen quality in stallion. Theriogenology 75: 1319-1326.

55. Brinsko SP, Varner DD, Love CC, Blanchard TL, Day BC, et al. (2005) Effect of feeding a DHA-enriched nutriceutical on the quality of fresh, cooled and frozen stallion semen. Theriogenology 63: 1519-1527.

56. Gottschalk M, Sieme H, Martinsson G, Distl O (2015) Analysis of breed effects on semen traits in light horse, warmblood, and draught horse breeds. Theriogenology 1: 1-7.

Epidemiological Studies on Ovine Lungworm Species in Northern Ethiopia

Andualem Yimer* and Abebe Desie

School of Veterinary Medicine, Wollo University, Dessie, Ethiopia

Abstract

A cross sectional study was conducted from November, 2015 to April, 2016 to determine the prevalence, associated epidemiological factors and identifying the species of ovine respiratory helminthes circulating in and around Wogera district. Modified Baermann technique was conducted to detect first stage larvae (L1) from 386 randomly sampled sheep kept under extensive and semi intensive management systems. Out of the total 386 faecal samples examined 180 were found to harboring one or more lungworm parasites with an overall prevalence of 46.6% (180/386). *Dictyocaulus filarial* (*D. filaria*) was the dominant lungworm species with prevalence of 18.9%, followed by *Mulliries capillaries* (*M. capillaries*) 14.2%, *Protostrongylus rufescens* (*P. rufescens*) 2.3% and Mixed infection with *D. filarial* and *M. capillaries* species (11.1%). In this study, animals with poor body condition (23.1%) were highly infected with significant difference (P<0.05) than medium (14.8%) and good body conditions (8.8%). There was statistical significant difference in susceptibility between different age groups (P<0.05), the young (25.1%) being more affected than adult (22.5%) animals. Significant differences (P<0.05) were found among areas of different altitude with an infection rate of 29% and 17.6% at higher and medium altitude areas respectively. Sheep kept under extensive management system and semi intensive management system also showed statistically significant variation (P<0.05) in infection rate with different lung worm species. The overall results obtained during this investigation showed that *D. filaria* is the most common lungworm species in its not only high prevalence rate, but also high degree of association with occurrence of clinical respiratory signs. The result of this study indicated that lungworms in sheep are common parasites which induce heavy economic loss that needs greater attention due to its impact on sheep production of the study area.

Keywords: Epidemiological factors; Ethiopia; Lungworm; Prevalence; Wogera district

Introduction

Ethiopia possesses over 25 million sheep and 21 million goats [1], parallel to its diverse ecology, production systems and ethnic communities. The CSA of Ethiopia estimated [1] that farmers in Amhara region, north eastern Ethiopia, had a total of 6.4 million sheep which are representing 25% sheep population of the country. According to FAO [2], 25% of the total annual meat production of the country comes from sheep. At the national level, sheep and goat account for about 90% of the live animal/meat and 92% of skin and hide export trade value of the country [2]. Small ruminants in Ethiopia are well adapted to local climatic and nutritional conditions and contribute greatly to the national economy however; poor animal management coupled with infectious and parasitic disease had reduced productivity of small ruminants [3].

Helminth parasites are among the causes of substantial productivity losses in ovine production of the country [4]. Respiratory diseases resulting from helminthes parasites are of a great economic concern in sheep production in the highlands of Ethiopia where sheep are important livestock units [5,6]. The three respiratory parasites that cause a significant damage in small ruminant production are *D. filaria*, *P. rufescent* and *M. capillarius*. From those lungworms particularly *D. filaria* can suppress the immunity of the respiratory tract and causes death, poor weight gain or loss of body weight as well as greatly affects the potential productivity of sheep in the areas where it is prevalent [7].

Few studies have been conducted in some areas of Ethiopia indicated high prevalence of lungworm infection in sheep population and its economic importance of the infection in certain areas of the country. Prevention and control of these parasites are therefore, essential for releasing the potential of sheep production in the country. However, in order to lay down lungworm control strategy at local and regional level, detailed investigation of current epidemiological situation and infection rate of lungworm infection in sheep population in the present study area is necessary, where sheep are important assets to the local farmers. Therefore, the objectives of this study were, to determine the prevalence of lungworm infection in sheep, identifying the major lungworm species circulating in and around Wogera district and epidemiological factors affecting the prevalence.

Materials and Methods

Study area

The study was conducted in Wogera district starting from November 2015 to April 2016. Wogera is one of the districts of North Gondar Administrative Zone, in Amhara regional state, located at 782 km northern of the capital city, Addis Ababa, in between 37.36°E and 12.46°N longitude and at an altitude of 2900 m.a.s.l in the northern highlands of Ethiopia. The rainfall pattern of the district is bimodal, with a short rainy season from March to May, followed by a long rainy season from June to September. It has an average annual rainfall of 700 mm and the mean annual temperature is 12.7°C [8].

Study population

Indigenous sheep reared under small holder farming system of

***Corresponding author:** Andualem Yimer, Assistant Professor, School of Veterinary Medicine, Wollo University, PO Box 977, Dessie, Ethiopia
E-mail: anduylmer007@gmail.com

extensive and semi intensive management system in the study area from two agro ecological areas (highland and midland) with different sex, age, and body condition score (poor, medium and good) [9] were used during the study period. The age of the animals was estimated by stage of dentition [10], based on these animals were categorized into young age groups (<1 years) and adult aged groups (>3 years). Sheep those have clinical respiratory sign as shown by coughing and nasal discharge were examined and recorded before sample taking and apparently healthy animals were also isolated and recorded before sampling. The risk factors were assessed for the presence of possible significant association with presence of lung worm infection.

Study design and sampling method

A cross-sectional study to determine the prevalence of lungworm infestation and stratified random sampling techniques were used to collect the data. Out of 25 of peasant association of Wogera district, 6 peasant association of the district were selected by considering the difference in altitude. From the selected peasant associations, households were randomly selected. Sheep from each selected household of peasant association was examined with equal sample size from each peasant association.

Sample size determination

Simple random sampling strategy was followed to collect feces from the individual animals and a total of 386 fecal samples were collected and examined for lung worm nematodes, from purposively selected 6 peasant association of the district. To calculate the total size, the sample size was decided based on the formula described by Thrusfield [11]. The previous prevalence report of lung worm infection in sheep in Wogera district was reported to be 67.69% [12]. Therefore, an expected prevalence of 67.69% will be taken to estimate the sample size. Taking 95% confidence level, 5% precision and 336 sheep was need to establish the prevalence. However, 50 sheep were added in the study to increase the level of precision and randomness, and 386 sheep was sampled.

Sample collection and parasitological examination

Fecal samples were collected directly from the rectum of each sampled animal with strict sanitation and placed in air and water tight sample vial, while collecting fecal samples, necessary parameters (date of sampling, sex, age, body condition, respiratory symptoms, altitude and management system) were properly recorded, and brought to Gondar University Veterinary Parasitology Laboratory. When samples were reached in the laboratory they were immediately stored in the refrigerator (4°C) until they were processed.

For coproscopic examination of the fecal samples, a modified Baermann technique as described by Charles and Robinson [13] was employed to identify first stage larvae (L1) of lung worms. Briefly, 3 g of fecal sample was enclosed in gauze, fixed on to string rod and submerges in clean beaker filled with tape water and left for 24 hrs. The larvae in the feces migrate to the gauze and settle at the bottom of the beaker. After siphoning of the supernatant, the sediment was examined under stereo microscope, when L1 larvae of lung worms were observed under the microscope, a drop of 1% iodine solution was added to the sediment to immobilize the larvae for species identification [14]. Finally, first stage larvae (L1) were morphologically differentiated and identified [15].

Data analysis

Data collected from the study were entered to MS Excel sheet and analyzed by using SSPS version 20 software. Descriptive statistics was used to determine the prevalence of lung worm nematodes and Pearson chi square test was used to assess the degree of association between each risk factor such as sex, age, body condition, altitude, management system and respiratory syndromes with lung worm infection. In all analyses confidence level was held at 95% and P-value less than 0.05 was considered as significant.

Results and Discussion

Of the total 386 sheep examined over the study period, 180 were positive for lung worm infections and the study indicated an overall lungworm infection prevalence of 46.6% in Wogera district, northern Ethiopia. First stage larvae of *D. filaria* (18.9%), *M. capillaris* (14.2%), and *P. rufescens* (2.3%) were observed as single and mixed infections. Mixed infections were formed and observed between *D. filaria* and *M. capillaries* in 11.1% of sheep. This finding almost coincides with previous reports of overall prevalence rate of lung worm infection 48% in Addis Ababa by Mezgebu [16], 43.33% in Dessie zuria by Basaznew et al. [17] and 42% in North Gondar Zone by Yitagel et al. [18]. However, it was higher than reports of Muluken [19] in and around Bahir Dar, Kassa and Abdu [20] in Bahir Dar and Gebreyohannes et al. [21] in Mekedella Woreda, south east Ethiopia who reported prevalence of 18.16%, 20.2% and 28.6% respectively. With regard to the species of lungworms, it was observed that *D. filarial* was the predominant lung worm species in the study area followed by *M. capillaries* and *P. rufescens* in sampled sheep. This finding is more or less agrees with the previous findings of Nibret et al. [12] in Wogera district, northern Ethiopia, Tefera and Mekuria [22] in Debre Birhan Town who reported *D. filarial* is the dominant species to cause lung worm infection in sheep. However, in contrast to the present finding higher proportion of *M. capillaries* species was identified by Yitagel et al. [18] in North Gondar zone and Asaye and Alemneh [23] in and Around Bahir Dar City. The possible explanation for such variation in the prevalence of lung worm infection in different study areas could be attributed variation in agro-ecology of the study areas which favor or disfavor the survival of parasites larvae in general and/or the presence or absence of snail intermediate host in case of *P. rufescens* and *M. capillaris* in the study sites. Moreover, according to Bradford [24], the occurrence of lungworms is associated with time of sampling, methods followed to detect the parasitic larvae, level of immunity of sampled animals, management practice of the animal and expansion of veterinary services (Table 1).

In relation to the prevalence of lung worm infection in different age groups, 25.1% of young examined sheep were infected with different species of lung worm while, 22.5% of adult sheep were found infected with different species of lungworm. There is statistically significant difference in age susceptibility, the young age group being more affected by *D. filaria* (10.4%). This is in agreement with reports of Feseha and Gebrenegus [25], Teffera et al. [26] and Yohannes [27] in different part of Ethiopia who reported young animals are significantly more affected by different lung worm species than adult sheep. In contrast, this finding Besaznew et al. [17] in Dessie Zuria District, northeastern Ethiopia, reported higher prevalence of lung worm infection in adult animals. This variation in prevalence among different age groups might be due to the fact that there is development of acquired immunity in the adults due to previous exposure to the parasite and sheep that have recovered from previous infection have better protection (immunity against) re-infection [15].

In the present finding both sexes showed insignificant difference in susceptibility to infection with lungworms, even though the prevalence in female (32.4%) relatively higher than male (14.2%). This

Factors	Animals examined (%)	Prevalence of lungworm species (%)					X^2	P-value
		D. filaria	*M. capillaries*	*P. rufescens*	Mixed infection	Total positive		
Age							15	0.00
Young	170(44)	40(10.4)	27(7)	4(1)	26(6.7)	97(25.1)		
Adult	216(56)	33(8.5)	28(7.3)	5(1.3)	17(4.4)	83(22.5)		
Sex							4.6	0.33
Male	124(32.1)	27(7)	12(3.1)	4(1)	12(3.1)	55(14.2)		
Female	262(67.9)	46(11.9)	43(11.1)	5(1.3)	31(8)	125(32.4)		
Body Condition							48	0.00
Poor	127(32.9)	37(9.6)	23(6)	4(1)	25(6.5)	89(23.1)		
Medium	147(38.1)	20(5.2)	21(5.4)	4(1)	12(3.1)	57(14.8)		
Good	112(29.0)	16(4.1)	11(2.8)	1(0.3)	6(1.6)	34(8.8)		
Management System								
Extensive	340(88.1)	65(16.8)	51(13.2)	9(2.3)	41(10.6)	166(43)	7.1	0.01
Semi intensive	46(11.9)	8(2.1)	4(1)	-	2(0.5)	14(3.6)		
Location							6.5	0.04
Highland	206(53.4)	43(11.1)	34(8.8)	6(1.6)	29(7.5)	112(29)		
Midland	180(46.6)	30(7.7)	21(5.4)	3(0.8)	14(3.6)	68(17.6)		
Total	386(100)	73(18.9)	55(14.2)	9(2.3)	43(11.1)	180(46.6)		

Table 1: Lungworm infestation in sheep by age, sex, body condition, management system and altitudes taken as risk factors for infestation.

finding was in agreement with studies reported by Desta et al. [28] in Ambo District, Eyob and Matios [29,30] in Asella province and Gebreyohannes et al. [21] in Mekedella district, South Wollo, Ethiopia. This higher prevalence rate of lung worm infection in female animal could be due to the fact that the resistance to infection is abolished at the time of parturition and during early lactation in female animals. However, this result contradicts with the findings of Nibret et al. [12] in Wogera District; Weldesenebet and Mohamed [30] in Jimma, who reporter higher prevalence of lung worm infection in males than female animals. These variations may be due to the improper distribution of sample selection between the two sexes [31], and most of the sampled sheep are not in preparturient period during the study time.

With regard to the physical body condition the prevalence was significantly higher (P<0.05) in sheep with poor body conditions (23.1%) than in those with medium (14.8%) or good body conditions (8.8%). The current finding is in agreement with studies reported by Selam et al. [32], Mihreteab and Aman [33] they reported higher prevalence rate in animals with poor body condition, but disagree with the finding of Weldesenebet and Mohamed [30] who reported higher prevalence rate in animals with good body condition. The variation in prevalence among the different body conditions might be associated with immune suppression in sheep with poor body conditions and concurrent infection by other parasites including gastrointestinal tract helminthes and/or malnutrition [33]. Poorly nourished sheep appear to be less competent in getting rid of lungworm infection and the infestation with a parasite by itself might results in progressive emaciation of the animals [34,35] (Table 2).

There was high significant difference between the prevalence rate of lung worm infection of sheep in the two management systems (P<0.05). It was found that 43% prevalence rate of lung worm infection was observed in animals under extensive management system, while very low prevalence rate, 3.6% was found in semi intensive management system. The current findings are in accordance with previous results of Yitagel et al. [18] in North Gondar Zone who reported prevalence rate of, 51.8% and 24.5% in extensive and semi intensive management system respectively. This could be due to the fact that sheep in extensive management system have a chance of grazing in the field contaminated with intermediate host for *P. rufescens* and *M. capillaries* or they possibly infested with larvae as well as easily obtained *D. filarial* from the herbage [36]. However, it contradicts with the result of Weldesenebet and Mohamed [30] who reported higher prevalence of lung worm infection in sheep under semi intensive management system (28.6%) than in extensive management system (26.0%).

The result of this study has shown that prevalence rate of lungworm infection in the study animals was significantly increase (P<0.05) with altitude, accordingly prevalence of 29% in high land and 17.6% in mid land areas was observed. This result is in agreement with the result reported by Alemu et al. [5] Mireteab and Aman [33] who found significant difference among the various agro-ecology (P<0.05) in their result. This might be due to the effect of altitude is attributable to climatic parameters. That is the survival and development of lungworm larvae is favored by low moisture content and high humidity [15].

The result of this study also showed that, 19.17% of those apparently healthy sheep and 27.46% of those showing clinical respiratory signs were infected with different lungworm species, with statistically significant variation (P<0.005) in prevalence rate. Similarly, with higher statistically significant variation (x^2=32.21, P=0.00) *D. flaria* was the dominant prevalent species in sheep with respiratory signs from the other lung worm species as clearly indicated in Table 2. The result coincides with the observation of Alemu et al. [5], Desta et al. [28], Eyob and Matios [29] and Hasen et al. [37] in different parts of the country. This might probably due to the fact that during the end of prepatent phase of the parasite post patent parasitic bronchitis, which is responsible for clinical respiratory sign, developed and caused by immature lungworm in the air ways and cellular infiltration of the epithelium [24].

Conclusion

The result of present study indicated that lungworm is one of the major helminthosis of sheep in and around Wogera district, which is affecting the health and production performance of sheep. The prevalence of lung worm infection is significantly higher in young and animals under extensive management system but very low prevalence rate was observed in sheep kept under semi intensive management system. *Dictocaulos flaria* is the dominant lungworm species responsible for clinical manifestation of respiratory sign and higher prevalence rate of lungworm infection was observed in animal

Lungworm Species	Apparently healthy animals (n=240) Prevalence (%)	Animals with respiratory sign (n=146) Prevalence (%)	X^2	P-value
D. filaria	32(8.3)	41(10.6)	32.21	0.00
M. capillaries	23(6)	32(8.3)	8.74	0.00
P. rufescens	5(1.3)	4(1)	0.87	0.32
Mixed infection	14(3.6)	29(7.5)	18.05	0.01
Total	74(19.17)	106(27.46)	60.5	0.00

Table 2: Lungworm infection in relation to respiratory signs manifested.

with poor body condition and sheep sampled from relatively higher altitude areas. Therefore, emphasis should be given towards improving the overall health, nutritional conditions and management system of sheep in the study areas.

References

1. Central Statistical Authority (2006) Ethiopian agricultural sample survey. Vol II. Report on livestock and livestock characteristics. Statistical Bulletin 388. CSA, Addis Ababa, Ethiopia.
2. FAO (2004) Livestock sector brief: Ethiopia. Livestock information, sector analysis and policy branch (AGAL), FAO, Rome, Italy.
3. Taylor M, Coop R, Wall R (2007) Veterinary parasitology. 3rd edn. Black Well Publishing, IOWA, USA, pp: 94-97.
4. Ahmed EF, Markvichitr K, Tumwasorn S, Koonawootrittriron S, Choothesa A, et al. (2007) Prevalence of Fasciola spp infections of sheep in the Middle awash River Basin, Ethiopia. Southeast Asian J Trop Med Public Health 38: 51-52.
5. Alemu S, Leykun EG, Ayelet G, Zeleke A (2006) Study on small ruminant lungworms in northeastern Ethiopia. Vet Parasitol 142: 330-335.
6. FAO (2006) International scheme for the coordination of dairy development and International meat development scheme. Report of a mission to Ethiopia, May 27-June 28; Working paper 23; Rome, Italy.
7. Gelagay A, Leakemariam Y, Esayas G, Selam T, Kassahun A (2005) Study on the prevalence of lung worm infection in Gondar town. Ethiopian Vet J 9: 75-76.
8. Wogera Woreda Rural and Agricultural Office (WWRAO) (2007) Weather and Climate for casting Office.
9. ESGPIP (2007) Control of Internal Parasites in Sheep and Goats. Technical Bulletin 3. Ethiopia Sheep and Goat Productivity Improvement Program.
10. FAO (1993) Ethiopian Livestock sector development project. Preparation Report, FAO, Rome, Italy 1: 51.
11. Thrusfield M (2007) Veterinary epidemiology. 3rd edn. BlackWell Science Ltd. Cambridge, USA, pp: 225-228.
12. Moges N, Bogale B, Chanie M (2011) Dictyocaulus Filaria and Muellerius capillaris are Important Lungworm Parasites of Sheep in Wogera District, Northern Ethiopia. Int J Anim Vet Adv 3: 465-468.
13. Hendrix CM, Robinson E (2006) Diagnostic veterinary parasitological for veterinary technicians. 5th edn. Mosby Inc., St. Louis, Missouri, USA, p: 243.
14. Zajac AM, Conboy GA (2006) Veterinary Clinical Parasitology. 8th edn. Australia Blackwell publishing, pp: 11-14.
15. Urquhart G, Armour J, Duncan A, Jennings F (1996) Veterinary Parasitology. 2nd edn. Blackwell Science, Scotland, pp: 39-58.
16. Mezgebu M (1995) A survey on ovine fascioliasis and lungworm infection in Addis Ababa and the surrounding highland areas. DVM Thesis, Faculty of Veterinary Medicine, Addis Ababa University, Debre-Zeit, Ethiopia.
17. Bogale B, Ebre A, Melaku A (2012) Ovine Lungworm Infection: Prevalence, Species Composition and Associated Risk Factors in Dessie Zuria District, Northeastern Ethiopia. Afr J Basic Appl Sci 4: 73-76.
18. Terefe Y, Tafess K, Fekadie G, Kebede N (2013) Prevalence of lungworm infection in small ruminants in North Gondar zone, Amhara National Regional State, Ethiopia. J Parasitol Vector Biol 5: 40-45.
19. Muluken Y (2009) Prevalence of ovine lungworms in and around Bahirdar. DVM thesis, college of Agriculture and Veterinary Medicine, School of Veterinary Medicine, Jimma University, Jimma, Ethiopia.
20. Tamire K, Mohamed A (2013) Prevalence of Ovine Lung Worms-Around Bahir Dar, East Africa, Ethiopia. Acta Parasitol Glob 4: 71-79.
21. Gebreyohannes M, Alemu T, Kebede E (2013) Prevalence of Ovine Lungworms in Mekedella Woreda, Ethiopia. J Anim Prod Adv 3: 208-214.
22. Tefera Y, Mekuria S (2016) Lungworm Infection in Ovine: Prevalence and Associated Risk Factors in Debre Birhan Town Ethiopia. J Vet Sci Technol 7: 303.
23. Asaye M, Alemneh T (2015) Prevalence of Lungworm Infection of Small Ruminants in and Around Bahir Dar City, Amhara Regional State, Ethiopia. J Vet Sci Technol S12: 002.
24. Bradford P (2002) Large Animal Internal Medicine. In: Veterinary Medicine: A text book of the disease of Cattle, Sheep, Pigs, Goats and Horse. 9th edn. Mosby. Inc., pp: 1452-1455.
25. Feseha G, Gebrenegus M (2004) Epidemiology of *Dictyocaulus filaria* in and around Debre Zeit, Modjo and a note in its prevalence at Alemaya 1976-1977. Report to the Ministry of Agriculture (MOA), Addis Ababa, Ethiopia, p: 16.
26. Teffera S, Melaku K, Asmamaw R (2006) The prevalence of ovine lungworm around Dessie and Kombolcha. DVM thesis, Faculty of Veterinary Medicine, Addis Ababa University Debreziet, p: 65.
27. Yohannes G (2006) Epidemiological study and an anthelmintic treatment trial of ovine dictyocaulosis in Debre Tabor town. M. S. thesis, Addis Ababa University, Faculty of Veterinary Medicine, Debre Zeit, Ethiopia.
28. Beyene D, Nigussie S, Ayana D, Abunna F (2013) The prevalence of lungworms in naturally infected sheep of Ambo District, Oromia, Ethiopia. Glob Vet 10: 93-98.
29. Eyob E, Matios L (2013) The prevalence and risk factors associated with ovine lungworm infestation in the Asella province, Central Ethiopia. J Parasitol Vector Biol 5: 116-121.
30. Weldesenebet D, Mohamed A (2012) Prevalence of small ruminant lung worm infection in Jimma town. Glob Vet 8: 153-159.
31. Addis M, Fromsa A, Ebuy Y (2011) Study on the prevalence of lungworm infection in small ruminants in Gondar town, Ethiopia. J Anim Vet Adv 10: 1683-1687.
32. Tesfaye S, Hagos Y, Teklu A, Gugsa G, Gebrekidan B (2015) Ovine Lung Worm Infection and Associated Risk Factors in and Around Wukro, Eastern Tigray, Ethiopia. Eur J Biol Sci 7: 120-124.
33. Bekele M, Aman A (2011) Ovine Lungworms in Tiyo District, South East Ethiopia: Prevalence, Effect of Altitude and Major Host Related Risk Factors. Glob Vet 7: 219-225.
34. Dar LM, Darzi MM, Mir MS, Kamil SA, Rashid A, et al. (2012) Prevalence and Pathology of Lung Worm Infection in Sheep in Kashmir Valley, India. J Anim Sci Adv 2: 678-685.
35. Radostits OM, Gay CC, Hinchcliff KW, Constable PD (2007) Veterinary Medicine: A textbook of the diseases of cattle, sheep, pigs, goats and horses, 10th edn. New York: Elsevier Saunders, pp: 1541-1564.
36. Radostits O, Gay C, Blood D, Hinchclift K (1994) Disease associated with helminthes parasites. In: Veterinary Medicine: A text book of the disease of Cattle, Sheep, Pigs, Goats and Horse. 9th edn. Harcourt Publishers, Ltd. London, pp: 1564-1569.
37. Hasen A, Takele S, Simenew K (2013) Ovine lungworm infestation rate on fecal larvae recovery basis. Acta Parasitol Globalis 4: 29-33.

Phenotypic Characterization of Indigenous Sheep Types in Bale Zone, Oromia Regional State, Ethiopia

Belete Asefa[1*], Tadesse Abate[1] and Eshetu Adugna[2]

[1]*Department of Animal and Range Sciences, School of Agriculture, Madda Walabu University, PO Box 247, Bale Robe, Ethiopia*

[2]*Department of Animal and Range Sciences, Sinana District Livestock and Fishery Production, Ethiopia*

Abstract

This study was aimed to generate organized information on physical characteristics and prediction of live weight using linear body measurements of indigenous sheep types in five districts of Bale zone (Agarfa, Dinsh, Goba, Sawena and Dawe Kechan). The study was based on field measurements. Multistage purposive sampling was used for selection of districts. Three kebeles from each districts were sampled using simple random sampling techniques. About 600 matured sheep (540 female and 60 male) sheep were sampled for body measurements and qualitative character based on four age category (1 PPI, 2 PPI, 3 PPI and 4 PPI). Both qualitative and quantitative data were analyzed using Statistical analysis system. On the identified dimensions, the sheep population in highland district were found within the same region of space and were clustered with long tailed, no toggle, black and red coat color, no wattle, lateral ear form and forward and upright horn orientation while sheep in Sawena and Dawe kechan were characterized as patch coat color pattern with black and white color, polled horn, dropped ear form, fat rumped tail type, concave head profile and absence of toggle and presence of wattle. The highest correlation between chest girth and body weight both for male and female sheep indicate that chest girth is the best variable for predicting live weight than other measurements. The overall mean of body weight, body length, heart girth, wither height, pelvic width, ear length, rump height, rump length, rump width and head length were 26 Kg, 48.75 cm, 71.4 cm, 62.1 cm, 16.32 cm, 11.1 cm, 63.66 cm, 14.04 cm, 16.86 cm and 9.11 cm, respectively. The best predicted body weight (BW) Model for female sheep is -13.53+0.40HG+0.25BL-0.17HL and Model for male sheep (BW) is -13.66+0.41HG+0.39SC+0.27RL-0.11PW. The present phenotypic characterization reveals that, the existence of diversity of sheep genetic resource across different agro-ecologies. Arsi bale sheep breed is distributed in highland districts and black head Somali sheep is distributed in lowlands of bale zone.

Keywords: Bale zone; Characterization; Indigenous sheep types; Phenotypic traits

Introduction

Ethiopia has diverse indigenous sheep breeds, at least 9 breeds and 14 traditional sheep populations, distributed across diverse ecology, production systems and communities or ethnic groups [1]. As a result of their wide range of habitat, behavioral and reproductive adaptations, sheep have evolved into a large number of different geographically separate phenotypic forms or races varying in size, fleeces, conformation, muscling and coat color. Despite low level of productivity due to several factors such as genotype, environmental and institutional constraints [2] indigenous sheep breeds have a great potential to contribute more to the livelihood of people in low input, small holder and pastoral production systems [3].

Identification and characterization of livestock genetic resources and their production environment is vital for long-term genetic improvement and sustained use of available resources [4]. In Ethiopia, only few breeds have a fair description of their physical appearance [5]. Characterizing the existing sheep production systems and analyzing their production constraints are important tools to diagnose the status and trends of the system, and thus to identify areas for future interventions [6]. Classical description of breeds is based upon phenotype because an organism's phenotype is principally a manifestation of its genotype, and that it lends itself to direct measurement on the organism. As such, phenotypic characterization is therefore complementary to the powerful biotechnological techniques for measuring genetic diversity on the genome [5].

Information on body weight with several body measurements is necessary not only to monitor the growth of the sheep but also to estimate genetic correlations between body weight and body measurements. These measurements provide important evidences for the growth of the breed and the properties that change with environmental effects and feeding factors. In addition, body measurements are important data sources in terms of reflecting the breed standards [7] and are important in giving information about the morphological structure and development ability of the animals. Body weight is measured is also important to determine suitable medication dosage during health care and required feed amount of the animal [8] as indicator of breed standards great convenience for the prediction of body weight without weighbridges [9,10].

In general, Information on phenotypic traits of sheep type in the bale zone is limited despite its contribution and role as source of cash income and improving food security in both lowland and highlands of bale zone. Local breeds are also a source of genetic diversity needed by modern livestock production to ensure stability and continuity. In addition, if there are previous works supposedly done, updating of previous results is vital since genetic resources and production systems

***Corresponding author:** Belete Asefa, Department of Animal and Range Sciences, School of Agriculture, Madda Walabu University, PO Box 247, Bale Robe, Ethiopia
E-mail: beleteasefa@gmail.com

are not static, routine inventories and on-going monitoring. Thus, more detailed characterization study of Bale sheep and its production system are required. Hence, this study was attempted to physically characterize indigenous sheep types in Bale zone, Oromia Region, Ethiopia.

Materials and Methods

Description of study area

The study was conducted in three districts of bale highlands (Agarfa, Dinsho and Goba) and two districts of bale lowlands (Sawena and Dawe kechan) in year of 2015/2016. Bale zone have 9 highland districts, 9 lowland districts and two town administrative. The zone falls between latitude 5°22'-8°08'N and longitudes 38°41'-40°44'E. The total land area of the Zone is 69,661 km^2, which ranked the zone as the largest zone in Oromia National Regional States. The zone have about 2,825,215 cattle, 528,746 sheep, 1,405,715 goats, 300,077 horse, 49,657 mule, 170,153 donkey, 244,073 camel and 747,662 chicken [11].

Source of animal and management

All indigenous sheep type found in study districts of bale zone was used as source of animal. Since it is on farm characterization, animals in hands of farmers was used and data regarding body measurement and morphometric characteristics were collected early in the morning before animal release the burn and fed any feed.

Sample size and sampling techniques

For Morphological characters (qualitative) and body measurements (quantitative) about 600 sheep (540 female and 60 males) was selected based on sex and age of animals from sheep herds of 300 Household. Pregnant females (ewes) was excluded in sampling because of pregnancy have influence on body parameters. Animals should be selected from herds of sheep by considering distances between the herd and family houses to clearly get different animals. Each experimental animal was identified by sex, site, flock number and estimated age group. There is the effect of age and sex on body weight and linear body measurements. All age group sheep were classified into five age groups such as no pair of permanent incisor (1 PPI, 2 PPI, 3 PPI and 4 PPI).

Data collection

Data was recorded on the prepared format adopted from the standard description list developed by FAO [12] and of ILRI-OADB breed descriptor list [13]. All the data was taken early in the morning since body measurements are influenced by posture, motion and gut content of the animals.

Morphological characters like: coat color type and pattern, hair type, head profile, ears shape, ear orientation, wattle, horn shape, horn orientation, ruff and tail type was studied with naked eye observation. Body measurements (cm) such as Chest Girth (CG), Body Length (BL), Height at Wither (WH), Rump Height (RH), Rump Length (RL), Rump Width (RW), Pelvic Width (PW), Thoracic Depth (TD), Ear Length (EL), Horn Length (HL), Tail Length (TL), Tail Circumference (TC), Scrotum circumference (SC) and Teat Length (TL) were measured using tailors measuring tape with records taken to the nearest cm after restraining and holding the animal in an unforced position. Weight was measured in the morning before their release for feeding to minimize post-prandial gut variation and measured using suspended spring balance having 50 kg capacity with 0.2 kg precision (Figure 1).

Data management and statistical analysis

All the collected data were coded and recorded in Microsoft excel spread sheet. Qualitative data from individual observation was analyzed following the frequency procedures of SAS version 9.1, 2003). Chi-square test was employed to test the assumption of equal proportion between the categorical variables.

Observations on morphological characters were analyzed for male and female sheep using frequency procedure of Statistical Analysis System (SAS, release 9.1, 2003). Means, standard deviations, standard errors and coefficients of variation was computed for all the quantitative traits measured using the General Linear Procedure (GLM) of SAS statistical Analysis System (SAS, release 9.1, 2003). For adult animals, sex and age group of the experimental sheep was fitted as fixed independent variables while body weight and linear body measurements except scrotum circumference and was fitted as dependent variables. Scrotum circumference was analyzed by fitting age group as fixed factor. When analysis of variance declares significance, least square means was separated using adjusted Tukey-Kramer test. The model employed for analyses of body weight and other linear body measurements except scrotum circumference and teat length were:

$$Y_{ijk}=\mu_i+Ai+Dj+Dk+e_{ijk}$$

where, Y_{ijk}=the observed k (body weight or linear body measurements) in the ith age group, j^{th} Sex and k^{th} districts; μ_i=Overall mean; A_i = the effect of ith age group (i=1 PPI, 2 PPI, 3 PPI and 4 PPI); D_j=the effect of jth Sex (j=1 and 2); Dk=the effect of kth district (Goba, Agarfa, Dinsho, Dawe kachen and Sawena); $eijk$=random residual error.

Pearson's correlation coefficients for each trait were estimated between body weight and other body measurements within sex and age group (SAS, Release 9.1, 2003). Within each age group, stepwise regression procedure (SAS, release 9.1, 2003) was used to determine the best-fitted regression equation for the prediction of body weight from body measurements. Similar stepwise regression was employed for females within each age group by excluding SC from the model. Best-fitted models was selected based on coefficient of determination (R^2), mean square error and simplicity of measurement under field condition. The following models were used for the analysis of multiple linear regressions.

For male:

$$Yj=\alpha+\beta X1+\beta X2+\beta \ldots\ldots +\beta nXn+ej$$

Where: Yj=the response variable (body weight)

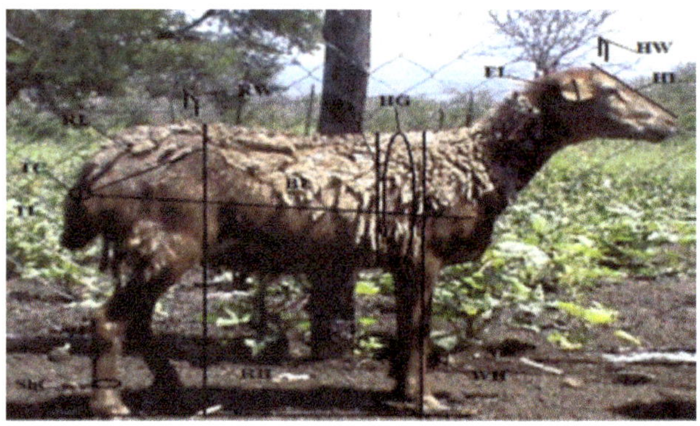

Figure 1: Morphometric variables studied and their reference points. Notes: BW: Body weight; HG: Heart girth; WH: Wither height; RH: Rump height; TD: Thorax depth; BL: Body length; TL: Tail length; TC: Tail circumference; HL: Head length; HW: Head width; ShC: Shin circumference; EL: Ear length; RW: Rump width; RL: Rump length.

α=the intercept

X1, X2, X3, X4, X5, X6 and *Xn*= are the explanatory variables (body length, height at wither, chest girth, tail length, tail circumference, scrotal circumference and body condition, respectively).

$\beta 1, \beta 2, ..., \beta_n$ is regression coefficient of the variables *X (X1, X2, ... , n)*

*e*j=the residual random error.

For female:

$Yj=\alpha+\beta X1+\beta X2+ ...... \beta_n X_n+ej$

Where: *Yj* = the dependent variable body weight

α=the intercept

X1, X2, X3, X4, X5 and X_n are the independent variables; body length, height at wither, chest, girth, tail length, tail circumference and body condition, respectively.

$\beta 1, \beta 2, ..., \beta n$ is regression coefficient of the variable $X1, X2, ... , X_n$

ej=the residual random error.

Results and Discussion

Characterization of physical traits

Physical body characteristics of sheep population in highland and lowland of bale zone are presented in Table 1 and Figure 3. The results show that the presence of clear morphological variations between and within these indigenous sheep types. According to the report of Solomon there are high morphological, ecological, ethnic and production systems diversity of indigenous sheep distributions in Ethiopia [14]. The result of Yakubu points out that phenotypes are an expression of genetic characteristics, modified by environmental conditions and that variance in both genetics and environment may affect phenotypic variance [15]. It is in the context of these assertions that this study exclusively depended on morphometric measurements, geographic locations and qualitative traits to unravel the characteristic of genetic diversity amongst sheep types, which is most relevant for managing the present and future genetic diversity of the breed.

There were varied coloration patterns amongst the sheep populations sampled with predominantly patch (67.8%) followed by spotty (20.2%) of various colors. The most dominant coat colors of sheep in highland (Agarfa, Dinsho and Goba) were red while for lowland (white on body part and black color on their head). Majority of sheep population have no horn (polled) (49.4%) of which about 79.7% were found in lowland. The predominant ear form is dropped (53.3%) followed by (46.5%). They are mainly characterized by absence of toggle (95.3%), absence of wattle (59.2%), absence of ruff (98%) and absence of muzzle (97.5%). They are also characterized as having flat head profile (82.5%). The main tail types were fat tailed (57%) of which about 95% are from highland. Sheep in low land (Sawena and Dawe Kachen) were characterized as fat rumped (100%).

A multiple correspondence analysis was carried out on the twelve qualitative traits recorded and a bi-dimensional graph representing the associations among the different categories of qualitative traits is presented in Figure 2. The interpretation is based on points found in approximately the same direction from the origin and in approximately the same region of the space. From the figure it can be seen that 18.4% of the total variation is explained by the first two dimensions (10.2%) by the first and (8.2%) by the second dimensions.

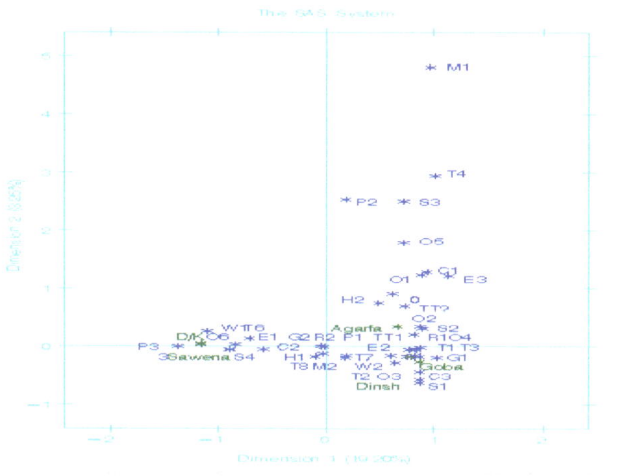

Figure 2: Bi-dimensional plot showing the associations among the categories of the different morphological variables.

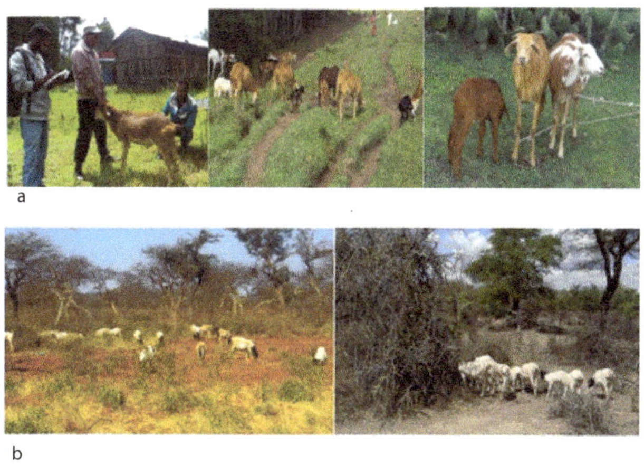

Figure 3: a) Typical example of bale highland sheep.b) Typical example of bale Lowland sheep.

On the identified dimensions, the sheep population in highland district were found within the same region of space and were clustered with fat tailed, no toggle, black and red coat color, no wattle, lateral ear form and forward and upright horn orientation while sheep in Sawena and Dawe kechan were characterized as patch coat color pattern with black and white color, polled horn, dropped ear form, fat rumped tail type, concave head profile and absence of toggle and presence of wattle. The result of qualitative characterization revealed that there were diversified sheep breeds in bale zone. Around highlands of Bale zone, Arsi Bale sheep were distributed while around lowlands Blackhead Somali sheep were distributed.

Correlation between body weight and linear body measurements

The association between body weight and linear body measurements for male and female sample sheep population was presented in Table 2. In male's positive and strong association were found between body weight and other linear body measurements. The associations are chest girth (r=0.82), wither height (r=0.74), body length (r=0.74). In females also chest girth (r=0.86), body length (r=0.74)), rump height (r=0.48), among the body measurements, chest girth was the most strongly correlated trait with body weight (r=0.96 for males; r=0.97 for females). This highest association of chest girth with body weight than

		District					
		Agarfa	Dinsho	Goba	Sawena	D/K	
Character	Attribute	N(%)	N(%)	N(%)	N(%)	N(%)	Overall
Coat color pattern	Plain	23(19.2)	20 (16.7)	29(24.2)	-	-	72(12)
	Spotted	38(31.7)	47(39.2)	36(30)	-	-	121(20.2)
	Patchy	59(49.1)	53(44.1)	55(45.8)	120(100)	120(100)	407(67.8)
	X^2-Value						269.25**
Coat color type	Black	10(8.33)	15(12.5)	9(7.5)	-	-	34(5.7)
	White	1(0.8)	6(5)	7(5.8)	3(2.5)	5(4.2)	22(3.7)
	Red	59(49.2)	33(27.5)	35(29.2)	-	-	127(21.1)
	Grey	5(4.2)	1(0.8)	10(8.3)	-	-	16(2.7)
	Bla+whit	11(9.2)	15(12.5)	26(21.7)	103(85.8)	92(76.7)	247(41.1)
	Bla+red	10(8.3)	11(9.2)	3(2.5)	-	-	24(4)
	Whit+red	24(20)	39(32.5)	30(25)	14(11.7)	23(19.1)	130(21.7)
	X^2-Value						352.35**
Hair Type	smooth	89(74.2)	87(72.5)	102(85)	106(88.3)	109(90.8)	493(82.2)
	curl	31(25.8)	33(27.5)	18(15)	14(11.7)	11(9.2)	107(17.8)
	X^2-Value						418.05**
Horn shape	Straight	28(23.33)	53(44.17)	62(51.67)	-	-	143 (23.8)
	Curved	47(39.17)	50(41.67)	36(30)	3(2.5)	1(0.8)	137(22.8)
	Spiral	10(8.33)	8(6.67)	6(5)	-	-	24(4)
	Polled	35(29.17)	9(7.5)	16(13.33)	117(97.5)	119(99.2)	296(49.4)
	X^2-Value						418.05**
Horn orientation	Backward	18(15)	13(10.8)	9(7.5)	-	-	40(6.7)
	Upward	36(30)	24(20)	23(19.17)	1(0.83)	-	84(14)
	Lateral	32(26.67)	58(48.33)	64(53.33)	2(1.67)	1(0.83)	157(26.2)
	Forward	-	11(9.17)	-	-	-	11(1.8)
	Downward	-	5(4.17)	8(6.67)	-	1(0.83)	14(2.3)
	Polled	34(28.33)	9(7.5)	16(13.33)	117(97.5)	118(98.33)	294(49)
	X^2-Value						467.21**
Ear form	Dropped	54(45)	7(5.8)	27(22.5)	117(97.5)	115(95.83)	320(53.3)
	Lateral	66(55)	112(93.33)	93(77.5)	3(2.5)	5(4.17)	279(46.5)
	Upward	-	1(0.83)	-	-	-	1(0.2)
	X^2-Value						341.72**
Toggle	Present	5(4.17)	11(9.17)	12(10)	-	-	28(4.7)
	Absent	115(95.83)	109(90.83)	108(90)	120(100)	120(100)	572(95.3)
	X^2-Value						24.95**
Ruff	Present	6(5)	4(3.33)	2(1.67)	-	-	12(2)
	Absent	114(95)	116(96.67)	118(98.33)	120(100)	120(100)	588(98)
	X^2-Value						16.27**
Muzzle	Present	15(12.5)	-	-	-	-	15(2.5)
	Absent	105(87.5)	120(100)	120(100)	120(100)	120(100)	585(97.5)
	X^2-Value						61.53**
Wattle	present	11(9.17)	2(1.67)	-	117(97.5)	115(95.83)	245(40.8)
	absent	109(90.83)	118(98.33)	120(100)	3(2.5)	5(4.17)	355(59.2)
	X^2-Value						518.56**
Head profile	Flat	108(90)	118(98.33)	114(95)	80(66.67)	75(62.5)	495(82.5)
	concave	12(10)	1(0.83)	6(5)	6(5)	6(5)	31(5.2)
	convex	-	1(0.83)	-	34(28.33)	39(32.5)	74(12.3)
	X^2-Value						132.95**
Tail type	Fat tailed	114(95)	110(91.67)	118(98.33)	-	-	342(57)
	Long tailed	6(5)	10(8.33)	2(1.67)	-	-	18(3)
	Fat rumped	-	-	-	120(100)	120(100)	240(40)
	X^2-Value						603.96**

N=Number of sheep exhibiting a particular qualitative character; **p<0.01; *P<0.05; ns=p>0.05; X^2=Pearson chi-square; D/K=Dawekechan

Table 1: Qualitative traits of sheep type in study area.

	BL	BW	HG	WH	PW	RH	RL	RW	HL	EL	TtL
BL		0.74**	0.64**	0.49**	0.24**	0.40**	0.042ns	0.45**	0.46**	-0.15ns	0.32**
BW	0.74**		0.86**	0.48**	0.31**	0.49**	0.07ns	0.51**	0.45**	-0.07ns	0.41**
HG	0.74**	0.82**		0.49**	0.32**	0.48**	0.11**	0.52**	0.52**	-0.08ns	0.48**
WH	0.60**	0.74**	0.70**		0.09ns	0.69**	0.25**	0.43**	0.41**	0.03ns	0.20**
PW	0.06ns	0.03ns	0.25ns	0.14ns		0.08ns	0.04ns	0.22**	0.41**	-0.18ns	0.06ns
RH	0.65**	0.69**	0.73**	0.82**	0.20ns		0.38**	0.46**	0.33**	0.10ns	0.23**
RL	0.16ns	0.41**	0.24ns	0.21ns	-0.14ns	0.47**		0.13**	0.09*	0.10ns	0.06ns
RW	0.36**	0.39**	0.48**	0.37**	0.01ns	0.47**	0.21ns		0.27**	0.07ns	0.29**
HL	0.09ns	-0.01ns	0.21ns	0.44**	0.31*	0.20ns	-0.10ns	0.17ns		-0.18ns	0.38**
EL	-0.58**	-0.30ns	-0.51**	-0.36ns	-0.36ns	-0.37ns	0.09ns	-0.19	-0.21		0.07ns
SC	0.63**	0.70**	0.62**	0.62**		0.59**	0.27*	0.30*	0.03ns	-0.40**	

**p<0.01; *P<0.05; ns=Non-significant; BW=Body weight, HG=Heart girth, WH=Height at Withers, BL=Body length, PW=Pelvic width, RH=Rump height, RL=Rump length, HL=Head length, EL=Ear length, TtL=Teat length, SC=Scrotal circumference

Table 2: Correlation coefficients among body measurements and weight of females and males of indigenous sheep in the study area (values above the diagonal are for females and below the diagonal are for males) (N=60 male; N=540 females).

other body measurements was in agreement with other results [16,17] and it can indicate that chest girth is the best variable for predicting live weight than other measurements. Ear length had lower and negative correlation coefficients with body weight and other linear body measurements. The result was agreement with the report of Bafowethu for zulu sheep, there is negative correlation of ear length with body weight and other linear body measurements [18].

Live body weight and linear measurements

Body measurements are considered as qualitative growth indicators which reflect the conformational changes occurring during the life span of animals. Although live body weight is an important growth and economic trait, it is not always possible to measure it due to mainly the lack of weighing scales, particularly in rural areas. Body measurement can also be used routinely in weight estimation and selection programmes based on its utility in determining breed evolution trends [7].

Sex effect: The least square means and standard errors for the effect of sex and their interaction on body weight and other body measurement are presented in Table 3. Body weight and some other linear body measurements does not show significant different between sexes. For trait showing significance difference female were larger than male. The result is agreement with the finding of Abera for sheep type in Selale area female have larger linear body measurements than male counterpart [16].

Age effect: The size and shape of the animal increases until the animal reach its maturity and the effect of age on body weight and other body measurements were also observed indifferent sheep breeds of Ethiopia [19]. Body weight and all body measurements were significantly affected by age group except horn length. All the body measurements were increased as the age increased from the intermediate age group (1 PPI) to the oldest 4 PPI and greater age group. Similar finding was reported by Fasae who noted that body weight and body measurements increased with age of ewes for the first three years and then decreased slightly for ewes above four years [20].

District effect: District had a significant effect on body weight and all other linear body measurements. The finding is agreement with the report of Mesfin [17]. Results for body weight and linear measurement shows that Agarfa district had significantly larger (P<0.05) linear measurements than others sheep population.

Body weight values in rams and ewes of sheep types in the study area were 25.64 kg and 26.36 kg, respectively. The finding was lower than the report of Solomon where the average adult body weight of Arsi-Bale sheep was 28.6 kg [21]. The weight of ewes in this study (26.36 kg) was comparable with the report of Wosseme for Hararghae highland sheep [22]. The overall mean of body length, heart girth, wither height, pelvic width, ear length, rump height, rump length, rump width and head length were 48.75 cm, 71.4 cm, 62.1 cm, 16.32 cm, 11.1 cm, 63.66 cm, 14.04 cm, 16.86 cm and 9.11 cm, respectively.

Regression analysis

The knowledge of livestock weight assessment remains the backbone on which all animal production management practices are hinged [23]. Multiple linear regression analysis was carried out to predict live body weight of an animal. Regression of body weight over independent variables, which have higher correlation with body weight, was done to set adequate model for the prediction of body weight separately for each sex.

Comparable R^2 values were obtained for all relationships existing between BW and other LBMs for both female and male sample sheep population. Thus under field conditions, live weight estimation using heart girth alone would be preferable to combinations with other measurements because of difficulty of the proper animal restraint during measurement and the low proportion of animals at each dentition classes as well.

In this study in order to develop the prediction equation, only three quantitative traits were selected in the prediction equation for ewes (CG+BL+HL) and only four linear body measurements were taken to be incorporated in to the model for male (CG+SC+RL+PW) (Table 4). The fitted prediction model was selected with smaller value of C (p) and higher R^2 values. Several authors in similar studies have concluded that heart girth can be used as a sole predictor of body weight due to high associate regression coefficients obtained [24]. The importance of HG in weight estimation demonstrated in the present study could be as a result of the fact that muscle, and some fat along with bone structure contribute to its formation [25]. From this study it is concluded that hear girth is the best sole predictors of body weight of sheep at farmers condition.

Conclusion

Planning of any breeding program including community based breeding strategy and /or breed improvement scheme needs the identification of genotypic and phenotypic traits of the particular sheep breed and also to know the genetic ability of that breed and the production environment that can influence productivity of the animal.

Effect and level	BW	BL	HG	WH	PW	EL
	LSM ± SE	LSM ± SE	LSM ± SE	LSM ± SE	LSM ± SE	LSM ± SE
Over all						
CV	26 ± 2.83	48.75 ± 3.28	71.4 ± 4.70	62.1 ± 3.87	16.32 ± 2.82	11.1 ± 1.08
	10.78	6.74	6.59	6.24	17.31	9.78
R2	0.12	0.29	0.18	0.13	0.20	0.18
District	*	*	*	*	*	*
AGARFA	27.25 ± 0.2a	50.25 ± 0.3a	73.50 ± 0.42a	65.00 ± 0.35a	17.68 ± 0.25a	10.74 ± 0.09c
DINSHO	26.96 ± 0.2a	50.55 ± 0.3a	72.65 ± 0.42a	61.04 ± 0.35b	16.25 ± 0.25b	10.44 ± 0.09d
GOBA	27.21 ± 0.2a	50.57 ± 0.3a	73.40 ± 0.42a	62.21 ± 0.35b	18.00 ± 0.25a	10.90 ± 0.09c
SAWENA	24.92 ± 0.2b	46.46 ± 0.3b	69.06 ± 0.42b	61.41 ± 0.35bc	14.00 ± 0.25c	11.54 ± 0.09c
DK	25.10 ± 0.2b	45.93 ± 0.3b	68.39 ± 0.42b	60.65 ± .35c	15.65 ± 0.25b	11.83 ± 0.09a
Sex	ns	ns	*	*	ns	ns
Male	25.64 ± 0.38a	48.28 ± 0.49a	68.47 ± 0.65b	60.76 ± 053b	16.90 ± 0.40a	10.83 ± 0.15a
Female	26.36 ± 0.2a	48.8 ± 0.16a	71.73 ± 0.21a	62.20 ± 0.17a	16.25 ± 0.13a	11.11 ± 0.05a
Age group	*	*	*	*	ns	*
1 PPI	24.82 ± 0.1c	47.26 ± 0.2c	68.74 ± 0.32c	61.17 ± 0.27b	16.39 ± 0.21a	11.01 ± 0.08b
2 PPI	26.57 ± 0.2b	49.19 ± 0.3b	71.86 ± 0.42b	61.56 ± 0.35b	16.75 ± 0.27a	11.39 ± 0.10a
3 PPI	27.15 ± 0.2ab	49.55 ± 0.2ab	72.88 ± 0.37b	62.76 ± 0.32a	16.08 ± 0.25a	11.11 ± 0.09b
≥ 4 PPI	27.85 ± 0.2a	50.25 ± 0.3a	74.44 ± 0.49a	63.62 ± 0.42a	15.97 ± 0.32a	10.80 ± 0.12b
Effect and level	RH	RL	RW	HL	SC	
	LSM ± SE	LSM ± SE	LSM ± SE	LSM ± SE	LSM ± SE	
Over all	63.66 ± 3.49	14.04 ± 1.22	16.86 ± 1.50	9.11 ± 0.81	24.65 ± 2.2	
CV	5.49	8.71	8.92	8.95	9.04	
R2	0.11	0.25	0.07	0.31	0.10	
District	*	*	*	*	*	
AGARFA	66.04 ± 0.31a	14.95 ± 0.11a	17.35 ± 0.13a	9.90 ± 0.07a	25.37 ± 0.64ab	
DINSHO	62.30 ± 0.31c	13.41 ± 0.11c	17.25 ± 0.13ab	9.13 ± 0.07c	25.58 ± 0.64a	
GOBA	63.48 ± 0.31b	13.00 ± 0.11d	16.97 ± 0.13b	9.45 ± 0.07b	24.54 ± 0.64ab	
SAWENA	63.65 ± 0.31b	14.50 ± 0.11b	16.47 ± 0.13c	8.77 ± 0.07d	23.75 ± 0.64b	
DK	62.84 ± 0.31bc	14.35 ± 0.11b	16.25 ± 0.13c	8.30 ± 0.07e	24 ± 0.64ab	
Sex	*	ns	*	ns		
Male	62.53 ± 0.47b	13.77 ± 0.18a	16.0 ± 0.19b	9.19 ± 0.12a	24.65	
Female	63.79 ± 0.15a	14.07 ± 0.06a	16.96 ± 0.06a	9.09 ± 0.04a	-	
Age group	*	*	*	*	ns	
1 PPI	63.20 ± 0.25b	14.15 ± 0.09a	16.44 ± 0.10c	8.80 ± 0.06c	24.42 ± 0.35a	
2 PPI	63.69 ± 0.32b	14.18 ± 0.12ab	16.87 ± 0.13b	9.33 ± 0.08ab	25.16 ± 0.65a	
3 PPI	63.64 ± 0.29b	13.86 ± 0.11b	17.15 ± 0.12ab	9.15 ± 0.07b	24.58 ± 0.92a	
≥ 4 PPI	64.75 ± 0.38a	13.89 ± 0.14ab	17.32 ± 0.15a	9.45 ± 0.09a	28 ± 2.92a	

Table 3: Live Body Weight and Linear Measurements in study area.

Sex	Model	I	b1	b2	b3	b4	b5	R^2	CP
Female	CG	-10.18	0.51	-	-	-	-	0.75	186.20
	CG+BL	13.69	0.39	0.25	-	-	-	0.81	10.38
	CG+BL+HL	-13.53	0.40	0.26	-0.17	-	-	0.82	5.76
Male	CG	-9.49	0.51	-	-	-	-	0.68	43.88
	CG+SC	-12.22	0.39	0.43683	-	-	-	0.74	27.98
	CG+SC+RL	-14.41	0.38	0.38463	0.33	-	-	0.77	19.53
	CG+SC+RL+PW	-13.66	0.41	0.39	0.27	-0.11		0.79	15.79

Table 4: Multiple linear regression analysis of live body weight on different LBMs for male and female sheep in the study area.

The study was conducted in Bale zone oromia regional state of Ethiopia. Even though the study areas are rich in livestock resources including small ruminants, nothing has been done to characterize, identify and document theexisting indigenous sheep types and its production system.

The characterization of sheep in this study was helpful to livestock farmers and researchers in preserving the genetic resources of some of the indigenous Ethiopian sheep breeds, as well as to farmers/ pastoralists and dealers in livestock products in the production, processing and marketing of livestock and livestock products. The present study reveal that there is polymorphism, both in qualitative and morphometric traits, among sheep types in highland and low land, inferring considerable genetic variability. However, whether the variations in these morphological traits are caused by adaptive or non-adaptive sources needs to be further verified by comparing between relative levels of population divergence in quantitative traits and neutral DNA markers.

Acknowledgements

First of all authors would like to thank Madda Walabu University for allowing and funding budget to undertake the research activities. Special appreciation and thanks goes to the farmers/pastoralists of Agarfa, Dinsho, Goba, Sawena and Dawe kechan districts of Bale zone for their time devotion, providing necessary data and allowing their animals for body measurements.

References

1. Solomon G, Sisay L, Komen H, van Arendonk JAM (2007) Estimates of genetic parameters and genetic trends for live weight and fleece traits in Menz sheep. Small Rumin Res 70: 145-153.
2. Markos T (2006) Productivity and health of indigenous sheep breeds and crossbreds in the central Ethiopia highlands. Swedish University of Agricultural Science (SLU), Uppsala, Sweden.
3. Kosgey IS, Okeyo AM (2007) Genetic improvement of small ruminants in low-input, smallholder production systems: Technical and infrastructural issues. Small Rumin Res. 70: 76-88.
4. Workneh A (1992) Preliminary survey of indigenous goat types and goat husbandry practices in southern Ethiopia. Alemaya University of Agriculture, Ethiopia, p: 153.
5. Workneh A, Ephrem G, Markos T, Yetnayet M, Rege EO (2004) Current State of Knowledge on Characterization of Farm Animal Genetic Resources in Ethiopia. Proceedings of the 11th Annual conference of the Ethiopian Society of Animal Production.
6. Getahun L (2008) Productive and economic performance of small ruminant production in production system of the highlands of Ethiopia. University of Hohenheim, Stuttgart-Hoheinheim, Germany.
7. Riva J, Rizzi R, Marelli S, Cavalchini G (2002) Body Measurements in Bergamasca Sheep. Small Rumin Res 2: 221-227.
8. Kunene NW, Nesamvuni AE, Nsahlai IV (2009) Determination of predict equations for estimating body weight of Zulu (Nguni) sheep. Small Rumin Res 84: 41-46.
9. Afolayan RA, Adeyinka IA, Lakpini AM (2006) The estimation of live weight from body measurements in Yankasa sheep. Czech J Anim Sci 51: 343-348.
10. Yakubu A (2009) Fixing collinearity instability in the estimation of body weight from morpho biometrical traits of West African dwarf goats. Trakia J Sci 7: 61-66.
11. BZWP (Bale Zone Woreda Profile) (2008) Bale Zone Woreda Profile.
12. FAO (Food and Agriculture Organization of the United Nations) (1986) Animal genetic resources data banks–2. Descriptor lists for cattle, buffalo, pigs, sheep and goats. Animal Production and Health Paper No. 59, Volume 2. Rome.
13. Workneh A, Rowlands J (2004) Design, execution and analysis of the livestock breed survey in Oromiya Regional State, Ethiopia. OADB (Oromiya Agricultural Development Bureau), Addis Ababa, Ethiopia, ILRI (International Livestock Research Institute), Nairobi, Kenya.
14. Solomon G, Komen H, van Arendonk JAM (2008) Selection on linear size traits to improve live weight in Menz sheep under nucleus and village breeding programs. Livest Sci 118: 92-98.
15. Yakubu A, Salako AE, Imumorin IG, Ige AO, Akinyemi MO (2010) Discriminant analysis of morphometric differentiation in the West African Dwarf and Red Sokoto goats. S Afr J Anim Sci 40: 381-387.
16. Abera B, Kebede K, Gizaw S, Feyera T (2014) On-Farm Phenotypic Characterization of Indigenous Sheep Types in Selale Area, Central Ethiopia. J Vet Sci Technol 5: 180.
17. Mesfin A (2015) On Farm Phenotypic Characterization of Indigenous Sheep Types and their Production System In Wolaita Zone, Southern Ethiopia. Haramaya University, Ethiopia.
18. Bafowethu SM (2012) Phenotypic characterization of Zulu sheep: Implications for conservation and improvement. University of Zululand.
19. Tesfaye G (2008) Characterization of Menz and Afar Indigenous Sheep Breeds of Smallholders and Pastoralist for Desighing Community Based Breeding Strategies in Ethiopia. Haramaya University, Dire Dawa, Ethiopia.
20. Fasae OA, Chineke AC, Alokan JA (2006) Relationship between some Physical Parameters of Grazing Yankasa Ewes in the Humid Zone of Nigeria. University of Agriculture, PMB 2240, Abeokuta, Nigeria.
21. Solomon G (2008) Sheep resources of Ethiopia: genetic diversity and breeding strategy. Wageningen University, The Netherlands.
22. Wossenie SH (2012) On-Farm Phenotypic Characterization of Hararghe Highland Sheep and their Production Practices in Eastern Hararghe Zone, Ethiopia. MSc Thesis, Haramaya University, p: 140.
23. Otoikhian CSO, Akporhuarho AM, Oyefia OP, Isidahomen CE (2008) Body measurement parameters as a function of assessing body weight in goats under on-farm research environment. African J Gen Agricult 4: 1595-6984.
24. Taye M, Abebe G, Gizaw, S, Lema S, Mekoya A, et al. (2010) Traditional management systems and linear body measurements of Washera sheep in the western highlands of the Amhara National Regional State, Ethiopia. Livest Res Rural Dev 22: 169.
25. Okpeku M, Yakubu A, Peters SO, Ozoje MO, Ikeobi CON, et al. (2011) Application of multivariate principal component analysis to morphological traits of goats in southern Nigeria. Acta Agric Slovenica 98: 101-109.

Investigation of the Use of Alternative Economic Indices and QTL-Assisted Selection for the Genetic Improvement of Production and Health Traits in Bangladeshi Dairy Cattle

Kabirul Islam Khan MD[1]* and Raphael A Mrode[2]

[1]*Department of Genetics and Animal Breeding, Chittagong Veterinary and Animal Sciences University, Chittagong, Bangladesh*

[2]*Animal and Veterinary Sciences, Scotland's Rural College, Roslin Institute Building, Easter Bush, Midlothian, Edinburgh, EH25 9RG, United Kingdom*

Abstract

The study was undertaken to investigate the use of several economic indices including QTL assisted selection for the improvement of production and health trait of dairy cattle under Bangladesh conditions. Five traits (lactation milk, fat, protein yield, somatic cell score (SCS) and direct mastitis) were simulated over 14 generations, considering three selection objectives (selection for direct mastitis; milk SCS; and the combination of direct mastitis and SCS). In addition the selection objective for SCS was simulated incorporating marker/QTL information. Genetic gains per generation for different traits were calculated by plotting the average true breeding values (TBVs) and estimated breeding values (EBVs) over generation. Selection of replacement bulls and cows were based on total merit. The genetic gains based on TBVs and EBVs of cows for milk, fat and protein yield in three selection objectives with no QTL information were similar, but gains were higher with QTL- assisted selection implemented for SCS. Genetic gains of cows for different traits based on TBVs were higher than bulls, but reverse results were obtained for bulls. The genetic trends for all traits in cows were similar in all selection objectives. However, for bulls distinct differences were observed between the QTL and no QTL-assisted selection schemes and also between SCS and the combination of SCS and direct mastitis selection objectives. Higher correlations between TBVs and EBVs for lactation milk and fat yield for both cows and bulls were found under QTL-assisted selection compared to the no QTL-assisted selection schemes. The QTL-assisted selection scheme showed higher rates of genetic gain for lactation milk, fat and protein yields than no QTL-assisted selection. However, it does not affect SCS and index values from any of the selection objectives or selection schemes. The QTL-assisted selection scheme has a positive effect on milk production and mastitis control.

Keywords: Mastitis; Breeding values; Quantitative trait loci; Selection schemes

Introduction

In Bangladesh, commercial dairy farming is increasing and the farmers rear mainly the Holstein breed and crossbreds between the Holstein and local breeds [1]. The increasing use of these breeds in farming systems is leading to higher prevalence of dairy related health problems, such as, mastitis and milk fever. Among the dairy related health problems, the prevalence of mastitis are from 19.9% (dry season) to 44.8% (wet season) in commercial dairy farming [2], while under government dairy farms it is about 25.5% [3]. Furthermore, Deshi improved varieties (Pabna and Red Chittagong cows) and local cows that produce more milk are also affected with mastitis.

Mastitis is one of the most frequent diseases affecting dairy cattle and it is a major problem in the dairy industry, leading to economic losses from the cost of treatment (antibiotics) and decreased production level (milk yield). It also increases labour and replacement costs. Mastitis is a complex disease which is caused by a number of pathogens such as, *Staphylococccus aureus* and *Streptococcus agalactiae* (both are contagious) and coliforms, streptococci and enterococci (all coming from the cows environment i.e., bedding, manure and soil). The pathogens can cause clinical mastitis, with changes in milk composition, an increase in somatic cell counts and even death. Health data in dairy cattle are routinely recorded in Denmark, Finland, Norway, and Sweden and the improvement for clinical mastitis have been included in their breeding programmes. In these countries, mastitis is indirectly selected for using somatic cell count (SCC) and also direct measures of mastitis [4].

However, the data on mastitis infection and the causal pathogen are not available in developing countries especially under Bangladesh dairy farming conditions. When real data are not available, a simulation study could be useful in designing future goals for the industry. Mastitis data was simulated by Carle´n et al. [5], they considered mastitis as a binary trait and distinguished between cows with at least one case of mastitis (1) and cows without cases (0).

The average daily milk yield of improved varieties of cattle (Pabna and Red Chittagong Cows) in Bangladesh is ranging from 2.5 to 5.0 litres [6-9]. Due to the unsystematic breeding and lack of adequate knowledge on herd management by the farmers, the population of these breeds of cattle and their productivity is decreasing. However, increasing the population number and the productivity of these breeds, the available options are better management, feeding, animal health care and breeding. Among these options the breeding is a permanent and stable solution, but it requires an objective breeding goal for

***Corresponding author:** Md. Kabirul Islam Khan, Department of Genetics and Animal Breeding, Chittagong Veterinary and Animal Sciences University, Chittagong-4202, Bangladesh, E-mail: kik1775@yahoo.co.uk

the whole industry [1]. Recently the government of Bangladesh has started a genetic improvement programme for increased production of milk in the subsistence farming with a traditional (progeny-testing programme) selection and mating approach. However, this method is time consuming, costly and require proper recording. But there is no well-developed recording system for dairy cattle genetic evaluation and improvement [9]. However, this improvement programme is focused only on milk yield with no attention on health traits. Among the health traits, somatic cell count is one of the traits which is much easier to record compared to mastitis for instance. Thus, a study that examines the possible consequences of an improvement programme that ignores or includes somatic cell score (SCS) in the selection objective becomes very important in the Bangladesh situation. In addition, when mastitis records are not available, the efficiency of utilising SCS with the option of incorporating marker information could be more efficient.

The process of selection for a particular trait using genetic markers, is called marker assisted selection (MAS). MAS can accelerate the rate of genetic progress by increasing the accuracy of selection and by reducing the generation interval [1,10]. However, the benefits of MAS are greatest for traits with low heritability. Marker identification and use should enhance future prospects for breeding of such traits as tolerance or resistance of the environmental stresses, including diseases [11]. In addition, more benefits could be expected from MAS with more specific applications, such as early selection of animals, or by the application of dynamic procedures, i.e., letting the respective weights to QTL and polygenic values in the selection criterion vary across generations. However, before incorporation of markers in a breeding programme, careful assessment is required for the potential benefits of MAS and of the design of the breeding programme [12].

Several simulation studies on the impact of using QTL information has been reported in the literature (e.g., Meuwissen and van Arendonk, [13]; Ruane and Colleau [14]; Spelman and Garrick [10]; Spelman et al. [15]; Abdel-Azim and Freeman [11]. Out of them, Spelman et al. [15] tests the additional genetic gains of MAS, and they observed limited benefit (1.8% genetic gain) of MAS in conventional progeny testing schemes through a deterministic approach. The available studies in the literature have used simple breeding structures and small populations with selection for a number of non-overlapping generations, however, deterministic simulation includes more realistic population structure and overlapping generations. The deterministic simulation studies reported that QTL responses from MAS schemes were higher than those from non-MAS schemes. A few studies of genetic research related to lactation and udder health has been reported [16].

Currently the experimental analysis of industry herd information is difficult due to lack of data, as there is no systematic genetic improvement programme for dairy cattle in Bangladesh. Therefore, the use of stochastic computer simulation models, according to SØrensen et al. [17], Carle´n et al. [5] would be helpful in examining the future potential genetic improvement for milk yield traits by using MAS or quantitative trait loci (QTL) assisted selection. For the achievement of this the aim of the current study was (i) to simulate a multi dairy trait model under three selection objectives using a stochastic approach; (ii) to incorporate marker/QTL information for the genetic improvement of dairy cattle; and (iii) to evaluate the different economic selection indices under QTL-assisted and no QTL- assisted selection schemes.

Materials and Methods

Simulation of breeding values and phenotypic values of each trait

A stochastic simulation study was used for multi dairy traits with mastitis liabilities under Bangladesh conditions and Pabna cattle considered as model breed. The methodology was used in developing the current simulation model (1) is based on Falconer and Mackay [18], Verrier [19] and Carle´n et al. [5].

$$Y_{ijk}=\mu+L_i+a_j+P_j+e_{ijk} \quad [1]$$

Where, Y_{ijk} is the individual trait value;

μ is the overall mean;

L_i is the effect of ith lactation;

a_j is the cows additive genetic value;

P_j is the permanent environmental effect; and

e_{ijk} is the temporary environmental effects.

The effect of dominance and epistasis was not considered in this model.

In this study, a herd consisting of 400 cows, the progeny of 80 bulls were simulated using FORTRAN 95 to mimic a situation for the improvement in a large dairy herd of Bangladesh, as data recording across herds is not established. Five traits (total lactation milk, fat and protein yields, somatic cell score and direct mastitis resistance) were simulated over 14 generations (from year 3.5 to 50 year) considering three selection objectives of milk yield (selection for direct mastitis resistance, milk somatic cell score, and the combination of direct mastitis resistance and somatic cell score), assuming an infinitesimal model. In addition somatic cell score (SCS) was simulated assuming QTL which accounted for 15% of the genetic variance. The phenotypic mean with standard deviations of five different traits and the economic values of the respective traits are presented in Table 1. The data were derived from 270 days lactation yield and the milk payment system was on milk volume only. The direct mastitis resistance was simulated as a binary traits with underlying normally distributed liability with phenotypic means of zero and standard deviation of 1.0 (i.e., ~N (0, 1). The (co)variance matrices for the additive genetic (breeding values) and environmental effects (temporary and permanent) were calculated for the base population from the parameters shown in Table 2.

The phenotypic values for the cows were created as the sum of the mean, the animal breeding value and the environmental values for the respective traits. The progeny breeding values were the sum of the sample half from each parent plus the Mendelian sampling term (which was calculated as the product of Cholesky decomposition matrix of genetic (co) variance matrix, and Φ_i is a vector of randomly selected pseudo-normal deviates). The base population was assumed unrelated. Seventy five percent of the base cows were selected randomly for the next lactation. The phenotypic records of cows with lactations two and three were simulated to have an increase of 20% and 25% in temporary environmental effects, respectively, compared to that of lactation one. After the third lactation, all the older cows were culled and replaced by the two years old young animals (both bulls and cows) and were used for mating and offspring production.

Mating strategy and production of offspring

Three population structures for considering direct mastitis resistance, SCS and a combination of direct mastitis resistance and SCS objectives, were simulated. The calving interval and generation interval for the cows were maintained at 1.3 and 3.5 years, respectively. From fourth to later generations (up to 14), 30% cows were culled in each generation and replaced with the replacement heifers. A total of 40

Traits	Mean with standard deviations	Economic values (US$)	References
Milk yield (Kg)	1782.29 ± 262.5	0.39	Khan et al.
Fat yield (Kg)	77.74 ± 9.1	-0.52	Khan
Protein yield (Kg)	71.42 ± 8.7	-0.29	
Somatic cell score	3.09 ± 0.6	-3.97	Wolfová et al.
Mastitis	0 ± 1.0	-3.97	Carle´n et al.

Table 1: Mean with standard deviations and economic values (US$) of different traits.

	[1]MY	[1]FY		[1]PY		[2]SCC	[3]Mastitis
MY	**0.26**		0.63		0.59	-0.13	0.2
FY	0.57	**0.27**		0.79		0	0
PY	0.46	0.82		**0.25**		0	0
SCS	0.14	0		0		**0.08**	0.07
Mastitis	0.36	0		0		0.67	**0.03**

Table 2: Heritabilities (bold), genetic correlations (lower diagonal) and phenotypic correlations (upper diagonal) of the different traits.

bulls (12 older bulls and 28 young bulls) were used for mating from fourth to later (up to 14) generations by natural mating.

The matings was random, hierarchical straight breeding. In all generations, the calving rate and survivability for bulls and cows were maintained at 65% and 90%, respectively. The sex ratio for the offspring was maintained as 1:1 for males to females.

Genetic evaluation, construction of selection index and calculation of genetic gains

Estimated breeding values (EBVs) were obtained from a multi-trait animal repeatability model according to Meuwissen et al. [20] and Mrode [21] and the model of analysis can be presented as:

$$Y = Xb + Za + Wpe + e \quad [2]$$

where, Y is the traits yield;

e is the vector of error terms;

a is the vector of animal breeding value, random;

b is a vector of fixed effects (lactation), used in the simulation model;

pe is the vector of random permanent environmental effect and non-additive genetic effects, which are independently distributed with means of zero and variance σ^2_{pe} and σ^2_e, respectively;

X, Z and W are incidental matrices relating records to fixed, animals and permanent environmental effects; respectively.

var (pe)=P where P is the (co)variance matrix between permanent environmental effects

$var(e)=I\sigma^2_e=R$

var(a)=AG, where G is the (co)variance matrix and;

$$var(y) = ZAZ'G + WPW + R$$

and the mixed model equation become:

$$\begin{bmatrix} X'X & X'Z & X'W \\ Z'X & Z'Z + A^{-1}G & Z'W \\ W'X & W'Z & W'W + P \end{bmatrix} \begin{bmatrix} \hat{b} \\ \hat{a} \\ pe \end{bmatrix} = \begin{bmatrix} X'y \\ Z'y \\ W'y \end{bmatrix}$$

Selection was based on the computed total economic index values, for bulls, heifers and cows. In the case of young animals (heifers and bulls) selection was based on the total economic index using parent averages. The total economic merit was the sum of the product of EBVs and the economic value (Table 1) for all traits: Total economic merit $(T)=\Sigma a_i G_i$, where, a_i's and G_i's are the economic and the breeding values, respectively, for the different traits, expressed in dollar (US$).

The asymptotic genetic gain for this population was derived by calculating the generation-by-generation change in the averages of phenotypic and genetic values (based on true and estimated breeding values).

Selection of males and females using different scenarios

In this study, the milk yield, fat yield, protein yield, somatic cell scores (SCS) and directs mastitis resistance was simulated. The selection of males and females to be parents was done according to 6 scenarios: (1) Considering milk yield, fat yield, protein yield and SCS in the index and observing the change in mastitis resistance as it was in the simulation, but not selected for in the objective; (2) Considering milk yield, fat yield, protein yield and mastitis resistance in the index and observing the change in SCS as it was in the simulation, but not selected for in the objective; (3) Considering milk yield, fat yield, protein yield, SCS and mastitis resistance in the index; (4) Considering milk yield, fat yield, SCS and QTL explaining 15% of the additive variance in SCS in the index and observing the change in mastitis resistance as it was in the simulation, but not selected for in the objective; (5) Considering milk yield, fat yield, SCS and QTL explaining 25% of the additive variance in SCS in the index and observing the change in mastitis as it was in the simulation, but not selected for in the objective; and (6) Considering milk yield, fat yield and protein yield and observing the change in SCS and mastitis resistance as they were in the simulation, but not selected for in the objective.

Comparison of selection objectives and selection schemes by Pearson correlation coefficient

The comparison of three different selection objectives and QTL-assisted and no QTL-assisted selection schemes was done by the Pearson correlation coefficient between true breeding values (TBVs) and estimated breeding values (EBVs). Furthermore, the average values for TBVs and EBVs for different traits on both cows and bulls were plotted over generations to estimate the response (genetic gains). These estimated rate response values were also used for comparing the different selection objectives and selection schemes.

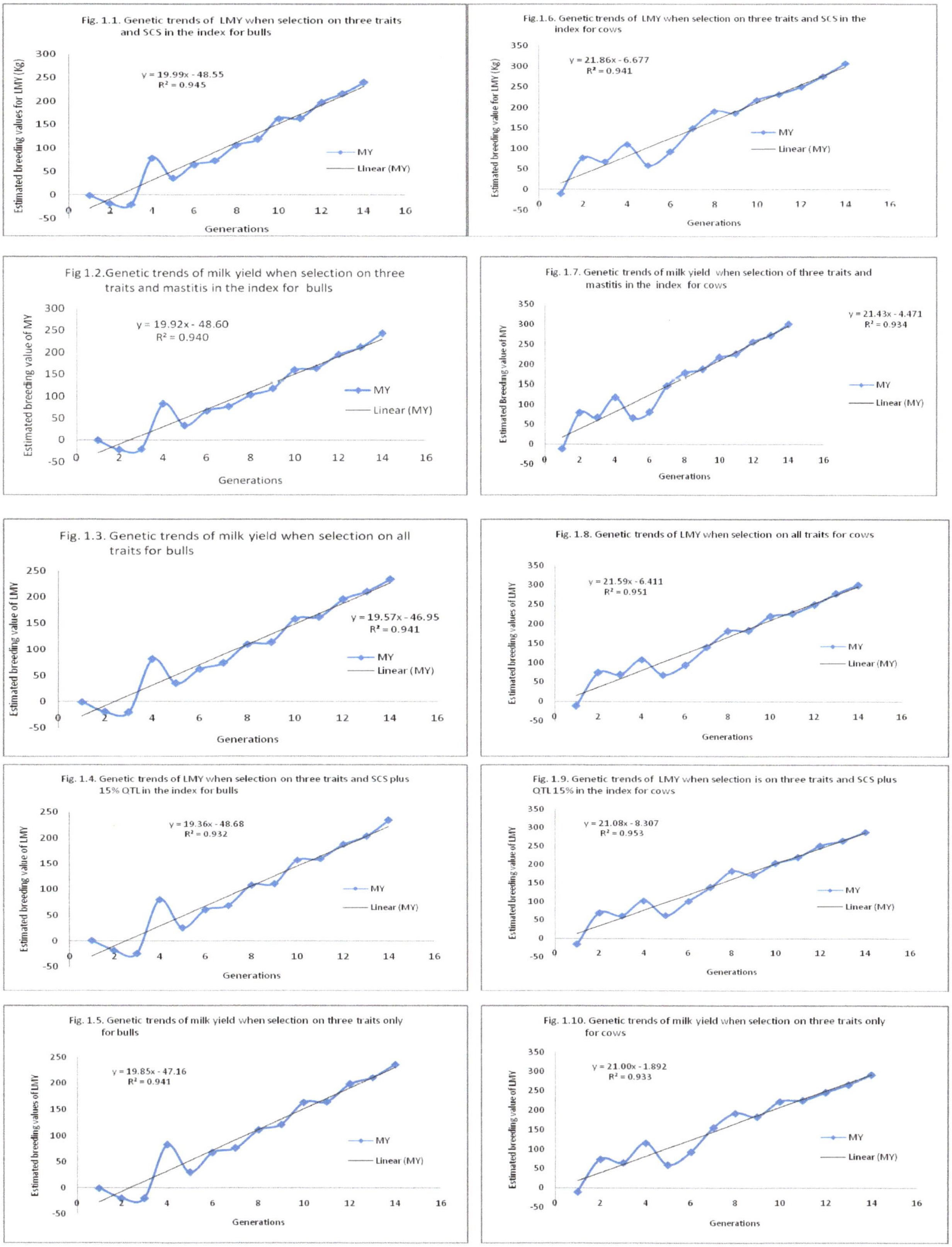

Figure 1: Genetic trends of lactation milk yield (LMY) when selecting on production (milk, fat and protein yields), mastitis resistance and somatic cell score (SCS) with or without QTL assisted selection for bulls and cows per generation, based on different selection scenarios.

Statistical Analysis

All combinations were simulated with ten replicates. From this data the average genetic merit for animals born within a generation was calculated. Results from all simulation models were analysed by using Proc GLM and Proc MIXED of SAS (SAS v.9.2, 2008). The differences of values between different mastitis liabilities scenarios and selection schemes were tested with the probability value of $P \leq 0.05$.

Results and Discussion

Means with standard errors of phenotypic and genetic gains (σ_g) in Kg per generation, based on true breeding values (TBVs) and estimated breeding values (EBVs) for the different traits, under three different mastitis liabilities, with total merit (economic selection index) in QTL-assisted and no QTL assisted selection schemes as selection objective, for cows and bulls, respectively, are presented in Tables 3 and 4.

Table 3 indicates that the phenotypic gains for all the traits of cows in the three different selection objectives under the no QTL-assisted selection scheme were similar. The phenotypic gains for all traits under the selection objective SCS of cows of the different selection schemes, were similar, therefore the selection schemes no QTL-assisted and QTL-assisted selection had no significant differences ($P<0.05$) with regards to genetic gains in the different traits (Table 3). However, based on EBVs, the genetic gains for all the traits were higher than the values based on TBVs and phenotypic values, but statistically no significant differences were found for cows as well as bulls. Based on EBVs, the genetic gains for milk yield, fat yield and protein yield were higher than the gains that were calculated for the selection based on TBVs and phenotypic values, for both cows and bulls, but no statistical significant differences were observed. Genetic gains were differed by the differences of selection objectives were reported by SØrensen et al. [22], Lessen et al. [23].

However, the gains based on EBVs for milk yield, fat yield and protein yield was higher in the no QTL-assisted selection scheme than the 15% and 25% QTL-assisted selection schemes when selecting for low SCS, but no significant differences were observed. Similarly, under the QTL-assisted selection scheme the genetic gains of all the traits for bulls were higher than when no QTL is fixed for SCS, but no significant differences were obtained. The genetic gains for milk yield under no QTL-assisted selection per year in the three different selection objectives were from 0.75 to 0.79% for cows and 0.73 to 0.85% for bulls. These values were lower than those published by Lee et al. [24]; Andrabi and Moran [25,26]. They obtained annual genetic progress for milk yield of 1 to 2%. The genetic gains for the economic index were similar in all selection objectives and also for both the QTL-assisted and no QTL-assisted selection schemes. The genetic gains of SCS were found to be similar for the QTL-assisted and no QTL-assisted selection schemes and between the three different selection objectives. The genetic gains for economic merit of all selection objectives and also between the QTL-assisted and no QTL-assisted selection schemes were statistically similar. The higher genetic gains in the different traits under the QTL-assisted selection scheme were attributed to the effect of polygenes and QTL. Abdel-Azim and Freeman [26] found that QTL-assisted selection was superior to no QTL assisted selection.

The genetic gains of bulls for the different traits based on TBVs (Table 4) were higher compared to that of the cows (Table 3) under the no QTL and QTL assisted selection schemes, but reverse scenarios was found for selection based on EBVs. However, although higher gains was found for selection based on EBV compared to that based on TBVs for cows, similar genetic gains were observed for bulls for the same scenarios. The differences in genetic gains for the different traits between selection based on TBVs or EBVs, might be due to the effects of inclusion of fixed and random factors, and also taken into account when using true breeding vales in the animal model for the estimation of breeding values. Furthermore, the differences of genetic gains in the different traits between cows and bulls might be due to the differences of sexes and also the effects of differences in selection intensity. The genetic gains can be differed by the animal model parameters, selection intensities and with the differences of sexes were mentioned by other researchers (Israel and Weller [27], Ntombizakhe Mpotu et al. [28]).

The changing genetic gain of a particular generation born cows and bulls (all) in average phenotypic values, average true breeding values, average estimated breeding values (Kg) and average economic merit (US$), when selection was based on estimated breeding values, for the different traits were plotted. The trends for all the traits in all three mastitis liabilities scenarios under QTL-assisted and no QTL-assisted selection schemes were similar. Therefore, for example, only the lactation milk yield, total economic merit, direct mastitis resistance and somatic cell score trends over 14 generations of selection and mating for both cows and bulls based on EBVs, are shown in Figures 1-4.

From Figure 1 (Figure 1.6-1.10), it can be seen that the trends for lactation milk yield in all three selection objectives under the QTL-assisted and no QTL-assisted selection schemes for cows, were similar. In the first three generations, the genetic gains were negative and in the fourth generation a sharp increased rate can be observed, followed by a decreased rate in the fifth generation. However, from generations 6 to 14 a steady increased genetic rate can be seen. The base cows were used for the progeny production up to generation 3 and in generation 4 all the base cows were replaced by the replacement heifers. Thereafter, 30% of the cows were replaced each year up to 14 generations. This might be the cause for the fluctuations in the genetic gain with the increases of generation number. Similar causes were identified by Dzama et al. [29] for stochastic simulation studies.

In the cases of bulls (Figure 1.1-1.5), the rate of genetic gains was negative in generation 1, but in generation 2 a rapid increase and from generations 3 to 5 a fluctuating rate can be observed. However, from generation 6 onwards steady increase can be seen. The fluctuation of the genetic gains might be due to the bulls used in those years. In the first 2 years, the base bulls were used and in generation 3 selected young bulls were used. The higher genetic gains were obtained in generation 4 onwards might be the effects of specific sire and dam matings in those generations. That sire and dam have a positive effect on increase in genetic gain, were reported by Dzama et al. [29]; Andabi and Moran [25].

The average total economic merit (Figure 2) and the genetic gains for direct mastitis resistance (Figure 3) for both cow and bull trends, were similar to that of Figure 1 for lactation milk yield, in all the mastitis scenarios under both QTL-assisted and no QTL-assisted selection schemes. The fluctuations in the trend might be attributed to similar causes as that of the genetic gains in Figure 1. However, the trend pattern for the genetic gains of somatic cell score were different for cows and bulls under the no QTL-assisted selection scheme and it also differed between the QTL-assisted and no QTL-assisted selection schemes (Figure 4). Under the no QTL-assisted selection scheme, for cows the somatic cell score rate of genetic gains between somatic cell score and the combination of direct mastitis resistance and somatic cell score mastitis resistance scenarios were similar, but it was different from the QTL-assisted selection scheme of somatic cell score mastitis

Based on	Selection scheme	Traits	Selection objectives		
			Direct Mastitis	SCS	Combination of direct mastitis and SCS
			Δg	Δg	Δg
True Breeding Values (TBV's)	No QTL –assisted	MY	25.98 ± 3.304	26.29 ± 2.634	25.98 ± 3.637
		FY	0.38 ± 0.164	0.40 ± 0.145	0.40 ± 0.211
		PY	0.21 ± 0.155	0.29 ± 0.176	0.26 ± 0.188
		Mas	0.019 ± 0.010	0.019 ± 0.011	0.018 ± 0.011
		SCS	0.009 ± 0.007	0.010 ± 0.011	0.007 ± 0.008
		EIndex	9.80 ± 1.250	9.92 ± 1.028	9.75 ± 1.318
	QTL-assisted (15%)	MY		25.06 ± 2.694	
		FY		0.39 ± 0.115	
		PY		0.26 ± 0.148	
		Mas		0.017 ± 0.006	
		SCS		0.008 ± 0.006	
		EIndex		9.49 ± 1.108	
	QTL-assisted (25%)	MY		26.50 ± 3.229	
		FY		0.41 ± 0.198	
		PY		0.32 ± 0.211	
		Mas		0.017 ± 0.006	
		SCS		0.010 ± 0.006	
		EIndex		10.03 ± 1.294	
	QTL-assisted	MY		25.48 ± 3.129	
		FY		0.34 ± 0.194	
		PY		0.21 ± 0.194	
		Mas		0.018 ± 0.009	
		SCS		0.009 ± 0.007	
		EIndex		9.70 ± 1.151	
Estimated Breeding Values (EBV's)	No QTL- assisted	MY	30.01 ± 4.262	27.99 ± 2.972	30.23 ± 4.402
		FY	0.46 ± 0.142	0.43 ± 0.107	0.46 ± 0.176
		PY	0.28 ± 0.131	0.29 ± 0.129	0.31 ± 0.155
		Mas	0.011 ± 0.003	0.011 ± 0.004	0.011 ± 0.004
		SCS	0.008 ± 0.005	0.008 ± 0.007	0.006 ± 0.006
		EIndex	11.33 ± 1.628	11.55 ± 1.349	11.39 ± 1.641
	QTL-assisted (15%)	MY		29.52 ± 3.257	
		FY		0.47 ± 0.105	
		PY		0.32 ± 0.141	
		Mas		0.011 ± 0.003	
		SCS		0.008 ± 0.005	
		EIndex		11.18 ± 1.301	
	QTL-assisted (25%)	MY		30.92 ± 3.848	
		FY		0.48 ± 0.163	
		PY		0.34 ± 0.192	
		Mas		0.012 ± 0.002	
		SCS		0.008 ± 0.006	
		EIndex		11.71 ± 1.507	
	QTL-assisted	MY		29.41 ± 2.691	
		FY		0.42 ± 0.169	
		PY		0.26 ± 0.153	
		Mas		0.011 ± 0.003	
		SCS		0.007 ± 0.005	
		EIndex		11.18 ± 1.028	

MY=Milk yield, FY=Fat yield, PY=Protein yield, Mas=Direct mastitis resistance, SCS=Somatic Cell Score, EIndex=Economic selection index, and QTL=Quantitative trait Loci; Means with superscript a and b are different at 5% level of significance between selection objective with in a generation and between selection schemes within selection objectives.

Table 3: Mean with standard error of genetic gain (Δg) in Kg per generation for different traits under three different mastitis liabilities with total merit in QTL-assisted and no QTL assisted selection schemes as selection objective, for cows.

Based on	Selection scheme	Traits	Selection objectives		
			Direct Mastitis	SCS	Combination of direct mastitis and SCS
			Δg	Δg	Δg
True Breeding Values (TBV's)	No QTL assisted	MY	28.27 ± 2.255	28.35 ± 2.759	27.93 ± 2.821
		FY	0.42 ± 0.140	0.43 ± 0.112	0.43 ± 0.142
		PY	0.25 ± 0.112	0.29 ± 0.126	0.28 ± 0.129
		Mas	0.018 ± 0.006	0.009 ± 0.008	0.019 ± 0.009
		SCS	0.008 ± 0.005	0.018 ± 0.009	0.007 ± 0.005
		EIndex	10.66 ± 0.835	10.71 ± 1.025	10.49 ± 1.033
	QTL-assisted (15%)	MY		27.75 ± 2.310	
		FY		0.45 ± 0.101	
		PY		0.29 ± 0.127	
		Mas		0.017 ± 0.007	
		SCS		0.007 ± 0.006	
		EIndex		10.51 ± 0.924	
	QTL-assisted (25%)	MY		28.46 ± 2.216	
		FY		0.45 ± 0.142	
		PY		0.33 ± 0.173	
		Mas		0.017 ± 0.006	
		SCS		0.008 ± 0.006	
		EIndex		10.77 ± 0.893	
	QTL-assisted	MY		28.22 ± 3.304	
		FY		0.40 ± 0.178	
		PY		0.24 ± 0.154	
		Mas		0.018 ± 0.008	
		SCS		0.007 ± 0.006	
		EIndex		10.73 ± 1.216	
Estimated Breeding Values (EBV's)	No QTL assisted	MY	27.87 ± 3.010	27.99 ± 2.972	27.40 ± 3.363
		FY	0.41 ± 0.130	0.43 ± 0.107	0.42 ± 0.133
		PY	0.25 ± 0.113	0.29 ± 0.129	0.27 ± 0.122
		Mas	0.011 ± 0.003	0.011 ± 0.004	0.01 ± 0.003
		SCS	0.007 ± 0.004	0.008 ± 0.007	0.006 ± 0.004
		EIndex	10.54 ± 1.144	10.58 ± 1.109	10.32 ± 1.258
	QTL-assisted (15%)	MY		27.11 ± 2.781	
		FY		0.43 ± 0.105	
		PY		0.26 ± 0.123	
		Mas		0.010 ± 0.003	
		SCS		0.006 ± 0.005	
		EIndex		10.28 ± 1.103	
	QTL-assisted (25%)	MY		28.00 ± 2.885	
		FY		0.42 ± 0.142	
		PY		0.30 ± 0.175	
		Mas		0.011 ± 0.002	
		SCS		0.007 ± 0.005	
		EIndex		10.62 ± 1.134	
	QTL-assisted	MY		27.80 ± 2.831	
		FY		0.39 ± 0.161	
		PY		0.24 ± 0.145	
		Mas		0.010 ± 0.003	
		SCS		0.006 ± 0.005	
		EIndex		10.57 ± 1.065	

Traits descriptions are same as footnote on Table 3; Means with superscript a and b are different at 5% level of significance between selection objective within a generation and between selection schemes within selection objectives.

Table 4: Means with standard errors for genetic gain (Δg) in Kg per generation for different traits under three different mastitis liabilities with total merit as selection objective, for bulls.

Selection scheme	Traits	Cow			Bull		
		Selection objectives			Selection objectives		
		Direct mastitis	SCS	Combination of direct mastitis and SCS	Direct mastitis	SCS	Combination of direct mastitis and SCS
No QTL assisted	MY	0.9	0.89	0.89	0.94	0.92	0.92
	FY	0.77	0.76 ± 0.01	0.77 ± 0.01	0.82 ± 0.01	0.79 ± 0.01	0.76 ± 0.01
	PY	0.72	0.72	0.72	0.76 ± 0.01	0.74 ± 0.01	0.66 ± 0.02
	Mas	0.67 ± 0.01	0.67 ± 0.01	0.67 ± 0.01	0.70 ± 0.01	0.71 ± 0.01	0.71 ± 0.01
	SCS	0.57 ± 0.01	0.59 ± 0.01	0.57 ± 0.00	0.51 ± 0.03	0.62 ± 0.02	0.56 ± 0.01
	EIndex	0.9	0.9	0.9	0.94	0.92	0.92
QTL-assisted (15%)	MY		0.9			0.92	
	FY		0.77			0.79 ± 0.01	
	PY		0.71 ± 0.01			0.73 ± 0.01	
	Mas		0.64 ± 0.01			0.67 ± 0.02	
	SCS		0.54 ± 0.01			0.59 ± 0.02	
	EIndex		0.9			0.92	
QTL-assisted (25%)	MY		0.9			0.92	
	FY		0.77			0.79 ± 0.01	
	PY		0.72 ± 0.01			0.70 ± 0.02	
	Mas		0.66 ± 0.01			0.70 ± 0.01	
	SCS		0.55 ± 0.01			0.63 ± 0.02	
	EIndex		0.9			0.92	
QTL-assisted (Milk, fat and Protein)	MY		0.9			0.93	
	FY		0.76 ± 0.01			0.75 ± 0.01	
	PY		0.70 ± 0.00			0.67 ± 0.01	
	Mas		0.68 ± 0.01			0.70 ± 0.02	
	SCS		0.59 ± 0.01			0.53 ± 0.02	
	EIndex		0.9			0.93	

Traits descriptions are same as footnote on Table 3; Means with superscript a and b are different at 5% level of significance between selection objectives within a generation and between selection schemes within selection objectives and between cows and bulls.

Table 5: Correlations for the estimated breeding values of different traits under three different selection objectives for cows and bulls.

liabilities scenario. Up to generation 4 the rate was similar, after that a steady increased rate can be observed, but at generation 14, the rate suddenly dropped. In the case of bulls, distinct differences were observed between the QTL-assisted and no QTL-assisted selection schemes and also between somatic cell score and the combination of somatic cell score and direct mastitis liabilities scenarios. The differences in the rate of genetic gains for somatic cell score might be due to the QTL-assisted selection that was considered on the somatic cell score basis. Traits that considered QTL-assisted selection have an impact on genetic gains, as were reported by Abdel-Azim and Freeman [11].

Correlations for the estimated breeding values of different traits under the three different selection objectives for cows and bulls under quantitative trait loci (QTL) assisted (15% and 25%) and no QTL-assisted selection schemes are presented in Table 5. The correlations for milk yield (0.89 to 0.94), fat yield (0.76 to 0.82), protein yield (0.66 to 0.72), direct mastitis resistance (0.67 to 0.71), somatic cell score (0.51 to 0.62) and for the economic selection index (0.90 to 0.94) for all selection objectives and selection schemes were similar for both cows and bulls (Table 5). The correlations of different traits in cows and bulls was hierarchical among traits, that is milk yield>fat yield>protein yield>direct mastitis resistance>SCS, except for the combination of direct mastitis resistance and SCS in bulls where direct mastitis resistance correlations were higher than that of protein. The correlations of the economic selection index between the different selection objectives of cows and bulls are similar, but bulls had higher values than cows for both the QTL and no QTL assisted selection schemes. Furthermore, the correlations of the economic selection index under SCS between no QTL and QTL assisted selection are also similar. The higher correlation value indicated that the bulls were superior to cows. On the other hand Carlen et al. [5] observed the correlation for lactation was 0.76 for and for 150 days milk yield but these values are lower than the t value for milk yield in this study.

Conclusion

It can be seen that the rate of genetic gains for milk -, fat and protein yields were similar for cows and bulls in the three different selection objectives under the no QTL-assisted and QTL-assisted selection schemes. However, direct mastitis resistance differed between the selection objectives and schemes. In this study, the QTL-assisted selection scheme has a low impact somatic cell scores. This might be due to low phenotypic variation with low heritability for somatic cell scores. However, the QTL-assisted selection scheme has a positive effect on milk production and mastistis control. This study offered an opportunity to utilise somatic cell score as an indirect trait for mastitis control, which leads to a higher milk yield and increase the genetic gains. However, this study can be widely used under practical situations for genetic improvement of dairy cows.

Acknowledgements

The authors are very much grateful to the Commonwealth Scholarship Commission for providing the fellowship to the first author. They also like to thanks to the Scottish Agricultural College, Edinburgh, United Kingdom for their active cooperation and support to pursue this study.

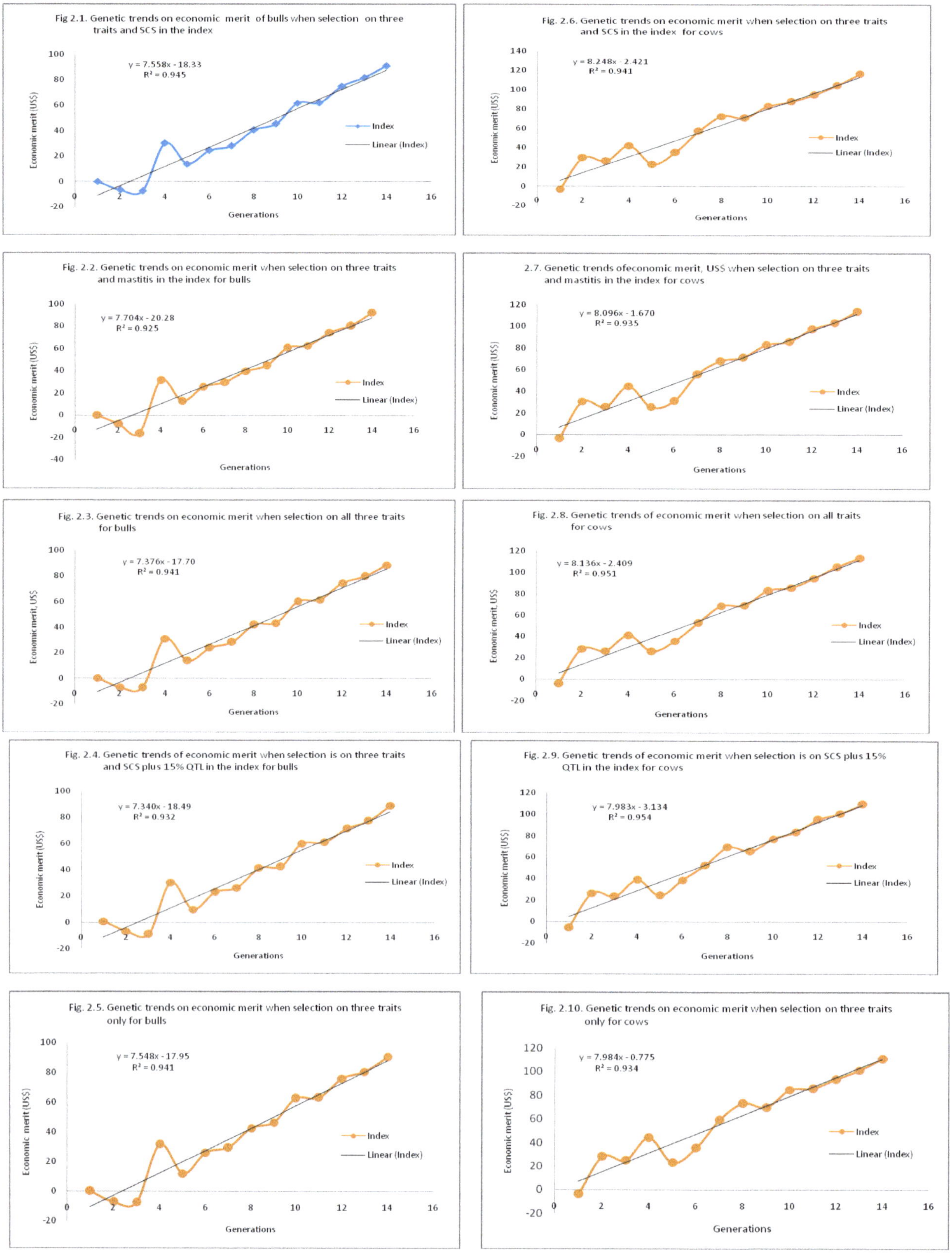

Figure 2: Genetic trends of average total economic merit (US$) when selecting on production (milk, fat and protein yields), mastitis and somatic cell score (SCS) with or without QTL assisted selection for bulls and cows per generation, based on different selection scenarios.

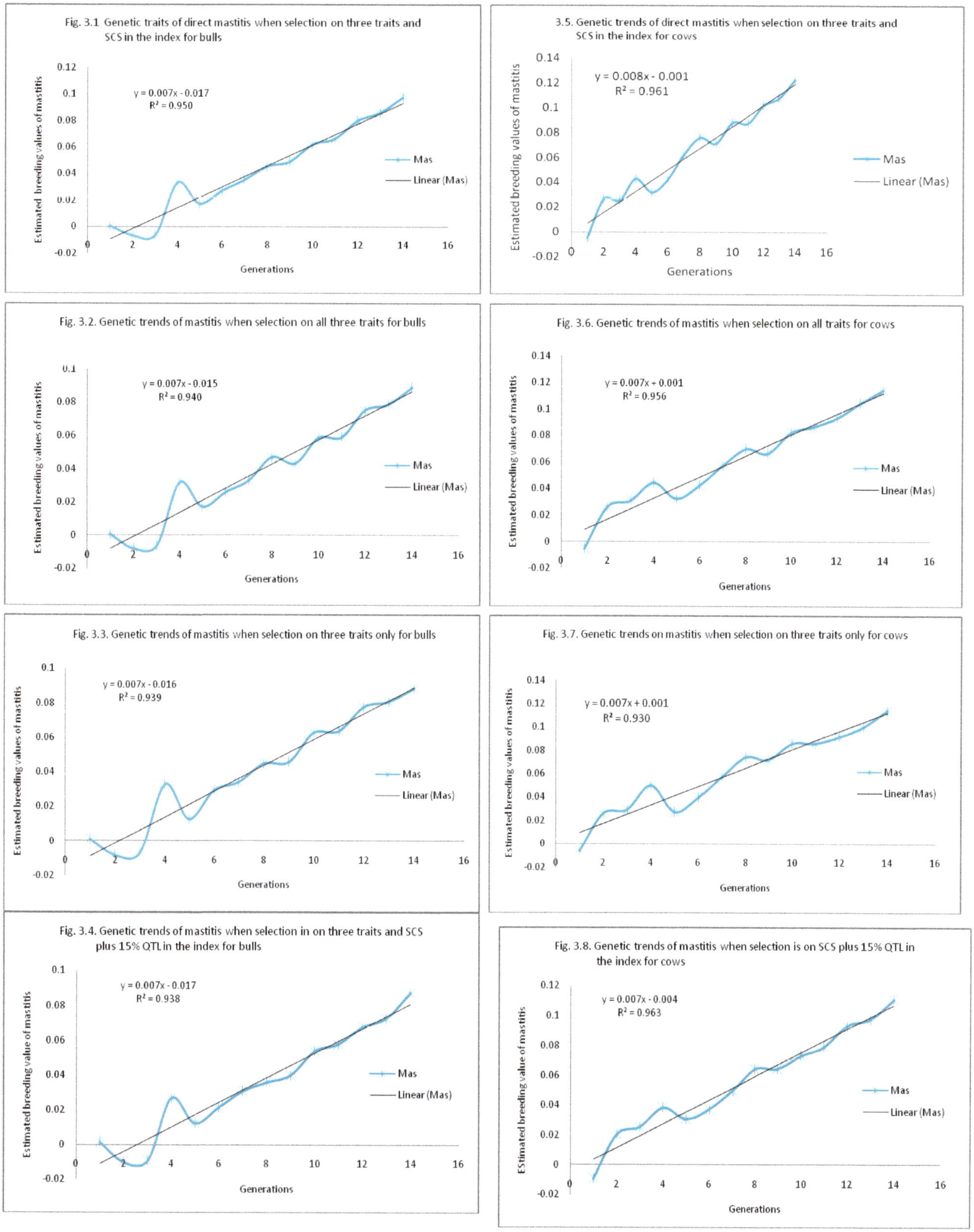

Figure 3: Genetic trends of direct mastitis resistance when selecting on production (milk, fat and protein yields), mastitis and somatic cell score (SCS) with or without QTL assisted selection for bulls and cows per generation, based on different selection scenarios.

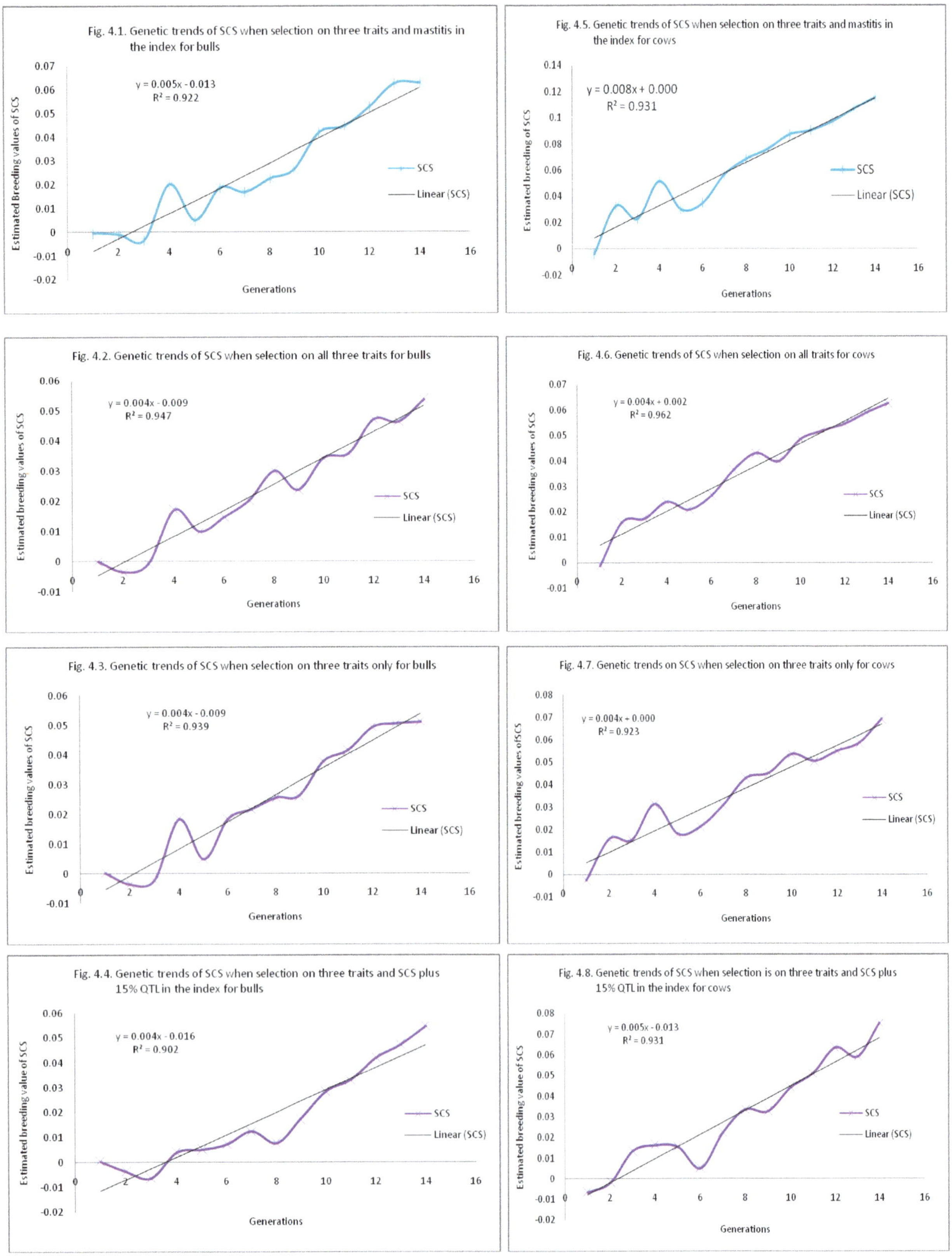

Figure 4: Genetic trends of somatic cell score when selection on production (milk, fat and protein yields), mastitis and somatic cell score (SCS) with or without QTL assisted selection for bulls and cows per generation, based on different selection scenarios.

References

1. Khan MKI, Blair HT, Lopez-Villalobos N, Johnson PL (2005) Productive, reproductive and economic performance of dairy cattle in Bangladesh. Proc Assoc Advance Anim Breed Genetic 16: 124-127.
2. Rhaman MA, Bhuiyan MMU, Kamal MM, Shamsuddin M (2009) Prevalence and risk factors of mastitis in dairy cows. Bangladesh Veterinarian 26: 54-60.
3. Uddin MA, Kamal MM, Haque ME (2009) Epidemiological study of udder and treat diseases in dairy cows. Bangladesh J Vet Medicin 7: 332-340.
4. Charfeddine N, Alenda R, Groen AF, Carabaño MJ (2000) Genetic parameters and economic values of lactation somatic cell score and production traits. J Dairy Sci 83: 84-91.
5. Carle´n E, Emanuelson U, Strandberg E (2006) Genetic evaluation of mastitis in dairy cattle using linear models, threshold models, and survival analysis: A simulation study. J Dairy Sci 89: 4049-4057.
6. Majid MA, Nahar TN, Talukdar AI, Rahman MA (1998) Reproductive performance of purebred F_1, F_2 and F_3 cows raised in Savar dairy farm. Bangladesh J Livest Res 2: 63-71.
7. Khan MKI, Huque KS, Miah AG, Khatun MJ (2000) Study on the performance of Red Chittagong cows under different production system. Pakistan J Biol Sci 3: 318-319.
8. Bhuiyan AKFH, Shahjalal M, Islam MN, Rahman AKMA, Keown JF, et al. (2008) Characterzation, conservation and improvement of Red Chittagong Cattle of Bangladesh. In Proceeding of the USDA Project Review Workshop. Vol. 1, pp: 26-28.
9. Khan MKI, Blair HT, Lopez-Villalobos N (2012) Lactation curves of different cattle breeds under cooperative dairying conditions in Bangladesh. J Appl Anim Res 40: 179-185.
10. Spelman RJ, Garrick DJ (1997) Utilisation of marker assisted selection in a commercial dairy cow population. Livest Prod Sci 47: 139-147.
11. Abdel-Azim G, Freeman AE (2002) Superiority of QTL-assisted selection in dairy cattle breeding schemes. J Dairy Sci 85: 1869-1880.
12. Dekkers JCM (2007) Estimation of economic values for dairy cattle breeding goals: bias due to sub-optimal management policies. Livest Prod Sci 29: 131-149.
13. Meuwissen THE, van Arendonk JAM (1992) Potential improvement in rate of genetic gain from marker-assisted selection in dairy cattle breeding schemes. J Dairy Sci 75: 1651-1659.
14. Ruane J, Colleau JJ (1996) Marker assisted selection for a sex limited character in a nucleus breeding population. J Dairy Sci 79: 1666-1678.
15. Spelman RJ, Garrick DJ, van Arendonk JAM (1999) Utilisation of genetic variation by marker-assisted selection in commercial dairy cattle populations. Livest Prod Sci 59: 51-60.
16. Shook GE (2006) Major advances in determining appropriate selection goals. J Dairy Sci 89: 1349-1361.
17. SØrensen JT, Kristensen ES, Thysen I (1992) A stochastic model simulating the dairy herd on a PC. Agric Syst 39: 177-200.
18. Falconer DS, Mackay TFC (1997) Introduction to quantitative genetics. 4th edn. Longmans Green, Harlow, Essex, UK, pp: 122-159.
19. Verrier E (2001) Marker assisted selection for the improvement of two antagonistic traits under mixed inheritance. Genet Sel Evol 33: 17-38.
20. Meuwissen THE, Hayes B, Goddard ME (2001) Prediction of total genetic value using genome-wide sense marker maps. Genet Sel Evol 28: 161-176.
21. Mrode MR (2005) Use of genetic markers in prediction of breeding values. Linear models for the prediction of animal breeding values. 2nd edn, pp: 163-191.
22. SØrensen MK, Berg P, Jensen J, Christensen LG (2006) Stochastic simulation of breeding schemes for total merit in dairy cattle. Interbull Bulletin 23: 183.
23. Lassen J, SØrensen MK, Madsen P, Ducrocq V (2007) A stochastic simulation study on validation of an approximate multitrait model using pre-adjusted data for prediction of breeding values. J Dairy Sci 90: 3002-3011.
24. Lee KL, Freeman AE, Johnson IP (1998) Estimation of genetic change in the registered Holstein cattle population. J Dairy Sci 68: 2629-2638.
25. Andrabi SMH, Moran C (2007) Selection of dairy cow bulls for artificial insemination. Intl J Agric Biol 9: 175-178.
26. Abdel-Azim G, Freeman AE (2003) Effects of including a Quantitative Trait Locus in selection under different waiting plans of young bulls. J Dairy Sci 86: 667-676.
27. Israel C, Weller JI (2000) Effect of misidentification on genetic gain and estimation of breeding value in dairy cattle populations. J Dairy Sci 83: 181-187.
28. Ntombizakhe M, Charles S, Edward BB (1993) Breeding strategies for genetic improvement of dairy cattle in Zimbabwe. I. Genetic Evaluation. J Dairy Sci 76: 1163-1172.
29. Dzama K, Walter JP, Ruvuna F, Sanders JO, Chimonyo M (2001) Index selection of beef cattle for growth and milk production using computer simulation modelling. South African J Anim Sci 31: 65-75.

Serum Concentrations of Strontium, Lead, Nickel, Vanadium and Aluminum in Horses

Saeed Nazifi[1]*, Neda Eskandarzade[2], Mahsa Khosravi[1], Maryam Haddadi[1] and Mojtaba Rahsepar[1]

[1]Department of Clinical Studies, School of Veterinary Medicine, Shiraz University, Shiraz, Iran
[2]Department of Basic Sciences, School of Veterinary Medicine, Shahid Bahonar University, Kerman, Iran

Abstract

Providing data on the serum concentration of some important heavy metals in horses of different age and sex is an indicator of short-term exposure and also help to understand influence of these factors in metals intoxication. We reported serum concentrations of some elements in healthy horses and assessed any relationship with age and sex. Fifty-three samples from horses were analyzed by atomic absorption. Mean serum concentrations (µg/ml) ± SD values for strontium were (0.25 ± 0.15), vanadium (0.20 ± 0.02), aluminium (0.71 ± 0.16), nickel (0.10 ± 0.08) and lead (0.09 ± 0.04) µg/ml. No significant correlations were noted between measured elements with age, however, a significant correlation was detected between age with concentration of lead ($P<0.05$). We concluded that older horses had more ability to absorb this element from their environment, or ability to detoxify lead decreased with increase in age.

Keywords: Strontium; Aluminum; Vanadium; Nickel; Lead; Horse

Introduction

Heavy metals are widely spread in human and animal environments by sources like industries and can cause some biological malfunctions. For example, absorbed Ni changes membrane properties and balance of oxidation/reduction systems. It has great affinity for cellular structures like chromosomes and its toxicity is teratogenic and carcinogenic [1-3]. This element is excreted mainly via the urine and to a lower extent in breast milk. Milk and dairy products are one of the main contributors to the chronic dietary exposure to nickel (Ni) in humans [4]. Lead (Pb) has been one of the most common toxicants encountered in veterinary practice and peripheral neuropathy, intermittent colic, and mild anemia are common features of acute toxicosis with this element in general [5]. Equines are food and milk-producing animals in many countries, therefore determining status of toxicants in equine biological components is relevant to human health, and therefore should not be underestimated [6,7]. However, the toxic doses of elements in animals have not been known yet because there is disagreement between results of published studies, and still the physiological mechanisms involved in mineral poisoning are also not yet understood. Finding correlations between some physiological parameters such as age and level of elements accumulation in blood helped underestanding this criteria.

Although there are several studies which revealed that quantities of metals in horse biological components were good bio-indicator for environmental pollution and nutritional status [8-11] there is still limited reference about influence of age and sex on blood elements concentrations in these animals. This study was conducted to evaluate the amounts of some important elements such as strontium (Sr), aluminum (Al), vanadium (V), nickel (Ni) and lead (Pb) in the blood of horses of different age and sex in Shiraz which could be used in disease assessment of human and equine and better understanding the physiological parameters attributed to these elements intoxication.

Materials and Methods

This study was conducted on a group of 53 horses which belonged to two farms around Shiraz. The horses were considered healthy based on physical examination. There were 22 males, 31 females. Animals were divided into 3 groups regarding age <5 years (n=16), 5-10 years (n=26), >10 years (n=11).

Sampling

Blood samples were taken aseptically from jugular veins, placed into tubes without any anticoagulant and put in the water-bath at 37°C to coagulate. After clotting, the samples were centrifuged and sera were obtained. Samples were kept at -20°C until chemical analysis.

Animal ethics

The experiment was performed under the approval of the state committee on animal ethics, Shiraz University, Shiraz, Iran (IACUC no: 4687/63). Also, the recommendations of European Council Directive (86/609/EC) of November 24, 1986, regarding the protection of animals used for experimental purposes were considered.

Preparation of the samples

The serum samples were analyzed by 700 µl hydropercloric acid 98% and nitric acid 65% added to 300 µl of serum and kept for 16-20 hours in 80°C water-baths. The prepared samples were analyzed by atomic absorption spectrometry (Shimadzu AA-670, Japan).

Measurement of the elements

Trace elements were analyzed by flame and air-C_2H_2 for Pb, Sr, Ni and N_2O-C_2H_2 for Al and V. Primarily, the atomic absorption was set to a special wavelength, 217 nm for Pb, 232 nm for Ni, 309.3 nm

***Corresponding author:** Dr. Saeed Nazifi, Professor of Veterinary Clinical Pathology, Department of Clinical Studies, School of Veterinary Medicine, Shiraz University, Shiraz, Iran, E-mail: nazifi@shirazu.ac.ir

for Al, 460.7 for Sr and 318.4 nm for V; the machinery was calibrated by injecting 5-6 standard solutions with different concentrations in normal range of each element, solutions were injected to the machinery and element concentration was measured in μg/ml.

Statistical analysis

Statistical analysis was performed using SPSS software (version 18). The effect of age on the concentration of the analyzed elements in the serum of horses was determined by Kruskal-Wallis H except for Ni, which was analyzed by one-way ANOVA. The effect of sex on the concentration of the analyzed elements in the serum of horses was determined by Mann-Whitney U test except for Ni, which was analyzed by Independent-Samples t-test. $P<0.05$ was considered as statistically significant. The relationship between the amount of serum concentrations of individual elements and different age and sex was calculated using Spearman correlation analysis.

Results and Discussion

Serum concentration of analyzed elements (μg. mL^{-1}) in different categories with regard to sex and age are presented in Tables 1 and 2. All heavy metals evaluated were present in the blood of the horses and serum concentration of the analyzed elements followed the order Al>Sr>V>Ni>Pb. The different age and sex studied here did not influence the serum contents of Ni, Al and V ($P>0.05$) although significant correlation between age and concentration of Pb was detected ($P<0.05$).

Strontium (Sr)

In our study Sr concentration in females (0.3 ± 0.02 μg/ml) was more than in males (0.18 ± 0.03 μg/ml) which was not consistent with a study done by Pablack et al. [12] that showed no gender differences in Sr concentration existed in liver and kidney of horses. The reason for this difference is not clear and no information is available in this regard. So, more investigations are required for better understanding of this finding. According to Table 2, No significant correlation between concentrations of Strontium with age was seen which was in agreement with a study carried out by Pablack et al. [12] which showed no age-dependent differences in Strontium concentration in liver and kidney of horses. Although Sr concentration in animals with age more than 10 years old (0.20 ± 0.07 μg/ml) was lower than horses with age 5-10 years (0.27 ± 0.02 μg/ml) and <5 years old (0.25 ± 0.02 μg/ml) ($P<0.05$). This is probably because of higher absorption of strontium from the intestines of younger horses than adults. In the body, strontium behaves very much like calcium and will accumulate in bones. Excess stable strontium causes problems with growing bone. For this reason, children are more susceptible to the effects of stable strontium than adults who have mature bone [13]. Studies in humans suggested that the elimination rate of strontium is strongly affected by age and sex, due to differences in bone metabolism [14].

Lead (Pb)

As lead is an important environmental contaminant, in this context, reports on lead poisoning exist for horses and other livestock in contaminated areas [15-17]. Pourjafar and his coworkers in 2008 confirmed usability of horse hair as a test bio-indicator for Pb envirmental pollution [9]. However, there was no decisive agreement on intoxication of horses by this heavy metal. For example, in a study carried out in India with 288 horses from three different areas (industrial, highway adjacent and rural zone) no clinical signs associated with intoxication by lead were detected in the studied animals [18]. On the other hand, a study conducted with horses living on farmland in the vicinity of non-ferrous metal smelters in China showed signs of intoxication by lead in horses [19]. Lead concentrations in the blood and organs of horses indicated lead concentrations in equine by-products. The lead toxicity values in the blood for farm animals have been always lower than those in humans [20] and in horses, the concentration of 0.25 μg mL^{-1} is accepted as maximum limit [21]. According to our results, contents of Pb in 100% of samples analyzed present levels below the detection limits. As shown in Table 1, in males, Pb concentration (0.1 ± 0.00 μg/ml) was significantly higher than females (0.08 ± 0.01 μg/ml). As shown in Table 2, although all of the horses used here were in the same environment, there is significant increase in Pb concentration in group with more than 10 year-old horses (0.1 ± 0.00 μg/ml) compared to the other two groups. Also, Pb concentration increased with increasing in age, so there is a correlation between age with concentration of Pb ($P<0.05$). It seemed that ability to detoxify lead decreased with increase in age or older horses had more ability to absorb this element from their environment, however, further investigations are needed to confirm this hypothesis. Present data was in agreement with a research done by Rudy which indicated that contamination of meat of cattle by Pb clearly depends on the age of these animals and older cattles had more Pb concentrations [22]. But our finding is not in agreement with Asano et al. [23] who reported that there was no age-dependent correlation in Pb concentration of mane hair in male and female racing horses. In present study, the mean serum Pb concentration in 53 horses was (0.09 ± 0.04) μg/ml which was lower than the values reported by De Souza et al. [24] (1.058 μg/ml).

Nickel (Ni)

If we consider presence of high amount of Ni in legumes such as

Sex	Ni (μg mL^{-1})	Pb (μg mL^{-1})	Sr (μg mL^{-1})	Al (μg mL^{-1})	Va (μg mL^{-1})
Male	0.096 ± 0.01	0.1 ± 0.00^{a}	0.18 ± 0.03^{a}	0.72 ± 0.03	0.20 ± 0.00
Female	0.115 ± 0.01	0.08 ± 0.01^{b}	0.30 ± 0.02^{b}	0.70 ± 0.02	0.20 ± 0.00

Values that have a different superscript (a, b) differ significantly from each other ($P<0.05$).

Table 1: Concentrations (μg/ml) of strontium (Sr), aluminum (Al), vanadium (Va), nickel (Ni) and lead (Pb) in the serum of horses, depending on the sex of the animals (Male: n=22; Female: n=31).

Age	No	Ni (μg mL^{-1})	Pb (μg mL^{-1})	Sr (μg mL^{-1})	Al (μg mL^{-1})	Va (μg mL^{-1})
<5	16	0.09 ± 0.02	0.08 ± 0.02^{a}	0.25 ± 0.02^{a}	0.71 ± 0.04	0.2 ± 0.00
5-10	26	0.11 ± 0.01	0.09 ± 0.00^{b}	0.27 ± 0.02^{a}	0.69 ± 0.03	0.2 ± 0.00
>10	11	0.1 ± 0.01	0.1 ± 0.00^{c}	0.20 ± 0.07^{b}	0.75 ± 0.04	0.2 ± 0.00

Values that have a different superscript (a, b, c) differ significantly from each other ($P<0.05$).

Table 2: Concentrations (μg/ml) of strontium (Sr), aluminum (Al), vanadium (Va), nickel (Ni) and lead (Pb) in the serum of horses, depending on the age.

alfalfa which is in equine diet the importance of evaluating this element in these animals is evident. However, reference values of blood Ni concentrations were not common in the literature and no toxicity studies were identified for horses. Besides, according to the European Food Safety Authority, contribution of foods of animal origin with high exposure to Ni to human diet is not insignificant [25]. In the present study, there is no significant difference in Ni concentration in all of the groups and the different age and sex studied here did not influence the contents of this element (P>0.05). This was the same as the findings revealed by Asano et al. [23] who reported that there was no age dependent correlation in Ni concentration of mane hair in male and female racing horses. In present study, the mean serum Ni concentration in 53 horses was (0.10 ± 0.08) μg/ml which was higher than the values reported by De Souza et al. [24] (0.006 μg/ml).

Vanadium (V)

Vanadium and related compounds are known to exert potent toxic effects on a wide variety of biological systems mediated by oxygen-derived free radicals [26]. Concentration of this element in blood was the most suitable indicator of the body burden and was better tolerated by small animals including rats and mice than by larger animals, such as horses [27]. Acute toxicity value for vanadium is considered highly species-dependent [28,29]. Reference value of blood V concentration was not common in the literature. Based on Tables 1 and 2, difference in age and sex had no significant influence on vanadium status and there was no age-related correlation in vanadium concentration between groups (P>0.05).

Aluminum (Al)

Aluminium was classified as metalloestrogens because it increased estrogen-related gene expression in human breast cancer cells cultured in the laboratory [30]. In our investigation the contents of this toxic metal in the blood analyzed was not influenced by sex and age, therefore, there was no age-related correlation in Al concentration (P>0.05) which was in agreement with an investigation performed by Asano et al. [23] who reported that there was no age-dependent correlation in Al concentration of mane hair in male and female racing horses. In present study, the mean serum Al concentration in 53 horses was (0.71 ± 0.16) μg/ml which was lower than the values reported by Asano et al. [23] (64.5 ± 77.0) μg/g in the mane hair of horses.

Conclusion

We concluded that contamination of blood of horse by lead depends on the age of these animals although further investigations are needed to confirm this hypothesis.

Acknowledgments

The authors would like to thank the Research Council of Shiraz University and School of Veterinary Medicine, Shiraz University for financial and technical support of this study.

Funding

This study was funded by Shiraz University (Grant number: 71-GR-VT-5).

Conflict of Interest

The authors declare that they have no conflicts of interest.

References

1. Buttice C (2015) Nickel compounds. In: Colditz GA. The SAGE encyclopedia of cancer and society (second edition) SAGE publications, Inc., pp: 828-831.
2. Costa M, Sutherland JF, Peng W, Salnikov K, Broday L, et al. (2002) Molecular biology of nickel carcinogenesis. Mol Cell Biochem 222: 205-211.
3. Samal S, Mishra C (2011) Significance of Nickel in Livestock Health and Production. Int J Agro Vet Med Sci 5: 349-361.
4. Tabinda AB, Zafar S, Yasar A, Munir S (2013) Metals Concentration in Water, Fodder, Milk, Meat, Blood, Kidney and Liver of Livestock and Associated Health Impacts by Intake of Contaminated Milk and Meat. Pakistan J Zool 45: 1156-1160.
5. Ciobanu C, Slencu BG, Cuciureanu R (2012) Estimation of dietary intake of cadmium and lead through food consumption. Rev Med Chir Soc Med Nat Iasi 116: 617-623.
6. Kucera E (1988) Dogs as indicators of urban lead distribution. Environ Monit Assess 10: 51-57.
7. Kozak M, Kralova E, Sviatko P, Bilek J, Bugarsky A (2002) Study of the content of heavy metals related to environmental load in urban areas in Slovakia. Bratisl Lek Listy 103: 231-237.
8. Kapron B, Nowakowicz-debek B, Wnuk W, Martyna J, Saba L, et al. (2010) Effect of living conditions on heavy metal contents in Polish Konik horses coat hair and blood serum. Ochr Oerod Zas Nat 44: 66-71.
9. Pourjafar M, Badiei KH, Shakhse-Niaie M (2008) Horse Hair as an Indicator of Pb Pollution Around Shiraz Oil Industry Iran. J Environ Sci Technol 1: 42-46.
10. Topczewska J (2012) Effects of seasons on the concentration of selected trace elements in horse hair. J Cent Eur Agric 13: 671-680.
11. Topczewska J, Krupa W (2013) Influence of horse breed and housing system on the level of selected elements in horse's hair. J Elem 18: 287-295.
12. Pablack N, Mainzer B, Lahrssen-Wiederholt M, Schafft H, Palavinskas R, et al. (2014) Concentrations of strontium, barium, cadmium, copper, zinc, manganese, chromium, antimony, selenium and lead in the equine liver and kidneys. Springer Plus 3: 343-353.
13. ATSDR (Agency for Toxic Substances and Disease Registry). Public Health Statement: Strontium. Cdc.gov. Agency for Toxic Substances and Disease Registry, 2016.
14. Shagina NB, Bougrov NG, Degteva MO, Kozheurov VP, Tolstykh EI (2006) An application of in vivo whole body counting technique for studying strontium metabolism and internal dose reconstruction for the Techa River population. J Physics 41: 433-440.
15. Lemos RA, Driemeier D, Guimarães EB, Dutra IS, Mori AE, et al. (2004) Lead poisoning in cattle grazing pasture contaminated by industrial waste. Vet Hum Toxicol 46: 326-328.
16. Palacios H, Iribarren I, Olalla MJ, Cala V (2002) Lead poisoning of horses in the vicinity of a battery recycling plant. Sci Total Environ 290: 81-89.
17. Rodriguez-Estival J, Barasona JA, Mateo R (2012) Blood Pb and δ-ALAD inhibition in cattle and sheep from a Pb-polluted mining area. Environ Pollut 160: 118-124.
18. Dey S, Dwivedi SK (2004) Lead in blood of urban Indian horses. Vet Hum Toxicol 46: 194-195.
19. Liu ZP (2003) Lead poisoning combined with cadmium in sheep and horses in the vicinity of non-ferrous metal smelters. Sci Total Environ 309: 117-126.
20. Marcal WS, Villegas-Navarro A, Nascimento MRL, Guerra AP, Fujihara CJ, et al. (2003) Bovinos e eqüinos como bioindicadores da poluiçao ambiental. Rev Brasil Ciencia Vet 10: 16-20.
21. Gilman A (1991) Heavy metals and their antagonists. In: The pharmacological bases of Clocks. Eds. Guanabara Koogan, Rio de Janeiro, pp: 1061-1065.
22. Rudy M (2009) Correlation of lead, cadmium and mercury levels in tissue and liver samples with age of cattle. Food Addit Contam Part A Chem Anal Control Expo Risk Assess 26: 847-853.
23. Asano R, Suzuki K, Otsuka T, Otsuka M, Sakurai H (2002) Concentrations of toxic metals and essential minerals in the mane hair of healthy racing horses and their relation to age. J Vet Med Sci 64: 607-610.
24. De Souza MV, Ferreira Fontes MP, Alves Fernandes RB (2014) Heavy metals in equine biological components. R Bras Zootec 43: 60-66.
25. EFSA CONTAM Panel (EFSA Panel on Contaminants in the Food Chain) (2015) Scientific Opinion on the risks to animal and public health and the environment related to the presence of nickel in feed. Eur Food Safety Authority J 13: 4074-4076.

26. Aureliano M, Crans DC (2009) Decavanadate and oxovanadates: Oxometalates with many biological activities. J Inorg Biochem 103: 536-546.

27. WHO (World Health Organisation) (1988) Vanadium. Environmental Health Criteria 81. World Health Organization Geneva.

28. Hudson TGF (1964) Vanadium: Toxicology and biological significance. In: Browning E (ed.), Elsevier Monographs on Toxic Agents, Amsterdam, Elsevier Publishing Company, pp: 67-78.

29. Kucera J, Lener J, Mnukova J, Bayerova E (1998) Vanadium exposure tests in humans: Hair, nails, blood, and urine. In: Nriagu JO (ed.), Vanadium in the environment. Part 2: Health effects, New York, John Wiley & Sons, pp: 55-73.

30. Darbre PD (2006) Metalloestrogens: an emerging class of inorganic xenoestrogens with potential to add to the oestrogenic burden of the human breast. J Appl Toxicol 26: 191-197.

Study on Prevalence of Ruminant Fasciolosis and its Associated Risk Factors in Kombolcha, North East Ethiopia

Shimels Tikuye*

EIAR, National Agricultural Biotechnology Research Center, Holleta, Ethiopia

Abstract

A cross sectional study was conducted to determine prevalence and risk factors associated with ruminant fasciolosis in Kombolcha, Amhara regional state from October 2010 to March 2011. For the purpose of the study fecal samples were taken from a total of 420 ruminants (168 cattle, 149 sheep and 103 goats) and subjected to coprological examination, specifically sedimentation technique. Based on the coproscopic examination the prevalence of fasciolosis was found to be 9.52% (n=16) in cattle, 37.58% (n=56) in sheep and 6.8% (n=7) in goats. Among the ruminants the prevalence of fasciolosis showed statistically significant variations (χ^2=53.6095, P=0.000), being very high in sheep and low in goats and poor body condition 45 (60%). This study revealed the presence of statistical significant differences (χ^2=103.08, P=0.000) between the three body conditions, the prevalence recorded in poor condition animals was very high. On the contrary there was no significance difference (P>0.05) in sex and age groups. In conclusion fasciolosis was found to be important ruminant disease in the study area, thus to control the disease and reduce the economic loss in this area, appropriate control strategies should be given.

Keywords: Coprology; Fasciolosis; Kombolcha; Prevalence; Ruminant; Sedimentation

Abbreviations: %: Percent; °C: Degree Celsius, *F. gigantica*: *Fasciola gigantica*; *F. hepatica*: *Fasciola hepatica*; *L. natalansis*: *Lymnaea natalansis*; *L. truncatula*: *Lymnaea truncatula*; masl: meters above sea level; mm: millimetre; SPSS: Statistical Package for Social Science; USD: United States Dollar; EIAR: Ethiopian Institute Agriculture Research; Km: Killo meter; χ^2: Pearson chi square.

Introduction

Fasciolosis is among the important parasitic worm infection which limits productivity of animals due to mortality, reduced growth rate, reduction in weight gain and unthriffines, reduction in working power, condemnation of large number of infected liver, increased susceptibility to secondary infection and expense due to control measure. The parasite is caused by the common liver fluke *Fasciola hepatica* and *F. gigantica*. The disease is a plant-borne trematode zoonosis [1] and is categorized under a neglected tropical disease [2].

The genus Lymnea in general, species of *L. truncatula* and *L. natalensis* are the most common intermediate hosts for *F. hepatica* and *F. gigantic* respectively. These species of snail was reported to have a worldwide distribution [3]. *F. gigantica* is found in most continents, primarily in tropical regions [4].

The parasite is the most prevalent helminthes infection of ruminants found in most parts of the world including Ethiopia. *F. hepatica* is found in areas with altitude of 1200 to 2560 masl while, *F. gigantica* is found at altitudes bellow 1800 masl but both species co-exist in areas where altitude ranging between 1200 to 1800 masl [5].

According to Yilma J, Malones JB the economic losses of fasciolosis are mostly caused by mortality, morbidity, reduced growth rate, condemnation of liver, increased susceptibility to secondary infection and the expense of control measures [5]. According to Fufa and Rokni the average loss of *Fasciola* was 6300 USD and 4000 USD per annum in Jimma and wolayta soddo municipal abattoir respectively [6,7].

Coprological examination from faces by using standard sedimentation technique is used for the diagnosis of fasciolosis for detection of *Fasciola* eggs [8]. In the study area, ruminants are important asset to farmers but the data regarding to Ruminant fascioliosis are not well documented. Therefore, the objectives of this study were to determine the prevalence and to asses with the risk factors of ruminant fasciolosis in Kombolcha.

Materials and Methods

Study area

Kombolcha is a town in North- Eastern Ethiopia located in the south Wollo zone of the Amhara regional state, located 375 km North East of Addis Ababa, between 11° 084' 49" latitude and 0.39° 737' 46" longitude of with an elevation between 1500-1840 meter above sea level. Kombolcha experiences bimodal rainfall which is the short rainy season occurs usually from March to May and the long rainy season extends from June to September. The minimum and maximum mean annual rainfall ranges from 750 to 900 mm, the annual temperature ranges from 11.8°C to 26°C and the relative humidity varies from 23.9% to 79%.

Study animals

A total of 420 indigenous breeds of ruminants (cattle, sheep and goat) managed extensively were randomly selected and subjected to qualitative coproscopic examination by standard sedimentation technique to determine the prevalence rate of *Fasciola* in the study area. The selected animals were from different species, age, sex and body condition groups.

***Corresponding author:** Shimels Tikuye, EIAR, National Agricultural Biotechnology Research Center, Holleta, PO Box: 249, Ethiopia
E-mail: shimelstk@gmail.com

Study methodology

Coproscopy was used to determine positivity of the animals for fasciola. Fecal samples for parasitological examination were collected directly from the rectum of each species, using disposable plastic gloves and placed in clean screw capped universal bottle and each sample was clearly labeled with animal identification, species, sex, age and body condition score. Fecal samples were preserved with 10% formalin solution to avoid the eggs developing and hatching. In the laboratory, coproscopic examinations were performed to detect the presence of *Fasciola* eggs using the standard sedimentation techniques. A drop of methylene blue solution was added to the sediment to differentiate it from eggs of paramphistomum. Eggs of *Fasciola* species show yellowish color while eggs of paramphistomum species stain by methylene blue [9].

Sample size

For estimation of *Fasciola* prevalence, the sample size was determined by assuming the expected prevalence to be 50%, the statistical Confidence Interval level was 95% while the desired precision was 5% and a sample size of 384 ruminants (cattle, sheep and goat) was determined based on the formula given by Thrusfield [10]. However, a total of 420 ruminants were taken to increase the precision of the study.

$$n = \frac{Z^2 P_{exp}\left(1 - P_{exp}\right)}{d^2}$$

where, n=sample size,

P_{exp}=expected prevalence,

d^2=desired precision,

Z=constant from normal distribution table at a given confidence level.

Data analysis

All raw data generated from the study were coded and entered in MS Excel database system. Using SPSS version 16 computer program, data were analyzed by using Chi-square (χ^2) test to determine the variation in infection, prevalence between species, sex, age and body condition score. Statistical significance was set at P<0.05 to determine whether there are significant differences between the parameters measured between the groups.

Results

Coproscopic examination was conducted from October 2010 to March 2011 showed that from a total of 420 indigenous ruminants managed extensively examined for the presence of *Fasciola* by using sedimentation technique, 79 ruminants revealed *Fasciola* egg in their faces with an over all prevalence of 18.81%.

The prevalence rate was higher in ovine (37.58%) and lower in bovine (9.52%) and caprine (6.80%) species respectively. Infection rate was statistically significant (P<0.05) (Table 1).

Prevalence of fasciolosis in male and female animals was 22.91% and 15.77% respectively. However, no significant difference (P>0.05) was observed between sexes (Table 1).

The highest prevalence was recorded in ruminants aged 1<x<3 years (20.41%) and >3 years (20.00%). Meanwhile, low prevalence was observed in less than 1 year with value (15.45%). But this difference was not statistically significant (p>0.05) (Table 1). Where X- represent age in terms of years

The prevalence of ruminant fasciolosis in animals with a poor body condition (60%) was higher than animals with medium (12.5%) and good body condition (7.10%) respectively. Significant difference (P<0.05) in prevalence was observed among body condition of the study animals (Table 1).

Discussion

Fasciolosis in ruminants was found with prevalence rates of 9.52% (n=16) bovine, 37.58% (n=56) ovine and 6.79% (n=7) of caprine and with over all prevalence rate of 18.81% of ruminants from coproscopic result. It showed a statistically significant difference (p<0.05) between bovine, ovine and caprine. This difference may be due to species sensitivity to *Fasciola*, thus animals, like cattle's have a moderate to high degree of resistance to primary infection. But sheep and goats do not develop a protective immunity to re-infection while cattle's develop immunity to defend infections and develop protection against re-infection with *Fasciola* [11]. Caprines have lowered prevalence of fasciolosis when compared with bovine and ovine. This may be due to the fact that goats are browsers. These differences could be due to difference in management system, grazing habit and resistance to parasitic infection. Similar result support the present finding is reported by Henok [12] in and around Hirna town.

The prevalence rate of bovine fasciolosis was 9.52% (n=16) in the study area. This was lowered when compared with 41.41% in and around Woreta [13], 34.04% in Turkey but the present study was higher than 4.9% in Soddo [7,14]. This variation may be due to the agro-ecological and climatic differences between the localities, although differences in the management systems and sample size.

The prevalence of ovine fasciolosis was found to be 37.5% (n=56) in the study area. This finding was lower when compared with previous reports in different parts of the country by Molalegne [15] 49% in and around Dawa-Cheffe, [16] 56.3% in Upper Awash River Basin, but higher than that of Ahmed [17] 13.2% in Middle Awash River Basin. These variations may be due to differences in temperature, moisture, humidity and soil for multiplication of intermediate host.

The prevalence of caprine fasciolosis was found to be 6.8%. This result is lower when compared with Adediran [18] 9.1% in Ibadan, Nigeria. This may be due to difference in climatic conditions, geographical regions and sample size of the study.

The prevalence of *Fasciola* in male and female ruminants was recorded as 22.91% and 15.77% respectively. There was non-significant difference (P>0.05) between the two sexes indicating that sex have no effect on disease prevalence. This may be probably due to that grazing habit of both sex groups in similar pasture land. Similar findings that strengthen the present result are reported by Mulualem and Ashenafi [19,20]. But, Balock indicated that high prevalence rate in the male than female [21]. This may be due to the management system with more time exposure of male to the field while females are kept in door system during pregnancy and lactation period.

The prevalence of ruminant fasciolosis among >3 years (20%) and 1<x<3 years (20.41%) was higher than that of <1 year (15.45%), but this difference was not statistically significant. The higher infection rate in 1<x<3 years and >3 years animals could be due to long time exposure to disease entity and their grazing habit close to submerge areas [22].

Prevalence of ruminant fasciolosis was also carried out based on the basis of body condition. Poor body condition animals were significantly higher (P<0.05) than that of medium and good body condition animals

Risk factors	No. examined	No. positive	Prevalence (%)	χ^2	p-value	CI
Species						
Bovine	168	16	9.52	53.6095	0.000	95%
Ovine	149	56	37.58			
Caprine	103	7	6.80			
Total	420	79	18.81			
Sex						
Male	179	41	22.91	3.4262	0.064	
Female	241	38	15.77			
Total	420	79	18.81			
Age						
<1 year	123	19	15.45	1.2958	0.523	
1<x<3 years	147	30	20.41			
>3 years	150	30	20.00			
Total	420	79	18.81			
Body condition						
Poor	75	45	60	103.0842	0.000	
Medium	176	22	12.50			
Good	169	12	7.10			
Total	420	79	18.81			

Table 1: Prevalence of Ruminant fasciolosis and its association with various risk factors in Kombolcha.

respectively. This indicates that the importance of fasciolosis in causing loss of appetite and poor utilization of food, which results in a loss of body weight. This finding agrees with [17] in Middle Awash River Basine, [23] in Adigrat and [24] in Yilmana Densa district.

Conclusion

Fasciolosis is one of the major helminth infections for ruminant production in the study area. This prevalence found in the study area could be also due to the water lodgment from Borkena River which increased irrigated land masses and ponds at grazing areas of animals and the trend of livestock owners to graze their animals in these areas at the time of feed scarcity. The Observed differences in the prevalence of parasitic infections between species were probably due to differences in grazing habit and host susceptibility to infection. Therefore, Strategic anthelmentic treatment with appropriate fluckcidal drugs, a combination of control measures including drainage, fencing and mulluscicides and awareness creation should be implemented to control the helminthes infection.

Acknowledgements

I would like to express my heartly thanks to Dr. Mullugeta Tefera for his technical advice, over all guidance and valuable comments on my draft documents to appear in the present form. My special thanks go to my families with their advice, moral and financial support during the study period. Lastly but not least I would like to express my thanks to Kombolcha Regional Veterinary Diagnostic Laboratory for their logistic support.

References

1. Mas-Coma S, Bargues MD, Valero MA (2005) Fascioliasis and other plant-borne trematode zoonoses. Int J Parasitol 35: 1255-1278.
2. Farrar J, Hotez P, Junghanss T, Kang G, Lalloo D, et al. (2013) Manson's Tropical Diseases. J Elsevier Health Sciences.
3. Urquhart GM, Duncan J, Armour L, Dunn J, Jennings AM (1996) Veterinary parasitology second edition, Black well science, UK.
4. Dalton JP, Spithil TW (1998) Progress in development of liver fluke vaccine. Trends Parasitol 14: 224-228.
5. Yilma J, Malones JB (1998) A geographical information system forces model for strategic control of fasciolosis. In: Ethiopia Vet Parasitol 78: 103-127.
6. Taddele T, Worku T (2007) The prevalence and economic significance of bovine fasciolosis at Jimma abattoir, Ethiopia. Internet J Vet Med 3: 15.
7. Fufa A, Loma A, Bekele M, Alemayehu R (2009) Bovine fasciolosis: coprological, abattoir survey and its economic impact due to liver condemnation at Soddo municipal abattoir, Southern Ethiopia. Trop Anim Health Prod 42: 289-292.
8. Rokni MB, Massoud J, Kia EB (2003) Comparison of Adult Somatic and cysteine proteinase antigens of Fasciola gigantica in Enzyme linked Immunosorbent Assay for diagnosis of bovine Fasciolosis. In: DIE seminar on biotechnology, proceeding November 9-13, Tehran, Iran.
9. Hanson J, Brian P (1994) The epidemiology, diagnosis and control of helminthes parasites of ruminants. A hand book, Rome: Food and Agricultural Organization of the United Nations. Pp: 72.
10. Thrusfield MV (2005) Veterinary Epidemiology. 3rd ed., Blackwell Science, Oxford, pp: 234-238.
11. Soulsby EJL (1982) Helminthes, Arthropods and protozoa of domesticated Animals, seventh edition, Balliere. Tindall and London, UK; pp. 40-52.
12. Henok M, Mekonnen A (2011) Study on the Prevalence and Risk Factors of Fasciolosis in Small Ruminants in and around Hirna Town, Ethiopia. Global Veterinaria 7: 497-500.
13. Binyam T, Hanna A, Sisay G (2012) Study on coprological prevalence of Bovine fasciolosis in and around Woreta, Northwestern Ethiopia. J Vet Med Anim Health 4: 89-92.
14. Avcioglu H, Guven E, Balkaya I, Kaynar O, Hayirli A (2014) Evaluation of Coprological and Serological Techniques For Diagnosis of Bovine Fasciolosis. Israel J Vet Med 69: 203-210.
15. Molalegne B, Nuradis I, Nahili A (2010) Study on the prevalence of Ovine fasciolosis in and around Dawa-Cheffa, Kemissie. African J Agric Res 5: 2981-2985.
16. Michael A, Beyene P, Yilma J, Don P, Yoseph S, et al. (2004) Infection prevalence of ovine fasciolosis in small irrigation schemes along the Upper Awash River Basin. Ethiopia Vet J 9: 19-26.
17. Ahmed EF, Markvichitr K, Jumwasorn S, Koonawooththtin S, Achoothesa JS (2007) Prevalence of fasciola Species infections of sheep in the middle awash river basin, Ethiopia. Southeast Asian J Trop Med Publ health 38: 51-52.
18. Adediran OA, Adebiyi AI, Uwalaka EC (2014) Prevalence of Fasciola species in ruminants under extensive management system in Ibadan southwestern Nigeria. Afr J Med Med Sci 43: 137-141.
19. Mulualem E (1998) Epidemiology of bovine, Fasciolosis in woredas of south Gonder administrative zone bordering Lake Tana. Ethiopian Vet J 2: 1-13.
20. Ashenafi K, Birhan T, Alemu A, Biniam T (2016) Prevalence of fasciolosis in small ruminants and associated risk factor in and around Kombolcha. J Adv Parastol 3: 61-65.

21. Balock FC, Arthur RJ (1985) A Survey of fasciolosis in beef cattle killed at abattoir in Southern Queen land. Australian Vet J 62: 320-326.

22. Tasawar ZU, Minir CS, Hayat M, Lashari H (2007) The prevalence of Fasciola hepatica in goats around Multan. Pak Vet J 27: 5-7.

23. Eyerusalem G, Yeshitila A, Mihreteab B (2012) Prevalence of Ovine Fasciolosis in Adigrat, North East Ethiopia. Global Veterinaria 9: 92-96.

24. Basaznew B, Abeje M, Mersha C (2012) Pervasiveness of Fasciolosis in Sheep in YilmanaDensa District, West Gojjam Zone, Amhara Region, Northwestern Ethiopia. Acta Parasitological Globalist 3: 34-37.

The Effects of Iron Supplementation on the Growth Rate and Antioxidant Activity of *Trichomonas vaginalis*

SM Razavi[1], E Foroudi[1], E Rakhshandehroo[1], F Nejati[1] and S Nazifi[2*]

[1]*Department of Pathobiology, School of Veterinary Medicine, Shiraz University, Shiraz, Iran*
[2]*Department of Clinical Studies, School of Veterinary Medicine, Shiraz University, Shiraz, Iran*

Abstract

Trichomonas vaginalis is a common protozoan parasite found in females and males worldwide. The parasite causes mild to severe inflammations in the urogenital tract. This study was conducted to evaluate the effect of iron excess on the growth rate and the activity of antioxidant enzymes in *T. vaginalis*. The parasite was cultured in Diamond's Trypticase Yeast Maltose (TYM) media with and without iron supplementation and assessed at 2, 3, 5, 7, 9, 11, 13 and 15 days post inoculation (dpi). The results showed significant higher numbers of the parasite in medium with iron supplementation. Furthermore, our findings revealed higher activities of antioxidant enzymes (SOD, GPX and CAT) in parasites cultured with iron supplementation. In conclusion, the present experiment showed that iron increased not only the multiplication rate but also the antioxidant activities of *T. vaginalis*. It seems that iron could protect *T. vaginalis* from toxic oxygen metabolites during tissue invasion and helps the parasite to maintain its pathogenicity for the host.

Keywords: *Trichomonas vaginalis*; Iron; Growth; Antioxidant enzymes

Introduction

Trichomonas vaginalis, a flagellated protozoan parasite, causes a prevalent sexually transmitted disease worldwide. The parasite mainly affects the urogenital tract of both men and women. In women, symptoms are heavier which range from mild to severe inflammation with a frothy malodorous discharge and severe irritation [1]. The parasite can invade the squamous epithelium and associates with vaginitis, low birth weights and many perinatal complications [2].

T. vaginalis lacks the ability to synthesize many of the macromolecules *de novo*. Therefore, the uptake of nutrients is from the vaginal secretions or through the host and/or bacterial cells [3]. This implicates that *T. vaginalis* is required to include many of the essential macromolecules in culture media. Among those molecules, vitamins and minerals such as iron seem very important for the survival of the parasite [4].

Iron is required to maintain maximal levels of ferredoxin and pyruvate-ferredoxinoxido reductase activity [5]. Also, it appears that resistance to complement-mediated lysis is dependent upon a high concentration of iron [6]. Iron has been demonstrated to upregulate the expression of cysteine proteinases, which have been found to degrade the C3 portion of complement on the surface of the organism which allows the organism to evade complement-mediated damage [6]. In addition, the pathogenesis of *T. vaginalis* is differentially modulated by iron [7]. Considering the role of iron for the pathogenesis *Trichomonas* in the host, it can be assumed that this element could have a significant effect on the growth rate of the parasite.

Free radicals are very reactive chemical substances which can cause oxidative damages to the living organisms. Under normal physiological conditions, there is a critical balance in the generation of free radicals and antioxidant defense systems against free radical injury [8,9]. The imbalance between free radical production and antioxidant defense creates a condition known as oxidative stress. Clinical observations and experimental evidence suggest that oxidative stress plays a dominant role in the host's defense against parasitic infections [10].

The function of antioxidant enzymes has to some extent been studied in ruminant hosts infected with the blood protozoan parasites [11-13]. The presence of superoxide dismutase (SOD) and NADH oxidases was reported in *T. vaginalis* [14,15]. However, the mechanisms of cellular protection against adverse effects of oxygen metabolites have not been investigated well in trichomonads. Therefore, this study was conducted in order to investigate the status of the iron supplementation on the growth rate and the activity of major antioxidant enzymes (glutathione peroxidase (GPX), superoxide dismutase (SOD) and catalase (CAT) in *T. vaginalis*.

Materials and Methods

T. vaginalis cultivation

A *T. vaginalis* isolate, kindly obtained from Shiraz University of Medical Sciences, Shiraz, Iran was routinely cultured in Diamond's TYM medium [16], composed of 150 mg of Tryptone, 12 g of yeast extract, 5.5 g of glucose, 2.5 g of sodium chloride, 0.5 g of L-cysteine, 0.5 g of sodium thioglycolate, 80 mg of Gentamicin, 2 mg of Amphotericin B, Penicillin G (1 × 10^6 SI), 120 ml of horse serum and 0.75 g of agar. The medium was constituted per 1000 ml of distilled water and its pH was set at 6.2.

The parasites were recultured in TYM media with and without iron supplementation and kept at 37°C. Each group consisted of 48 microtubes containing 1.2 ml culture media and 10 µl media containing about 3000 *T. vaginalis* organism. In Iron-supplemented group, ferrous sulfate was also added to adjust a final Fe concentration on 400 µM [7]. Six microtubes from each group were removed and followed at 2, 3, 5,

***Corresponding author:** Dr. Saeed Nazifi, Professor of Veterinary Clinical Pathology, Department of Clinical Studies, School of Veterinary Medicine, Shiraz University, Shiraz, P.O. Box: 1731- 71345, Iran
E-mail: nazifi@shirazu.ac.ir

7, 9, 11, 13 and 15 days post inoculation (dpi). The cultured specimens were centrifuged at 3000 g for 3 min; the pellet was resuspended in 1 μL of sterile distilled water, shaken thoroughly and examined by a Neubauer cell chamber to calculate the parasite numbers per ml. Finally, the contents of each micro tube were kept at -20°C until the biochemical assays were performed.

Biochemical assays

Glutathione peroxidase (GPx) activity: The activity of GPx was evaluated with GPx detection kit (Ransel kit produced by Randox Co., UK) according to the manufacturer's instructions. GPx catalyze the oxidation of glutathione (GSH) by cumene hydroperoxide. In the presence of glutathione reductase (GR) and NADPH, the oxidized glutathione (GSSG) is immediately converted to the reduced form with a concomitant oxidation of NADPH to NADP+. The decrease in absorbance at 340 nm against blank was measured spectrophotometrically. One unit (U) of GPx activity was defined as the amount of enzyme that converts 1 μmol of NADPH to NADP+ per minute. The GPx activity was expressed as unit per mg of protein (U/mg protein).

Superoxide dismutase (SOD) activity: SOD detection kit (Ransod®, Randox Co., UK) was used to evaluate total SOD activity. This method employs xanthine and xanthine oxidase (XOD) to generate superoxide radicals which react with 2-(4-iodophenyl)-3-(4-nitrophenol)-5-phenyltetrazolium chloride (INT) to form a red formazan dye. The SOD activity is then measured by the degree of inhibition of this reaction. One unit of SOD is that which causes 50% inhibition of the rate of reduction of INT under the conditions of the assay. SOD levels were recorded at 505 nm and through a standard curve, and expressed as unit per mg of protein (U/mg protein).

Catalase (CAT) activity: Tissue catalase activity was assayed spectrophotometrically by monitoring the decomposition of H_2O using the procedure of Aebi [17]. Briefly, 0.5 ml of 30 mmol/l H_2O solution in 50 mmol/l phosphate buffer (pH=7.0) and 1 ml of 1:10 diluted tissue supernatant was added and the consumption of H_2O was followed spectrophotometrically at 240 nm for 2 min at 25°C. The molar extinction coefficient was 43.6 l/mol per cm for H_2O. Catalase activity was expressed as the unit that is defined as μmol H_2O consumed/min per mg of protein. In order to achieve the average activity of each enzyme in the whole parasite population, the values measured for each case were divided into the parasite number.

Statistical analysis

Student's *t* test was used to compare the effects of iron supplementation on the evaluated parameters. All data were analyzed using the Statistical Package for Social Sciences (SPSS, 16.0) and the significance was set at P<0.05.

Results

The pattern of alterations in the parasite number of both culture media is presented in Figure 1. Our data showed that although the parasites number was increased in both media from the start of the study toward the end, it was overall higher in iron-rich medium. Significant elevations of parasite number were seen at 2, 5, 7 and 15 days post inoculation (dpi) in iron-rich medium compared to usual Diamond's TYM medium. The alterations in the activity of antioxidant enzymes in different days are presented in Figure 2. The results revealed that the activity of GPx was significantly higher in parasites cultured in iron-rich medium. These differences were recorded at 2, 3, 5, 7, 11, 13

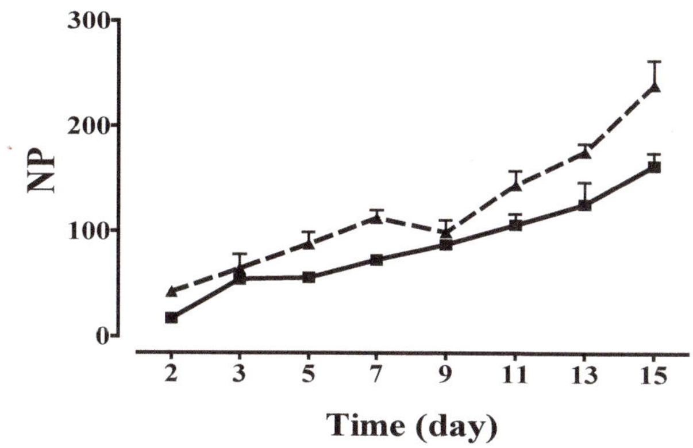

Figure 1: Number of *T. vaginalis* cultured in Diamond's Trypticase Yeast Maltose (TYM) media with (▲) and without iron supplementation (■) during 15 days post inoculation. NP: Number of Parasites ((organism/ml) × 10000).

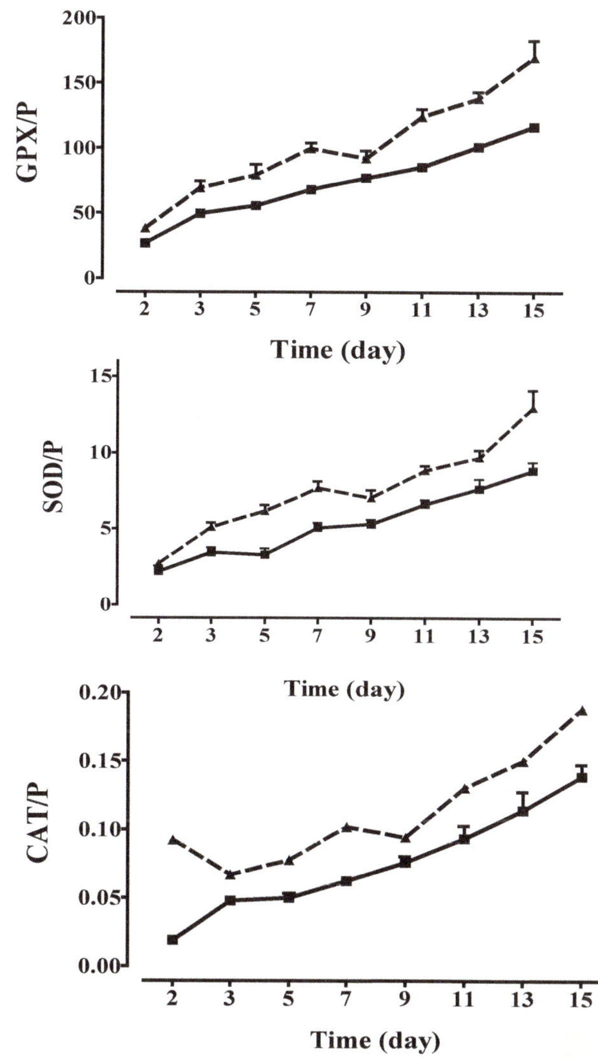

Figure 2: The activity of antioxidant enzymes (as unit/mg) in *T. vaginalis* cultured in Diamond's Trypticase Yeast Maltose (TYM) media with (▲) and without iron supplementation (■) during 15 days post inoculation. Note that the average activity of each enzyme in the whole parasite population was divided into the parasite number.

and 15 dpi; however, no significant difference was observed at 9 dpi.

A remarkable increase in GPx activity was evident in *T. vaginalis* cultured in iron-rich condition at 2, 3, 5, 7, 11, 13 and 15 dpi, but no significant difference was recorded at 9 dpi. Remarkable elevations were also observed in SOD activity in *T. vaginalis* grown in iron-rich medium at all samplings except for 2 dpi. The pattern of changes in the activity of Catalase (CAT) was different from that of GPx. According to our data, a significant increase in CAT activity was evident at 5, 7, 11, 13 and 15 dpi but not at 2, 3 and 9 dpi.

Discussion

In the present study, the growth rate of *T. vaginalis* grown in the presence of iron was significantly higher compared to those cultured in medium with no iron supplementation. These observations reinforce the idea that increasing the level of iron favors the multiplication of the parasite, thus exacerbating the symptoms of the disease. Similarly, previous reports confirmed that *T. vaginalis* essentially requires iron for its growth in the human vagina, where the iron concentration is changing. This element could increase the parasite multiplication in different culture media [5,18]. It seems that iron is an important nutrient for the growth of different protozoan genera such as *Entamoeba*, *Leishmania*, *Plasmodium* and Trichomonads. *Leishmania* and *Plasmodium* can use haemoglobin as a source of iron by catabolism of the haem group [19]. *Leishmania chagasi* also expresses a NADPH-dependent iron reductase capable of converting oxidized Fe^{3+} into the more soluble Fe^{2+} form [20]. In addition, the ability of *Tritrichomonas foetus* for the uptake of iron from the host environment may be a critical factor for its pathogenicity and virulence [21]. The parasite grows in the bovine vagina where lactoferrin is available and also invades the bovine uterus, where abundant transferrin exists [22].

Corroborating our data, Lehker and Alderete [18] assessed the responses of *T. vaginalis* to iron depletion or iron excess to evaluate the regulatory role of this element on certain properties of the parasite. They stated that, in comparison with organisms grown in excess iron, iron restriction resulted in greater than or equal to 80% lower rates of protein synthesis, greater than or equal to 3-fold decreases in cell densities and 2.5-fold longer generation time.

The role of iron in *T. vaginalis* has been shown to be associated with the virulence of the parasite in mice [7]. In addition to the increased virulence, iron also enhances the level of adherence and the cytotoxicity of Trichomonads [7].

High metabolic rate of the rapidly growing and multiplying parasites will produce large amounts of toxic by-products in the cells. Excessive *in vivo* generation of these products can adversely affect the cell functioning. The accumulation of high concentrations of free radical, mainly the reactive oxygen species (ROS), could damage the cell phospholipid membranes and vital macromolecules [23]. This condition is considered as oxidative stress which is indicated by impairment of antioxidant systems [24]. The balance between free radicals and antioxidants may be disrupted in many diseases. Previous studies show that protozoan parasite infections such as *Plasmodium* sp. [25], *Trypanosoma* sp. [26], *Trichomonas foetus* [27] and some nematodes [28,29] can induce oxidative stress in the host. However, defense mechanisms operating against reactive metabolites of molecular oxygen in *T. vaginalis* have not been studied in detail.

The results obtained here corroborate that iron has significant effect on the antioxidant activity of *T. vaginalis in vitro*. We revealed that the activities of GPx, SOD and CAT were significantly higher in iron-supplemented media. Higher numbers of parasites along with the increased amounts of antioxidant activities in the parasites grown in the presence of iron clearly indicate that this element enhances the strength of *T. vaginalis* to resist the vaginal defense mechanisms. Corroborating our data, Razavi et al. [30] studied the status of the activity of antioxidant enzymes in *Trichomonas gallinae* cultured in aerobic and anaerobic media. They revealed higher activities of GPx, SOD and CAT activities in *Trichomonas* cultured in both environments. These conditions stimulate the production of those protective enzymes at early and late stages of cultivation, depending upon the presence of oxygen in culture media. In contrast to these results, Ellis et al. [31] stated that *T. vaginalis* trophozoites lack the major peroxide-reducing enzymes, catalase and glutathione peroxidase. However, the presence of glutathione reductase and SOD activity suggested that some detoxification mechanisms may operate in *T. vaginalis*. This controversy is likely due to the sensitivity of *T. vaginalis* to oxygen above physiological levels which led to the lack of adequate peroxide reducing enzymes.

Antioxidant defense mechanisms have been indicated in other protozoans. Incubation of *E. histolytica* isolates under different culture conditions with an oxygen radical generating system induces an increase in SOD activity [32]. Therefore, it was suggested that regulation of SOD may support the parasite from invasion by oxygen metabolites. Although the specific activity of FeSOD in *E. histolytica* is reduced in the presence of a ferrous iron chelator (1, 10-phenanthroline), the total activity was found to be increased substantially. It was hypothesised that at low Fe^{2+}-levels in *E. histolytica*, the iron molecule in FeSOD may be replaced by an alternative divalent cation, like Mn^{2+}. Also, it can be argued that the affinity of iron to the enzyme is much higher than to the repressor molecules.

In conclusion, it can be noted that iron-supplemented media stimulate not only the higher growth rates but also the higher activity of antioxidant enzymes (SOD, GPX and CAT) in different days post inoculation for *T. vaginalis*. These observations could suggest that positive regulations of antioxidant enzymes in the presence of iron may contribute to protect *T. vaginalis* from oxygen free radicals during tissue invasions.

Acknowledgement

The authors would like to thank the Research Council of Shiraz University and School of Veterinary Medicine, Shiraz University for financial and technical support of this study (Grant No.71-GR-VT-5).

Conflict of Interest

The authors declare no conflicts of interest.

References

1. Wölner-Hanssen P, Krieger JN, Stevens CE, Kiviat NB, Koutsky L, et al. (1989) Clinical manifestations of vaginal trichomoniasis. JAMA 261: 571-576.
2. Petrin D, Delgaty K, Bhatt R, Garber G (1998) Clinical and Microbiological Aspects of *Trichomonas vaginalis*. Clin Microbiol Rev 11: 300-317.
3. Heine P, McGregor JA (1993) *Trichomonas vaginalis*: a reemerging pathogen. Clin Obstet Gynecol 36: 137-144.
4. Diamond LS (1986) *In vitro* cultivation of the Trichomonadidae: a state of the art review. Acta Univ Carol Biol 30: 221-228.
5. Gorrell TE (1985) Effect of culture medium iron content on the biochemical composition and metabolism of *Trichomonas vaginalis*. J Bacteriol 161: 1228-1230.
6. Alderete JF, Provenzano D, Lehker W (1995) Iron mediates *Trichomonas vaginalis* resistance to complement lysis. Microb Pathog 19: 93-103.
7. Ryu JS, Choi HK, Min DY, Ha SE, Ahn MH (2001) Effect of iron on the virulence of *Trichomonas vaginalis*. J Parasitol 87: 457-460.

8. Poli G (1993) Liver damage due to free radicals. Br Med Bull 49: 604-620.

9. Ramakrishna V, Jailkhani R (2007) Evaluation of oxidative stress in insulin dependent diabetes mellitus (IDDM) patients. Diagn Pathol 2: 22.

10. Schirmer RH, Schöllhammer T, Eisenbrand G, Krauth-Siegel RL (1987) Oxidative stress as a defense mechanism against parasitic infections. Free Radic Res Commun 3: 3-12.

11. Nazifi S, Razavi SM, Kianiamin P, Rakhshandehroo E (2011) Evaluation of erythrocyte antioxidant mechanisms: antioxidant enzymes, lipid peroxidation and serum trace elements associated with progressive anemia in ovine malignant theileriosis. Parasitol Res 109: 275-281.

12. Razavi SM, Nazifi S, Bateni M, Rakhshandehroo E (2011) Alterations of erythrocyte antioxidant mechanisms: Antioxidant enzymes, lipid peroxidation and serum trace elements associated with anemia in bovine tropical theileriosis. Vet Parasitol 180: 209-214.

13. Esmaeilnejad B, Tavassoli M, Asri-Rezaei S, Dalir-Naghadeh B, Malekinejad H, et al. (2014) Evaluation of antioxidant status, oxidative stress and serum trace mineral levels associated with *Babesia ovis* parasitemia in sheep. Vet Parasitol 205: 38-45.

14. Linstead DJ, Bradley S (1988) The purification and properties of two soluble reduced nicotinamide: acceptor oxidoreductases from *Trichomonas vaginalis*. Mol Biochem Parasitol 27: 125-134.

15. Ellis JE, Cole D, Lloyd D (1992) Influence of oxygen on the fermentative metabolism of metronidazole-sensitive and resistant strains of *Trichomonas vaginalis*. Mol Biochem Parasitol 56: 79-88.

16. Diamond LS (1957) The establishment of various trichomonads of animals and man in axenic cultures. J Parasitol 43: 488-490.

17. Aebi H (1984) Catalase *in vitro*. Methods Enzymol 105: 121-126.

18. Lehker MW, Alderete JF (1992) Iron regulates growth of *Trichomonas vaginalis* and the expression of immunogenic trichomonad proteins. Mol Microbiol 6: 123-132.

19. Wilson ME, Britigan BE (1998) Iron acquisition by parasitic protozoa. Parasitol Today 14: 348-353.

20. Wilson ME, Lewis TS, Miller MA, McCormick ML, Britigan BE (2002) *Leishmania chagasi*: uptake of iron bound to lactoferrin or transferrin requires an iron reductase. Exp Parasitol 100: 196-207.

21. Kulda J, Poislova M, Suchan P, Tachezy J (1998) Enhancing effect of iron on experimental infection of mice by *Tritrichomonas foetus*. Parasitol Res 85: 692-699.

22. Tachezy J, Kulda J, Bahníková I, Suchan P, Rázga J, et al. (1996) *Tritrichomonas foetus*: iron acquisition from lactoferrin and transferrin. Exp Parasitol 83: 216-228.

23. Wiseman H, Halliwell B (1996) Damage to DNA by reactive oxygen and nitrogen species: role in inflammatory disease and progression to cancer. Biochem J 313: 17-29.

24. Hirotomo K, Horie T, Ishikawa S, Tsuda C, Kawakami S (2010) Oxidative stress in skeletal muscle causes severe disturbance of exercise activity without muscle atrophy. Free Radical Biol Med 48: 1252-1262.

25. Becker K, Tilley L, Vennerstrom JL, Roberts D, Rogerson S, et al. (2004) Oxidative stress in malaria parasite-infected erythrocytes: host-parasite interactions. Inter J Parasitol 34: 163-189.

26. Docampo R, Moreno SN (1984) Free radical metabolites in the mode of action of chemotherapeutic agents and phagocytic cells on *Trypanosoma cruzi*. Rev Infect Dis 6: 223-238.

27. Kitchener KR, Meshnick R, Fairfield A, Wang CC (1984) An iron-containing superoxide dismutase in *Tritrichomonas foetus*. Mol Biochem Parasitol 12: 95-99.

28. Jong EC, Mahmoud AA, Klebanoff SJ (1981) Peroxidase-mediated toxicity to schistosomula of *Schistosoma mansoni*. J Immunol 126: 468-471.

29. Kazura JW, Fanning MM, Blumer JL, Mahmoud AA (1981) Role of cell generated hydrogen peroxide in granulocyte-mediated killing of schistosomula of *Schistosoma mansoni in vitro*. J Clin Invest 67: 93-102.

30. Razavi SM, Changiz S, Rakhshandehroo E, Nejati F, Nazifi S (2016) An investigation on the pattern of antioxidant enzymes activities in *Trichomonas gallinae* cultured in aerobic and anaerobic conditions. Sci Parasitol 17: 36-42.

31. Ellis JE, Yarlett N, Cole D, Humphreys MJ, Lloyd D (1994) Antioxidant defences in the microaerophilic protozoan *Trichomonas vaginalis*: comparison of metronidazole-resistant and sensitive strains. Microbiol 140: 2489-2494.

32. Bruchhaus I,Tannich E (1994) Induction of the iron-containing superoxide dismutase in *Entamoeba histolytica* by a superoxide anion-generating system or by iron chelation. Mol Biochem Parasitol 67: 281-288.

Camel Calf Husbandry Practices and Health Problems in Fafem Zone, Ethiopian Somali Region

Abdi Hassan Rirash, Befekadu Urga Wakayo* and Hassan Abdi

College of Veterinary Medicine, Jigjiga University, Jigjiga, Somali Regional State, Ethiopia

Abstract

Background: Calf mortality represents a major production and livelihood constraint in the Somali region of Ethiopia. Disease was incriminated as a major underlying cause. However, epidemiology of major calf diseases in the region is not well documented.

Methods: Cross-sectional study was conducted between October 2014 and March 2015 to explore major camel calf (≤ 1 year) diseases and associated drivers in Gursum and Kebribeya districts of Somali region. Participatory survey of calf husbandry and diseases was conducted on 51 camel holdings. Clinical and laboratory examination of health problems was performed on 189 camel calves.

Results: Camel holding size showed inter-herd and geographical variability. Calves accounted to 13.5% of average camel herds. Peak camel calving period was between October and March. Calving usually (86.3%) occurred from late-afternoon to night hours. Majority (90.2%) of producers restricted early colustrum intake and 78.4% restricted milk suckling after 1 month. Further suckling restriction, introduction of green forages and herd mixing were practiced after 3 months of age. According to producers young (<6 months) calves were commonly affected by diarrhea (100%), orf (92.2%), respiratory illness (33.3%), plant poisoning (25.5%) and camel pox (7.9%). Major problems reported in older (6-12 months) calves include; mange (94.1%) and tick (86.3%) infestations, ring worm (62.7%); camel pox (56.9%); trypanosomosis (51%) and respiratory illness (9.8%). Calf health investigation detected Sarcoptes scabie var cameli (16.4%) and mixed tick (*H. dromedary, H. truncatum* & *R. pulchelis*) (12.7%) infestation, diarrhea (3.7%) and respiratory illness (1.1%). Mange infestation and plant poisoning were higher in Gursum district whereas tick infestation was higher in small herds.

Conclusion: Camel calves were exposed to different debilitating and/or life threatening diseases. Potential risk factors include; inadequate colustrum feeding, under-nutrition, and premature exposure to endemic pathogens, vectors and harmful plants. Further epidemiological and intervention studies are recommended.

Keywords: Calves; Camel; Colustrum; Diseases; Ethiopia; Husbandry; Poisoning

Introduction

The one humped camel (*Camelus dromedarius)* is multi-functional farm animal species uniquely adapted to arid and semi-arid zones. Ethiopia is home to an estimated 2.4 million camels found mainly in the arid to semi-arid regions [1]. For pastoralist and agro-pastoralist communities residing in these harsh environments, the camel represents a vital source of food, income and other services [2,3]. Developing camel production could offer a suitable alternative for meeting chronic and often escalating challenges of food insecurity in eastern Africa [4]. However, performance and hence livelihood and economic contribution of regional camel populations is very low owing to complex constraints such as; poor husbandry systems, widespread feed shortage and diseases, inadequate health and extension services, etc. [5].

Under east African pastoral/agro-pastoral production systems, heavy pre-weaning calf mortality represents a major impediment to camel herd growth and production potential. This is further compounded by low reproduction rates attributed to delayed maturation, long gestation period and long inter-calving intervals [6-8]. High camel calf mortality rate of up to 53.1%, before 1 year, has been reported in eastern Ethiopia [9]. Widespread diseases, malnutrition due to household competition for milk and predators accounted for the major share of these losses [5,6,10] Studies in east Africa indicate that camel calves are susceptible to a wide range of diseases including; diarrhea, pox, contagious ecthyma, contagious skin necrosis, pneumonia, tick and mite infestations and internal parasites [11-13]. Withholding colostrum from neonates due to belief of many pastoralists that it causes fatal scouring was an important risk factor to heavy disease losses [4,14].

Epidemiological information on magnitude, causes and important risk factors of major camel calf diseases in the Somali region of Ethiopia is, at best, patchy. Therefore, the study attempted to describe major camel calf health problems and associated husbandry constraints in selected districts of the Ethiopian Somali region.

Methodology

Study area

The study was conducted in Gursum and Kabribayah Districts of Fafen zone in the Ethiopian Somali Region. The altitude of Fafem zone

***Corresponding author:** Befekadu Urga Wakayo, College of Veterinary Medicine, Jigjiga University, Jigjiga, Somali Regional State, Ethiopia
E-mail: fikeurga@gmail.com

ranges between 1,500-1,800 m.a.s.l and the topography ranges from of flat to gentle slope, hilly and mountainous. The average annual rainfall ranged from 300 mm to 500 mm and average monthly temperature ranges 16 to 20°C. Fafem zone is divided into three separate Food Economy Zones (FEZs), namely, sedentary agriculturalists (9.1%)., agro pastoralists (56.8%) and pastoralists (34.1%) [15]. It has eight administrative districts, namely Jigjiga, Kebribeyah, Harshin, Babile, Awbare, Gursum, Tullu Guled and Gololchen. Of these, Gursum and Kebribeya districts were selected for the study by considering accessibility of camel herds and representation of different production systems in the zone.

Study design

Participatory survey of camel producers and clinical examination of corresponding camel calf (<12 months) stocks was conducted Gursum and Kebribeya districts from October 2014 to March, 2015. The study aimed to identify major health problems affecting camel calves and to describe corresponding animal, husbandry, and environment related risk factors in the study area.

Sampling

A total of 8 kebele's were selected by random lottery method from a sampling frame of all Kebele's in the two study districts. Subsequently, camel producers and corresponding calf stocks were sampled systematically by including every 5th consenting household during field visit to selected kebele's. Taking logistic constraints in to account, a total of 51 camel rearing households and 189 calves aged ≤ 12 months were included in the study.

Data collection

Participatory interview survey was conducted on selected camel producers. Information pertaining to camel holding pattern, age related calf husbandry practices (early colustum feeding, milk suckling, feeding forages, and housing/herding), and priority calf health problems was recorded using a semi-structured format prepared for the specific purpose. Local disease names were cross-checked against reported symptoms to confirm disease identity.

Calves (aged ≤ 12 months) in selected camel holdings were examined e for clinical health status based on history and physical examination. Local disease names and corresponding clinical symptoms were triangulated to establish identity of calf health problems as outlined below.

- **Diarrhea/Scour:** Watery off smelling feces and soiled perineum in recently born calves. Leads to drastic weight loss, sunken eye and often death.
- **Contagious ecthyma/Orf:** Small swelling and hard scabs around mouth sometimes depressed and avoid feeding.
- **Respiratory illness:** Cough and nasal discharge, progressive loss of condition.
- **Plant poisoning:** Sudden death following grazing in rangelands.
- **Camel mange:** Itching, reddening of skin, hair loss and crusts on neck shoulder abdomen and inside of legs. Affected animals are sometimes reluctant to feed properly and gradually lose body condition.
- **Tick infestation:** Visible parasites usually inside of thighs and tail base, progressive lose body condition in severe cases.
- **Ring worm/Dermatophytes:** Circular hair loss around head neck and back without any sign of itching.
- **Camel pox:** General illness, small soft swellings mainly around eyes and head, nasal and/or ocular discharge enlarged lymph nodes.
- **Camel trypanosomosis:** Progressive weight loss even during or shortly after rainy season and edema of lower body.

Visible Ticks were manually collected from their attachment sites and placed in a universal bottle pre-filled with 70% alcohol. Skin scraping was collected from suspected cases of mange/mite infestation (exhibiting scales, crusts, alopecia and/or itching) in universal bottles pre-filled with 10% formalin according to [16]. All sample containers were properly labeled (household and animal id #, date, specimen type) and transported in an ice box to laboratories at College of Veterinary Medicine - Jigjiga University for analysis.

Tick species were identification based on standard procedure and morphological criteria as described by [17]. Skin scrapings were liquefied by adding KOH on petridish and examined under low power microscopy to identify species using a morphological key [18].

Statistical analysis

Participatory survey, clinical investigation and laboratory analysis data were entered on Microsoft Excel spreadsheets and analyzed using SPSS - 20 (SPSS inc). Numerical and categorical data were summarized using descriptive statistics (Mean ± SE and percentage (%)), frequency tables and graphs. Chi square test and comparison of means (independent-t and ANOVA tests) were used to draw inferential contrasts on camel holding patterns, calf rearing practices and health problems. Camel/calf holding sizes and calf age estimates were not normally distributed. Therefore, contrasts were made using natural logarithm (Ln) and reported in back transformed values. Statistical significance was determined at $p<0.050$.

Results

Camel holding pattern

Total herd size varied from 7 to 90 heads of camel with an average of 24.44 ± 1.08 camels/herd. Meanwhile, the size of calf stocks in herds varied from 1 to 11 and averaged 3.27 ± 1.07 calves/herd. Average total herd camel ($p=0.016$) and calf holdings ($p=0.002$) sizes were higher in Gursum (31.6 ± 3.14 camels and 4.23 ± 0.34 calves per herd) compared to Kebribeya (22.45 ± 2.7 camels and 2.85 ± 0.32 calves per herd) district.

Calving calf rearing practices

Calving trends: According to surveyed camel producers, camels usually calved in late afternoon - evening hours 24 (47.1%) or during night time 20 (39.2%), and less commonly in the morning 7 (13.7%). Meanwhile, the calving month of calculated from reported calf age estimates showed higher ($p<0.050$) calving frequency during the long (Jilal) dry season (October -March) compared to the short (Haga) dry season as well as the Dira Gu (April-May) and Karan Gu (August-September) rainy periods (Figure 1a). Calving outside the long-dry season was comparatively more frequent ($X^2=7.8$, $p=0.039$) in Gurusm (34.8%) than Kebribeya (17.5%) district (Figure 1b).

Colustrum provision: Only 5 (9.8%) of surveyed camel producers allowed full suckling of colustrum by the newborn calf on its first day of life. Remaining producers restricted initial colustrum intake by

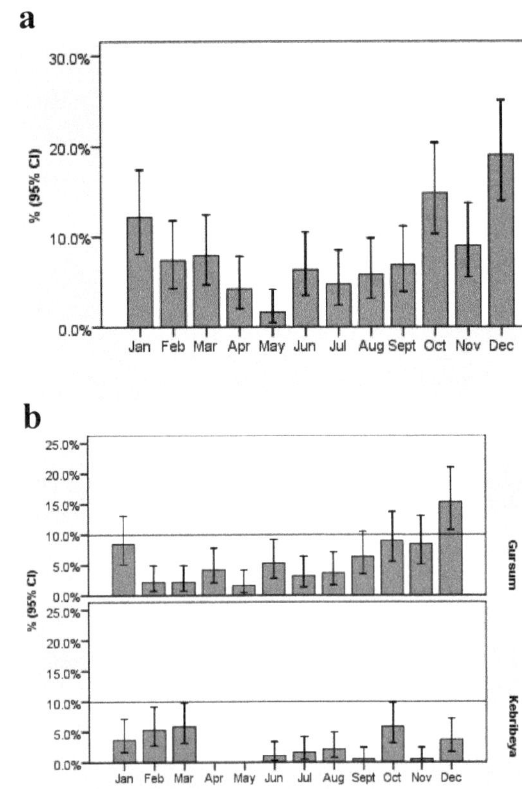

Figure 1: Annual distribution of camel calving months (%); total (a) and according to study district (b).

limiting suckling 28 (54.9%) or partially milking colutsrum before the calf suckles 18 (35.3%). The practice was always associated to risk of fatal scouring. Frequency of full suckling, restricted suckling and milking - suckling - hand feeding in Gursum (9.7%, 51.6% and 38.7%, respectively) and Kebribeya (10%, 10% and 80%, respectively) districts showed variation (X^2=9.7, p=0.003).

Feeding and watering: All participants reported that calves were given only milk during the 1st months and milk plus water until 3 months of life thereafter. During the 1st month of life daily milk suckling frequency ranged from ≥ 5 (94.1%) to ≤ 4 (5.9%) per day. Until the 3rd month, 21.6% and 78.4% producers allowed ≤ 5 and ≤ 3 suckling per day, respectively. After the 3rd month, suckling was reduced to 3 (7.8%) and ≤ 2 (92.2%) times per day. Producers gradually initiated hand feeding fresh-cut green grass/forages 12 (23.6%) or grazing on nearby range plants 39 (76.5%) after latter age.

Housing/Herding: Majority of producers 42 (82.4%) kept the newborn camel calf with its dam around homesteads during day and in separate night enclosure until 3 months of age and 9 (17.6%) started mixing neonates with older calves before latter age. After 3 months of age, all mixed newborn calves with older immature herd mates for daytime nearby range foraging and/or in night calf enclosures.

Calf health problems

Participatory survey: Overall, surveyed camel producers identified nine major calf health problems showing (except for respiratory illness) age-group related variations. Accordingly, the most frequently reported young camel calf (<6 months) problems were; diarrhea 51 (100%), contagious ecthyma/orf 47 (92.2%), respiratory illness 17 (33.3%), plant poisoning 13 (25.5%) and camel pox 4 (7.9%). Meanwhile, mange 48 (94.1%) and tick 44 (86.3%) infestations; ring worm/dermatophytes (alopecia and scaliness) 32 (62.7%); camel pox (general illness plus popular lesions around head) 29 (56.9%); trypanosomosis 26 (51%) and respiratory illness 5 (9.8%) were frequently reported problems in older growing (6-12 months) calves (Figure 2).

Plant poisoning in young (<6 months) calves was only reported in Gursum (38.7%) district (p=0.001). Reporting frequency (RF) of mange/mite infestation was higher (p=0.019) in Gursum (100%) compared to Kebribeya (80%) district (Figure 3).

Field calf investigation: Examination of camel calves detected 64 (34.9%) apparent health problems including; *Sarcoptes scabie var cameli* 31 (16.4%), tick infestation 24 (12.7%), diarrhea/scour 7 (3.7%) and respiratory illness (nasal discharge and recent history of cough) 2 (1.1%). Tick infestations involves *H. dromedary* 22 (11.6%), *R. pulchelis* 19 (10.05%) and *H. trancatum* 16 (8.4%) species mainly as mixed species affections (Table 1).

Mean age (months) of camel calves exhibiting diarrhea was higher (p=0.000) than that of healthy calves or calves facing tick and mange/mite infestation or respiratory illness (Figure 4). Prevalence of mange/mite infestation was higher in Gursum 28 (21.2%) compared to Kebribeya 3 (5.3%) district calf flocks (Table 2). Meanwhile, tick infestation was more prevalent in small (<25 camel) 12/56 (21.4%) compared to medium (25-50 camels) 8/106 (7.5%) or large (>50 camels) 4/27 (14.8%) herds (p=0.037).

Discussion

Overall camel holding pattern showed high variability among

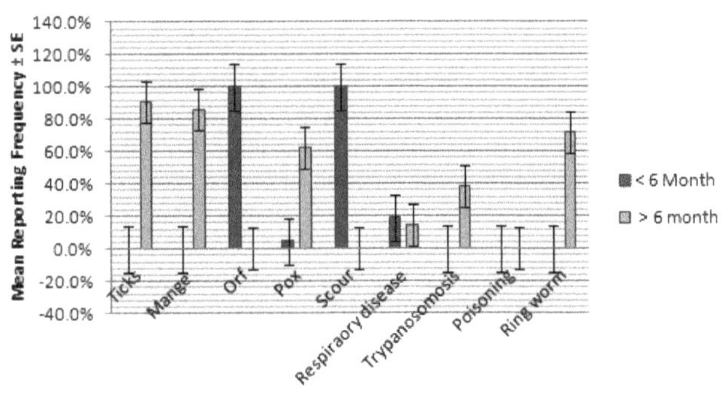

Figure 2: Reporting frequency (RF) of major health problems relative to calf age group.

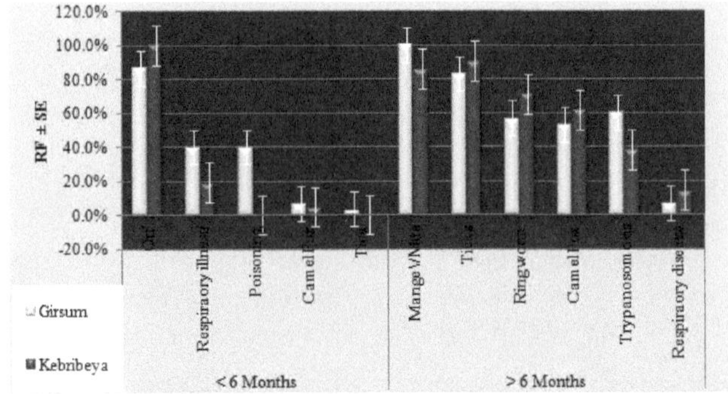

Figure 3: Reporting frequency (RF) of major camel calf health problems according to study districts.

Tick Species	N	%
H. dromedary	2	1.1%
R. pulchelis	2	1.1%
H. dromedary+H. trancatum	3	1.6%
H. dromedary+R. pulchelis	5	2.6%
H. dromedary+H. trancatum+R. pulchelis	12	6.3%

Table 1: Frequency of tick infestation pattern according to species composition.

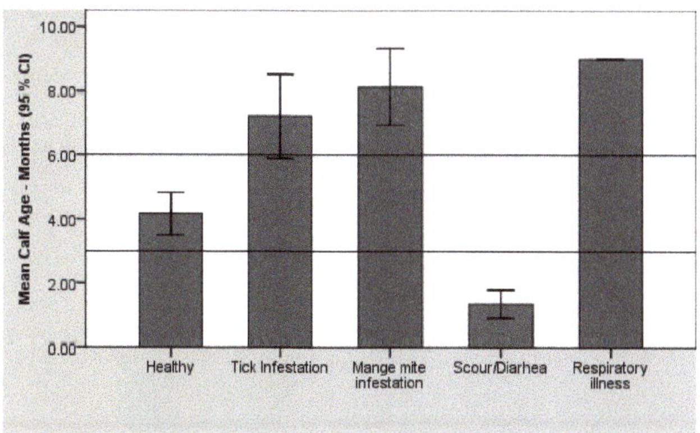

Figure 4: Average age of calves according to health status.

Health Problems	Districts		*Fishers>p value*
	Gursum (132)	Kebribeya (57)	
Mange/mite infestation	28 (21.2)	3 (5.3)	*0.004*
Tick infestation	15 (11.4)	9 (15.8)	*0.261*
Diarrhea/Scour	7 (5.3)	-	*0.077*
Respiratory illness	-	2 (3.5)	*0.090*
Total	**50 (37.9)**	**12 (21.1)**	***0.017***

Table 2: Frequency (n (%)) of camel calf health problems relative to districts.

households and the average camel herd size was 24.4 ± 1.1 animals. This was comparable to average camel herd size of 25.7 ± 29.8 previously reported from Somali region of Ethiopia [19]. Calves aged ≤ 12 months accounted for 13.5% of average camel holding reflecting slow herd growth rate. This was probably attributed to slow reproduction and/or high calf mortality rates. In agreement, [6] reported that camels in the study area had late (>5 years) first calving and long (around 2 years) inter-calving interval. This was compounded by high pre (61.5%) and pos (33.5%) weaning calf mortality [20]. Spatial variations in average camel holding size could reflect differences in agro-ecological and market potentials. Gursum district has higher precipitation and vegetation cover as well as better access to milk market chains supplying Jigjiga town and Somali land.

Traditional east African camel pastoralists control breeding time in such way as to ensure calving during growing months as well as year round milk supply [7,21]. Similarly, current findings indicate a seasonal camel calving tendency with higher percentage of camels giving birth between October and January. In the study area, this represents earlier parts of the long Jilal dry season immediately following Karan (Gu) rains [15]. The period offer abundant plant growth and milder weather which favor both milk production and reduces risk of extreme neonatal losses due to extreme weather. Moreover, the next growing period after Dira (Gu) rains (April-May) coincides with age of calf introduction to green forages. Parturition outside the peak calving months was more common in Gursum compared to Kebribeya district which probably reflects longer rain and growing intervals in the former. Meanwhile, 39.2% of camel calving was reported to occur at night. This complicates timely detection and management of calving difficulty which represents a common problem in the species [21].

Camel calves are born with an immature immune system. So they require immediate passive immune transfer through colustral (first-milk) IgG intake within 24 hours of birth [22]. In contrast, majority (90.2%) of producers in the current study restricted early colustrum intake by limiting suckled volumes (54.9%) or by milking portions of the first-milk before calf is allowed to suckle (35.3%). The latter practice was frequent in Kebribeya district and could indicate more serious colustrum restriction as it denies any unobserved suckling opportunity in the first 24 hours of life. Camel pastoralists in Somali [10] and Borana [11] areas of Ethiopia and adjacent areas in eastern Africa [4,21,23] were widely recognized for restricting early colustrum intake. In contrast, [20] reported that up to 46.4% of camel producers in adjacent areas allow full colustrum suckling by camel newborns which could be attributed to difference of production systems covered by the study. In accordance with previous studies [4], the main reason for restricting early colustum intake was a fear of fatal scour. In fact, camel colustrum is known to have powerful laxative effects attributed to its high total protein (15.8-19.5%) and mineral (1.4-2.8%) content [24]. However, risk of scour could be mitigated by dividing the optimum colostrum intake in to multiple feeding episodes mainly within 4 hours of birth as recommended for bovine calves [25].

Camel newborns were totally dependent on milk for nutrition during the first 3 months of life. However, milk suckling frequency was substantially restricted by majority of producers (78.4%) after the 1st month of life. In addition, after age of 1 month camel producers were reported to limit the number of teats a calf is allowed to suckle using various forms of physical barriers [20]. Widespread practice of suckling frequency and teat access restrictions probably reflect magnitude of calf - human (household/market) competition for milk. Such early milk restrictions hold substantial negative implications to survival and growth of newborn camel calves. Others suggested that conflicting trends of rising consumer demand and stagnantly-low productivity was tipping competition for camel milk against calves and contributing to heavy mortality losses in eastern Africa [21,26].

The age of 3 months was a particularly critical transition phase for camel calves in the study area. At this age, all producers mixed calves with older herd-mates and gradually introduced green forages wherein milk suckling frequency was further restricted by most (92.2%) producers. Newborn calves are very prone to trauma, predation, poisoning and diseases when prematurely mixed to older animals in rangelands or night enclosures. Experiences from modern bovine farming systems emphasize crucial need of segregating calves by age and maintaining sanitation in housing facilities [25]. In contrast to the current finding, communities around the study area were previously reported to initiate green feeds at younger age of 1 month [20]. Meanwhile, [23] indicated that Somali camel calves in Kenya began grazing at 3-4 months of age which was comparable with the current observation. On the other hand, [7] indicated that, in Ethiopia, camel calves were exclusively fed on milk until the age of 6 months and weaning ensued thereafter. The age and manner of weaning is predicated on existing levels of milk production, consumer demand (domestic and market) and intended use of calves. Early introduction of forage/grazing could pose additional negative pressure on nutrition and health of camel calves having inadequately developed digestive tracts.

According to surveyed producers the diseases commonly affecting camel calves in the study area were; diarrhea, orf, mange and tick infestations, ring worm, camel pox, trypanosomosis, respiratory illness and plant poisoning in the given order. These were comparable to range of diseases reported from different areas in Ethiopia [6,7] and neighbouring countries [12,13,23,27]. Cross-sectional field investigation of camel calf (≤ 12 months) diseases detected mange *(Sarcoptes scabie var cameli)* infestation (16.4%), mixed tick *(H. dromedary, H. truncatum* and *R. pulchelis)* infestation (12.7%), diarrhea (3.7%) and respiratory illness (1.1%). Ecto-parasite infestation and diarrhea were recognized to be the principal camel calf health problems in the study area [20]. A higher prevalence of mange (Sarcoptes scabiei) infestation has been reported for camels aged ≥ 1 year [28]. Meanwhile, a longitudinal study (covering all major seasons) of camel calf diseases in Borana reported higher prevalence of *sarcoptic mange* (47.9%) and tick (25.6%) infestations, diarrhea (5.1%) and respiratory infections (4.5%) [11]. Observed and/or reported frequency of plant poisoning and mange infestation were higher in Gursum compared to Kebribeya district which was probably attributed to agro-ecological variations. Heavy mange and tick infestation in camel calves reflects potentially substantial direct morbidity losses as well risk of tick borne diseases. Considering availability of reasonably effective and affordable control strategies, prevailing camel calf ecto-parasite infestation challenges reflect critical gaps in animal health services and/or producers awareness

Major camel calf diseases demonstrated distinct age dependent predisposition trends. Accordingly, diarrhea, orf and plant poisoning were more common in younger (<6 months) calves. In contrast, mange and tick infestation, ring worm, pox and trypanosomosis mainly affected older growing (6-12 months) calves. Newborn camel calves have little natural immunity [22]. In the face of inadequate early colustrum intake and poorly hygienic husbandry practices, camel neonates would be highly exposed to diverse environmental and contagious pathogens associated with diarrhea. Owing to absence of colustral passive immune transfer, contagious ecthema/orf most commonly affects very young animals in endemic areas. Meanwhile, introduction of lush green forages to young calves lacking well developed foregut and intestines could also predispose digestive disorders like diarrhea. Likewise, premature range grazing could force small calves (having limited browsing reach) to consume potentially poisonous low-growing shrubs like *Lantana camara* which was abundant in Gursum district. On the other hand, mange and tick infestation, ring worm and trypanosomosis were contact/vector transmitted endemic problems having chronic and progressive nature. Therefore, these conditions are likely to surface some time after young camel calves start mixing with older potential infected herd-mates and grazing in vector infested rangelands. Meanwhile, camel pox has been characterized as strong maternal passive immune transfer and transmitting by tick (*H. dromedary*) vectors [29]. Therefore, risk of infection would naturally increase when contact with potentially infected animals and/or vectors increase after maternal antibodies in circulation had dwindled.

Camel calves in the study area face different health problems including contagious and environmental infections; ecto-parasite infestation, vector borne diseases; and plant poisoning. Inadequate early colustrum feeding, poor health and hygiene management, and premature herd mixing and release to rangelands could be important epidemiological determinants. Effect of health problems could be compounded by nutritional disorders associated to premature milk restriction and forage/grazing introduction. Successful rearing of camel calves requires improved husbandry and health care practices matched to the physiological need of animals and local distribution of disease agents. This demands deeper and more comprehensive epidemiological characterization of important camel calf health problems in different agro-ecological settings.

Acknowledgments

The authors would like to thank the College of Veterinary medicine - Jigjiga University for facilitating logistic and laboratory facilities.

References

1. FAO STAT (2011) Food and Agriculture Organization of the United Nations statistical databases.
2. Abbas B, Al-Qarawi A, Al-Hawas A (2000) Survey on camel husbandry in Qassim region, Saudi Arabia: herding strategies, productivity and mortality. Mag Anim husbandry Vet Med Tropic Countries 53: 293-298.
3. Tura I, Kuria G, Walaga HK, Lesuper J (2010) Camel Breeding Management among the Somali, Sakuye, Gabbra and Rendille Pastoralists of Northern Kenya. Tropentag, Zurich, Switzerland.
4. Schwartz HJ, Dioli M (1992) The One-Humped Camel in Eastern Africa: A Pictorial Guide to Diseases, Health Care and Management. Verlag Josef Margraf, Scientific Books, Weikersheim FR, Germany.
5. Yesihak Y, Bekele T (2003) Growth pattern of one humped camel (Camelus dromedarius). Proceeding of the 11th Annual Conference of the Ethiopian Society of Animal Production (ESAP), Addis Ababa, Ethiopia.
6. Keskes S, Ibrahim M, Tessema TS, Tamir B, Regassa F, et al. (2013) Production systems and reproductive performances of Camelus dromedarius in Somali regional state, eastern Ethiopia. J Agric Environ Int Dev 107: 243-266.
7. Tefera M (2013) The Ethiopia Camel. Haramaya University.
8. Al-Juboori A, Baker MM (2012) Studies on Common Reproductive Disorders in Dromedary Camels (Camelus dromedarius) in United Arab Emirates (UAE) Under Field Conditions. 3rd Conference of theInternational Societyof Camelid Researchand Development, Muscat.
9. Getahun T, Kassa B (2002) Camel Husbandry Practices in Eastern Ethiopia: The Case of Jijiga and Shinile Zones. Nomadic Peoples 6: 158.
10. Tadesse Y, Urge M, Abegaz S, Kurtu MY, Kebede K, et al. (2014) Husbandry and breeding practices of dromedary camels among pastoral communities of Afar and Somali regional states, Ethiopia. J Agric Environ Int Dev 108: 167-189.
11. Megersa B (2014) Major Diseases of Camel Calves in Borana of Southern Ethiopia. Afr J Basic Appl Sci 6: 159-165.
12. Gilbert K, (2012) A Study to Determine Factors Affecting Health and Productivity of Camel Calves in Marsabit District of Kenya, A Thesis, University of Nairobi.
13. Kuria SG, Tura I, Amboga S, Walaga HK, Lesuper J (2011) The current status of camel (Camelus dromedarius) calf management among pastoral communities of northern Kenya, Livest Res Rural Dev 23.
14. Kamber R, Farah Z, Rusch P, Hasig M (2000) The supply of newborn camel foals (Camelus dromedaries) with mmunoglobulin G. Schweiz Arch Tierheilkd 142: 581-588.
15. Save the Children-UK/SC-UK (2004) Somali Regional State, Ethiopia: Livelihood Zone (LZ) Map: Source: Field Surveys conducted by SCUK/DPPB. Food Security Monitoring and Early Warning Programme – Revised 2004 Pastoralism in Ethiopia: Its total economic values and development challenges. Project Evaluation Report: Oxfam Canada, December 2007, Addis Ababa, Pp: 1-33.
16. Walton SF, Currie D (2007) Problems in diagnosing scabies, a global disease in human and animal populations. Clin Microbiol Rev 20: 268-279.
17. Walker AR, Bouattour JL, Estrad-Pena IG, Horalk AA, Pegram RG, et al. (2003) Ticks of domestic animals in Africa: A Guide to identification of Species. Bioscience and Reports, Edinburgh, UK. pp: 262.
18. Wall R, Shearer D (1997) Veterinary Entomology. Arthropod ectoparasites of veterinary importance, Chapman and Hall, London, pp: 2-5.
19. Seifu E (2009) Analysis on the contributions of and constraints to camel production in Shinile and Jijiga zones, eastern Ethiopia. J Agric Environ Int Dev 103: 213-224.
20. Awoke K, Ali SM (2015) Traditional Husbandry Practices and Major Challenge of Young Stock (Camel Calf) in Fafen Zone, Ethiopian Somali Regional State, Ethiopia. J Environ Anal Toxicol 5: 321.

21. Farah KO, Nyariki DM, Ngugi RK, Noor IM, Guliye AY (2004) The Somali and the Camel: Ecology, Management and Economics. Anthropologist 6: 45-55.

22. Bishr AM, Magdub AB, Abuzweda ABR (2013) The Appropriate Time Required for Newborn Calf Camel to Get Optimal Amount of Colostrums Immunoglobulin (IgG) with Relation to Levels of Cortisol and Thyroxin, World Academy Sci Eng Technol 7: 03-21.

23. Njanja JC (2007) Major factors associated with high morbidity, mortality and poor performance of camel calves, kids and lambs in the Rendille and Samburu pastoral herds in Marsabit District Kenya. PhD Thesis University of Nairobi.

24. Yagil L (1994) The camel in today's world: A Handbook of Camel Management. GIFRID/ Welthungerhilfe, Wageningen, The Netherlands. 74p.

25. Kumaresan A, Layek SS, Mohanty TK, Patbandha T, Prasad S (2012) Managing Calf Scours - A Herd health approach. Intas Polivet 13: 8-14.

26. Wilson RT (1998) Camels, the Tropical Agriculturalists (CTA). Macmillan Ltd., In: Yagil R (ed.), 1982. Camels and camel milk. FAO Animal Production and Health Paper, Food and Agriculture Organization.

27. Gluecks IV (2007) The Prevalence of Bacterial and Protozoal Intestinal Pathogens in Suckling Camel Calves in Northern Kenya. Free University of Berlin, Germany.

28. Feyera T, Admasu P, Abdilahi Z, Mummed B (2015) Epidemiological and therapeutic studies of camel mange in Fafan zone, Eastern Ethiopia. Parasit Vectors 8: 612.

29. OIE Terstrial Mannual (2014) Chapter 2-9-2. Camel Pox.

Prevalence of Avian Tuberculosis in Domestic Chickens in Selected Sites of Ethiopia

Aweke Kindu[1] and Gashaw Getaneh[2]*

[1]*College of Veterinary Medicine, Addis Ababa University, Debre Zeit, Ethiopia*
[2]*Faculty of Veterinary Medicine, Unit of Biomedical Science, University of Gondar, Gondar, Ethiopia*

Abstract

This study was conducted on 282 domestic chickens of Bahir Dar, Yilimana densa woreda, and Bishoftu by using avian tuberculosis diagnosis procedures such as single intradermal avian tuberculin test, post mortem examination, and Ziehl-Neelsen (Z-N) staining from tissue samples of naturally infected Domestic chickens (*Gallus domesticus*). The overall of this disease current prevalence was determined based on tuberculin skin test results supported by Z-N stain and post mortem lesions and it was 4.26% (12/282) (95% CI: 1.9-6.6), with higher prevalence in semi-intensively reared exotic chickens (5.85%) than backyard reared indigenous local chicken. This indicates the occurrence of this disease has a statistical significance association both with the breed and production system, both having a p-value of 0.03. Twelve strong positive reactor chickens have shown a swelling of greater than 5 mm in diameter 48 h. of post injection with different variety results, some with edematous swelling, and others with firm erythematic nodular swelling. Typical tuberculous lesions were seen mostly on the liver and spleen. From 12 tuberculi reactor slaughtered chickens, a total of seven (58.3%) chickens had gross lesions on different visceral organs, of which three (42.9%) examined chickens have manifested gross lesions on more than one organ. On acid fast staining five (41.67%) with grossly discernible lesions revealed acid-fast rods. For culturing, Lowenstein-Jensen (L-J) media was used as it yields more positive cultures, greater numbers of colonies on positive tubes, and shorter incubation times. None of the samples shown colonial growth till 8 weeks of incubation period and this may be due to the slow growth nature of mycobacterial species (especially when the infection was due to *Mycobacterium avium* subspecies *paratuberculosis* which needs a considerable long time for growth) and/or the current incubation temperature (37°C) may not be optimal as it does not fit the natural hosts internal body temperature and still the culture result is under process to see any growing colony. Therefore, this finding signaling an urgent need for intervention program to control the disease in domestic chickens and prevent zoonotic transmission.

Keywords: Avian tuberculosis; *Mycobacterium avium* complex; Prevalence; Avian tuberculin skin test; Domestic Chicken

Introduction

The total chicken population in Ethiopia were estimated to be 42 million and with regard to breed, 40.63 million (96.61%), 231,478 (0.55%) and 1.19 million (2.84%) of the total chicken were indigenous, hybrid and exotic, respectively [1]. From the total chicken population of Ethiopia, 99% are raised under the traditional backyard/scavenging system of management, while 1% is reared under intensive management system [2]. Recently, the increased demand for chicken meat and egg consumption in the country level resulting an increase in the number of chickens reared under intensive and semi-intensive management system. The traditional backyard poultry management system is characterized by minimal human care, with birds scavenging in the backyard for food, with poor management and nutrition. The impact of domestic chicken in the national economy of developing countries and its role in improving the nutritional status, income, food security and livelihood of many small holders is significant. Several factors have been suggested for high mortality and low production characteristics of domestic chicken. In Ethiopia, poultry diseases are considered the most important factor responsible for reducing both the number and productivity of chickens. Avian tuberculosis is one of the most important diseases that affect domestic and pet birds [3]. Several *Mycobacterium* spp. can be involved in the etiology of avian tuberculosis [4]. Species of Mycobacteria other than *M. bovis, M. leprae* and *M. tuberculosis* are often referred to as "atypical mycobacteria". The most commonly encountered pathogens among the atypical mycobacteria are species of the *M. avium* complex (MAC). *M. avium* complex consists of two species: *M. avium* and *M. intracellulare*; because these species are difficult to differentiate, they are also collectively referred to as *M. avium-intracellulare* (MAI) [5]. There are over 20 recognized serotypes within the *M. avium* complex. According to the current taxonomy, *M. avium* species contains four subspecies; *M. avium* subspecies *avium* (*M. avium avium)* of serotypes 1, 2, 3, and 6, *M. avium hominissuis* of serotypes 4 to 6, 8 to 11 and 21, *M. avium paratuberculosis*, and *M. avium silvaticum*. *M. avium avium* (often simply called *M. avium)* belonging to serotypes 1, 2, 3, and 6 are the principal cause of avian tuberculosis in wild, domestic and captive birds [6,7]. In addition to *M. avium*, other mycobacteria including *M. genavense, M. intracellulare, M. scrofulaceum, M. fortuitum, M. tuberculosis,* and *M. bovis* can also cause avian tuberculosis, but the incidences are rare [4,7].

M. avium, the major cause of avian tuberculosis, considered as "atypical mycobacteria", comprises aerobic, non-spore forming, and non-motile rod shaped bacteria that vary in length from 1-3 μm [6]. They are weakly Gram-Positive and stained specifically by acid fast staining method, due to its high levels of lipids in Mycobacterial cell wall. *M. avium* is highly resistant to environmental challenges and can

***Corresponding author:** Gashaw Getaneh, University of Gondar, Faculty of Veterinary Medicine, Unit of Biomedical Science, P.O. Box 196, Gondar, Ethiopia
E-mail: gashaw_getaneh@ymail.com or gashaw296@gmail.com

survive in soil up to 4 years, and this makes eradication of the organism difficult [7,8].

The most common route of infection for susceptible birds is the alimentary tract [6,7]. The disease is transmitted to the susceptibles bird by ingestion and inhalation of aerosolized infectious organisms. Infected birds, as they shed large amounts of organism into the environment and contaminated water and soil as the Mycobacteria can survive for several times in the environment, are the main source of infection [9]. The bacilli are exuded from ulcerated lesions of the intestine and are voided in droppings. The disease is more prevalent in places with high population density, poor sanitation, and unhygienic conditions [10]. The disease in the affected individual results unthriftiness, atrophy of the breast muscle, decreased egg production, and increased mortality, which culminates into severe economical losses.

Mycobacterium avium complex is the most commonly associated with human disease. MAC is primarily a pulmonary pathogen that affects individuals who are immune compromised (e.g., from AIDS, hairy cell leukemia, immunosuppressive chemotherapy). In humans, *M. avium* is capable of inducing a progressive and disseminated type of disease that is relatively refractory to treatment both in HIV/AIDS patients [11] and in normal hosts [12]. *M. avium* is the isolate in more than 95% of patients with AIDS who develop *M. avium* complex infections (MAC). MAC lung disease occurs rarely in immunocompetent hosts. *M. intracellulare* is responsible for 40% of such infections in immunocompetent patients [5].

Diagnosis of avian tuberculosis in chickens depends on detection of specific immunological response, in live birds [13] or isolation of *M. avium* by culturing tissue samples of killed birds. The most widely used test in live domestic fowl, and the only test for which an international standard for the reagent exists, is the tuberculin test [4]. This test is used to determine whether an individual has been infected in the past with the causative agent of avian tuberculosis or not. The test result is determined based on Office International Des Epizooties (OIE) 2008 guideline and accordingly this, a positive test reaction is any swelling at the injected site, from a small firm nodule approximately 5 mm in diameter to gross oedema extending to the other wattle and down to the neck. No clinical signs will be provoked in uninfected birds [4].

When clinical signs of the disease are seen in a flock or typical lesions of tuberculous are present at necropsy, demonstration of acid-fast bacilli in smears or histopathologic sections made from affected organs is regarded as sufficient for positive diagnosis [13]. If acid-fast bacilli are not found, but typical signs or lesions are present in the birds, culture of the organisms on artificial media such as Lowenstein-Jensen (L-J), Stonebrink, and Middlebrook agar must be attempted [14,15]. L-J yields more positive cultures and greater numbers of colonies on positive tubes, and incubation times is shorter, should be incubated for at least 8 weeks [4].

Despite the fact that traditionally reared indigenous local chicken account for a greater proportion of chicken population in Ethiopia, some research has been carried out on them and no organized research at all has been conducted yet on semi-intensively reared commercial chicken on the prevalence of avian tuberculosis. In Ethiopia, avian tuberculosis has been reported previously in indigenous local chickens of Adama, Sebeta, and Debre Birhan with a prevalence of 6.3% [16] and recently a prevalence of 4.23% of avian tuberculosis was reported in indigenous local chickens of Shashemene district [17]. However, there is no information about the epidemiology and significance risk factors for avian tuberculosis in north-western part of Ethiopia (particularly around Bahir Dar area) and in commercial poultry farms of Bishoftu. Therefore, the Objectives of this study were:

- To investigate the prevalence of avian tuberculosis using single intradermal avian tuberculin test on domestic chickens in three selected sites of Ethiopia.
- To identify the possible etiological agents responsible for avian tuberculosis in those avian tuberculin reactor chicken.

Materials and Methods

Geographic description of the study area

This study was conducted in three selected sites of Ethiopia, in Amhara Region (around Bahir dar area and in Yilmana densa Woreda) and in Oromia Region (in Bishoftu town). Bahir dar is located in north-western part of Ethiopia, 487 Kms from Addis Ababa. Bahir dar has a latitude of 11°36'N and longitude of 37°23'E, and has an elevation of 1,830 meters above sea level. Total annual rainfall ranges from about 1100-1530 mm/year. The mean monthly temperature of the area is about 19°C, with monthly mean maximum temperature of 27.3°C and monthly mean minimum temperature of 11.5°C [18].

The second district is Yilmana densa Woreda of Amhara Region and it's Center (Adet) has a latitude of 11°17'N and longitude of 37°43'E and has a distance of about 445 Kms from north of Addis Ababa and 42 Kms south of Bahir dar. It has M-25, Tepid moist cool mountains and plateau agro-ecology. Yilmana densa Woreda has an altitude which ranges from 1500 to greater than 3000 m.a.sl. It have only one rainy season, which extends from mid-may to October and all the remaining months (November to mid-may) are categorized as dry season and have estimated average annual minimum and maximum air temperatures of 9.27°C and 25.74°C, and 860.2 mm and 1770.5 mm rainfall, respectively [19].

The third district is Bishoftu which has a latitude of 8°45'N and longitude of 38°59'E, about 47 Kms southeast of Addis Ababa at an altitude of 1850 meters above sea level. The average annual temperature in Bishoftu is 18.7°C with average annual minimum and maximum air temperatures of 14°C and 26°C and have average annual rainfall is 866 mm. The driest month is December with 5 mm. Most precipitation falls in July, with an average of 232 mm [20].

Animal study procedure

Study animal: The poultry management pattern in Bahir Dar and Yilmana densa Woreda from which some part of this study has been conducted were entirely free-ranging traditional backyard production system of the local indigenous chickens. Generally, this traditional poultry production system is characterized by minimal human care, with birds scavenging in the backyard for food, a few handfuls of local grain, and possibly simple night shades, but no veterinary medical attention. Whereas the poultry production system in Bishoftu from which some part of this study has been conducted were semi-intensively reared commercial chickens and all flocks live together in a small, crowded and unhygienic area and fed grains by the owners. A total of 292 chicken from both sex and above the age of 20 weeks were selected for single intradermal avian tuberculin test. In Bishoftu, at least 50 chickens per farm were selected from four commercial layers farms while in backyard indigenous local chickens 25% of the flock were selected depending on the population in each flock. Age of the chicken was determined by using information from the owners.

Study design and sample size determination: To determine the sample size, an expected prevalence of 50% was taken since there is no previous organized research conducted on the prevalence of avian tuberculosis on commercial chickens and indigenous local chickens of these selected sites. The desired sample size (N) for this study was calculated using the formula given by Thrusfield [21];

$$N = \frac{1.96^2 P_{exp}(1 - P_{exp})}{d^2}$$

Where, N=required sample size, Pexp=expected prevalence, d=desired absolute precision. Using this formula, the estimated sample size was 384 chickens. But due to the poor availability of the reagent (avian PPD), a total of 292 chickens were sampled despite of their sex, age, and health status to avian tuberculosis to find the present prevalence of avian tuberculosis. To come up with this, a cross-sectional study was conducted and then chickens have been selected by using simple random sampling method.

Avian tuberculin skin test: Before undergoing any examination procedures, each chicken were given an identification number (ID No) using ink on wattle/comb and/or legs. A total of 292 apparently healthy chickens were assessed for avian tuberculosis by using single intradermal avian tuberculin test, the most widely used test in domestic fowl. It is recommended that avian tuberculin should contain the equivalent of at least 25,000 IU/mL, giving a dose for practical use of 2500 IU/0.1 mL [4]. In this test, 0.1 mL of avian tuberculin, PPD (AVITUBAL-25000 IU/ml, Czech Republic) extracted from the *M. avium* (strain D.4 ER) were injected into the wattle using 1 mL of insulin needle intradermally on to a randomly selected 52 indigenous local chickens in Bahir Dar town and its surrounding sites, 31 indigenous breed chickens in Yilmana densa Woreda, and 209 exotic chickens in Bishoftu. The study in Bishoftu was conducted on randomly selected Bovans brown chickens from four semi-intensive commercial farms, Farm 1 (n=53), Farm 2 (n=53), Farm 3 (n=52), and Farm 4 (n=51).

The tuberculin skin test is based on a delayed hypersensitivity reaction. This test is used to determine whether an individual has been infected in the past with the causative agent of tuberculosis or not. A previously infected individual would harbor reactive T-cells in their blood. Avian tuberculin skin test results were read after 48 h. of post injection. The test result was determined based on OIE 2008 guideline and accordingly this, a positive test reaction is any swelling at the site, from a small firm nodule approximately 5 mm in diameter to gross oedema extending into the other wattle and down the neck. No clinical signs will be provoked or the test antigen does not provoke any response at the injection site in uninfected birds and the test was considered as negative for avian tuberculosis [4].

Postmortem gross pathological examinations: For postmortem examination, 12 strong avian tuberculin reactor chickens were purchased and then slaughtered in the poultry post mortem class at College of Veterinary Medicine and Agriculture (CVMA) of Addis Ababa university. At necropsy, all internal organs were examined, any observed gross lesions were recorded, tissues from any organs showing pathologic gross tuberculous lesions were collected; however, tissues from liver, spleen, and intestine at different segments were sampled regardless of the presence or absence of lesions since they can be highly affected by the MAC group. Tuberculosis suspected tissue samples that were collected from different organs by using sterile universal bottles each containing normal saline solution (0.9%) were labeled and kept in a deep freeze (-20°C) in the microbiology laboratory at the College of Veterinary Medicine and Agriculture, Bishoftu until being transported to Aklilu Lemma Institute of Pathobiology (ALIPB-AAU) tuberculosis research laboratory, Addis Ababa, for culturing. During transportation, these tissue samples were transported in cold chain using icebox packed with ice packs to keep low temperature.

Mycobacteriologic culture and ziehl-neelsen staining: At ALIPB Tuberculosis laboratory, two slant types of Lowenstein-Jensen (L-J) media were prepared; one was enriched with 1% sodium pyruvate and the other was enriched with glycerol. Then tissue samples were macerated in sterile Petridish to get fine pieces by using sterile scissor and forceps, and then each sample was homogenized using sterile mortar and pestle for 10 min in 5 mL of normal saline solution. Seven mL of homogenate from each sample was transferred to centrifuge tube and decontaminated by adding an equal volume (7 mL) of 4% NaOH by centrifugation at 3,000 rpm at 4°C for 15 min. After centrifugation, the supernatant was discarded, while the sediment was neutralized with 10% HCl with phenol red as an indicator. Neutralization was achieved when the color of the solution changed from purple to yellow. Thereafter, 0.1 mL of suspension (one to three drop) from each sample was spread on to two slant types of Lowenstein-Jensen (L-J) medium. Cultures were then incubated aerobically at 37°C for up to 8 weeks with weekly observation for growth of colonies.

On the meantime of tissue processing for culturing on L-J media, the remaining sediment portion of the homogenated tissue were smeared and stained using the Ziehl- Neelsen staining technique for direct microscopic examination. Smears were heat-fixed, flooded with concentrated carbon fuchsin, heated gently to steaming for 5 minutes. Then the stain was poured off and the smears were washed with tap water and decolorized with 3% HCl in 95% alcohol for 1 min., with slides being washed under running tap water between each step. The smears were then counter stained with methylene blue for 1 min., air-dried and examined under the 100x oil immersion object of a light microscope for the presence of Acid Fast Bacilli (AFB).

Statistical analysis

The data collected were analyzed using STATA version 11.0 for Windows (Stata Corp. College Station, TX, USA). The prevalence of avian tuberculosis is defined as the number of avian tuberculin skin test reactor chickens from the total number of avian tuberculin injected chicken results expressed in percent. The variation of prevalence in relation to different risk factors was analyzed using chi-square (χ^2) statistical test. Both Postmortem examinations and Ziehl-Neelsen staining of samples which was taken from characteristic post mortem lesions were used to support the prevalence rate. District, altitude, sex, age, breed, Body condition, purpose of keeping, and production system dependent prevalence were compared and analyzed by the χ^2 statistical test. In the analyses, the confidence interval was 95% and $p<0.05$ was set for significance.

Results

Avian tuberculin skin test results

From the total of 292 avian tuberculin injected chickens, 282 chickens were followed up for the test result on the second and third day of post injection while the rest 10 chickens were not seen for the test result by different reasons such as death, sell, get away from the nearby house. Of the 282 observed chickens for the test result, 12 chickens were positive, reactors to avian tuberculin skin test, having a swelling greater than 5 mm in diameter with different variety results, some with edematous swelling, the others with firm erythematic nodular swelling and the prevalence was, therefore, 4.26% (95% CI: 1.9-6.6). Individual reactor chicken observation shown that swelling seen starting 24 h. post- PPD injection increase in size on the second and third day of post injection (as indicated in the Figures 1 and 2). A total of 29 (10.28%) avian tuberculin injected chickens have shown bluish discoloration around the injection site without any visible swelling resulting doubtful interpretation which still needs further investigation (Figure 3).

Assocation of the risk factors with avian tuberculin positivity showed that exotic breed of chicken had higher rate of avian tuberculin positivity than local breed and the difference was statistically significant (χ^2 =4.7076, Pr =0.03). Similarly, chicken managed under intentsive system had higher tuberculin positivity rate than those in backyard traditional system of production and the difference was ststaistically significant (χ^2–4.7076, Pr=0.03) (Table 1). All the other risk factors considered showed no statistically significant difference among the groups compared in each category with respect to their positivity to tuberculin test (Table 2).

Gross pathological findings

From 12 tuberculin positive slaughtered chickens, a total of seven (58.3%) chickens had gross lesions on different visceral organs (liver, intestine, proventriculus and uterus) (Figures 4 and 5), of which three (42.9%) examined chickens have manifested gross lesions on more than one organ. A total of five (41.67%) of 12 avian tuberculin reactor chickens haven't shown any visible lesion on the visceral organs. The typical tuberculous lesions were grayish-yellow to grayish-white, pin-point to irregularly round, and few to innumerable small nodules and pin-point whitish nodules were observed in liver (Figure 4) and uterus showed extensive disminated lesions with nodular lesions. Calcification was not seen in the nodules. Organs such as the spleen and liver were enlarged; especially spleen was enlarged to about twice of the normal size. Adhesion of the intestinal tract to one unit, and uterus with other reproductive organs were encountered. On Ziehl-Neelsen staining from the total of 12 slaughtered chickens, five (41.67%) with grossly discernible lesions revealed acid-fast rods. From seven chickens with grossly discernible lesions, two of them (28.57%) were negative for acid fast staining.

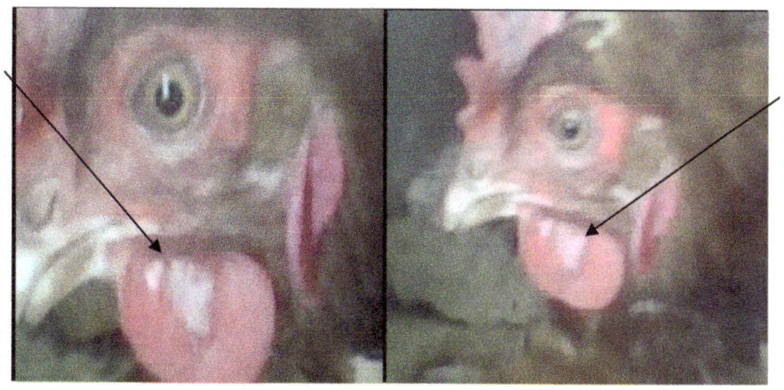

A B

Figure 1: Edematous swelling observed at the left wattle at (A) 48 h and (B) 64 h of post injection of avian tuberculin.

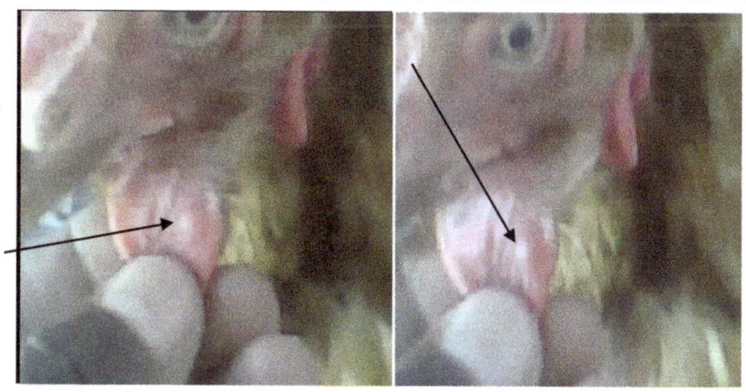

Figure 2: Firm erythematic nodular swelling observed at 48 h of post injection of avian tuberculin.

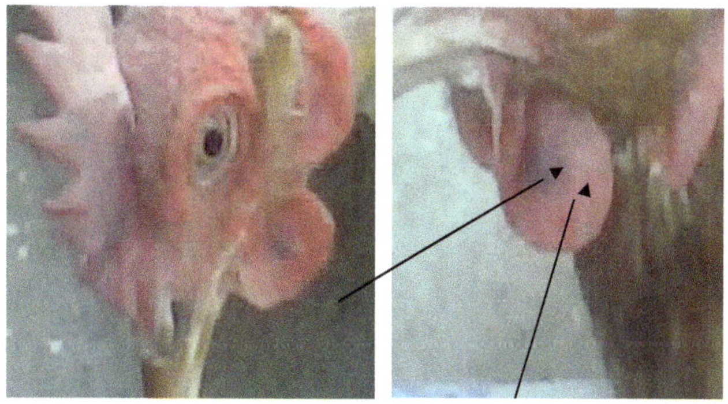

Figure 3: Bluish discoloration after injection of tuberculin shown by the tip of the arrow.

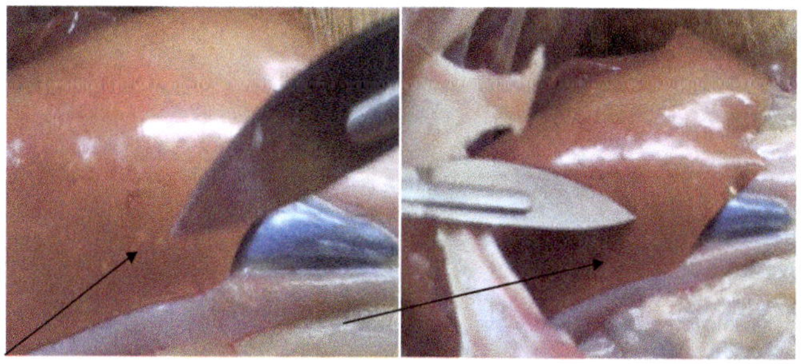

Figure 4: Small whitish nodular tuberculous lesions on the liver of chickens during post mortem examination (indicated by the tip of the arrow).

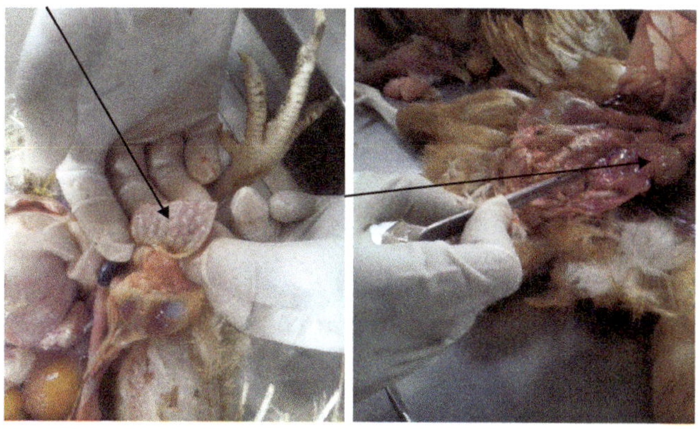

Figure 5: Gross pathological lesions on the (A) proventriculus and (B) uterus.

Mycobacteriologic culture results

From the total of 34 cultured samples (17 on sodium pyruvate enriched L-J slants and the other 17 on glycerol enriched L-J slants) those taken from different organs of 12 slaughtered tuberculin reactor chickens, none of them have shown colonial growth up to 8 weeks of incubation period with weekly observation basis.

Discussion

The present study revealed that the overall prevalence of avian tuberculosis was 4.26% (95% CI: 1.9-6.6) in domestic chickens in

Variables	Categories	No. of examined chickens (%)	No. of tuberculin skin test positive (%)	Chi-square (χ^2)	p-value (Pr)
District	Bahirdar	48(17.0)	0	4.7076	0.095
	Yilmana Densa	29(10.3)	0		
	Debre zeit	205(72.7)	12(5.85)		
Altitude	mid land	253(89.7)	12(4.74)	1.4366	0.231
	high land	29(10.3)	0		
Sex	male	18(6.4)	0	0.8545	0.355
	female	264(93.6)	12(4.54)		
Age	young	89(31.6)	2(2.24)	1.2866	0.257
	adult	193(68.4)	10(5.18)		
Breed	local	77(27.3)	0	4.7076	0.030*
	exotic	205(72.7)	12(5.85)		
Body condition Production Purpose	Poor good layer	167(59.2) 115(40.8) 265(94.0)	12(4.53) 7(4.19) 5(4.34)	0.8040 0.0040	0.370 0.949
	broiler	17(6.0)	0		
Production system	extensive	77(27.3)	0	4.7076	0.030*
	intensive	205(72.7)	12(5.85)		

*Altitude: high altitude >2500 meters & mid altitude >=1500-2500 meter above sea level.

Table 1: Association of risk factors to avian tuberculin skin test results.

Chicken ID NO-	Goss pathological lesions observed at different organs				Z-N stain result
	Liver	Spleen	GIT	Others	
B_1	✓Y	✓Y	Y(Pro)	n	Positive
B_2	✓Y	✓Y	n	n	Negative
B_3	✓Y	n	n	n	Positive
B_4	n	n	n	n	Negative
MU_1	✓Y	✓Y	n	n	Positive
MU_2	n	n	Y(SI)	Y(UA)	Positive
MU_3	n	Y(Sp)	Y(Pro)	n	Positive
ME_1	n	n	n	n	Negative
ME_2	n	n	n	n	Negative
ME_3	n	n	n	n	Negative
ME_4	n	n	Y(AIT)	n	Negative
ME_5	n	n	n	n	Negative

Key of the table: Y=Small pin-point nodular lesions or other pathological lesions, n=no lesions observed by visualization, Pro=proventriculus, SI=Small Intestine, UA=Uterus Adhered, Sp=Splenomegaly, AIT=Adhesion of Intestinal Tract.

Table 2: Post-mortem findings and acid fast staining results.

selected sites of Ethiopia. This study pointed out the presence of avian tuberculosis in semi-intensive reared exotic chickens in bishoftu (5.85%) for the first time by using single intradermal avian tuberculin test. The study also shown that the disease is not much important in indigenous local chickens at Bahir dar area and Yilimana densa woreda that are kept in backyard reared scavenging production system even if the sampled size were small. With respect to the overall prevalence of this disease occurrence, it was agreed with the previous study in other part of central Ethiopia [16] (6.3%); [17] (4.23%) and comparable with the findings of greater prevalence in the mid-lands than high-lands.

The study indicated that semi-intensively reared chickens are constantly exposed to overcrowding, high contact rate with them selves and to the small space of the floor within unhygienic housing system and that may serve as sources of infection. Overcrowding within a flock brings in stress, which in turn could affect the nature and number of lesions occurring [22]. So in this study, the main risk factors for avian tuberculosis occurrence and transmission are breed and production system. This indicates the occurrence of this disease has a statistical significance association with both the breed and production system, both having a p-value of 0.03. Bovans brown chickens that reared in semi-intensive production system have a higher prevalence of the disease than indigenous local chickens which is reared in backyard system. In semi-intensive commercial chicken production system large number of chickens were kept in one small house as a result they share the same floor (mostly ground soil) for standing and constant movement, and use the same feed and water trough, and share the same atmosphere. That's the risk of exposure of other healthy chickens from one infected chicken is greater in semi-intensive production system than extensive ones.

Sex, purpose of keeping, and age variation on the occurrence of avian tuberculosis was recoded; but all of them had not a statistical significant association. High prevalence of the diseases was shown in Bovans brown adult female chickens that are kept for layer purpose than any other classes. Female chickens are allowed to live longer time than their male counterparts (broiler purpose) because of keeping them for need of egg production and this gives a better chance for bacilli to establish infection over a long period of time and to be shed in the external environment from which other chickens can easily get the bacilli. Thus, older chickens by contaminated the environment could act as a source of infection to other members in the flock especially in unhygienic semi-intensive production system where there is greater number of chickens per unit area than that of extensive production system.

Moreover, the study also attempted to further isolate the possible etiologic agents of avian tuberculosis using culture, postmortem examinations, and Ziehl-Neelsen staining in addition to the prevalence finding by single intradermal avian tuberculin skin test. The variation of swelling with regard to its size and/or time of occurrence after injection of avian tuberculin is due to the variation of individual chickens specific immune response ability to the injected PPD. In the present study granulomatous lesions were found on the liver, spleen, gastrointestinal tract and also in the uterus. Some of the chickens that were positive for avian tuberculin skin test during ante mortem examination don't show any observable lesion at time of post mortem examination and this may be due to the false positivity of the tuberculin skin test or missing of the lesions because it may not still well develop. Chickens that have negative avian tuberculin skin test do not necessarily mean it's free of tuberculosis infection because the test may have false negativity. Because of the false positivity or negativity of the test, the prevalence of this disease may be recorded as little below or above than the exact figure of prevalence within the population.

The reason we obtained no colonial growth up to eight weeks of incubation time may due to culturing still requires longer duration of incubation time as *Mycobacterium* growths slowly and/or the current incubation temperature(37°C) may not be optimal and may cause retardation of growth since it does not much the hosts(chickens) internal body temperature at which the *M. avium* complex growths bestly. This does not necessarily mean cultured sample results are negative on L-J media as mycobacterial colony growth may not shown up to 16 weeks, especially when the infection was due to *M. avium* subspecies *paratuberculosis* which needs a considerable longer time for growth [4].

Conclusions and Recommendations

This study showed an overall avian tuberculosis prevalence of 4.26% in domestic chickens in three selected sites of Ethiopia using avian tuberculin skin test, the most widely used test in domestic fowl [4] with a higher prevalence in semi-intensive reared commercial exotic chickens (5.85%) in bishoftu (the major sources of chickens meat, egg for Addis ababa) for the first time. Some studies [11,12] indicated that there is a zoonotic transmission of *M. avium* complex to human populations, signaling an urgent need for intervention program to control this disease. Based on the above conclusion, the following recommendations were forwarded:

- The sensitivity and specificity of avian tuberculin skin test on local indigenous chickens of Ethiopia should be investigated to validate and verify its use for large scale diagnosis of avian tuberculosis in the country.
- It is suggested that government and policy makers should work together with poultry farm owners and Veterinarians to design methods for the control of avian tuberculosis in semi-intensive commercial farms.
- During chicken flock replacement, the original sites should be thoroughly disinfected and repopulated chickens should not contact with other farm chickens.
- As treatment of infected chicken is not recommended because of the high cost and prolonged time of treatment, control and prevention of the disease before entry is the best option suggested to saving economic losses due to this disease and to prevent Zoonotic transmission.
- Cultural taboos like giving of raw liver of chicken before cooking (immediately after slaughtering) to children for feeding purpose should be prevented.

Acknowledgement

The authors would like to thank Akililu lemma institute of pathobiology in general and sub-thematic Avian TB project in particular for their funding all financial matters required for this study and the aothors also heartfully thank all of the veterinarians working at the ALIPB for their support of necessary equipments and reagents and their knowledge sharing. The authors also gratitude all of the local chicken and poultry farm owners for their willing to do this thesis on their chickens. We acknowledge Bahir Dar Regional Veterinary Laboratory for their contribution Interms of facilities.

References

1. Central Statistics Authority (2009) Agricultural sample survey 2009/10. Report on livestock and livestock characteristics. Volume II. Statistical Bulletin No. 468, Addis Ababa, Ethiopia.
2. Tadelle D, Kijora C, Peters KJ (2003) Indigenous chicken ecotypes in Ethiopia: growth and feed utilization potentials. Int J Poult Sci 2: 144-152.
3. Abubakar MB, Ambali AG, Tamjdo T (2007) Rural chicken production: Effects of gender on ownership, and management responsibilities in some parts of Nigeria and Cameroon. Int J Poult Sci 6: 413-416.
4. OIE (2008) OIE Terrestrial Manual for Avian tuberculosis. Office International des Epizooties. Chapter 2.3.6, p: 497-506.
5. Koirala J (2012) Mycobacterium Avium-Intracellulare. Medscape reference.
6. Fulton RM, Thoen CO (2008) Tuberculosis. In: Diseases of Poultry. Saif YM, Barnes HJ, Glisson JR, Fadly FM, Mc Dougald LR, et al. (eds.) Iowa State University Press, Ames, IA, USA, pp: 836-844.
7. Dvorska L, Matlova L, Ayele WY, Fischer OA, Amemori T, et al. (2007) Avian tuberculosis in naturally infected captive water birds of the Ardeideae and Threskiornithidae families studied by serotyping, IS901 RFLP typing, and virulence for poultry. Vet Microbiol 119: 366-374.
8. Thoen CO (1998) Tuberculosis. In: A Laboratory Manual for the Isolation and Identification of Avian Pathogens. Swayne DE, Gilson JR, Jackwood MW, Pearson JE, Reed WM (eds.). American Association of Avian Pathologists, Philadelphia, USA, pp: 69-73.
9. Tell L, Woods L, Cromie R (2001) Mycobacteriosis in birds. Rev Sci Tech 20: 180-203.
10. Dhama K, Mahendran M, Tomar S (2007) Avian tuberculosis: an overview. Poultry Punch 24: 38-52.
11. Horsburgh CR, Hanson DL, Jones JL, Thompson SE (1996) Protection from *Mycobacterium avium* complex disease in human immunodeficiency virus-infected persons with a history of tuberculosis. J Infect Dis 174: 1212-1217.
12. Iseman MD (1989) *Mycobacterium avium* complex and the normal host. N Engl J Med 321: 896-898.
13. Office International des Epizooties (2000) OIE manual for standards of diagnostic tests and vaccines. Book Review. Office International des Epizooties (OIE): 4th edn. pp: 364-389.
14. Baron EJ, Peterson LR, Finegold SM (1994) Bailey and Scott's Diagnostic Microbiology (9th edn). Mossy-Yearbook, Missouri, USA, pp: 590-633.
15. Karlson AG, Thoen CO (1991) Tuberculosis. In: A laboratory manual for isolation and identification of avian pathogen. Purchase HG, Domermuth CH, Arp LA, Pearson JE (eds.). 3rd edn. Iowa: Kendall/ Hunt Publishing.
16. Tadesse S, Woldemeskel M, Molla B, Tibbo M, Kidane D, et al. (2004) Avian mycobacteriosis in domestic chickens from selected agro-climatic regions in Ethiopia. J Appl Res Vet Med 2: 17-25.
17. Abda S (2013) Prevalence of avian tuberculosis and associated risk factors in domestic chickens at Shashemene district, Ethiopia. MSc Thesis in Tropical Veterinary Microbiology. College of Veterinary Medicine and Agriculture, Addis Ababa University, Bishoftu, Ethiopia, pp: 1-48.
18. Central Statistics Agency (2008) Ethiopian Agricultural sample survey, diagnosis of bovine fasciolosis. Vet Parasitol 105: 337-343.

19. Adet Agricultural Research Center (2014) Ambo Plant protection Research Center. Ethiopian Institute of Agricultural Research.

20. National Metrological Service Agency (2005) National Metrological Service Agency. Rainfall and temperature data, Addis Ababa, Ethiopia.

21. Thrusfield M (1995) Veterinary Epidemiology. 3rd edn. Blackwell Science, London, pp: 225-228.

22. Gross WB, Falkinham III JD, Payeur JB (1989) Effect of environmental-genetic interactions on Mycobacterium avium challenge infection. Avian Dis 33: 411-415.

PERMISSIONS

All chapters in this book were first published in JVST, by OMICS International; hereby published with permission under the Creative Commons Attribution License or equivalent. Every chapter published in this book has been scrutinized by our experts. Their significance has been extensively debated. The topics covered herein carry significant findings which will fuel the growth of the discipline. They may even be implemented as practical applications or may be referred to as a beginning point for another development.

The contributors of this book come from diverse backgrounds, making this book a truly international effort. This book will bring forth new frontiers with its revolutionizing research information and detailed analysis of the nascent developments around the world.

We would like to thank all the contributing authors for lending their expertise to make the book truly unique. They have played a crucial role in the development of this book. Without their invaluable contributions this book wouldn't have been possible. They have made vital efforts to compile up to date information on the varied aspects of this subject to make this book a valuable addition to the collection of many professionals and students.

This book was conceptualized with the vision of imparting up-to-date information and advanced data in this field. To ensure the same, a matchless editorial board was set up. Every individual on the board went through rigorous rounds of assessment to prove their worth. After which they invested a large part of their time researching and compiling the most relevant data for our readers.

The editorial board has been involved in producing this book since its inception. They have spent rigorous hours researching and exploring the diverse topics which have resulted in the successful publishing of this book. They have passed on their knowledge of decades through this book. To expedite this challenging task, the publisher supported the team at every step. A small team of assistant editors was also appointed to further simplify the editing procedure and attain best results for the readers.

Apart from the editorial board, the designing team has also invested a significant amount of their time in understanding the subject and creating the most relevant covers. They scrutinized every image to scout for the most suitable representation of the subject and create an appropriate cover for the book.

The publishing team has been an ardent support to the editorial, designing and production team. Their endless efforts to recruit the best for this project, has resulted in the accomplishment of this book. They are a veteran in the field of academics and their pool of knowledge is as vast as their experience in printing. Their expertise and guidance has proved useful at every step. Their uncompromising quality standards have made this book an exceptional effort. Their encouragement from time to time has been an inspiration for everyone.

The publisher and the editorial board hope that this book will prove to be a valuable piece of knowledge for researchers, students, practitioners and scholars across the globe.

LIST OF CONTRIBUTORS

Fahimeh Golestani and Tahereh Naji
Department of Basic Sciences, Faculty of Pharmacy, Pharmaceutical Sciences Branch, Islamic Azad University (IAUPS), Tehran, Iran

Homayoun Hosseinzadeh Sahaifi
Iranian Fisheries Science Research Institute, Agricultural Research, Education and Extension Organization, Tehran, Iran

Abdulhakim Albe and Teka Feyera
College of Veterinary Medicine, Jigjiga University, Jigjiga, Ethiopia

Kefyalew Gebeyew
College of Dry Land Agriculture, Department of Animal and Range Science, Jijiga University, Ethiopia

Chalachew Kassahun, Ahmed Adem, Mebrie Zemene and Kassahun Berrie
Department of Veterinary Pharmacy, Faculty of Veterinary Medicine, University of Gondar, Gondar, Ethiopia

Gashaw Getaneh
Department of Biomedical Science, Faculty of Veterinary Medicine, University of Gondar, Gondar, Ethiopia

Mohsin Ali Gazi and Makhdoomi DM
Division of Surgery and Radiology, Sheri Kashmir University of Agricultural Sciences and Technology Kashmir, Jammu and Kashmir, India

Mir SA
Division of Pharmacology and Toxicology, Sheri Kashmir University of Agricultural Sciences and Technology Kashmir, Jammu and Kashmir, India

Sheikh GN
Division of Epidemiology and Preventive Medicine, Sheri Kashmir University of Agricultural Sciences and Technology Kashmir, Jammu and Kashmir, India

Helen Louton, Elke Rauch, Michael Erhard and Shana Bergmann
Department of Veterinary Sciences, Chair of Animal Welfare, Ethology, Animal Hygiene and Animal Husbandry, Faculty of Veterinary Medicine, LMU Munich, Veterinaerstraße 13/R, 80539 Munich, Germany

Sven Reese
Department of Veterinary Sciences, Chair of Anatomy, Histology and Embryology, Faculty of Veterinary Medicine, LMU Munich, Veterinaerstraße 13, 80539 Munich, Germany

Masri Junihardy, Maskur M, Soegeng Prasetyo, Muhamad Ali and Sulaiman N Depamede
Postgraduate Study Program of Management and Livestock Resources, Faculty of Animal Science, Mataram University, Jalan Majapahit 62 Mataram, NTB-83125, Indonesia

Boon Allwin
Department of Wildlife Science, Madras Veterinary College, TANUVAS, Chennai, Tamil Nadu, India

Kalignan PA
Zoo Veterinarian, Bannerghatta Zoological Park, Karnataka, India

Pradeep Nag BS and Gopikrishnan D
Department of Gynecology, Madras Veterinary College, TANUVAS, Chennai, Tamil Nadu, India

Nishit S Gokarn
Department of Surgery, Madras Veterinary College, TANUVAS, Chennai, Tamil Nadu, India

Ararsa Duguma
Haramaya University, College of Veterinary Medicine, Ethiopia

Ian Scott
Laboratorio de Biología Celular Aplicada, Escuela de Medicina Veterinaria, Núcleo de Investigación en Producción Alimentaria, Facultad de Recursos Naturales, Universidad Católica de Temuco, Chile

Jorge Parodi
Laboratorio de Biología Celular Aplicada, Escuela de Medicina Veterinaria, Núcleo de Investigación en Producción Alimentaria, Facultad de Recursos Naturales, Universidad Católica de Temuco, Chile
Laboratory Research and Education Tonalli Ltd., Chile

Alfredo Ramirez-Reveco
Cryobiology and Spermatozoa Functionality Analysis Laboratory, Institute of Animal Sciences, Faculty of Veterinary Sciences, Universidad Austral de Chile, Valdivia, Chile

Alison N Beloshapka and Hannah D Holscher
Department of Animal Sciences, University of Illinois, Urbana, IL, USA

Kelly S Swanson
Department of Animal Sciences, University of Illinois, Urbana, IL, USA
Division of Nutritional Sciences, University of Illinois, Urbana, IL, USA

Genevieve M Forster
Department of Clinical Sciences, Colorado State University, Fort Collins, CO, USA

Elizabeth P Ryan
Department of Clinical Sciences, Colorado State University, Fort Collins, CO, USA
Department of Environmental and Radiological Health Sciences, Colorado State University, Fort Collins, CO, USA

Zineddine Esma and Bereksi Reguig Karima
Département de Biologie/Université UDL de Sidi-Bel-Abbès, Algéria

Carlos F Agudelo and Shachar Dvir
Small Animal Clinic, University of Veterinary and Pharmaceutical Sciences Brno, Czech Republic

Zeki Yilmaz and Meric Kocaturk
Uludag University, Veterinary Teaching Hospital, Internal Medicine Department, 16059, Gorukle, Bursa-Turkey

Anteneh Hailu Tegegn
Semeral Veterinary Regional Laboratory, Afar, Ethiopia

Aklilu Feleke
College of Veterinary Medicine and Agriculture, Addis Ababa University, PO Box 34, Bishoftu, Ethiopia

Wesinew Adugna
VSF Suisse, Addis Ababa, Ethiopia

Simenew Keskes Melaku
College of Agriculture and Natural Resources, Dilla University, PO Box 419, Dilla, Ethiopia

Temesgen Tesfaye, Chala Mohammed, Lama Yimer and Misgana Duguma
School of Veterinary Medicine, Wollega University, Nekemte, Ethiopia

Mammo Mokonnen
Bako Agricultural Research Center, Ethiopia

Prerna Vohra and Kuldeep Singh Khera
Department of Zoology, College of Basic Sciences and Humanities, Punjab Agricultural University, Ludhiana, Punjab, India

Fufa Abunna, Tekeste Abriham, Takele Beyene, Ashenafi Feyisa, Dinka Ayana, Bedaso Mamo and Reta Duguma
College of Veterinary Medicine and Agriculture, Addis Ababa University, PO Box 34, Bishoftu, Oromia, Ethiopia

Fikru Gizaw
College of Veterinary Medicine, Semera University, PO Box 132, Samara, Ethiopia

Terefe Simon Juta
Department of Parasitology and Pathology, Jigjiga University, Jigjiga, Ethiopia

Nigussu Fasil and Dessie Sheferaw
School of Veterinary Medicine, Hawassa University, Ethiopia

Yidersal Erega and Solomon Tsegaye
College of Agriculture, Woldia University, P.O. Box 400, Woldia, Ethiopia

Sherif Mohamed Shoieb
Veterinary Teaching Hospital, Faculty of Veterinary Medicine, Mansoura University, Mansoura 35516, Egypt

Hussam Mohamed Mohamed Ibrahim and Sabry Ahmed El-khodery
Department of Internal Medicine and Infectious Diseases, Faculty of Veterinary Medicine, Mansoura University, Mansoura 35516, Egypt

Mohamed Sayed-Ahmed
Department of Internal Medicine and Infectious Diseases, Faculty of Veterinary Medicine, Mansoura University, Mansoura 35516, Egypt
Department of Clinical Pharmacy, College of Pharmacy, Jazan University, Jizan 45142, Saudi Arabia

Guluma Assefa, Ahmed Nur and Lamessa Keno
East Shoa Zone Livestock and Fishery Resource Office, Adama, Ethopia

Birhanu Abera, Diriba Lemma and Eyob Eticha
Asella Regional Veterinary Laboratory, Asella, Ethiopia

Gebeyehu Chali
Ilu Aba Bor Zone Livestock and Fishery Resource Office, Mattu, Ethioipia

Mahammed Hussen
Buno Bedelle Zone Livestock and Fishery Resource Office, Bedelle, Ethiopia

Barrilli LNE and Maiorka A
Animal Science Department, Federal University of Paraná (UFPR), 80035-050, Curitiba, Paraná, Brazil

Silva BAN and Raidan FSS
Institute of Agricultural Sciences/ICA, Federal University of Minas Gerais (UFMG), 39404-547, Montes Claros, Minas Gerais, Brazil

Falleiros FT and Silva CC
DSM Nutritional Products, Av. Engineer Billings 1729, 05321-010, São Paulo, Brazil

Araújo WAG
Animal Science Unit, Federal Institute of Education, Science and Technology Northern Minas Gerais (IFNMG), 39480-000, Januária, Minas Gerais, Institute of Agricultural Sciences/ ICA, Federal University of Minas Gerais (UFMG), 39404-547, Montes Claros, Minas Gerais, Brazil

Ayalew Nesgash, Belay Yaregal, Tesfamariam Kindu and Endalkachew Hailu
Faculty of Veterinary Medicine, College of Medical and Health Science, University of Gondar, PO Box 196, Gondar, Ethiopia

Caridad Suárez Machín and Carmen Amarilys Guevara Rodríguez
Cuban Research Institute of Sugar Cane (ICIDCA), Avenue White 804, Corner Central Road, San Miguel del Padrón, Havana, Cuba

Juan Miguel Gómez Cama
Universidad Nacional Autónoma de Honduras, UNAH, Havana, Cuba

Iannetti S
Veterinary Medicine, Istituto Zooprofilattico Sperimentale of Abruzzo and Molise G. Caporale, Campo Boario Teramo, Italy

Cioci D and Colangeli P
Computer Science, Istituto Zooprofilattico Sperimentale of Abruzzo and Molise G. Caporale, Campo Boario Teramo, Italy

Falcone MG
Veterinary Medicine, Ministry of Health, Office III DGSAF, Rome, Italy

Silva BAN
Institute of Agricultural Sciences/ICA, Federal University of Minas Gerais (UFMG), 39404-547, Montes Claros, Minas Gerais, Brazil
INRA UR 143 Zootechnical Research Unit, F-97170 Petit Bourg, Guadeloupe, France

Gourdine JL
INRA UR 143 Zootechnical Research Unit, F-97170 Petit Bourg, Guadeloupe, France

Corrent E and Primot Y
Ajinomoto Eurolysine S.A.S. 153, Rue de Courcelles, F-75817 Paris Cedex 17, France

Mourot J and Noblet J
INRA, UMR Breeding Systems, Animal and Human Nutrition INRA UMR 1079, 35590 St Gilles, France

Renaudeau D
INRA UR 143 Zootechnical Research Unit, F-97170 Petit Bourg, Guadeloupe, France
INRA, UMR Breeding Systems, Animal and Human Nutrition INRA UMR 1079, 35590 St Gilles, France

Hideyuki Takahashi, Atsuko Matsubara, Ouanh Phomvisith, Akari Shiga, Ha T Mai, Tetsuji Etoh, Yuji Shiotsuka, Ryoichi Fujino, Mitsuhiro Furuse and Takafumi Gotoh
Kuju Agricultural Research Center, Kyushu University, 878-0201 Kuju-cho, Oita, Japan

Akira Saito
Zenrakuren, Shiba 4-17-5, Minato-ku, 108-0014 Tokyo, Japan

Toshihisa Sugino
Graduate School of Biosphere Science, Hiroshima University, Higashi-Hiroshima, Higashi-Hiroshima-shi, 739-8528 Hiroshima, Japan

Christopher D McMahon
AgResearch Ltd, Private Bag 3123, Hamilton, New Zealand

Melaku Taye
South West Shoa Livestock Development and Fishery Office, Woliso, Oromia, Ethiopia

Teshome Jagema
Oromia Livestock Development and Fishery Office, Finfinne, Oromia, Ethiopia

Asefa Tadese
Ambo University, College of Agriculture, Ambo, Oromia, Ethiopia

Endalu Mulatu
Bedelle College of Agriculture and Forestry, Mettu University, Bedelle, Oromia, Ethiopia

Kumela Lelisa
National Institute for Control and Eradication of Tsetse Fly and Trypanomosis, Addis Ababa, Ethiopia

Delesa Damena
National Animal Health Diagnostic and Investigation Center, Sebeta, Oromia, Ethiopia

Rajion MA and Ebrahimi M
Department of Veterinary Preclinical Sciences, Universiti Putra Malaysia, 43400 Serdang, Selangor, Malaysia

Meng GY
Department of Veterinary Preclinical Sciences, Universiti Putra Malaysia, 43400 Serdang, Selangor, Malaysia
Institute of Tropical Agriculture, Universiti Putra Malaysia, 43400 Serdang, Selangor, Malaysia

Jafari S
Department of Veterinary Preclinical Sciences, Universiti Putra Malaysia, 43400 Serdang, Selangor, Malaysia
Department of Poultry Science, Faculty of Agriculture, Tarbiat Modares University, PO Box 14115-336, Iran

Torshizi MAK
Department of Poultry Science, Faculty of Agriculture, Tarbiat Modares University, PO Box 14115-336, Iran

Awol Ibrahim
Dawe Kechen District Pastoral Area Development Office, Ethiopia

Dagmar Nölkes
College of Veterinary Medicine, Haramaya University, Dire Dawa, Ethiopia

Elias Gezahegn
Bale Zone Pastoral Area Development Office, Ethiopia

Mekuriya Taye
Mede Welabu District Pastoral Area Development Office, Ethiopia

Keerthy AJ
Directorate of Animal Husbandry, Kerala, India

Omprakash AV
Poultry Research Station, Madhavaram Milk Colony, Chennai, Tamil Nadu, India

Churchil RR
Institutional Livestock Farm Complex, Veterinary College and Research Institute, Orathanadu, Than-javur, Tamil Nadu, India

Hudson GH
Department of Poultry Science, Madras Veterinary College, Chennai, Tamil Nadu, India

Megan Wilson and Anke Twigg-Flesner
Performance in Equestrian Sport Research Group, Hartpury University Centre, Hartpury College, Gloucestershire, GL19 3BE, UK

Andualem Yimer and Abebe Desie
School of Veterinary Medicine, Wollo University, Dessie, Ethiopia

Belete Asefa and Tadesse Abate
Department of Animal and Range Sciences, School of Agriculture, Madda Walabu University, PO Box 247, Bale Robe, Ethiopia

Eshetu Adugna
Department of Animal and Range Sciences, Sinana District Livestock and Fishery Production, Ethiopia

Kabirul Islam Khan MD
Department of Genetics and Animal Breeding, Chittagong Veterinary and Animal Sciences University, Chittagong, Bangladesh

Raphael A Mrode
Animal and Veterinary Sciences, Scotland's Rural College, Roslin Institute Building, Easter Bush, Midlothian, Edinburgh, EH25 9RG, United Kingdom

Saeed Nazifi, Mahsa Khosravi, Maryam Haddadi and Mojtaba Rahsepar
Department of Clinical Studies, School of Veterinary Medicine, Shiraz University, Shiraz, Iran

Neda Eskandarzade
Department of Basic Sciences, School of Veterinary Medicine, Shahid Bahonar University, Kerman, Iran

Shimels Tikuye
EIAR, National Agricultural Biotechnology Research Center, Holleta, Ethiopia

SM Razavi, E Foroudi, E Rakhshandehroo and F Nejati
Department of Pathobiology, School of Veterinary Medicine, Shiraz University, Shiraz, Iran

S Nazifi
Department of Clinical Studies, School of Veterinary Medicine, Shiraz University, Shiraz, Iran

Abdi Hassan Rirash, Befekadu Urga Wakayo and Hassan Abdi
College of Veterinary Medicine, Jigjiga University, Jigjiga, Somali Regional State, Ethiopia

Aweke Kindu
College of Veterinary Medicine, Addis Ababa University, Debre Zeit, Ethiopia

Gashaw Getaneh
Faculty of Veterinary Medicine, Unit of Biomedical Science, University of Gondar, Gondar, Ethiopia

Index